Business Mastery

Fifth Edition

A Guide for Creating a Fulfilling, Thriving Practice, and Keeping It Successful

Cherie Sohnen-Moe

Business Mastery

A Guide for Creating a Fulfilling, Thriving Practice, and Keeping It Successful

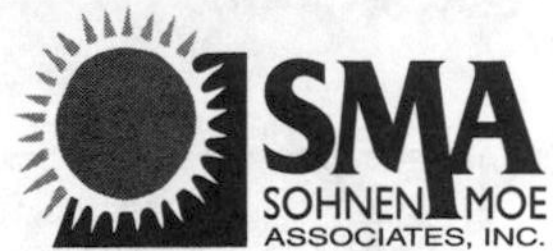

Published by Sohnen-Moe Associates, Inc.
PO Box 86913
Tucson, Arizona 85754-6913
520-743-3936
www.Sohnen-Moe.com

Publisher's Cataloging-in-Publication
(Provided by Quality Books, Inc.)

Sohnen-Moe, Cherie, author.
Business mastery : a guide for creating a fulfilling, thriving practice, and keeping it successful / Cherie M. Sohnen-Moe. -- Fifth edition.
pages cm
Includes bibliographical references and index.
LCCN 2015916334
ISBN 9781882908059
E-Book ISBN 9781882908035
1. Small business--Management--Handbooks, manuals, etc. I. Title.

HD62.7.S64 2015 658.02'2
QBI15-600200

Cover design: Deanna Sylvester
Illustrations: Deanna Sylvester
Editors: Terri Osborne, Deanna Sylvester, Nancy Triplett
Fifth Edition, 2016

Book/Interior Design: James Moe
www.BusinessMastery.us
Printed in the United States of America
Last digit is the print number: 9 8 7 6 5

Preface

Introduction

Mastering business is like bringing a rainbow down to earth. It involves taking dreams, principles, goals, and ideals, and turning them into something real that you and others can see and appreciate. In the approach taken in this book, mastering business is not about taking steps one-two-three and you're there. Instead, this approach asks you to recognize that many colors fill the rainbow of success, and you blend these colors into the shades that best suit you.

For the past 3 decades, *Business Mastery* has supported business owners in all realms to reach new levels of success. This book is written specifically for wellness professionals. If you're a massage therapist, chiropractor, counselor, acupuncturist, homeopath, Rolfing® practitioner, nutritional consultant, naturopath, herbalist, Reiki practitioner, esthetician, psychiatrist, Polarity therapist, physician, aromatherapist, personal trainer, reflexologist, physical therapist, yoga instructor, or a practitioner of any of the numerous allied healthcare professions, this book is for you!

This edition of *Business Mastery* includes updated information and new topics of interest. You can find valuable bonus material on the *Business Mastery* website (www.BusinessMastery.us), such as resource books, website links, forms, and information on select topics. Please visit the site regularly as we continually update it. I hope you find this edition of *Business Mastery* even more valuable and fun to use.

Business Mastery takes an in-depth look at how to build and maintain a successful practice. Depending on your level of business experience and expertise, you may find that you only need to concentrate on certain sections of this book. Some of the topics may not be relevant to you now, yet may become so in the future. These business skills are fundamental to your success—whether you work for someone else or are self-employed. Whatever path you choose, you can count on *Business Mastery* to help make your dreams a reality.

I wish you great happiness, health, prosperity, success, and balance!

About the Author

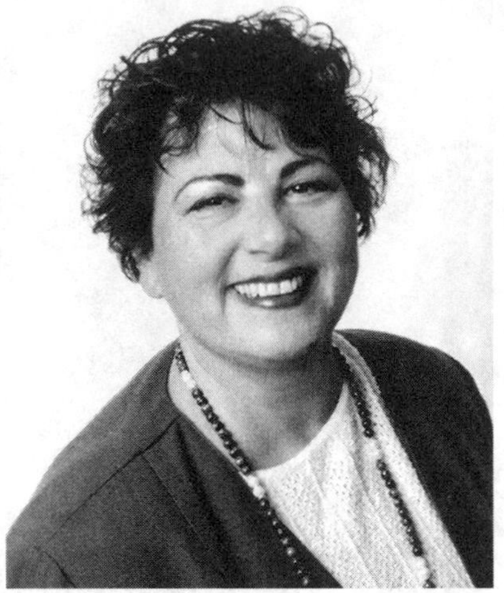

Cherie Sohnen-Moe is an author, business coach, international workshop leader, and successful business owner since 1978. Before shifting her focus to education and coaching, she was in private practice for many years as a massage and holistic health practitioner. Her background is diverse and she has worked with individual therapists, to small wellness centers, to day spas that have multiple locations, to businesses in retail and the hospitality industry. Cherie holds a degree in psychology from UCLA and has extensive experience in the areas of business management, training, and creative problem solving.

Cherie has served as a faculty member at the Desert Institute of Healing Arts, the Arizona School of Acupuncture and Oriental Medicine, and Clayton College of Natural Health. She has written more than 100 articles and is the author of the books *Business Mastery*, *Present Yourself Powerfully*, and *The Art of Teaching*. She is the co-author of *The Ethics of Touch*, a contributing author of *Teaching Massage*, and was interviewed for a chapter of *SAND TO SKY: Conversations with Teachers of Asian Medicine*. Her most popular workshops are Marketing from Your Heart, The Four Keys to Publicity, The Ethics of Touch, Therapeutic Communications, Present Yourself Powerfully, Profit with Products, and Creative Teaching Techniques.

Cherie's honors include: the Distinguished Service Award and the Professional Achievement Award from the American Society for Training and Development (ASTD); the Outstanding Instructor Award at the Desert Institute of the Healing Arts; the MO AMTA President's Award; and the Massage Therapy Hall of Fame.

Cherie is a firm believer in education and as such serves on the exam committee of the Federation of State Massage Therapy Boards (FSMTB). She is a founding member of the Alliance for Massage Therapy Education (AFMTE), has served on the board of directors for many years, and is the current President.

Cherie lives in Tucson, Arizona, with her husband, Jim, and their dog, Cinder. She is dedicated to assisting people reach the success they desire: personally, financially, and professionally.

Acknowledgments

So many people have supported me in making this book a reality. Much of the material for this book has been developed and refined over the past 40 years in my coaching practice, in courses and seminars I've facilitated, and through my process of personal and professional development. The team for this 5th edition is stellar! I am thankful to Terri Osborne and Nancy Triplett, whose writings, reviews, research, and editing have enriched and added clarity to this project. I am honored that Stephanie Beck overhauled the Online Presence chapter and shared so much of her content. I am so thankful to Lynda Solien-Wolfe for our numerous collaborations on retailing. I thank Bill Barren, Julie Goodwin, Tad Hargrave, Helene Jewell, Julie Onofrio, Diana Thompson, Ruth Werner, and Jan Zobel, for content and expertise. Thanks to Jim Moe for his beautiful interior book design. I give special appreciation to Deanna Sylvester for her outstanding coordination of this project, editorial assistance, and graphic design.

Many people were involved in the previous editions of *Business Mastery*. I am grateful for the suggestions, editing assistance, artistic creation, inspiration, content, and general support I received from Jada Ahern, Dominick Angiulo, Margaret Avery Moon, Simi Aziz, Barb Baun, Terry Belville, Ben Benjamin, Phyllis Bloom, Barbara Buchanan, Nikki Charns, Jacque Dailey, Robert Decker, Umanga deSilva, C. Diane Ealy, Rich Foster, Julie Goodwin, Reagan Hatch, Janice Hollender, Helene Jewell, Andrea Kartch, Jamie Lee, Maryanne LaBrash, Kathy Lynn Lee, Kathy Liddiard, Whitney Lowe, Jon Lumsden, Virginia Mahoney, Beth Mayer, Jim Moe, Shaye Moore, Daz Moran, Mark Moseley, Melissa Mower, Terri Osborne, Nancy Parker, Sheri Piper, Christine Rosche, Bob Sexton, Diana Thompson, Ravensara Siobhan Travillian, Karen Wilhelmsen, Neil Wilkinson, Tracy Williams, Kalyn Wolf, and Jan Zobel. Thank you all!

I acknowledge all of my friends who encourage me to pursue my dreams and keep me laughing. Most of all, I am so thankful for my wonderful husband, Jim. He has assisted in every phase of this book. His unconditional love and total support for whatever I choose to do has given me the courage to follow my heart.

How to Use this Book

No matter where you are in your career, if you're willing to take a new look at your life and challenge some of your old thought patterns, you'll find that reading this book from beginning to end is an incredibly valuable process.

Business Mastery has been designed to follow a pattern—the chapters build upon each other. It's intended for use both by practitioners in training and by professionals in the field. To fully assimilate the material in this book, it's best to read and study one chapter, or even one section, at a time. Although each chapter is self-contained, I suggest reading Sections 1 and 2 first. You may need to read a specific chapter and then go back to the beginning of the book. For instance, if you're considering going into partnership, proceed directly to Chapter 15, Business Start-up. Maybe you've been in practice for a while now; you have a business plan, you know what you want out of life, and you still aren't accomplishing your goals. In that case, you may want to start with Chapter 3, Success Strategies. Some sections include aspects of business that may not pertain to you—such as product sales, group practice, employees, or working for someone else. Just review them (someday, you may decide to incorporate those areas) and complete the sections that are appropriate to your career path. Many of the chapters include useful activities and thought-provoking Points to Ponder for personal exploration. While you can do these on your own, they're much more valuable when you discuss them with peers and colleagues. This isn't a book to read and put on a shelf. *Business Mastery* is a handbook—a resource tool for you to use regularly. It helps you create the success that you truly deserve!

Free Downloadable Workbook

Get the most out of *Business Mastery* by doing the activities and regularly referring to them. We've made it easier by creating the *Business Mastery Workbook*, that includes chapter highlights, all of the activities from this book (plus more), reproducible forms, an expanded glossary, and a graduate success checklist. I also recommend that you make this a journal to track your thought processes throughout this book and throughout your career. In the workbook, you can keep your responses to the activities, record your thoughts on the Points to Ponder, and document your progress. To download your free copy, go to https://sohnen-moe.com/bm5-workbook-request/.

Special Features of the Digital Edition

The digital edition of *Business Mastery* is interactive. On each chapter title page, the headings are hyperlinked to the corresponding section. Throughout the chapters, the margin guides take you to the referenced chapter and page number, and the web addresses take you directly to the referenced website. Each endnote superscript takes you to the appropriate endnotes page. Click away and have fun! Order the digital edition from VitalSource: https://www.vitalsource.com/publisher/products/business-mastery-cherie-sohnen-moe-v9781882908035?term=business+mastery.

Special Note for Students

Program durations vary from school to school: from several months to several years. Sometimes the business course is taught midway and other times near the end of the program. Some schools include 15 hours of business education, others 100. To download a checklist of action steps to prepare you for success when you graduate, and for other resources visit https://sohnen-moe.com/resources/resources-students/.

Teacher Resources

We offer a multitude of free teaching resources to schools requiring *Business Mastery*:

- A guide on the Art of Teaching Business
- Lesson Plan Builders (goals, objectives, and activities) for each chapter
- A Test Bank
- 600+ Slides and Handouts
- Videos and More!

Visit https://sohnen-moe.com/resources/resources-educators/ for more information.

Pictograph Glossary

The following icons signal tips, resources, related information, and activities.

Icon	Name	Description
	Activities	Most of the exercises involve writing. This is your cue to get out your journal or go to your computer.
	Idea	Quick tips or suggestions for other ways to utilize the information.
	Publication Resources	Books, magazines, and other publications with more information on specific topics.
	Internet Resources	Links to related websites, articles, e-books, and other resources.
BMW	Business Mastery Workbook Resource	Refers to forms, checklists, and resources in the *Business Mastery Workbook*.
→	Point Forward	Lets you know where you can find related information in a subsequent section.
←	Point Back	Reminds you to refer to an earlier section.
"	Inspirational Quotes	Quotes from historical figures and thought-leaders.
§	Section	Standard typographic symbol for a section. Similar to an octothorpe (#) for indicating a number.

What's In a Name?

For consistency and simplicity, the term practitioner is used throughout this book to refer to all types of wellness professionals. Some scenarios refer to specific professions, yet are relevant to almost every field. It's my hope that everyone can easily relate to the examples provided.

The term "client" is used instead of "patient" throughout this book, primarily to recognize that the relationship between a practitioner and client is a partnership. This approach assures that the best interests of the client are served. It also honors the client's role as an active participant rather than a passive recipient of wellness services.

Throughout most of history the male gender has been used exclusively to denote the generic pronoun when referring to women, as well as men. As our culture and language have evolved, we've struggled to find the appropriate way to refer to all persons equally. Unfortunately, in English at least, a gender neutral pronoun doesn't exist and thus there's no simple way to accomplish this except by using clumsy terms like s/he, his or her, himself/herself, or they/their. I chose to alternate the use of the female and male pronouns when a singular pronoun is required because grammatically, it's not yet acceptable to use "they." I intend for the principles illustrated by the examples to apply to all genders. I hope that by the time we work on a sixth edition, better options will exist.

Table of Contents

§1

Set a Strong Foundation

As you work to make your career dreams a reality, Section 1 of *Business Mastery* explores how to set a strong foundation. It prepares you to make decisions about your career based on a clear sense of who you are and what you want to accomplish.

Chapter 1 looks at ways to increase your self-awareness and make self-knowledge into a powerful ally for the work ahead of you. This chapter mainly consists of activities to help you assess your current state, identify your strengths and challenges, and clarify your values. The chapter finishes with an exploration of your ideal future.

Chapter 2 helps you transform the insights you gained from Chapter 1 into the activities of goal setting, strategic planning, and follow-through. These three key activities form the common denominator among successful people in all fields. This chapter assists you in developing a mission statement and goals—and translating them into activities vital to the daily, weekly, and monthly growth of your business. We then look at how savvy business people use strategic planning to create a roadmap to success.

Chapter 3 helps you define what success means to you, and supports you in a fearless examination of roadblocks that may stand in your way. You'll also find tips on how successful people manage their time, track results, and handle risks wisely.

Chapter 4 looks at how to ensure that your career lasts for the long term and grows as you do. It identifies time-tested ways to enhance career longevity and avoid burnout. The chapter also explores ways to develop a strong support system to help you stay on track and true to your vision.

1

Getting Started

"What lies behind us and what lies before us are tiny matters compared to what lies within us."

—Oliver Wendell Holmes

Self-Awareness is Key

Values Clarification

Your Ideal Future

Key Terms

Creative Visualization
Morals
Personal Assessment
Personality Types
Principles
Professionalism
Self-Awareness
Values

Achieving success in the business world while staying true to the principles of healing and service to others may, at times, seem like a paradox. The business world is often portrayed as being heartless, as indeed it can be if you don't know the rules. The exciting thing is that once you do learn the rules, you can choose which ones you want to incorporate in your life and determine how to circumvent the ones you don't like.

> "A journey of a thousand miles begins with a single step.
> —Lao Tzu

Many people who choose a career as a wellness practitioner don't enjoy the business facets and, thus, don't take the time to learn the rules for success. Unfortunately, that attitude rarely leads to success. On the other hand, those who take the time to master basic business knowledge and build solid career skills often enjoy a smooth road to success and prosperity.

To do the work you love, it's crucial to develop the business savvy that gives you the knowledge, tools, and insights you need to make informed career choices—choices that best support your financial and professional growth. Always remember why you chose your profession and stay grounded in the experience of the difference you make.

In the inspiring article titled "In the Service of Life," Rachel Naomi Remen, M.D., states:[1]

> *Service rests on the basic premise that the nature of life is sacred, that life is a holy mystery which has an unknown purpose. When we serve, we know that we belong to life and to that purpose. Fundamentally, helping, fixing and service are ways of seeing life. When you help, you see life as weak, when you fix, you see life as broken. When you serve, you see life as whole. Lastly, fixing and helping are the basis of curing, but not healing. Only service heals.*

Self-Awareness is Key

One of the most essential traits that successful people have in common is the dedication to knowledge. Knowledge is power, and self-awareness is the foundation of that knowledge. Before you even begin to create or update a plan for your career or business, it's vital that you assess your current state.

The first step is to get a clear picture of your own personality style and unique quirks. You can easily do this by taking a personality quiz in any of several books (or on many websites) about personality types or social styles. What book or system you choose to work with isn't as significant as finding material that rings true for you. The best books on personality types and communication styles offer a balance of conceptual and practical information, and include plenty of stories about how differences play out in day-to-day interactions.

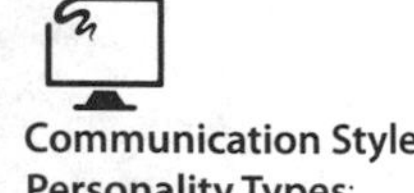

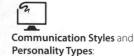

Communication Styles and **Personality Types**:

www.myersbriggs.org
www.discprofile.com
www.enneagraminstitute.com
https://similarminds.com
www.keirsey.com
www.personalitylab.org
www.personality-project.org
www.41q.com
www.humanmetrics.com

Figure 1.1 Wheel of Life Example

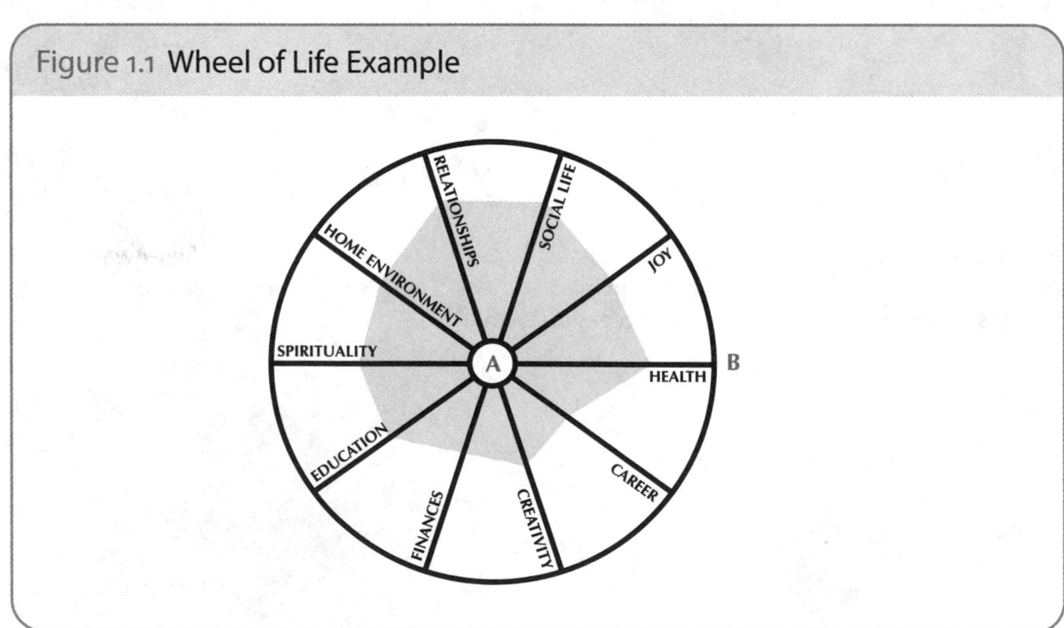

It's extremely difficult to get to your destination if you don't know where you are. Include the personal aspects of your life, as well as the professional ones, when assessing yourself. You're a whole being and your career is only one—albeit a very significant—part of your life. This chapter contains several activities to assist you in assessing yourself and visualizing your future.

Figure 1.1 is a completed example of an exercise called the "Wheel of Life." Its purpose is to support you in evaluating your life in a visual manner. Imagine that the center point (A) is the least desirable state and the outside of the circle (B) is the most desirable state.

§1

Wheel of Life Exercise

Print a blank copy of the Wheel of Life. Look at each category. Take a moment to think about where you are right now. Where is that in relation to where you want to be? Then mark along the line for each of the 10 categories where you feel you are right now. Finally, connect the dots. Do you have a balanced wheel or does it look like a starburst? Keep in mind that it's very difficult to smoothly roll through life when your wheel (life) isn't balanced.

You also might mark the "spokes" with an arrow in the direction that you see that particular spoke going. For example, if you're in school, then the education dot is an arrow pointing to the outside. If there's no particular activity in that spoke, then just put a dot.

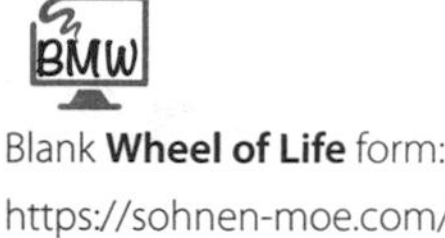

Blank **Wheel of Life** form: https://sohnen-moe.com/bm5-workbook-request/

Consider this wheel from two points of view. First, notice any categories that are proportionately nearer the center than others. Those are the areas on which you need to concentrate on improving. The object is to bring more balance to your wheel. The second aspect is to enhance all the categories so that they're toward the outside (most desirable) of the circle. I recommend that you do this exercise every few months. It's a great way to chart your progress! You can also utilize this tool to make a Wheel of Life that represents your ideal life situation. On a blank Wheel of Life write activities on each spoke that enable you to grow or maintain your position in each area of your life.

The next activities involve assessing yourself personally and professionally. These activities help you identify your strengths, challenges, and desires. We start with a personal assessment.

Personal Assessment

Write a biographical sketch spanning from your birth to the present. Include personal and family information as well as the following:

- Your major accomplishments
- Your talents and abilities
- The 3 things you do best
- Your challenges
- The obstacles you've overcome
- The 3 things you do the least well
- The 3 things for which you want to be remembered
- The memories you treasure most
- How you would like others to describe you
- The 3 things you want to accomplish in your life

The following activity explores your career. It's mainly designed for people who are currently in practice and are using this book to support them in moving to the next level. If you're using this book to help you start a new career, you may simply answer the last question in the list.

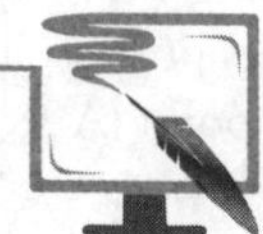

Career Assessment

Describe the current state of your career or business experience. Include length of time in your field, average yearly income, and number of clients. In addition, list the following:

- What are the 3 attributes of your practice of which you're the most proud?
- What is working well?
- What isn't working well?
- What changes would you like to see occur?
- What would you like people to say about your business?

The next activity is for students. Reflect upon your previous jobs or career tracks. Even if you haven't had a job, you probably have gained insight into your preferences and learned transferable skills by doing volunteer work or being active in extracurricular school activities. Also, these questions encourage you to think about aspects of your career that you may not have considered before. Your responses can help you determine how to pursue your career after graduation.

Assessment for Students

Highlight your previous job experience, education, and background that can contribute to your success in this career field. In addition, list the following:

- What previous jobs/work experiences have you most enjoyed?
- What previous jobs/work experiences have you least enjoyed?
- Do you feel comfortable reporting to others?
- Do you like to manage your own time or prefer someone else setting priorities and schedules?
- What kinds of people (clients or coworkers) do you prefer to work with?
- Do you enjoy or genuinely dislike paperwork?
- Do you like performing a variety of business tasks each day and week?
- How many hours do you work or want to work each week?
- Do you think you"ll prefer to spend the majority of time working with clients?
- Do you have marketing experience? Do you enjoy it?
- Do you want to offer other services besides your primary training? What other modalities/knowledge do you want to learn?
- Are you a disciplined, self-starter with an interest in running a business? What life experience has given you the opportunity to know this about yourself?
- Do you enjoy teaching?
- Do you enjoy doing research?
- Do your family and friends support your career goals?
- Who has given you career guidance already or might be a mentor for you?

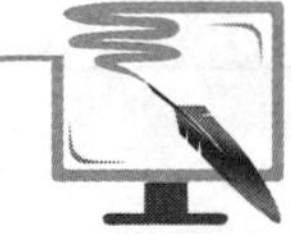

Self-Reflection

What did you learn about yourself in the previous four self-assessment exercises? Were you surprised by anything? How can you use this awareness to develop confidence about your previous accomplishments and determination toward the areas that need attention?

Values Clarification

A satisfying and balanced life occurs when your values are in synchrony with the way you live your life and run your business. Values are beliefs about what is intrinsically worthwhile or desirable, rather than what is right and correct. For example, if you have a strong value of making your services accessible to everyone, regardless of their economic means, you may be motivated to incorporate a sliding scale into your fee structure. This doesn't mean that you feel a moral obligation to have a sliding scale, to avoid acting unethically; you just view this as a better, more worthwhile arrangement. Individuals don't necessarily agree on what is important as a value, and may even change their value structures many times over the course of their lives.

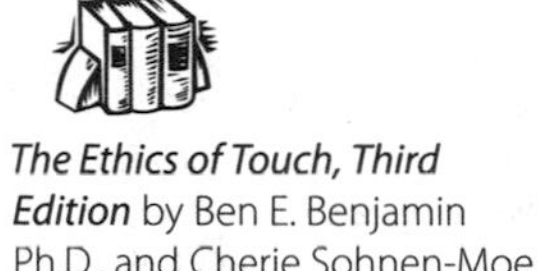

The Ethics of Touch, Third Edition by Ben E. Benjamin Ph.D., and Cherie Sohnen-Moe

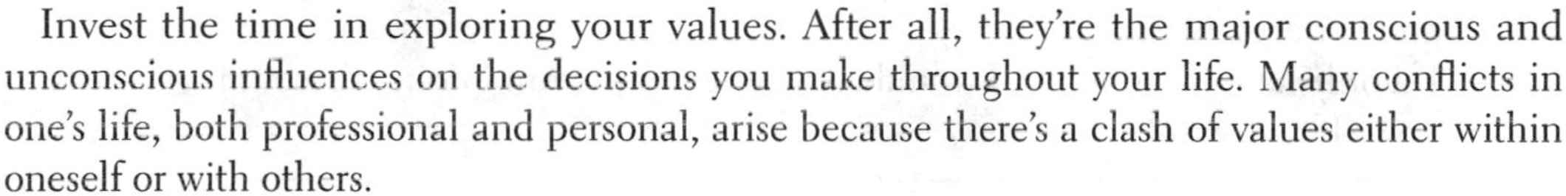

Invest the time in exploring your values. After all, they're the major conscious and unconscious influences on the decisions you make throughout your life. Many conflicts in one's life, both professional and personal, arise because there's a clash of values either within oneself or with others.

The following activities are designed to help you clarify your core values. Ask yourself the following questions and write down your responses, taking time to carefully consider each one. When you finish these lists, we recommend you discuss it with a fellow student, friend, or colleague. Engaging in a dialogue with others is another way to more fully explore your values.

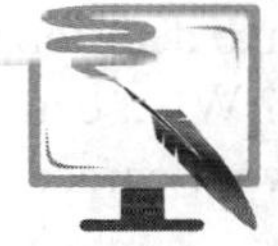

Questions to Clarify Your Professional Values

My Work Life

- My attitudes and beliefs about wellness are…
- My attitudes and beliefs about my profession are…

Professionalism

- How do my values enhance my professionalism and affect my work with clients?
- What are the most meaningful attributes of an effective practitioner in my field?
- Which of my personal values might conflict with professional rules of conduct?
- Which of my personal values might conflict with laws or regulation?

Core Values

- What are the most important personal characteristics for someone in my field?
- What are the key professional characteristics for someone in my field?
- When I look at my work life in perspective, the activities that have the most worth to me are…

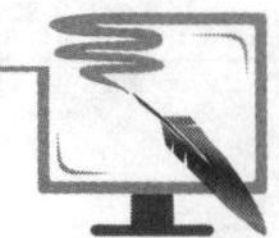

Questions to Clarify Your Personal Values

My Ideal Life

- What would I do with my life if I could do anything? Why?

Happiness

- The people I know who seem to be happy are happy because...
- I am happiest when I am...
- What is my most treasured memory? Why?

Relationships

- When I look at my home life, the activities that are the most worthy are...
- The things I most value in a relationship are...
- Who and what have been major influences in my values development?
- Who are the most important people in my life? What could I do to improve those relationships?

Core Values

- What values are most important to me?
- What are the character traits I deem essential?
- The most admirable things about me are...
- What is the greatest accomplishment of my life? What do I hope to do that is as great or even better?
- If I only had 1 year to live, I would concentrate on... Am I doing those things now? If not, why?

"What would you do if you weren't afraid?
—Spencer Johnson

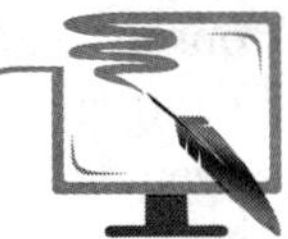

Values Reflection

Did you have trouble completing the values activities? How often do you make decisions and form relationships consistent with your personal and professional values? What can you do to keep your professional values in mind when making decisions for your career/business?

Your Ideal Future

Creative visualization is a powerful tool for career success. Envisioning your ideal future is one of the most enjoyable aspects of long-range planning. This section stimulates your imagination to visualize and manifest your ideal future. Allow yourself the freedom to state your desires, dreams, and goals. This is where you let your imagination roam free. Put aside any concerns about whether your vision is realistic or attainable. If you have any negative thoughts about your ability or worthiness to have this life, acknowledge those thoughts and continue with the exercise. Encompass all areas of your life, including your career, environment, relationships, finances, education, spirituality, health, and social life. If you prefer to visualize with your eyes closed, you may want to have a friend read you these questions, or you could make an audio recording of the exercise—leaving ample time for thought between questions.

Remember, this is about your IDEALS, not necessarily what you think is realistic. We forge some of these dreams into goals in the next chapter. Make any notes in your workbook journal.

"Ideals are like stars; you will not succeed in touching them with your hands. But like the seafaring man on the desert of waters, you choose them as your guides, and following them you will reach your destiny.
—Carl Schurz

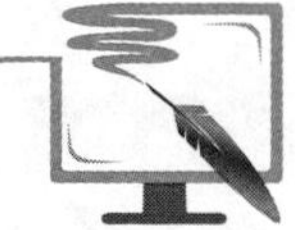

Visualizing Your Life and Career Success

Imagine that you're living the life of your dreams right now.

- Describe where you live: Where do you reside—what city, state, or country? What type of home do you live in? How is it furnished? What is the ambiance?
- Think about yourself: What do you look like? What are your attitudes toward life? How do you nurture yourself? How do you feel about yourself?
- Contemplate your relationships: Who are your friends? How do you interact with your family? How do you impact others? What are the important characteristics of your romantic relationship? What is your social life like?
- Now think about your career: What is your profession? What are your responsibilities and activities? What type of business atmosphere do you have? Who are your co-workers? What are your business relationships like? What is your financial status?
- Reflect upon your personal growth: What activities do you engage in to take care of your wellbeing? How are you furthering your education? What do you do to foster your spirituality? How do you spend your leisure time?
- Lastly, consider any other areas that are important to you: What do you do to make certain these things happen? What are your attitudes about them?

§1

See Chapter 3, pages 33-34 for information on how **visualization** works.

Another way to explore your ideal future is to ask yourself: "If I could be anywhere doing anything, where would I be and what would I be doing?" Be sure to note any realizations in your journal. Sometimes what's important are the qualities of life and not necessarily the specific activities. For instance, your future vision might not have "looked" dramatically different from your current status, but perhaps it "felt" different. Maybe you were more relaxed, energetic, and happier.

Does your ideal future look attainable? How do you feel about your abilities to work toward your dreams? If you have your doubts, remember that you need to be your own biggest cheerleader. Remain positive as you gather the requisite goal-setting tools found in the following chapters.

Now comes the difficult part—determining whether you're on the path to making your dreams become reality and deciding what you're willing to do to have your life be that of your dreams. It is perfectly okay to not work on everything at once—actually you will probably drive yourself (and those around you) crazy if you attempt to change too many things too quickly.

> "Courage is very important. Like a muscle, it is strengthened by use.
> — Ruth Gordon

You may also find that you aren't willing to take some of the required steps to achieve an aspect of your dream. Give yourself permission to set your own boundaries and priorities. This is where dreams differentiate from goals.

And thus, Chapter 2.

2
Life Planning

"The future belongs to those who believe in the beauty of their dreams."
— Eleanor Roosevelt

Goal Setting
- Setting Realistic Goals
- Purpose, Priorities, and Goals
- Goal Setting Techniques
- Goal Setting Enhancements
- Clarify Your Life Vision
- Ranking Goals

Strategic Planning

Follow-Through

Key Terms

Affirmations
Audio Recordings
Collage
Creative Visualization
Goal
Goal Setting
Mind Mapping Technique
Miniature Replica
Outline Technique
Picture Book
Picture Board
Priorities
Purpose
Reticular Activating System
SMARTER Goals
Strategic Planning
Vision Box

Now that you have assessed your current status and envisioned your ideal life, it's time to add substance to them by setting clear purposes, priorities, and goals for your life and your practice. As you work through this chapter, keep in mind that you may need to revisit it several times to work through all of the activities, particularly in regards to specific work environments. It takes time and patience to anchor your dreams into practical, everyday steps that lead to completed goals. Don't get discouraged if at times it seems overwhelming. Just take a break to re-energize, and come back to your goal setting when you're ready. Goal setting is a lifelong practice.

See Section 3 for details on **work environments**.

Goal Setting

Goal setting is the means of turning your dreams into reality. Many people imagine great things, yet very few accomplish their dreams. Dreams are similar to wishes: they are things we fantasize about, yet we do little to make certain they occur (but we're certainly ecstatic when they do). Goals are dreams to which you commit and take action to ensure their attainment.

Goal setting is tied into the reticular activating system (RAS), a network of neural tissue connecting the spinal cord and brainstem to the thalamus and cerebrum. The RAS regulates alertness and attention. It's also believed to be the center of arousal and motivation. Our senses (particularly sight) are constantly flooded with a vast amount of stimuli, yet we're consciously aware of only a fraction of that data because the RAS filters out what it deems insignificant information.[1] In essence, we have programmed directional signalers (or in some cases, blinders) in our brains. Although this may seem like an oversimplification, it's indeed how it functions.

For example, recall the last time you decided to get a new car. You finally chose the model and color, and it seemed like everywhere you went, you saw "your car." Of course all those people didn't just go out and purchase those cars when you did. Those cars were already on the road. You just hardly noticed them before because they weren't significant to you. This is the magnificence of goal setting. By establishing clear goals, you program your brain to be aware and notify your conscious mind of the information and opportunities that YOU DESIRE.

The inability to actualize goals is usually related to unclear goals, lack of commitment, conflict, or negative conditioning. Very few people write goals, and, of those who do, most don't always write their goals in a way that easily produces results. Sometimes they claim to want something, but what they really want is what that something represents. Occasionally conflicts exist in relation to the achievement of their goals. The attainment of one goal may preclude the fulfillment of another, or their immediate family or colleagues may not view the consequences favorably.

Setting Realistic Goals

> "If you have built castles in the air, your work need not be lost; that is where they should be. Now put foundations under them.
>
> —Henry David Thoreau

The first step is to set aside some time to think about your goals and put them into writing. It may be helpful to review your written goals to be sure they reflect your true desires—not what your spouse, parent, boss, or peers think you should want.

Sometimes it can be tempting to set unrealistic deadlines or goals that are dependent on other people. It's also easy to get caught up in a flurry of goal writing and generate pages and pages of goals, then hardly accomplish anything. At other times, we may get so bogged down in details that we lose sight of the big picture.

As you can see, setting realistic goals is often a balancing act. It requires careful thought. While you reach for your greatest potential, also ground your dreams in step-by-step actions that help you achieve your goals.

Profile: Whitney Lowe

Whitney Lowe is the director of the Academy of Clinical Massage and author of *Orthopedic Assessment in Massage Therapy and Orthopedic Massage: Theory & Technique*. He has been setting goals for many years. He is a very self-disciplined person, and once he learned about goal setting he took to it right away. He sets goals because:

> *I have found this to be an important part of the planning process as well as the process of measuring my success. When I set goals, it's the first step in giving me direction about how to get where I want to go. Once the goal is established, I can work backwards from there until I have identified all the smaller steps that are necessary to accomplish that goal. Unless some of the bigger goals are broken down into these smaller steps, it's very difficult to get started working on them. I feel that I have accomplished some very large tasks, such as getting a book finished and constantly meeting production deadlines for my bimonthly research newsletter. I have also set goals for myself in relation to my massage practice that are just as important. For example, I have found when I set small goals for studying and reviewing topics of anatomy, kinesiology or pathology, it was much easier to accomplish this study, and I really looked forward to it.*

§1

"The purpose of life is a life of purpose.
—Robert Byrne

Purpose, Priorities, and Goals

Goal setting is much more effective when it's connected to a larger picture. Instead of churning out a list of goals you want to achieve, consider a layered approach. Start by defining your purpose. Next, identify your major priorities. Then create goals that are aligned with the specific priorities.

Purpose

You need a context for your goals, something to connect them, otherwise they become chores. Most people do almost anything to avoid chores. **Purpose** provides that context. Purpose is very general—it's a direction, a theme. You can never actually complete a purpose; it's an ongoing process. Take a moment and think about what is really meaningful to you. Is there a common thread—one statement that encompasses your ideals, values, and dreams? You may have a purpose for your life and purposes for every major area of your life.

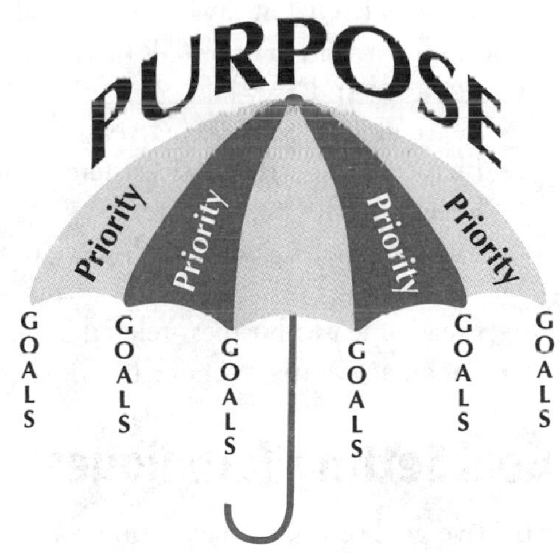

Overall Life Purpose Examples

- I make a positive difference.
- I'm happy.
- My life is an expression of love and joy.

You may find your life purpose shifting over time, becoming more refined. Remember, it isn't written in stone, though, in most instances, your priorities and goals are more likely to change, and not your life purpose. One of the most significant features of having a distinct life purpose is that it becomes easier to resolve any conflicting goals when you know the direction for your life.

"The secret of success is constancy to purpose.
—Benjamin Disraeli

Career Purpose Examples

- My career supports myself and others in being happy and healthy.
- I make a healthy difference.
- My career is a source of joy and prosperity.
- I'm innovative and successful in my career.
- My career is a joyous expression of who I am.

Priorities

Priorities are general areas of concern. They are less vague and not so all encompassing as purposes, yet not as specific as goals. Priorities are statements of intention that are connected with values. This is where you begin to make choices that support your overall purpose.

General Life Priorities Examples

- My relationships are nurturing and fun.
- I'm creative in all that I do.
- Each and every day I learn something new.
- My body is a manifestation of health and beauty.
- My communications are open and honest.

Career Priorities Examples

- My career is fulfilling and provides me with the income that I desire.
- I enjoy my work.
- I regularly participate with other colleagues.
- I continually expand my knowledge and skills.
- I'm creative in my work.
- My work environment is nurturing and professional.

Goals

"What you get by achieving your goals is not as important as what you become by achieving your goals.
—Zig Ziglar

Goals are very specific things, events, or experiences that have a definite completion, and you can objectively know when you've achieved them. Effective goals have the characteristics found in the acronym of SMARTER (see Figure 2.1).

Career Goal Examples

- I earn at least $40,000 per year.
- I have a wonderful music system in my office.
- I keep my client files current.
- I invest at least 5 hours each week in marketing.
- I review my business plan every 3 months.
- I read at least 1 business-related book each month.
- I'm an active member of 2 business groups.

Goal Setting Techniques

Effective goal setting is the groundwork for success. I advocate that you have written goals in addition to any other techniques you employ. The written word is so powerful! By inscribing your intentions, you say to yourself and the world that you know you deserve to have these things happen (see Figure 2.2). Sometimes people are afraid to write down their goals because they don't think they can achieve them, and thus they don't want a written reminder of their failures. Failure, per se, doesn't really exist in goal setting. Usually, when you don't accomplish a goal it's because you've set an inappropriate deadline, have inaccurate information, experience blocks, encounter conflicts, don't really want the goal, or are unwilling (or unable) to do what's required to accomplish the goal. Having written goals can only serve to support and teach you, enhancing your self-knowledge.

Figure 2.1 SMARTER

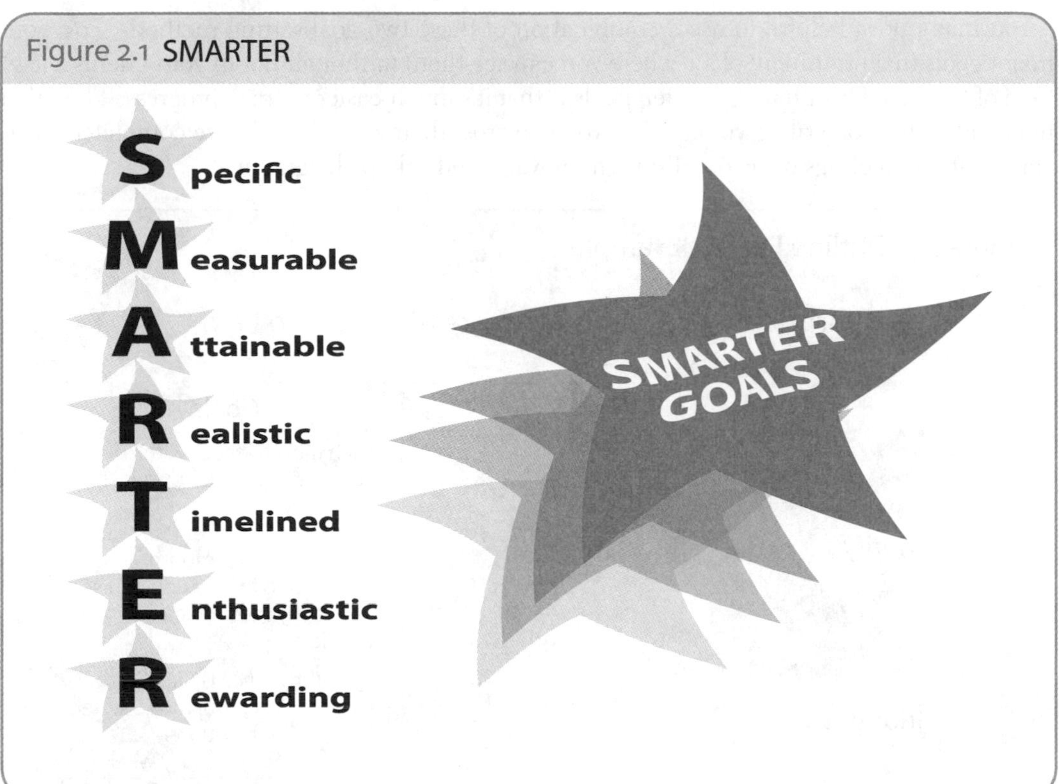

§1

"If one advances confidently in the direction of his dreams, and endeavors to live the life which he has imagined, he will meet with a success unexpected in common hours.
—Henry David Thoreau

Figure 2.2 Goal Setting Tips

- Always state your goals in the positive PRESENT TENSE. If you write in the future, they may remain in the future—never attained.
- Personalize your goals: use a pronoun (e.g., I, we, they, "your name") in every sentence.
- Make your goals real: something you know you can accomplish on your own without help or someone waving a magic wand over you.
- Don't use the terms "try," "will," "not," "never," "should," "would," "could" and "want."
- Include deadline dates whenever possible.
- Have fun!

Written Goals

Written goals are a powerful visual (and actually auditory) declaration of your intentions. The two most commonly used methods for goal setting are outline format and mind mapping. The **Outline** format is very effective for logical thinkers. When you use the outline format (see Figure 2.3), you write your purpose, priorities, and list the specific goals under each priority.

The **Mind Mapping** approach is excellent for visually oriented thinkers. In mind mapping, you actually write the purpose in the center of a page, attach spokes to the circle onto which you list the priorities, and extend lines off of each spoke onto which you write the specific goals. Another mind-mapping option is to draw an image in the middle of a page, such as an office filled with clients, a stack of money, or an umbrella (see Figure 2.4). Then, add related images as well as written priorities and goals.

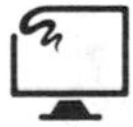

Online Mind-Mapping Tools

www.mindmeister.com
www.mind42.com
www.mindnode.com
www.mindgenius.com
toketaware.com/ithoughts-ios
www.mindmanager.com/en/

You may find it helpful to use a combination of these two goal-setting methods. Post your major goals in a prominent place where you can see them (although not in your clients' view). One of the benefits of having written goals is that it's much easier to track progress. The other major advantage of writing your goals is you can cross them out when they're completed—this contributes to feelings of accomplishment, reward, and acknowledgment.

Figure 2.3 **Outline Format Example**

Purpose: My career is an expression of who I am.

	Priority	Goals
Priority 1	I continually expand my knowledge and skills.	• Each month I meet with colleagues to share business experiences. • I read at least 2 business magazines each month. • I take a public speaking course before my second year in business.
Priority 2	My work environment is professional and nurturing.	• I paint my office by July 1. • I have a wonderful music system in my office by Aug 15. • I clean my office every week.
Priority 3	My career provides me with the income I desire.	• I earn at least $40,000 this year. • I take a 2-week vacation this winter. • I increase my client retention rate by at least 20%.

Figure 2.4 **Mind Mapping Example**

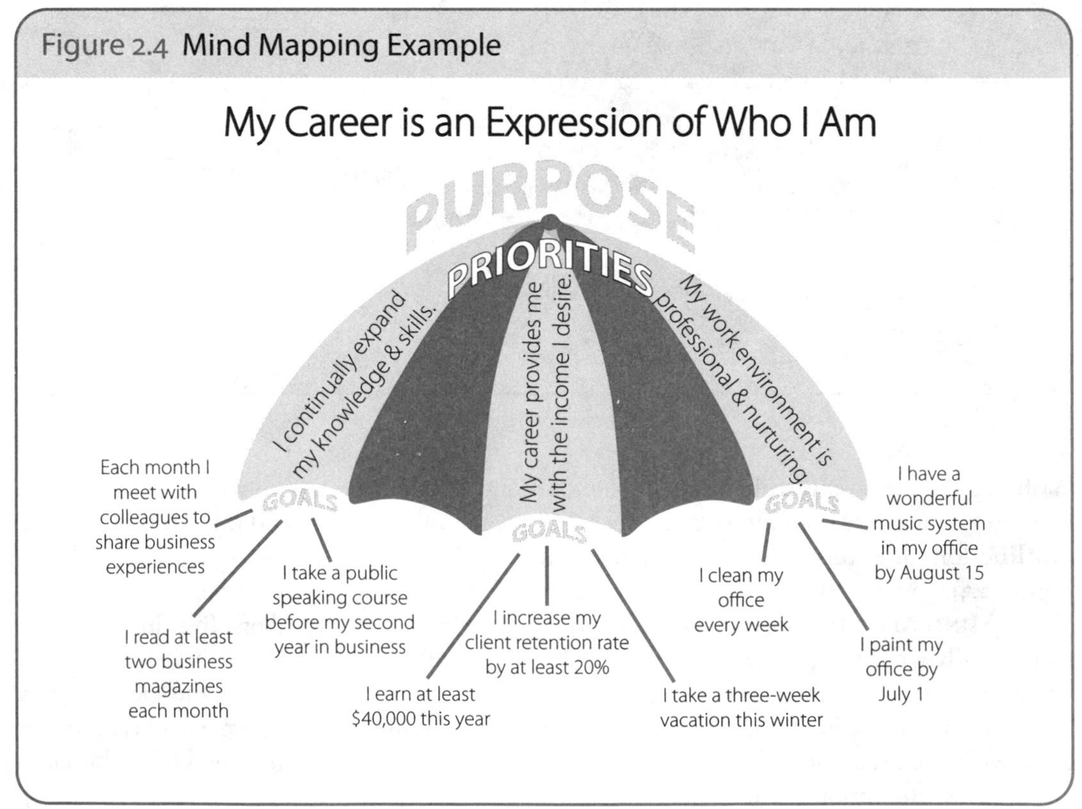

If you love technology, check out the many online tools (e.g., websites, software, apps) that are available for mind mapping and goal setting. Even if you use an online tool to help you visualize your intentions, you may want to print your creation so you have a physical representation to hold and look at as well.

When setting goals, use the format with which you feel the most comfortable and that proves to be the most effective. Include some type of written goals in addition to any other format, particularly for your career. You may want to use some of the other methods as a means of positive reinforcement or visualization. What is crucial is the way you actually state your goals and the individual steps necessary to accomplish them. Keep your goals SMARTER, follow the suggested goal setting techniques, and, most importantly of all, be sure they're YOUR goals. Setting goals can be creative and exciting. If you tend to use mainly one method, experiment with other techniques. Use as many of your senses as possible. Goal setting is a necessary component of success, but it doesn't have to be a burden. Remember, the purpose of setting goals is to make your dreams become reality.

> Opportunity is missed by most people because it is dressed in overalls and looks like work.
> —Thomas Edison

Goal Setting Enhancements

One of the ways to magnify the power of your goals is to involve as many of your senses as possible (particularly sight, touch, and sound) in the process. In addition to writing, you may want to use a variety of methods from visual illustration to audio recordings to physical representations.

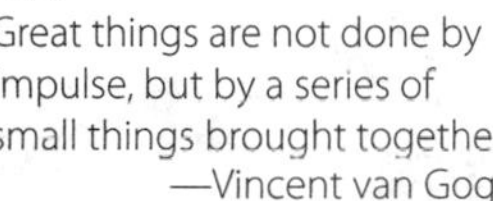

> Great things are not done by impulse, but by a series of small things brought together.
> —Vincent van Gogh

The more frequently you review your goals, the more likely you are to achieve them.

Make A Collage

Collages are a wonderful way to visually create your goals. To make a collage, get a large piece of poster board (22" x 28" is available in many colors at art supply stores). Set aside a couple of hours, get comfortable, put on some nice music, make yourself a cup of tea, get a stack of magazines, a pair of scissors and some glue, and prepare to have a fantastic experience! (By the way, this is a lot of fun to do with friends.) Decide the purpose of your collage—be it a representation of your whole life, your career, the next 6 months, or even just 1 major goal. Keeping your purpose in mind, go through the magazines and cut out pictures and words that appeal to you. Let your intuition be your guide. The items you choose may not be what you had anticipated. Don't worry about finding "perfect" pictures or words. They may be abstract or elicit a certain emotion. Remember, this is a representation of your dreams and goals.

Give yourself a time limit for cutting, or else you may find yourself there for days. After you've cut out plenty of pictures and words, glue them onto the poster board. You also may want to write some goals or affirmations on the board. Spend some time with your collage—allow yourself to experience the full impact. Finally, hang your collage in a place where you can see it every day.

See Chapter 3, pages 34-36 for more information on **affirmations**.

Compile a Picture Book

Picture Books are a good option if you don't have an appropriate place to hang a collage. The supplies needed are a large, 3-ring binder, a set of at least eight dividers, notebook paper, scissors, glue, and magazines. Use the dividers to arrange the categories of your goals, such as health, finances, education, and marketing. Follow the same directions for the collage, except glue the pictures and words by category onto notebook paper and then put the sheets in the binder. You can write your goals next to the pictures. The advantages of a picture book are that you can carry it with you and you can easily add more pages to it. The disadvantage is that you may not look at it as frequently as you would a collage.

Online tools for **visual goal setting.**

dreamitalive.com
www.pinterest.com

Create a Picture Board

Picture Boards are a combination of a collage and a picture book. Instead of gluing the pictures and words to paper or poster board, you pin them on a bulletin board. This technique makes it easy to literally shift your goals—put them in different perspective, add more goals, and take them down once they've been achieved. You can even create a virtual picture board to illustrate your goals, by using one of the many online services available for goal setting like DreamItAlive.com, VisionBoard.me, or the popular Pinterest.com.

> "You have to know what you want to get it.
> —Gertrude Stein

Assemble a Vision Box

Vision Boxes are another creative option to visually create your goals. The procedure is to find or make a box that is appealing. Cut out pictures and words from magazines and brochures that express your desires. Place those items, as well as any pictures or mementos that represent your goals, into the box. On the outside of the lid write "everything that is in this box is." Open the box every month or so to remove the items that have manifested, add new ones, and refocus on the ones remaining.

Record Your Goals

Audio Recordings of your goals are very effective. Write out your goals before you record them, following the suggested Goal Setting Techniques. The beauty of recording your goals is that you can listen to them at any time. It can be particularly beneficial to listen while sleeping for the subliminal effects. An interesting alternative is to have someone who is a positive authority figure, role model, or mentor record some of the goals. Experiment!

Pay attention to details. Make your replica as realistic as possible. Don't let a (perceived) lack of artistic proficiency limit your creativity in visualizing and expressing your goals. Be inventive and have fun!

Build a Miniature Replica

Physical Representations are excellent tools for depicting your goal(s). The idea is to create a 3-dimensional object that you can see and touch. This can be very powerful. It makes you really "look" at what you say you want. Generally it's a time-intensive endeavor, but it can be well worth it, particularly for the goals that are very meaningful to you and the ones you find difficult to achieve.

For example, if one of your goals is to remodel your office, you may want to build a miniature version of your office with all of the proposed changes. Get samples of the paint or wallpaper and put them on the walls. Make (or buy) miniature furniture. Create it as closely as possible to your plans. If one of your goals is to exercise regularly, you may want to make a sculpture of yourself exercising. If you cannot easily recognize yourself, attach a photo of your face to the sculpture.

The inclusion of scent adds another potent dimension. For example, if you've been telling yourself for the last few years that you'd really like to take a winter vacation in the mountains and you still haven't left the city, it may be that you need to make that goal more tangible. You might want to design a model of the desired location. Start by making a mini-mountain. Then construct a little cabin, and inside it put pictures of yourself and whomever else you want for company. Make some pine trees (using real pine needles if possible), and put pine essence on the trees. Now, every time you walk by your mountain, you see it, touch it, take in a deep breath, and smell the pine trees....

Clarify Your Life Vision

Before you even begin to consider developing or enhancing your practice, it's imperative to set a strong foundation by clarifying your life's purpose, priorities, and goals. Then, you can more effectively create your other plans. The following exercise guides you in writing your purpose, priorities, and goals for your overall life, the next 5 years, 3 years, 1 year, and 6 months. Your Wheel of Life and the previous exercises in this chapter and Chapter 1 can serve as guides. I recommend that you revisit this activity and add detailed career goals after you have worked through all of Section 1 and Section 2 of this book.

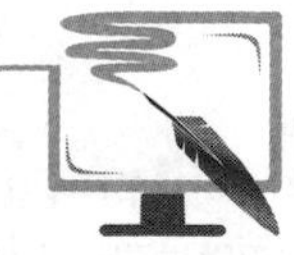

Life Planning

Take a few deep breaths, relax, and let your dreams and goals express themselves. Let them guide your mind, heart, and hands. For now, don't worry about "how" you write them. Let your creativity flow. You can go back later and rephrase your statements. Start by clarifying your life purpose. Review your Personal Assessment Exercises from Chapter 1. Think about your values, ideals, and dreams. Create a statement that reflects the essence of your life. Next, think about the aspects of life that are meaningful to you, and create priorities for those areas. Include all areas on the Wheel of Life. Then identify your life goals. Repeat this process for your 5-year, 3-year, 1-year, and 6-month plan.

Overall Life Plan

My purpose in life is:
My major priorities in life are:
My major goals in life are:

Five-Year Plan

My purpose for the next 5 years is:
My major priorities for the next 5 years are:
My major goals for the next 5 years are:

Three-Year Plan

My purpose for the next 3 years is:
My major priorities for the next 3 years are:
My major goals for the next 3 years are:

One-Year Plan

My purpose for the next year is:
My major priorities for the next year are:
My major goals for the next year are:

Six-Month Plan

My purpose for the next 6 months is:
My major priorities for the next 6 months are:
My major goals for the next 6 months are:

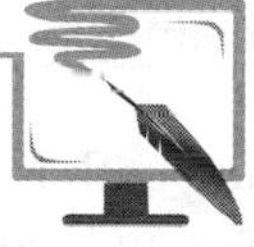

Reflection

Now that you've taken the time to clarify your purposes, priorities, and goals, it's time for reflection. Ask yourself the following questions:

1. What do I need to change in my life to accomplish these things?
2. What help from others do I need to achieve success in these areas?
3. Who are the people that can help me?
4. What problems do I anticipate when acting on these goals?
5. What will I achieve if I complete these goals?

Look Ahead

In the previous two activities, you set your intentions and reflected back on them to determine what you may need to work on next. What goals inspire you the most? What additional reflection questions can you ask yourself to determine your personal motivation toward creating a plan for your future? What do you see as your next step?

Ranking Goals

Congratulations! You now have written your intentions for your life and created your purposes, priorities, and goals. Having built this foundation puts you miles ahead of the general public and well on your path to success. Just writing some of your goals may be all the planning you need to do.

> "People who fail to plan, have planned to fail.
> —George Hewell

Not all goals or activities carry the same ultimate value. Some goals have a higher intrinsic worth, while others require more immediate action. This holds true whether you're planning your life, month, week, or day. Review your goal lists and rank them with an "A," "B" or "C." The "A" goals are the ones that are the most crucial for you to attain—the ones you can commit to right now. The "B" goals have importance to you, but aren't as significant as the "A" goals. The "C" goals are ones that would be nice if they actualized, but you aren't ready to commit to accomplishing them at this moment.

The next step in ranking your goals is to arrange them in terms of time priority. Start with your "A" goals. Make sure all goals have assigned target dates for completion. Then numerically rank each goal according to time priority (1 being the highest). Using the Sample Career Goals (in the previous section), your time priority list might look like this:

Online **Strategic Planning Tools**

www.planware.org
onstrategyhq.com/strategic-planning-software
www.gazelles.com/g/one-page-tools/strategy

7. I earn at least $40,000 per year.
5. I have a wonderful music system in my office.
2. I keep my client files current.
6. I review my business plan every 3 months.
1. I invest at least 5 hours each week in marketing.
4. I read at least 1 business-related book each month.
3. I'm an active member of 2 business groups.

Strategic Planning

We've all heard the cliché, "If you want to get something done, ask a busy person." This is because busy people have learned (often by necessity) how to plan and organize their lives. We can incorporate those skills into our lives so that we don't become overwhelmed or miss opportunities.

> "Great things are not done by impulse, but by a series of small things brought together.
> —Vincent van Gogh

Strategic planning benefits are numerous (see Figure 2.5). Planning helps renew enthusiasm, especially if a goal is tough to accomplish. Also, some goals may be very complex and require numerous sub-steps to be accomplished. This process of "divide and conquer" (i.e., breaking down a difficult problem into manageable chunks) is what strategic planning is about. Beware! This is also the stage that many people neglect to do and therefore become overwhelmed. Yet, whenever you reduce a goal to its component parts, the small steps toward reaching it are less overwhelming and more possible. You gain confidence with each little step forward.

Figure 2.5 Strategic Planning Benefits

- You're less likely to forget a major step.
- Creative ideas and brainstorming come easier.
- Goals become clarified and more real.
- You gain a better overall picture.
- You realize that some steps may require more immediate action than others.
- You gain knowledge of what is necessary to accomplish the goal.
- A more accurate timetable is developed.
- A written description of your intentions is a self-motivational tool.

§1

Strategic planning is a layered system: start with your major goal, analyze it, and break it into smaller goals and steps (see Figure 2.6). You may find that some of the "smaller" steps need their own strategic plan. I recommend that you make a master list of the activities required to achieve the major goal and use separate sheets for each project.

After you've completed your strategic planning for a major goal, transfer the target dates of the specific action steps to a calendar. This process helps you to visualize what it will take to accomplish that goal and discover any complications. You might find things such as: you have numerous target dates that are very close to each other and it would be difficult to accomplish all of them by the targeted time; the time to accomplish the specific steps will take longer than originally estimated and the completion date needs to be changed; other goals (not from this strategic plan) need to be accomplished in that same time frame; or you have conflicts due to other commitments. Determine if any of the target dates need to be adjusted and go back to your strategic plan, making any necessary changes to the specific steps or the overall goal itself. For complex strategic plans, I recommend using a spreadsheet, a Gantt chart, or project management software.

Project Management Tools

www.gantt.com
www.smartsheet.com
basecamp.com

Figure 2.6 **Action Steps for Strategic Planning**

1. List the current date and target date for accomplishing the goal.
2. Identify the major goal.
3. Describe the existing situation.
4. List the benefits of achieving the goal.
5. Brainstorm possible courses of action.
6. Choose the best solution.
7. Sketch a proposal outline.
8. Determine potential challenges and solutions.
9. Identify required resources.
10. Delineate specific action steps and target date for each step.
11. Transfer the target dates to a calendar.

Let's say that your vision is to do the following: work with 25 clients each week; practice in an office space with other wellness practitioners; share a front desk person who handles all the paperwork, bookkeeping, and scheduling; and net $45,000 per year. Of the many goals necessary to manifest this vision, the goal we use to illustrate the strategic planning process is to increase weekly clientele bookings from 15 to 25 clients within six months. See Figure 2.7.

In this strategic planning illustration, several of the goals need to have their own project sheet because of the many steps required to attain the goal (e.g., getting interviewed, doing the cooperative marketing projects). Other goals are more straightforward and self-explanatory, such as reading 3 business books and doing daily affirmations. If you experience any resistance or difficulty with any of your goals, break the goal down into as many specific steps as possible.

There is no such thing as an inappropriate goal, just a faulty time frame.

"The method of the enterprising is to plan with audacity, and execute with vigor; to sketch out a map of possibilities; and then to treat them as probabilities.

—Bovee

Figure 2.5 Strategic Planning Example

Today's Date: February 15
Target Date: August 15
Goal: I work with at least 25 clients per week.
Situation Description: I've been in practice for almost 2 years. I had a corporate account with ABC Electronics, but the company relocated. Now I average only 15 clients per week.
Benefits of Achieving This Goal: I can meet my lifestyle needs, pay off my school loans, take a vacation, and start a savings account.
Possible Courses of Action:

1. Get a part-time job at a clinic.
2. Hire an agent.
3. Actively market my practice.

Best Course: The most appropriate long-term solution is to actively market my practice, which could also include securing another corporate account.
Proposal Outline: To have 25 clients per week, I need a base of 100 active clients: five weekly, 15 biweekly, 40 monthly, and 40 occasional. I design a creative, fun marketing plan that includes increasing client retention.
Advantages: By augmenting my client list, I increase the odds of achieving my goal. Once my base is established, I won't have to put in as much effort into getting new clients because I incorporate client retention techniques.
Potential Conflicts/Disadvantages:

1. I don't really like marketing.
2. I'm not sure what to do.
3. There's a new company (with 4 therapists) offering corporate wellness care.

Solutions:

1. Do clearing exercises. Remind myself that marketing is simply sharing who I am and what I do. Do some of my marketing activities with colleagues.
2. Read books and magazines. Take marketing classes. Work with a business coach. Invest five hours per week on marketing.
3. Affiliate myself with the corporate wellness care company. Or, determine what my differential advantage is and pursue other accounts.

Action Required to Begin: Review my client files to determine session frequency. Set aside at least 2 hours to outline my marketing plan.
Resources Needed: Time, paper, pencils, and files. Ideally, samples of other practitioners' marketing plans.
Specific Steps to Achieve This Goal, Target Date

- I receive weekly wellness treatments, Starting 2/15
- I finalize my marketing plan (vision, goals, and analysis), 2/28
- I invest 5 hours per week to marketing for new clients, Starting 3/1
- I attend at least 2 networking functions monthly, Starting 3/1
- I do daily affirmations, Starting 3/1
- I invest 2 hours per week in client retention, Starting 3/1
- I do thorough intake interviews and treatment plans with all my clients, Starting 3/1
- For each of the next 6 months, I add 10 new clients to my client base, Starting 3/1

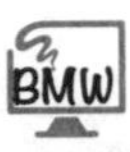

Strategic Planning
Blank copies of the Strategic Planning sheets:
https://sohnen-moe.com/bm5-workbook-request/

- I distribute at least 150 business cards monthly, Starting 3/1
- I do weekly client follow-up through calls and cards, Starting 3/1
- I redesign my brochures, 3/20
- I sponsor a fundraiser for my favorite charity, 3/20
- I join a business support group, 3/30
- I send a letter containing an incentive to non-current clients, 3/30
- I review and update my marketing plan monthly, Starting 3/31
- I distribute at least 100 brochures monthly, Starting 4/1
- I make at least 1 corporate wellness care proposal/presentation monthly, Starting 4/1
- I do at least 2 presentations/demonstrations monthly, Starting 4/1
- I contact at least 2 allied wellness practitioners monthly, Starting 4/1
- I send a welcome packet to all new clients, Starting 4/1
- I secure at least 1 corporate wellness care account, 4/30
- I read at least 3 business books, 4/1, 6/1, 8/1
- I send a newsletter to my clients, 4/20, 7/20
- I participate in at least 2 cooperative marketing projects, 5/15, 7/15
- I have a booth at the Wellness Expo, 5/20
- I develop a summer special for current clients, 5/25
- I get interviewed by the local paper, 5/31
- I'm a featured guest on 2 radio programs, 6/2
- I host a self-care booth at the Annual Street Fair, 6/15
- I appear on 4 television programs, 6/30
- I continue to add 4 new clients each month, Starting 9/1

Follow-Through

The most elaborate plan isn't going to create results if it isn't implemented. Transfer your goals and items from strategic planning sheets to a calendar, or create a simple tracking document on your computer (calendar programs make planning much less cumbersome). Refer to it often. It takes time, but long-term planning is time well invested. The clarity you acquire and the organization you create always save you at least the amount of time spent in actual planning.

A knowledge of the path cannot be substituted for putting one foot in front of the other.

—M.C. Richards

Crafting your life to be what you desire is a lifelong process. Putting your goals into writing is the first step. Increase the potential of achieving your goals by doing the following activities:

- Identify and clear obstacles.
- Take time to develop a strategic plan.
- Prioritize your daily activities.
- Track your goals.
- Develop a daily practice of using visualization and affirmations.

So far we have covered methods for self-exploration, goal setting, and strategic planning. Tracking goals and prioritizing your activities are techniques to assist you in staying on target. These topics, along with useful tools for achieving your goals (e.g., visualization, affirmation, clearing techniques, and some techniques to transform negative subconscious beliefs), are examined in Chapter 3.

See Chapter 18, page 253 for **technology ideas.**

3
Success Strategies

"Some men have thousands of reasons why they cannot do what they want to, when all they need is one reason why they can."

—Mary Frances Berry

What Is Success?
- Does Success Lead to Happiness?
- Self-Management

Barriers to Success
- Attitudes, Beliefs, and Perceptions
- How to Avoid Self-Sabotage

Tools for Actualizing Goals
- Creative Visualization
- Affirmations
- Breaking Old Habits
- More Than Positive Thinking

Time Management Principles
- The Pareto Principle
- Types of Time Needed to Run a Business
- High Priority Activities

Tracking
- Tracking Key Business Indicators
- Tracking Trends

The Art of Risk-Taking

Motivation
- Motivation Techniques

Key Terms

Acting As If
Affirmations
Attitudes
Barriers
Behavioral Theory
Beliefs
Clearing Techniques
Cognitive Theory
Continuing Education
Creative Visualization
Cross-lateral Movements
Defense Mechanism
Delegate
Dissolving Problems
Habits
Happiness
High Priority Activities
Humanistic Theory
Inner Critic
Key Business Indicators
Logistics
Marketing
Maslow's Hierarchy of Needs
Mental Contrasting
Motivation
Negative Conditioning
Pareto Principle
Perceptions
Perfectionist
Predetermined Goals
Procrastination
Professional Development
Psychoanalytic Theory
Psychotherapy
Reframing
Risk-Taking
Self-Management
Self-Motivation
Self-Sabotage
Sentence Completions
Social Cognition Theory
Social Learning Theory
Success
Success Markers
Time Management
Tracking
Trends
Values
Work Smarter—Not Harder

Thriving on chaos is a phrase that Tom Peters[1] has made common in the marketplace, and is also an apt description of how many of us lead our lives. But what is the price of our success through chaos? Have we excised ourselves (and our families) from our lives? It's easy to get enmeshed in our projects—telling ourselves that we will take time off next weekend, or maybe next month, well, at least sometime this year....

What Is Success?

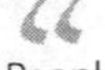

People are always blaming their circumstances for what they are. I don't believe in circumstances. The people who get on in this world are the people who get up and look for the circumstances they want, and, if they can't find them, make them.
—George Bernard Shaw

Quite often we have conflicting ideas of what it means to be successful and our requirements for success may vary greatly in the personal, business, and social realms. What does success really mean to you? Are you successful only if you earn a certain amount of money, perform miracles in your work, look a particular way, are in a perfect relationship, drive a great car, or live in the right neighborhood? In other words, what are your values? Is success a "thing" to achieve or a way of being?

In the book *Lead, Follow, or Get Out of the Way*, Jim Lundy describes success as the achievement of predetermined goals.[2] This means any goal! The key word is "predetermined." For instance, you may have accomplished something (possibly even something major) that you hadn't really intended, or even given much thought to, and somehow the victory seemed hollow. Most likely, that feeling was because you hadn't previously claimed it as a goal. Achievements are so much more fulfilling when they're planned. Thus, success is really a process—one that involves setting and achieving goals.

Does Success Lead to Happiness?

World Happiness Report
https://resources.unsdsn.org/world-happiness-report-2020

Happiness at Work Survey
https://fridaypulse.com/

Many people think that our successes will lead us to happiness. Often happiness is defined as one's personal satisfaction with life in general. We think, "I'll be happy as soon as I get that promotion" or "I'll be happy when I have my own private practice and don't have to work for so and so anymore." But researchers are finding that "happiness actually fuels success, not the other way around."[3] The truth is, if you practice positive thoughts and behaviors, you're more likely to be successful with many of your success markers (see Figure 3.1).

The World Happiness Report 2013 ranked 156 countries worldwide in terms of happiness. Denmark ranked number 1, Canada 6, and the United States ranked 17.[4] In the article "If You're Happy and You Know It..." Roy Saunderson reviewed that report and states, "Their findings suggest happy people live longer, are more productive, earn more, and are better citizens."[5]

Figure 3.1 Typical Success Markers

- Gross income
- Profit or salary
- Number of years in practice
- Number of years in current job
- Specialized knowledge and advanced techniques
- Total client base
- Number of clients seen each week
- Number of hours worked
- Amount of leisure time enjoyed
- Number of associates and employees
- Office location, square footage, or ambiance
- Prominence on a local, national, or international level

Harvard lecturer, author, and happiness expert, Shawn Achor, states that "the greatest competitive advantage in the modern economy is a positive and engaged brain." He goes on to suggest that you can train your brain for higher levels of happiness by adopting positive habits like these:[6]

- Write down 3 new things you're grateful for each day.
- Write for 2 minutes a day describing a positive experience you had that day.
- Exercise for 10 minutes a day.
- Meditate for 2 minutes, focusing on your breath going in and out.
- Write 1, quick email first thing in the morning thanking or praising a member on your team.

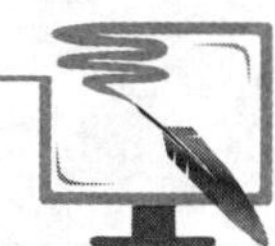

Identify Your Success Markers

List your success markers. Refer to the values exercises in Chapter 1 and explore how your values relate to your success. Identify what's truly important to you in terms of your overall life and then determine your career success markers. Only you can determine what success is for you—although others might attempt to influence you. As the saying goes, "One person's junk is another's treasure."

Explore The Happiness Factor

What and who are the people, places, or experiences in your life from which you derive satisfaction? Make a list divided into 2 columns, personal and professional items. How do the personal satisfaction items influence your professional life? How do the professional satisfaction items line up with the career purposes, priorities, and goals you delineated in the last chapter? Do you link happiness with success? How has one influenced the other at different times in your life? Take a look at your list of career success markers. Is this a list of things that will make you happy? Are you committed to pursuing happiness to positively affect your markers for success?

Self-Management

There is truly an art to being successful in the business world while staying balanced. It would be simple if our lives weren't filled with so many other meaningful activities. That just isn't the case. Most of us have a career or business, a family, social activities, and civic responsibilities. All of these are important. At times we may feel as though we're jugglers in a circus—keeping everything going, yet not fully enjoying any one aspect. So, what can we do? We certainly can't create a 30-hour day. The key to success is self-management. Self-management is artfully directing your life so that you easily and joyfully accomplish what you desire. It's about taking personal responsibility for every facet of your life and increasing personal productivity while staying true to yourself. Figure 3.2 highlights some of the components of effective self-management.

Figure 3.2 Effective Self-Management Components

- Knowing your values and living them
- Clarifying your purpose
- Setting priorities and goals
- Managing your time effectively
- Taking business risks wisely
- Staying inspired
- Balancing your personal and professional life
- Overcoming barriers to your success
- Committing to lifelong learning and professional development

Barriers to Success

To make the road to success a bit easier to travel, we take a look at some common barriers and what you can do to overcome them. Barriers to success can take varying shapes in our everyday lives and show up at the most inopportune times. Perhaps you've met the "Inner Critic," who stands ready to deliver a hefty dose of self-doubt or unhelpful criticism. Or, you may find yourself enjoying a career success moment and the next day you make some odd blunder that casts a shadow on what you previously accomplished. Perhaps you find yourself coming up with incredibly creative ways to procrastinate. If any of these scenarios sound familiar, rest assured that you aren't alone. These barriers to success, and others, are familiar to most successful professionals. They have wisely taken the time to understand the most common barriers and found effective ways to overcome them. Most barriers to success have their roots in negative conditioning. The good news is that you can change this conditioning.

Attitudes, Beliefs, and Perceptions

"Your attitude, not your aptitude, will determine your altitude.
—Zig Ziglar

Attitude plays a critical role in determining the difference between self-sabotage and success. Attitude is how one decides to approach something. Attitude is a choice. Attitude is the "lens" that colors how we view life experiences. All too often, when we encounter something new or challenging, we automatically have a negative attitude about it. If we choose to look at the new situation objectively and decide to stay open to learn more about it, our attitude already changes from a negative one to a positive one that is willing to adjust to the new circumstances.

Our attitudes stem from our beliefs. Ron Dalrymple, author of *The Inner Manager*,[7] states the following about false beliefs:

See pages 37-38 for **techniques to dissolve problems**.

> *As children, we are conditioned to believe many things and to adopt the arbitrary attitudes, emotions and behaviors of others. The delusions become our accepted reality. History is filled with examples of humankind's false beliefs, misperceptions and misguided behavior. Many of us limit and constrict ourselves daily with such notions. All of it's unnecessary.*
>
> *Perhaps the greatest thing to discover in life is that our potential for creativity, accomplishment and success is far greater than our imaginations allow. Motivational psychologists tell us if we can conceive it and believe it, we can achieve it. The power of thought, fueled by focused, positive emotions and consistent behavior, produces results of immense proportions. We must learn how the mind truly works and how we can best work with it, to get the most out of life and out of our practices.*

§1

The power of positive emotions is profound. Current research confirms that positive emotions are more than momentary good feelings; they broaden cognition, increase overall life satisfaction levels, and provide an enhanced ability to build skills and develop resources.[8]

While the ability to cultivate and maintain a positive attitude is a key to success, developing clear perception also keeps you on track to achieve your goals. Perception is much like attitude, although it's not always about choice. When we're faced with something new or challenging, we can choose to have a positive attitude toward it, but that doesn't mean that we automatically perceive it for what it is.

One of the wonders of life is the ability of people to "see" things in a different light. For instance, if you interview 10 people who have witnessed an event, you likely get 10 different depictions. Our perceptions are affected by our history, beliefs, and physiology. This is why it's vital to get feedback from trusted advisors. It's so easy to get tunnel vision and believe that your perception is the absolute truth.

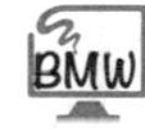

Perception Exercises

https://www.csus.edu/indiv/l/luenemannu/pdf/perception%20quiz.pdf

How to Avoid Self-Sabotage

If you find yourself slipping into negative self-talk, repeating errors, not learning from past mistakes, procrastinating, or surrounding yourself with inappropriate people, chances are a subtle undercurrent of self-sabotage is at work. Other common indicators of self-sabotage are blaming others for your misfortune or expecting failure.

The Inner Critic

Often the inner critic, that internal voice that tells us we're not good enough or that points out our faults and imperfections, becomes a formidable barrier to our success. This voice usually results from well-intended adults telling us as children what mistakes we were making. Unfortunately, when we internalized these comments as children, we had no filter in place to pick and choose which ones were useful and which ones weren't. So as adults, we're left with the whole bag. The inner critic can remind us to slow down when we're impatient. But it can also generate feelings of inadequacy as it nitpicks at everything we do, contributing to our barriers rather than our successes.

See the ***Business Mastery Workbook*** for Activity: "Establishing a Helpful Relationship with Your Inner Critic"

https://sohnen-moe.com/bm5-workbook-request/

Journaling is a great technique to tame your inner critic. Include your reflections from the activities in this book to start a journal. Follow up by writing in your journal on a regular basis (ideally daily). Include details of your daydreams, thoughts, conversations, interactions, and observations that spark something in you. In the article, "Journal to Retrain Your Inner Critic,"[9] Ann Hawkins says, "By creating even a brief opening in the day to pause, take stock, and reflect on thoughts and feelings in a journal, we establish a rich connection with ourselves in ways that can benefit us, our practice, and by extension, our clients."

> "We write to taste life twice, in the moment and in retrospection.
>
> —Anais Nin

Negative Conditioning

People are greatly influenced by events that have happened to them throughout their lifetime. Often we allow (subconsciously or consciously) our past mistakes, incompletions, and even our successes to obstruct the creation and accomplishment of new goals. We aren't always aware just how much impact our past has on our present and future.

The Journal Workshop

www.thejournalworkshop.com

We're a product of our experience. To cope with emotionally painful and difficult life events, it's common to respond with what is popularly referred to as "survival skills." The resulting beliefs and behavior tendencies, which may work well in the short term, can sometimes get in the way of living a happy and productive life. For instance, conclusions formed in the past may have been based upon false information or useful for a situation that was only valid at that time. Just because particular actions were effective in past situations, doesn't mean they will work equally well in the future. Simply stated, it's extremely difficult to be creative and spontaneous when shouldering the burden of the past.

Releasing negative thought patterns isn't always easy, but the results of doing so are worth the effort. When you're detached from those past beliefs and attitudes, you can replace them with new supportive thoughts that contribute to having your life be the way YOU want. Frequently, this clearing stage is overlooked (or worse, considered irrelevant or too time-consuming) and people attempt to move directly into repatterning. This is one reason why setting goals, writing affirmations, visualizing your goals, and listening to motivational recordings don't always work.

Tap Into Your Inner Power

> Nothing in life is to be feared. It is only to be understood.
> —Marie Curie

Sometimes lingering conflicts and negative conditioning need to be unearthed, acknowledged, and accepted before they can be replaced. For clearing to be truly effective, it must take place on all levels: mental, emotional, physical, and spiritual. The clearing process requires recognizing that a block exists and being willing to go through whatever it takes to fully release it, even if that means re-experiencing the buried negativity and pain.

Many people have used clearing techniques to pave the way to career success. Some well-known techniques include psychotherapy, bodywork/massage, yoga, rebirthing, some forms of martial arts, energy balancing, water flotation tanks, transpersonal counseling, hypnotherapy, meditation, cognitive therapy, psychic work, and written/verbal clearing exercises. Sometimes professional help is needed to break free from limiting beliefs rooted in the subconscious mind. This is particularly true if you find yourself bumping up against the same old behaviors and habits, confronting the same old thorny issues. Counselors trained in such methods as PSYCH-K and Emotional Freedom Techniques specialize in this type of personal growth work. Based on the body's subtle energies, these techniques have proven highly successful for many.

You may choose one or more techniques depending upon the issue. All of them aim to empower you to realize your deepest desires and to achieve career success. You may respond better to one type of clearing technique than another. Experiment!

Sentence Completions Clearing Technique

An example of one technique for releasing old thought patterns is called *sentence completions*. This clearing process is designed to elicit conscious and unconscious thoughts, attitudes, beliefs, and feelings so that they can be recognized and released, thus enabling you to be more free to achieve what you really desire.

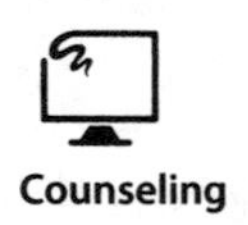

Counseling
counsellingresource.com
Mind-Body Clearing
www.psych-k.com

You can do these exercises in a written format by yourself, or verbally with a partner. If you want to do it verbally, have your partner ask you the questions and you let your answers come out uncensored. Your partner's role is to keep you moving through the process.

The directions for this type of exercise are: Designate 1 page for each question. At the top of the first page, write down the first question. Answer the question with the first thoughts that come to your mind. Don't try to figure out the "right" answers, as there are none. Let your thoughts and feelings come out uncensored.

Continue to list your thoughts. Fill the whole page. It isn't necessary to write complete sentences. Occasionally reread the question and list any new or different thoughts. Some of your answers may not make sense and that's okay. When you think that the list is finished, go over it again. Add any additional thoughts. For instance, with the clearing sentence of, "The things that are important to me are..." responses might be:

- Doing what I want
- Success
- Feeling good about myself
- Having fun
- Making a difference in the world
- Being healthy
- Friends
- Tacos
- Money
- Movies
- Traveling
- Happiness

Remember, it might not make sense—but if that's what's there, respect it.

Notice any unconscious defense mechanisms that may occur to distract you such as thoughts (e.g., the other things you really ought to be doing, how hungry you are, how silly this exercise is), daydreaming, falling asleep, or going blank. If you're experiencing these defenses, stop briefly, acknowledge to yourself what is happening and then continue with the exercise.

Do this same procedure for each question. It's common to find that some of your answers are the same or quite similar for different questions. Don't restrict any of the answers that come up.

You can create your own list of questions or refer to the additional activity in the *Business Mastery Workbook*.

§1

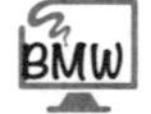

See the ***Business Mastery Workbook*** for Activity: "Sentence Completions"

https://sohnen-moe.com/bm5-workbook-request/

Procrastination

"Never put off until tomorrow what you can do today!" is the aphorism which makes every procrastinator cringe. Everyone has experienced putting off various duties, tasks, and responsibilities until the last possible minute (or longer). If this becomes a habit, it can be detrimental. According to business experts, this is the most common symptom of self-sabotage for a small business owner.

Procrastination brings to mind words such as lazy, unproductive, and inefficient, yet procrastination isn't necessarily a negative state. In fact, it's simply a signal that it's time to evaluate the status of the task in question and discover the reason(s) why it's staying at the bottom of the "to-do" pile.

The reasons for procrastination are numerous. Eliza Bergeson wrote an article called "Procrastination and The Art of Inner Feng Shui,"[10] stating that there are 6 common reasons we procrastinate:

- It's not in our best interests to do it and we know this on some level.
- It may not be the best time to do it or we're not ready.
- There's too much to do. We are overwhelmed or don't know what to do first.
- It's too hard or we don't know how to do it.
- It's boring. We'd rather do something else.
- It brings up strong emotions of grief, rage, fear, or panic.

> "It's not whether you get knocked down. It's whether you get up again.
> —Vince Lombardi

Perhaps one of the most common is setting such high, perfectionistic expectations for performance that accomplishing the task appears overwhelming, if not impossible. It's easy to set yourself up in this manner—to never feel quite good enough, continually dissatisfied with your performance, even though you got the job done. The delayed project then becomes a representation of your fear of failure and inadequacy.

Perfectionists believe that "adequate" or "sufficient" performance simply isn't good enough. "Adequate" and "inadequate" come to mean the same thing. Put these 3 words—perfection, adequate, and inadequate—in their proper perspective. Nothing is inherently wrong in having high standards but they need to be evaluated to determine if they're realistic. Perfection is impossible. To do a job adequately is to do what is needed. Inadequate means not meeting minimal requirements. If you feel fear about some task that you have to do, it could be you're setting perfectionistic standards for yourself that are difficult to meet.

> "Even if you're on the right track, you'll get run over if you just sit there.
> —Will Rogers

The main challenge for many perfectionists is that they believe that perfectionism is highly desirable. They see no reason to break their addiction to trying to be perfect. What they often fail to realize is that they're paying a high toll for maintaining their perfectionism. Creativity suffers greatly. In *The Woman's Book of Creativity*, Dr. Ealy notes that being tied to perfectionism sabotages creativity. "Creativity and perfection, like oil and water, don't mix. Expressing ourselves creatively requires us to assume risks, make mistakes, experiment with the unknown, and take leaps of faith. These activities occur only when we're energized by a spirit of adventure and curiosity."[11]

Oftentimes people can convince themselves that a task is critical when it isn't. It's prudent to evaluate whether a task is actually necessary. You must evaluate and rank your tasks (this may take the assistance of a consultant). If the task isn't something that you want to do and it isn't really necessary, you may take yourself off the hook.

> "Putting off an easy thing makes it hard, and putting off a hard one makes it impossible.
> —George H. Lonmer

Possibly you've agreed to do a certain task or activity that you really didn't want to do. If this is the case, it may not be too late to renegotiate. If you frequently find yourself having difficulty saying "No!" and procrastinate as a result, learn how to set limits and boundaries.

Sometimes procrastination is brought on by a lack of information. If you expect yourself to do a task without having the necessary knowledge, even the most routine task can become daunting. Before you begin a project, map out the technical, informational, and functional requirements. Once you have determined what supplies, information, and other resources are needed to complete the task, obtain them and begin your project. Being organized can make any task more palatable and run more smoothly. Additionally, give yourself permission to ask for the help you need. Asking for help can provide you with the energy and support to accomplish the task.

When procrastination simply comes down to having to do a task that must be done but is loathsome, or you're feeling a lack of creativity, here are some techniques that may help you move on: reframing; task breakdown and simplification; and delegation. Figure 3.3 gives a brief overview of each technique.

Figure 3.3 Tips to Overcome Procrastination

Reframing

Find an alternative way to view the project at hand. This may be done by creating a more pleasant environment to work on the task, such as listening to enjoyable music, sitting in a comfortable chair, sipping on your favorite beverage, or involving another person (preferably with a good sense of humor) in the task.

Put the task into perspective. For example, let's say you need to make 5 marketing calls, but you've been putting them off for weeks, telling yourself that you aren't good on the phone, you hate to do marketing, and you would rather just see your clients. At this rate the calls won't get done. Reframe the situation by asking yourself why you're making these calls. Remind yourself what you hope to accomplish and consider how these calls bring you closer to your goals. Reframing the situation and focusing on how doing a task may bring you closer to having what you want in your life can definitely bring more energy to tasks you have been avoiding.

Task Breakdown

Clarify action items and a timeline for a project by setting clear goals with target dates.

This is basically taking things one step at a time and keeping them as simple as possible. Doing this eliminates any question as to what exactly needs to be done, and also speeds up the whole process.

Delegation (or subcontracting)

Delegate tasks to colleagues or employees. Explore the possibilities. Determine if there are portions of the task (if not the whole thing) that can be done more easily and effectively by someone else. Consider trading tasks with a colleague. Remember, when you delegate or trade, you aren't handing over total responsibility for the finished product; you still need to oversee the tasks to assure their completion.

Procrastination isn't only a personal issue, it affects associates and staff as well. If you've discovered that you're a perfectionist, it can be extremely difficult to accurately gauge others' performance. You may be setting standards so high that not even you could attain them. Are you projecting your own perfectionism? Are you creating an atmosphere where people are afraid to take risks? Is it safe for your co-workers or employees to make mistakes?

If this is indeed the situation, discuss it with your associates and staff. Let them know that you're aware of your tendencies and address methods to improve working conditions. You need to set new standards—they can still be high, but not out of reach. If you can come to an agreement, everyone wins—you're happy, the people you work with won't feel as pressured, and the company gets higher quality work from the staff.

Procrastination in self and others is an issue that most people have to deal with at some point in their lives. Procrastination is a symptom. The important thing to remember is to listen to yourself. Find out what is behind the behavior. Evaluate the dynamics. Then you can alleviate the procrastination by making the necessary changes—be they internal or external.

> "Never put off a task until tomorrow if you can delegate it today.
> —Helen Reynolds

Figure 3.4 Strategies to Overcome Barriers

- Clarify your values and operate from them.
- Do clearing work or therapy.
- Set clear goals and devote yourself to them.
- Do visualizations and affirmations.
- Become a calculated risk-taker.
- Work smarter—not harder.
- Be informed and learn from your past mistakes.
- Refuse to be distracted by others or by your own delusions.
- See your detractors for what they are.
- Create a positive support system.
- Keep things in perspective and stay balanced.

Tools for Actualizing Goals

Now that you've made friends with your inner critic and learned how to avoid the pitfalls of negative conditioning and procrastination, it's time to explore two simple yet powerful tools for success: affirmations and creative visualization. Many successful people, from astronauts to Olympic athletes, have used these techniques to achieve daily success and high performance. We also look at some useful tips for breaking through blocks to creativity and dissolving thorny problems. All of these techniques are easy to learn and use. No special equipment needed!

> "Genius is one percent inspiration and 99 percent perspiration.
> —Thomas A. Edison

Creative Visualization

Creative visualization has inspired many people and accelerated their ability to change their lives and accomplish their goals. Yet, for others, it's a source of frustration. A popular saying goes "If you can't see it, you can't get it." That statement is true, but only in its purest sense.

According to Remez Sasson of Success Consciousness, creative visualization is:

> *...a mental technique that uses the imagination to make dreams and goals come true. Used in the right way, creative visualization can improve your life and attract to you success and prosperity. It is a power that can alter your environment and circumstances, cause events to happen, and attract money, possessions, work, people, and love into your life.*[12]

Creative visualization can help you stay inspired, energized, and on track to achieve your dreams and goals. However, not everyone "sees" the same way. Perhaps "experience" is a better word. When some people envision a goal, they don't actually see it, but they get a physical sensation or they hear the sounds associated with the goal.

For example, let's say you have a goal of going on a hike this weekend. You may actually see yourself waking up in the morning, getting dressed, and walking through the hills— fully seeing the surroundings. Another possibility is you might feel what it's like to be hiking: the stretching of your muscles, the smell of the flowers, and the emotional interaction you have with the environment. Finally, your "visualization" might be verbal. You may actually talk yourself through the day or even imagine the sounds of the animals, the wind, and the conversation of the others on the hike. Your visualization may also include a combination of sight, sound, smell, and sensation.

Creative Visualization: Use the Power of Your Imagination to Create What You Want in Your Life by Shakti Gawain

Indeed, the more senses you incorporate into your visualizations, the more powerful they become. You can visualize using the methods described under Goal Setting Techniques in Chapter 2 or create your own process. Another option is to carry a picture of the goal. For example, if you want a new car, have someone take a picture of you sitting in the exact model you desire or cut out a picture of the car from a brochure (and possibly glue on a picture of your face in the driver's seat). You could also use a graphic editing program to insert a photo of you into a photo of the car. It isn't necessary to "visualize" in any specific way. What works for one person may not for another. Do what works best for you.

Fortunately, creative visualization is such a powerful tool that practicing 5 minutes a day can balance out hours, days, or even years of negative patterning. Be patient. Even a few minutes a day will bear much fruit.

Acting As If

An extension of visualizing is the principle of "Acting As If." Essentially, this principle says that you increase the odds of obtaining your goals when you create the "feeling" of having the goal you visualize (or being what you visualize). Psychologists have been exploring this concept since the early 1900s. Numerous studies with athletes have proven the connection of mental practice on motor skill learning and performance. Other clinical studies have documented how changing the body can affect mood and attitude. For instance, the research article on *Treatment of Depression with OnabotulinumtoxinA: A randomized, double-blind, placebo controlled trial*[13] suggests that the brain continuously monitors the relative valence of facial expressions (by assessing the extent of facial muscle contractions and muscle tension by proprioception) and that mood responds accordingly.

> "You are never given a wish without also being given the power to make it true. You may have to work for it, however.
>
> —Richard Bach

In recent years, the concept of Acting As If has been popularized (and even mainstreamed) by books, films, and teachers talking about the "law of attraction" (e.g., like attracts like, thoughts create things, we get what we focus on). The pure Acting As If principle isn't based on magical reasoning; it's about the power of your mind to create results. A simplified example of this is as follows: You decide you want to be happy. You visualize yourself being happy. You think about how you would feel physically if you were happy. You imagine the kinds of thoughts you would have if you were happy. You do things that a happy person would do, such as smile and laugh. Soon, you just might discover that by acting as if you were happy, that you actually become happy.

Affirmations

An affirmation is a positive declaration that something is already so. It can be general or very specific. It's a constructive thought that you deliberately choose to place in your consciousness to produce a desired result. The purpose of writing or saying affirmations is to support you in actualizing your dreams and goals by replacing negative self-talk with positive self-talk.

Louise Hay is one of the most well-known authors on the topic of affirmations. She explains that when you state an affirmation, you're really saying to your subconscious mind: "I am taking responsibility. I am aware that there is something I can do to change."[14]

When you create affirmations, you essentially plant a seed for new beginnings. Avoid becoming attached to the specific details of "how" the affirmation will manifest. As with goal setting, always state your affirmations in the positive present tense and personalize them. Choose affirmations that feel good to you. What works for one person may not work for you. Affirmations can be used in many ways to produce powerful results. Experiment with some of the suggestions found in Figure 3.5.

Doubt, resistance, and physical discomfort are natural side effects of the affirming process. If you notice these feelings while you're creating an affirmation, don't fight them. Accept them, acknowledge them, and allow their expression. Sometimes these feelings are signals of deep conflicts that may require more (or other types) of clearing.

Keep in mind the power of your thoughts as you work with your favorite affirmations.

Affirmations are most effective when the path is clear of resistance. In the Law of Attraction, author and Neuro-Linguistic Programming (NLP) Practitioner, Michael J. Losier, suggests another way to steer clear of resistance when using affirmations. Instead of stating affirmations in the positive tense, which can stir up feelings of "That's just not true," Losier suggests that you simply rephrase affirmations to state that you're "in the process" of creating what you want. For example, "I'm in the process of growing a successful and prosperous business that supports my clients' sense of wellbeing and happiness."[15]

If you want to find out more about the connection between energy, our thoughts, and the world of "matter" around us, Losier suggests taking a look at the movie *What the Bleep Do We Know!?*,[16] a lively and sometimes humorous look at the world of quantum physics.

Figure 3.5 Affirmation Techniques

- Read your affirmations at least 3 times per day.
- Write each affirmation 10 to 20 times in succession.
- Write your affirmations while speaking them aloud to yourself.
- Write your affirmations in the first, second, and third person. For example: ***"I, Sue, am healthy." "You, Sue, are healthy." "She, Sue, is healthy."***
- Write your affirmations and tape them up (or use Post-it® notes) around your home, car, and office. Put them on the telephone, the refrigerator, your desk, mirrors, doors, over your bed, and on the dashboard.
- Make bookmarks with your affirmations on them.
- Record your affirmations and listen to them as you drive, exercise, and before you go to sleep.
- Meditate on your affirmations.
- Stand in front of a mirror and look at yourself while saying your affirmations.
- Take turns saying and accepting affirmations with a friend.
- Make flash cards with your affirmations and carry them with you.
- Design or buy clothes with affirmations on them.
- Sing or chant your affirmations.
- Create affirmation screen savers for your computer, phone, or tablet.

Figure 3.6 **Affirmation Examples**

Mind, Body, and Spirit

- I manifest my power with integrity and love.
- My life is a continual expansion of joy and aliveness.
- Everything I need is already within me.
- I trust my intuition.
- My life is filled with laughter and love.
- I'm the master of my life.
- I fully love and accept myself as I am.
- I live up to my own highest ideals.
- I communicate clearly and effectively.
- I'm a radiant, powerful being.
- I'm happy!
- I'm vibrantly healthy.
- My life is a joyous adventure.
- I'm creative in all that I do.
- My relationships are nurturing and fun.
- I'm aligned with the divine plan of my life.
- I appreciate the good in my life.
- I'm in an exciting, romantic relationship.
- I allow people to support me and they do.

Career and Finances

- My career is fulfilling and prosperous.
- The more abundance I have, the more I have to share.
- I'm well organized.
- I'm true to myself.
- My creativity is flowing and focused.
- I'm a dynamic public speaker.
- My career supports me in being who I am.
- I have the time, energy, wisdom, and money to accomplish my goals.
- Every dollar I circulate returns to me multiplied.
- I see the opportunities in life.

Breaking Old Habits

According to the Duke University study, "Habits—A Repeat Performance,"[17] 40% of your everyday actions are habitual. Dictionary.com defines a habit as an acquired behavior pattern regularly followed until it has become almost involuntary. Habits can be beneficial in that they streamline routine activities and free up your brain to concentrate on other activities. Unfortunately, a lot of habitual beliefs and behaviors can sabotage your efforts to be successful. It takes conscious thought and repetition to create the neurological pathways to alter old habits and replace them with new ones.

You may want to experiment with a fun and easy technique known as cross-lateral movement to break through blocks, increase your creativity, and generate useful ideas for your business. As Dr. Ealy explains in *The Woman's Book of Creativity*,[18] a cross-lateral movement cuts across an imaginary line splitting the body in half vertically. This happens when you swing the right arm across the body to the left side. Dr. Ealy proposes that these movements stimulate the learning centers of your brain while breaking up routine. At the very least, they get your blood pumping, and that's always a good thing!

Experience firsthand the benefits of this technique by taking a few moments to do the following exercise.

Basic Cross-Lateral Exercise

Give yourself plenty of room and take off your shoes. Start by standing up and swinging your left foot over your right. Then swing your right foot over your left. Repeat this action many times, establishing a rhythm. Now add your arms, swinging in the opposite direction from your legs. Establish your rhythm. Next follow your feet with your head so both are moving in one direction while your arms are going in the opposite direction. If you lose the pattern, stop everything, then start with the feet and build the movement.

To add interest, imagine yourself eating a favorite food, watching a colorful sunset, and petting your cat all at the same time. Have fun using images that are entertaining and relaxing for you. Maintain this movement and imagery for 5 minutes. Add music if you like. You may be pleasantly surprised to find yourself breathing vigorously and wanting to sit down after 5 minutes yet at the same time feeling exceptionally alert mentally.

Note: Cross-lateral movements can elevate your pulse, so pace yourself.

You can use this exercise for many issues. If you want to generate some new ideas for your business, set that intention before beginning the movements. As soon as you finish, begin writing what comes. If you're dealing with a specific problem, regardless of the type, embrace the problem then dance with it, using cross-laterals. Notice what has happened to it after you finish the movements. If you're engaged in a task that requires a lot of sitting, get up periodically and do some cross-lateral movements. You will find that you have increased your energy level and are mentally alert with ready access to your creativity. Have fun with this exercise!

> "Creative minds have always been known to survive any kind of bad training.
> —Anna Freud

More Than Positive Thinking

I don't want you to confuse the above techniques for mere positive thinking. Creative visualizations and affirmations are important, but alone they aren't as effective as when combined with what psychologist and researcher Gabriele Oettingen calls "mental contrasting." Her 20 years of research on motivation shows that it's not enough to simply dream about our goals, we must also visualize the obstacles to develop the motivation for overcoming them. In a recent *Entrepreneur* magazine interview, Oettingen suggests that we visualize our dream, picturing the desired outcome, and then contrast that visualization with the possible obstacles we may encounter in reality. When we do this, we're motivated to create our plan of action to overcome those obstacles. In fact, her research shows that we're more likely to achieve our dreams with mental contrasting, than when we dream of the positive outcomes alone. She calls her technique WOOP: Wish, Outcome, Obstacle, Plan. Remember this when you're implementing your tools for actualizing your goals and creating your strategic plans.[19]

Dissolving Problems

We all slip into negative thoughts from time to time. Sadness and anger are normal experiences. The key is to acknowledge these thoughts and feelings and then let them go. Sometimes this is an easy task and other times it's Herculean. Sentence completion exercises are an excellent method for releasing energy associated with negative conditioning. If you're having difficulties with a specific problem, first take an honest look to see if you're truly willing to resolve the problem. If you are, put aside approximately 2 hours and do the following clearing exercise.

Dissolving Problems

Take some notebook paper and write the following questions on the top of each sheet of paper, putting 1 question on each piece of paper and keeping them in the order given. Spend at least 5 minutes per page actually doing the exercise.

- What is the area you're having difficulty with? Describe in detail.
- What are your fears and attitudes regarding your problem?
- What aren't you getting?
- What are you getting that you don't want?
- What are you getting that you do want?
- Regarding this problem, how have you been trying to resolve it?
- Regarding this problem, what do you think you should be doing?
- What is it that you want?
- What is it that you should want?
- What are the benefits of not resolving this problem?
- What would you have to give up to resolve this problem?
- What would you have to realize to resolve this problem?
- What are you holding on to, or protecting, in regards to your problem?
- Who or what is limiting you?
- By solving this problem, what new problems will be created?
- What is it that you really want?
- What are the specific things you will do to resolve this problem?

Follow-Up: Did you get to the final question and develop a strategy for resolution? Why or why not? Did you tell the truth on every question? Did you have trouble discerning the truth for some questions?

Time Management Principles

Time Management Tools

www.franklincovey.com

Online Tools

www.rememberthemilk.com
www.evernote.com
www.toggl.com
www.mylifeorganized.net

Time management isn't about which appointment book you use. It's really about how well you use your time. It's based on realizing how much your time is worth and choosing activities that are the highest priority for you to achieve your goals. Time can either be an asset or a liability; it all depends on your attitudes. You can't alter time, only your attitudes and behaviors relating to time. Your attitudes toward time are influenced by conditioning and by your self-esteem.

What Is Your Attitude Toward Time?

- What thoughts and feelings do you have concerning time?
- How did your family relate to time?
- Do you respect yourself by taking the time to take care of yourself?
- Do you view time as your friend or your enemy?

Follow-Up: Will you continue to hold on to your beliefs around time, or are you interested in developing new skills and beliefs? How do you think those around you will respond as you make the necessary changes?

As you work to develop your time management skills and discover new ways to boost your personal productivity, you find many benefits.

Figure 3.7 **Effective Time Management Benefits**

- Doing the same work in less time.
- Increasing personal productivity.
- Earning more money.
- Decreasing frustration and stress.
- Having more time for planning.
- Devoting more time to your family.
- Spending more time with hobbies and recreation.
- Improving your health.
- Experiencing increased joy and success.

The Pareto Principle

The fundamental basis of time management is the **Pareto Principle**: The Pareto Principle states that 80% of your results are produced by 20% of your activities. And, conversely, 20% of your results are produced by 80% of your activities. Time management techniques are effective because most people spend a lot of time in activities that are not an efficient use of their time. These percentages vary for individual cases, but the principle holds. The more you learn to focus on these 20% activities and turn them into 40% or even 60%, the more productive, prosperous, and balanced you become.

Figure 3.8 **The Pareto Principle**

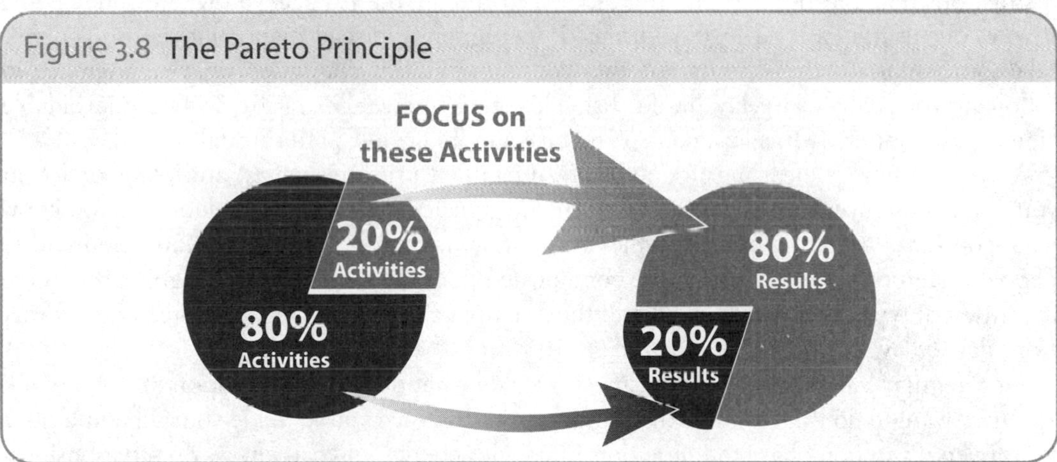

Figure 3.9 **Plan Like a Pro**

- Invest at least 10 minutes in daily planning.
- Focus on "A" goals first.
- Throughout the day ask yourself, "Is this the best use of my time?"
- Set specific times for taking and returning phone calls.
- Set a schedule and follow it.
- Review your master goal list at least once per week.
- At the end of the day, create the next day's goals and activities list.

Figure 3.10 Top 12 Time Management Tips

- Review goals and activities daily.
- Do your most challenging work during your peak performance cycles.
- Group similar activities together.
- Discourage interruptions.
- Learn to say "no."
- Track important data & activities.
- Avoid procrastination.
- Respect your body's and mind's cycles.
- Delegate whenever possible.
- Keep supplies stocked and easy to access.
- Take a quick stretch break every 20 minutes.
- Set an alarm to limit time-eating activities (e.g., Internet surfing).

Types of Time Needed to Run a Business

If you decide to become a business owner and intend to achieve optimal results, remember that you need to allot time for varied tasks. You need time to plan, work with clients, manage the business, continue your education, market your practice, communicate, develop ideas, take care of yourself, and have fun. Investing at least 10 to 15 minutes in daily planning is crucial to managing your time wisely.

Getting Things Done by David Allen

A common pitfall is to create an incredible to-do list, then let it fall to the wayside as everyday distractions pull you this way and that. Like a road map, the list gets you where you're going if you consult it as you navigate your day. If you ignore the road map, chances are you will take some unproductive detours. Another common pitfall is taking too rigid an approach to following your daily or weekly "to-do" list. This tends to create extra stress when unavoidable "side trips" require you to adjust course and take a more flexible path through your day.

When you have a clear purpose and have identified priorities, goals, and plans of action, you don't get so overwhelmed, even when the unexpected appears at your doorstep. You know what you have to do, the order in which to do it, and when it needs to be done. Sometimes people imagine things to be far more complicated than they really are. Recognize that there are different types of time you need and the amount of time spent in each category may vary from day to day.

Set a regular schedule for your business. Decide what days and what hours you will work. You may want to do this on a weekly or monthly basis. Once you've made your schedule, stick to it. Even if you don't have the time slots filled with clients, you can always do other business activities. It can be so tempting to look at your appointment book, not see anything scheduled for the afternoon and decide to go play. Occasionally this is fine, just be careful it doesn't become a habit.

Figure 3.11 Types of Time Needed to Run a Business

- Managing Business Logistics
- Working with Clients
- Professional Development
- Idea Development
- Marketing
- Having Fun
- Personal Wellness

§1

Work Smarter—Not Harder

The time you spend in planning is always well invested. When you first start planning, it may seem to take a long time; after doing it on a regular basis, you can plan your day very quickly. Remember, planning is to ultimately simplify your life—not make it more complicated.

The basis of productive planning is effective goal setting. The major element in planning (especially daily planning) is ranking. After you have written your daily plan, evaluate it. Decide which activities absolutely must get done today and rate them as Imperative. Review the other items and indicate the ones that need to be done very soon by labeling them as Important. Mark the rest of the activities (the ones that it would be nice if you accomplished them, but they're not of major significance) as being Desirable.

See Chapter 2, page 20 for more information on **prioritizing goals**.

Managing Business Logistics

We often forget to schedule appropriate time for the day-to-day tasks such as doing laundry, making phone calls, supervising staff (if you have any), keeping files, and purchasing supplies. All of these activities take time, often a lot more than anticipated.

Another aspect of managing your business has to do with respecting yourself and time in relation to bartering (or trading) services. Barter is usually a supplemental method of obtaining products and services that you prefer to not purchase with cash. The downside is that some people get so into bartering that they never earn any money. Be very clear about your reasons for trading. Before you do any type of bartering, ask yourself if you would spend money on that product or service if you had the cash. If not, don't trade. Remember, barter is considered taxable income in most countries.

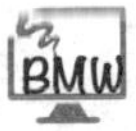

See the ***Business Mastery Workbook*** for a **Daily Plan** form.

https://sohnen-moe.com/bm5-workbook-request/

Working with Clients

The majority of your time is spent providing client services. Your ability to effectively schedule appointments greatly impacts your success and your stress level. Allot sufficient time between clients while not having large blocks of unproductive time. You may discover that you need to schedule an extra half hour for new clients and some ongoing clients who regularly need additional time. You may need a longer recuperation time after certain clients. Sometimes staying within the allotted session time can be difficult when you don't have anything else scheduled immediately after the session. While having the flexibility to extend a session is nice, be careful to respect the time boundaries of yourself and your client. The longer you're in practice, the more adept you become in judging how much time is necessary to spend with clients and between sessions.

In her article "How Much Time In Between Client Sessions Is Enough?"[20], Kristen Tammaro-Sparks says that "you will be able to save money and have more time for yourself by booking your clients very tightly together." She schedules no more than 15 minutes between clients because:

> *When I'm at work I'm fully involved in my work. That means I don't answer phone calls, texts, or emails. My only job is to make sure that the client is happy and they are receiving 100% of me. Everything else is systematized so I don't have to worry about it being done.*

> "A year from now you will wish you had started today.
> —Karen Lamb

One way to simplify scheduling is to set up a standing appointment with regular clients. For example, you may have a regular client scheduled for 10 a.m. each Wednesday. Both you and your client agree that this appointment stays in place each week unless the client calls to cancel. This approach creates a sense of comfort and ease for both practitioner and client.

If you work as an employee of a spa, group practice, or medical center, you may have little control over scheduling client sessions. However, in some cases, you can communicate scheduling preferences to an appropriate staff member who may agree to accommodate you whenever possible.

Professional Development

Continuing education is necessary to your career growth. Find ways to broaden your knowledge, particularly in the areas of interpersonal skills, product knowledge, technical skills, and business skills. Some ways to do that are reading magazines and books, taking classes, attending seminars, watching videos, and networking.

It's also helpful to be assessed periodically. This can be done by your clients and by colleagues. Some practitioners have every client fill out a form for every session and others go through this process only once or twice per year. Feedback is essential for your professional growth. This concept can seem a bit scary—the idea of being evaluated does have some ego risk involved, but how are you going to know which areas to enhance if no one tells you? Remember, knowledge is power. Since most work in this field is very individualized, it's recommended that you obtain as many evaluations as possible to get broader, more objective feedback. Many practitioners find evaluations highly beneficial. They are also a good way to get your clients more involved in their treatment.

> "
> The future has a way of arriving unannounced.
> —George F. Will

Getting assessed by your colleagues is essential. They can give you the kind of technical feedback that a client probably would not know. Again, it isn't necessary to be evaluated every time you work with your peers, but do it regularly. You can also make it fun. Your purpose isn't to "find fault" but to support each other in achieving excellence. This can be an enjoyable and cost-effective way to grow professionally.

Idea Development

Developing ideas is one of the most exciting and creative aspects of any business. Always be open to new opportunities. Brainstorm ways to streamline your procedures. Find methods to reduce your effort by diversifying your practice (e.g., hire employees, sell products, subcontract out work to other practitioners and take a percentage of the fees). Create ways in which you work with more than 1 client at a time (e.g., offer group sessions, give seminars, publish articles and books). The possibilities are bountiful!

Marketing

See Section 7, for more on **marketing**.

Marketing your practice is vital to your success. This is the aspect of business that most wellness practitioners neglect. When you first start your practice, you may spend more hours marketing than actually working with clients. Then, even when your business seems to be established, you still need to actively market yourself. People move, change practitioners, and try alternate methods of self-improvement. You can't rely on your clients to bring you more new clients. Marketing is necessary during all phases of your business. I have known several very successful practitioners whose businesses appeared to fall apart overnight. They were not marketing themselves well or tracking key business indicators, and they didn't notice the changes until it was too late. So they had to "start all over again." You can avoid this through regular marketing. It's critical that you invest at least 15% of your work time in marketing.

Having Fun

> "
> He who every morning plans the transactions of the day, and follows out that plan, carries a thread that will guide him through the labyrinth of the most busy life.
> —Victor Hugo

When your desire for success is strong, having fun can easily get pushed to the bottom of the list or get neglected altogether. It tends to be one of the least planned aspects of life. People are inclined to leave their enjoyment to chance. Think about the psychology of planning something to look forward to doing. For instance, knowing a special activity or vacation is on the horizon can give you a mental, emotional, and physical boost. Remember to balance your professional goals with your personal goals. Be sure to include fun in your life EVERY DAY!

Personal Wellness

Taking care of yourself is imperative, yet many people put themselves last. It's so easy to get caught up in your business and being there for others, that no time is left for you. Take care of yourself mentally, physically, emotionally, and spiritually. Make sure that every day you do at least 1 thing just for yourself. Respect your needs and wants. Create a support system for your business and personal life. Caregivers have a tendency to not allow themselves to be care-receivers. Don't let yourself fall into that syndrome. Allot as much time as needed to take care of you.

One major factor that influences your time is stress. If you don't handle stress productively, you can waste hours of time each day—not to mention time lost due to stress-related illness. Make certain that you exercise regularly, follow a healthy eating plan, and receive regular wellness care (e.g., massage, acupuncture, chiropractic). Take a quick stretch break every 20 minutes. Allot a 5-minute break every 2 hours to more thoroughly stretch your muscles, do some deep breathing, exercise your eyes, rest, and revitalize yourself.

See Chapter 4, pages 56-57 for information on **self-care and stress**.

High Priority Activities

High priority activities are the "20%" that produce 80% of your results. Before you can begin to increase the time spent in those important activities, you must identify them. The following exercise is designed to assist you in clarifying your high priority activities. The objective of this exercise is to begin concentrating your time and energy on items you've rated as being the most crucial to your success. You may be surprised at what you discover.

The more you focus on your high priority activities, the more productive you are. You may also discover some conflicts. If this happens, refer to your purpose, priorities, and goals. They usually provide direction. Sometimes you have to make difficult decisions and either delegate the other activities, simplify them, or eliminate them. It's also recommended that you show your list to a colleague. You might have overlooked something or you need to switch some of your priorities—and it's usually easier for someone else to be objective.

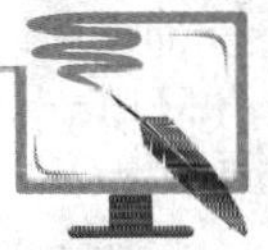

High Priority Activities

Make a copy of the High Priority Activities form found in the *Business Mastery Workbook* or draw 3 columns on a piece of paper, with the center column the widest. Label the left-hand column "Importance," the middle column "Activity" and the right-hand column "Time Spent." Think about the activities involved in your business. List at least 10 of the most important things you do in the center column. In the left-hand column, rate them in the order you think is most important to your success. In the right-hand column rate them in the order of how much time you spend in each activity. Do your importance rankings match up with your time-spent rankings? If not, what can you do to focus your energy on those higher priorities?

Business Mastery Workbook
https://sohnen-moe.com/bm5-workbook-request/

Tracking

Frequently, in business, we have no idea why things are going the way they are, including when they're going well. Was it that last ad? Could it have been that interview in the newspaper? Maybe it was the new brochure? Or was it due to extending office hours on Thursday? Even though it isn't always possible to know for certain the exact action that generated the desired results, you greatly increase your knowledge and optimize your efforts by tracking the important components.

> Results! Why, man, I have gotten a lot of results. I know several thousand things that won't work.
> —Thomas A. Edison

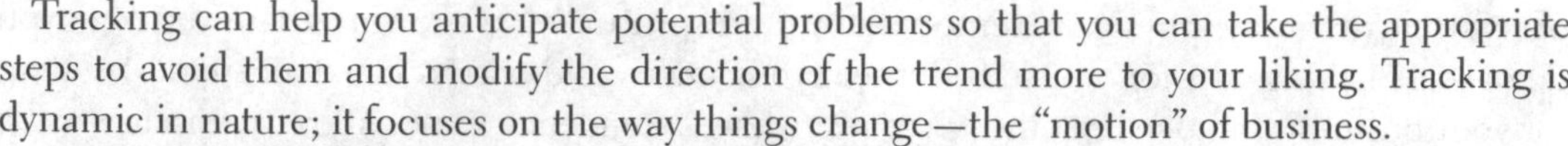

Tracking can help you anticipate potential problems so that you can take the appropriate steps to avoid them and modify the direction of the trend more to your liking. Tracking is dynamic in nature; it focuses on the way things change—the "motion" of business.

> Statistics are no substitute for judgment.
>
> —Henry Clay

Tracking is a documentation of items to identify trends such as marketing activities, client profiles, appointment bookings, and income levels. Closely monitor a broad range of activities because your appointment book, checkbook, and accounting journal don't always tell the whole story. A lot of critical data isn't included in those books and if you use them as your major reference point for judging your success, you may find yourself in a predicament. Oftentimes, things are not as they appear.

For example, imagine that you have been fairly well booked and have had a satisfactory level of income for the last few months, so you haven't been putting much attention into marketing. Then the next month goes by and you discover (to your dismay) that your client load has decreased and your income level has significantly dropped. You don't quite understand how this could happen—after all, everything seemed to be going so well.

Online tracking tools

www.simplekpi.com
www.klipfolio.com
www.toggl.com

You decide to carefully review your books and find that you've only had 3 new clients in the last 2 months, 4 clients have completed their work with you, and the time between sessions for the rest of your clients has been substantially increasing. Had you been keeping track of that kind of information on a summary sheet or a graph, you could have noticed the trend earlier and taken action (e.g., done some type of marketing) to rebuild your clientele. In any business, particularly one that's small, one slow month can be devastating.

Identifying seasonal trends is another helpful way to approach tracking. For instance, by tracking key business indicators, you may notice that for the last 3 years, your business dropped dramatically every October. Using that information, you can decide to increase your advertising and promotion in August and September, or you may just choose to take advantage of the slow period and plan a vacation for October. Conversely, it wouldn't be judicious for you to plan a vacation during your peak period.

A tip for becoming more proficient at time management is to keep a log of how you spend your time. Track all of your activities for several weeks—include everything, such as time spent on telephone calls, dealing with interruptions, taking breaks, working with clients, and so on. Tracking shows you where your time is being well spent or wasted.

Tracking Key Business Indicators

See Chapter 23, pages 336-338 for **when to alter your course.**

What is the best method for tracking key business indicators? You might use graph paper, computerized spreadsheets, custom-designed forms, online services, or simple notebook paper. Make the forms very clear and as straightforward as possible to fill out. Also, be certain to design your client forms so they provide you with information (e.g., how they heard about you), demographics, and session notes for your tracking sheets. Tracking methods are varied and the best method depends on what works easily for you. Consistency is key, so choose a method you feel comfortable with and that will not fall to the bottom of your priority list.

Experiment with tracking activities on a daily, weekly, monthly, or quarterly basis. Consistency is essential, particularly when tracking the results of marketing campaigns, since it often takes several months to discern those results. Additionally, you may discover that the results were due to a combination of factors. Thus, the measurable benefits of tracking are derived from the knowledge you develop over the long run.

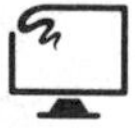

Practitioner's Journey Workbook and Stats Tracking Tool

practitionersjourney.com/tpj-workbook

Tracking is an essential component in making a business plan work. First, you must decide what you want to track. The list of items in Figure 3.12, your business plan, and your high priority activities are excellent places to begin. This data provides you with the information you need to assess the progress of your long-term goals and strategies. It will also enhance your decision making for future marketing campaigns and general business direction.

Studies show that tracking in itself increases your productivity. It's an excellent way to keep yourself motivated, evaluate your status, and help you determine the most appropriate areas in which to invest your time and money to build your practice. As with daily planning, it usually takes a little while to become adept at tracking. After you have experimented with various forms, you will discover the ones that are most appropriate for your needs and then it won't take you very much time at all to track (see Figures 3.13 and 3.14).

§1

Invest the time required for tracking—it's an information-rich and inspiring tool to help you run a productive and profitable business.

Figure 3.12 Useful Items to Track

- Client demographics
- Total number of active clients
- Total number of inactive clients
- Number of clients per day
- Types of clients
- Session time spent per client
- Time spent per client in adjunct support
- Time between sessions
- Type of techniques utilized
- Number of sessions per client
- Average cost of total treatment plan
- How your clients heard about you
- Referrals generated by specific marketing campaigns
- Time spent in all business activities
- Total income (e.g., daily, weekly, monthly)
- Total expenses

Tracking Trends

As you work to build a thriving wellness practice, keeping up to date with the latest trends is a vital skill. This requires paying attention to both consumer trends as well as industry trends. Fortunately, plenty of resources are available to help you gain insights into cultural, lifestyle, and industry trends. Best of all, it doesn't take a lot of time or money to keep your finger on the pulse of emerging trends.

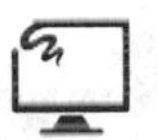

Track Trends
trendwatching.com

Trend watching can help identify a unique niche in the marketplace for you and keep you better attuned to the needs of your target markets. In the words of trend-watching guru, Reinier Evers, director of Trendwatching.com, "Knowing where the world of consumerism is heading will give you a point of view—a grip—and from that knowledge, you'll hopefully be able to come up with new goods, services, and experiences that appeal to your customers."

In short, trend watching can help spark new thinking that results in practical ways to reach new clients and retain existing clients. For instance, time-pressed, busy professional clients highly value convenience and stress reduction, yet they find it difficult to schedule daytime appointments. Based on this insight, you may decide to open your schedule for evening appointments several times a week. You may also decide to implement online scheduling so your clients can schedule appointments 24 hours a day at their convenience.

Tuning in to baby boomer trends—such as the avid preoccupation with healthy aging, maintaining a youthful appearance, and preventive wellness—may result in a more targeted brochure, a new line of antioxidant nutritional supplements, skin care products, or bodywork modalities geared toward satisfying this market's needs.

Other significant trends to track from an industry standpoint are legislative activity and educational standards. Knowing where you stand in relation to others in your industry, what certification or continuing education standards may be changing, and how you can best protect your business interests are key to managing your career and professional practice. Checking out online discussion groups can be useful in tracking trends from other professionals.

The best and simplest way to track consumer trends is to subscribe to the free Trendwatching newsletter. As for industry trends, trade journals often feature insightful articles about

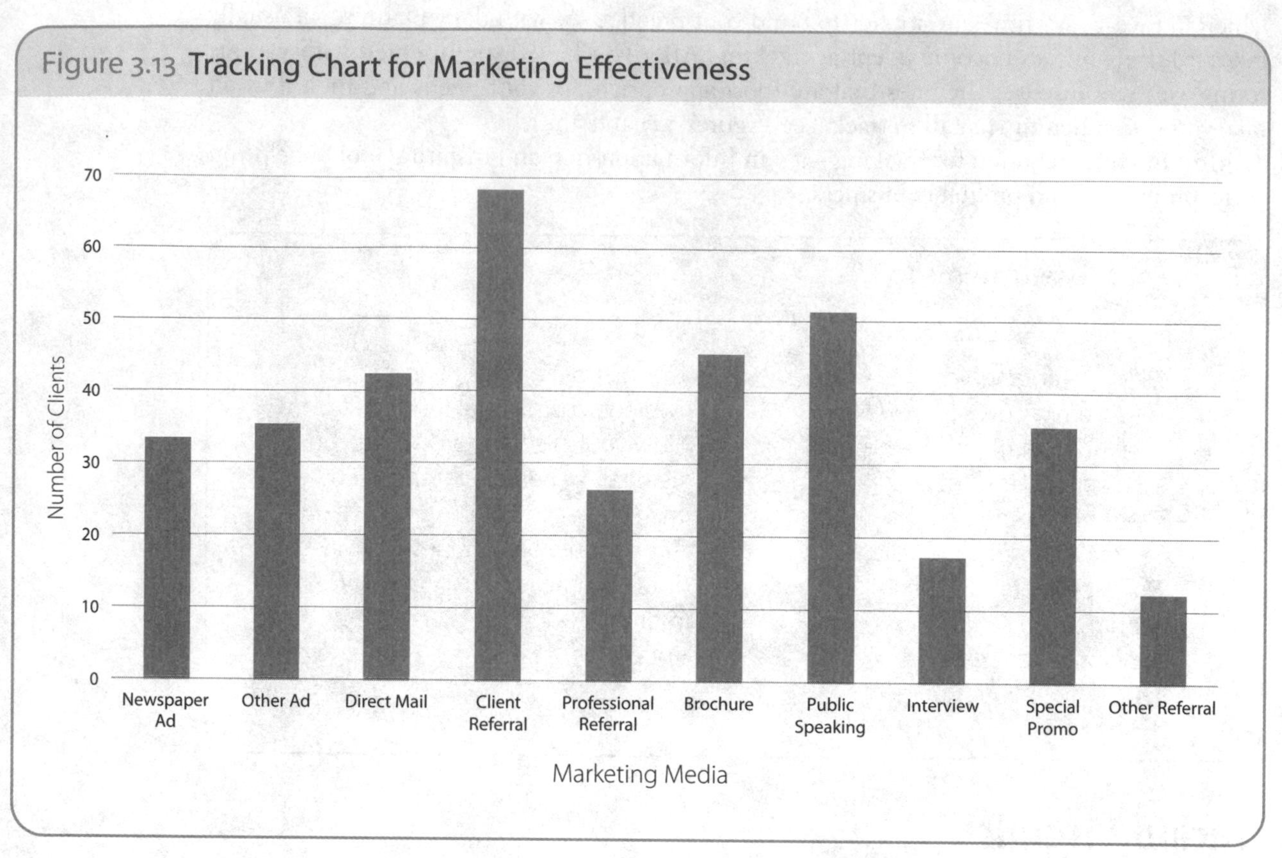
Figure 3.13 Tracking Chart for Marketing Effectiveness
Number of Clients
70
60
50
40
30
20
10
0
Newspaper Ad
Other Ad
Direct Mail
Client Referral
Professional Referral
Brochure
Public Speaking
Interview
Special Promo
Other Referral
Marketing Media

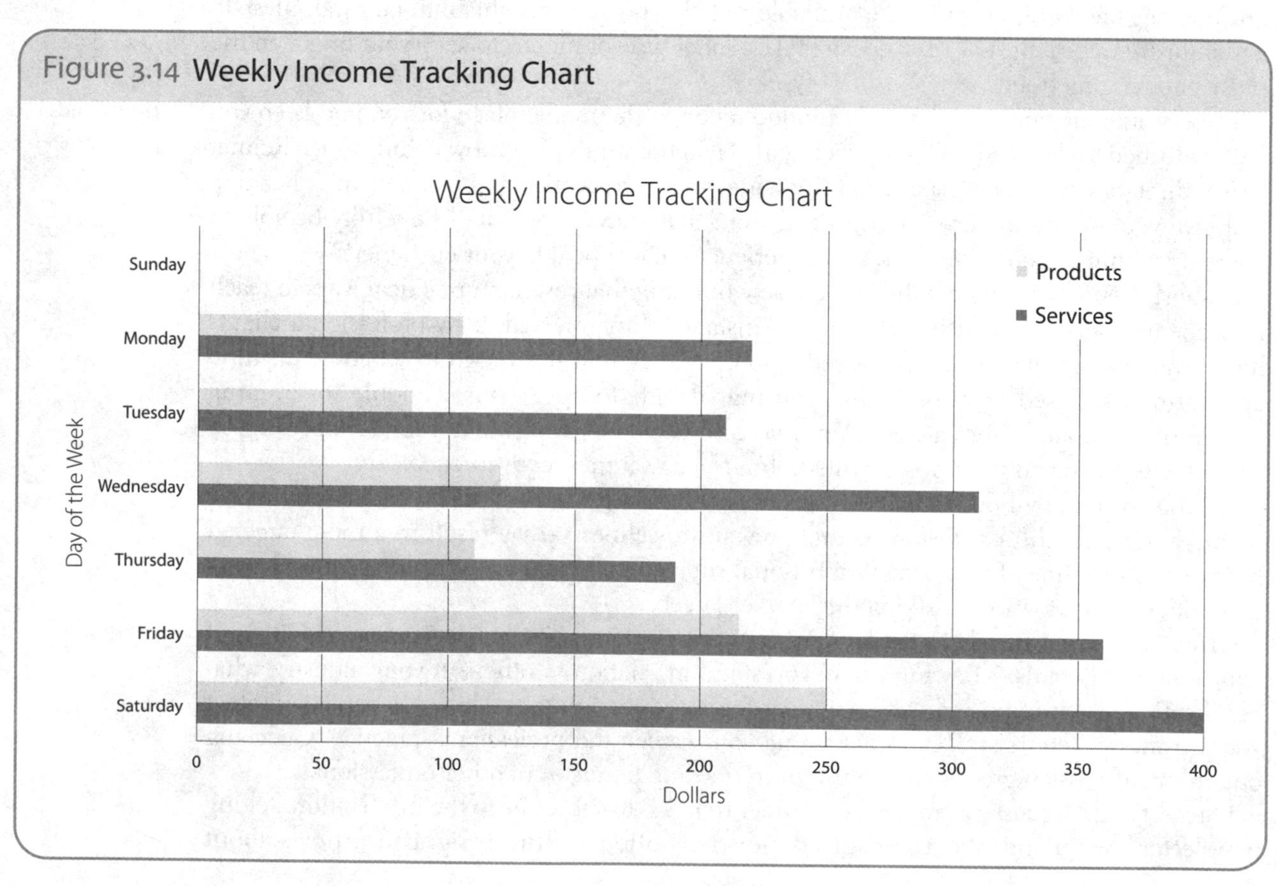
Figure 3.14 Weekly Income Tracking Chart
Weekly Income Tracking Chart
Sunday
Monday
Tuesday
Wednesday
Thursday
Friday
Saturday
Day of the Week
Products
Services
0
50
100
150
200
250
300
350
400
Dollars

consumer perspectives, legal trends, and educational standards. Browse a few trade journals and subscribe to the ones that most appeal to you. The information and insights you gain are well worth your investment. Build the habit of trend watching into your professional life by scheduling an hour or two each week to browse the Trendwatching newsletter and trade journals.

§1

Another valuable trend-watching resource is Ubercool, a site that tracks trends worldwide. If you have an extra half hour or so to spare, go to the website and search for "Fountain of Youth," for a brief look at baby boomer trends. According to Ubercool, baby boomers (born between 1946-1964) number 450 million in the Western world, and are the world's richest generation. Their forever-young attitudes substantially lift the beauty, wellness, and rejuvenation markets.

No introduction to trend watching would be complete without a look at the work of Faith Popcorn, respected trend watcher and author of *Clicking: 17 Trends That Drive Your Business—And Your Life.*[21] She asserts that for any business to be successful, it needs to click with at least 4 of the 17 trends. Visit her site to get more details.

Clicking Trends
www.faithpopcorn.com

The Art of Risk-Taking

Two commonly heard truisms are "nothing ventured, nothing gained" and "no guts, no glory." Taking risks is an integral part of life and especially true in business. It's the doorway to success. The art of risk-taking is knowing how to take smart risks. There's a difference between being a risk-taker and a daredevil. Taking risks is not about blindly jumping into any situation. To become proficient in taking risks, it's vital that you understand the components of risk taking, learn how to minimize your potential losses, and strengthen your risk-taking abilities.

The 2 major elements that influence your ability to successfully manage risks are the level of comfort you have in experiencing new or unusual situations and your self-esteem. Think about the source of your self-confidence. To what degree do you base it upon your opinions and values? How much do you look to others for validation? Is your behavior mainly motivated by external factors such as social approval and material consequences, or by internal considerations such as your beliefs and feelings?

> "Don't play for safety; it's the most dangerous thing in the world.
>
> —Hugh Walpole

In terms of self-esteem, the primary discomfort in taking risks stems from the fear of rejection. In considering your ability to feel confident in novel circumstances, the fundamental discomfort is usually due to inexperience. People take the safer routes so often that they haven't developed a bank of experiences from which to draw. Reflect upon your childhood. What messages were you given regarding the safety of your environment? How did your family deal with crises? What behaviors did you learn to adopt? You can alleviate a lot of anxiety by keeping your expectations realistic and embracing the opportunities for new experiences.

Risk-takers are achievers. They aren't content with the status quo. They prefer action to inaction and follow through on their goals with little hesitation. They are exhilarated by challenges rather than intimidated by them and proceed despite their fears. They also carefully evaluate risks and develop strategic plans of action. They distinguish facts from their emotions, which enables them to handle crises well and empowers their decision-making process. Risk-takers have a strong commitment to being and producing the best.

Another factor that impacts people's freedom to take chances is finances. Most people are overly concerned with money. The truth is that most successful business owners have failed at least once before finally making it. Again, you're the best judge of what's appropriate. You're the only one who can determine whether a risk is worthwhile. If you're considering taking a risk that has monetary ramifications, allot the time to thoroughly evaluate the possibilities. One step you can take now is to reduce your debt as much as possible. Often, what is more scary than the possibility of losing money is the potential for losing face.

Developing your skill in taking risks is a lifelong process. As you go through life, the stakes just seem to get higher. Build your repertoire of risk-taking experiences so that you successfully manage risks. By drawing upon your past experiences to see the similarities to the current situation, you can better determine an effective solution. Put yourself in situations that require you to exercise your creative problem-solving abilities. Start with low-risk situations, gradually increasing your confidence level so you feel more comfortable taking greater risks (see Figure 3.15).

> "Never test the depth of the water with both feet.
> —Kevin Coyne

The continual enhancement of your self-image is vital in cultivating risk-taking behaviors. Begin with positive self-talk. Fill your mind with thoughts about your potential. Become grounded in the knowledge that you are your own source of power and that this power is honorable. Expect to succeed. Release some of your conditioned apprehension and fear by doing the following clearing exercise.

Exploring Taking Risks

Think about a situation that makes you feel uneasy. Imagine what is the very worst thing that could possibly happen. Then evaluate the situation. Is it really that bad? Are your fears justified? Finally, visualize yourself being comfortable and confident while in that risky situation.

Follow-Up: In this activity, did you move past your thoughts on the worst thing that could possibly happen? Did you justify your fears honestly, without over-reacting, and get to a more comfortable feeling about the situation?

The following is an example of an effective risk assessment, with ideas for positive self-talk and appropriate risk-mitigating behaviors:

Risks:

The major risks to my earning potential are injury, long-term illness, or inaccurate income projections.

Mitigating Actions:

I take excellent care of my health: I eat well, take supplements, exercise regularly, take yoga classes 3 times per week, and receive at least 1 wellness treatment (e.g., massage, acupuncture, chiropractic) weekly. I maintain good body mechanics and use a hydraulic table. I also have a disability insurance policy.

I regularly review my business plan and make necessary adjustments. I invest at least 8 hours each week marketing my business. I set up a business support system with at least 1 other person within the next 4 months, and work with a business coach starting next month. I currently have an accountant who does my taxes and I know an attorney that I can consult with on legal matters.

Your attitudes about the world can greatly influence your facility in taking risks. Be enthusiastic about the present and future. Expand your view of life. Focus on the prospects for success and joy. Don't become immersed in the potentials for disaster. Accurately evaluate what would really happen if you were to take a risk and not succeed. Remember that success lies in taking action.

Figure 3.15 **The Do's and Don'ts of Risk-Taking**

The Do's of Risk-Taking
- Have a life plan with clear goals.
- Make sure the risk is aligned with your life plan.
- Evaluate potential gains and losses.
- Ask questions and research the situation.
- Know your strengths and limitations.
- Brainstorm several alternatives.
- List potential conflicts and solutions.
- Set a realistic timetable.
- Be flexible.
- Trust your intuition and instincts.
- Follow through and give it your best.
- Review and revise your strategy.
- Ask for support.
- Acknowledge the people who give you support.

The Don'ts of Risk-Taking
- Be unrealistic.
- Be a perfectionist.
- Deny your feelings.
- Ignore or minimize problems.
- Mistake emotions for facts.
- Rush.
- Procrastinate.
- Blame others for your mistakes.
- Give up too soon.
- Be afraid to cut your losses and move on.
- Trust blindly.
- Take risks just to prove yourself to others.
- Combine too many risks at once.

Motivation

Motivation is about satisfying desires and needs. The major theories of motivation are often described as behavioral, cognitive, psychoanalytic, social learning, social cognition, and humanistic. Listed below is a brief overview of each theory:

- The **Behavioral** point of view is based on observable behavior and states that biological responses to stimuli direct behavior (e.g., the famous Pavlov's dog experiments).
- The **Cognitive** approach is founded on the belief that making meaning is key to motivation and focuses on the impact of the structure and function of information processing.
- **Psychoanalytic** theory presumes that all action or behavior is a result of internal, biological instincts (e.g., Freudian analysis).
- **Social Learning** suggests that an individual's behavior can be motivated by observing the consequences that others experience.
- **Social Cognition** proposes that the environment, an individual's behavior, and the individual's knowledge, emotions, and cognitive development influence each other to determine motivation.
- The **Humanistic** view focuses on personal growth and interpersonal relationships, believing that people behave out of intentionality and values.

Abraham Maslow is one of the most well known researchers in the field of humanistic motivation. His original hierarchy of motivational needs had 5 divisions (see Figure 3.16). Recently, psychologists have taken his notes and modified the hierarchy to the following 8 levels: **physiological** (satisfaction of hunger, thirst, and sex); **safety** (security, shelter, and stability); **social** (belongingness and love); **esteem** (self-respect, power, competence, approval, recognition, and prestige); **cognitive** (knowledge, understanding, and exploration); **aesthetic** (symmetry, order, and beauty); **self-actualization** (find self-fulfillment and realize one's potential); and **transcendence** (connect to something beyond the ego or help others in their self-actualization). Maslow contends that people aren't compelled to reach a level until the needs of the level below are satisfied. Thus, it's extraordinarily difficult to be motivated toward self-actualization or transcendence if your safety or esteem needs aren't met.

> "This I have gained by philosophy: that I do without being commanded what others do only from fear of the law.
>
> —Aristotle

If you're unable to motivate yourself to do a particular task, find out what other needs you have that are not being met. You must appeal to the needs and desires that are the strongest at any given moment. Once you have satisfied those other needs, it's easier to complete the specific task.

Motivation Techniques

The two most common motivators are fear and incentive, both of which have serious shortcomings. Fear motivation is the oldest, easiest, and universally least effective means of motivation. It forces you to act out of fear of the consequences. Parents frequently use this technique with young children. The primary limitation of this style of motivation is that most people (particularly children) quickly build up a tolerance to fear. Since the repercussions are rarely enforced, they usually aren't taken seriously.

Incentive motivation promises a reward for behavior. This method is often used in business as a way to increase productivity and is also frequently used by people in the process of altering habits. The problems associated with this motivation system are that the rewards have to keep escalating to merit the same impact and withholding the reward represents a punishment. Incentive motivation doesn't satisfy your desire for achievement.

The most effective motivation is self-motivation, being inspired by the pure joy of accomplishment. Approaching life from this point of view is extremely empowering to yourself and to those around you. It can be very freeing to not need outside stimulus to induce action. This can be difficult because the results of your actions are often intangible or may not be realized for a long time.

Figure 3.16 Maslow's Modified Hierarchy of Motivational Needs

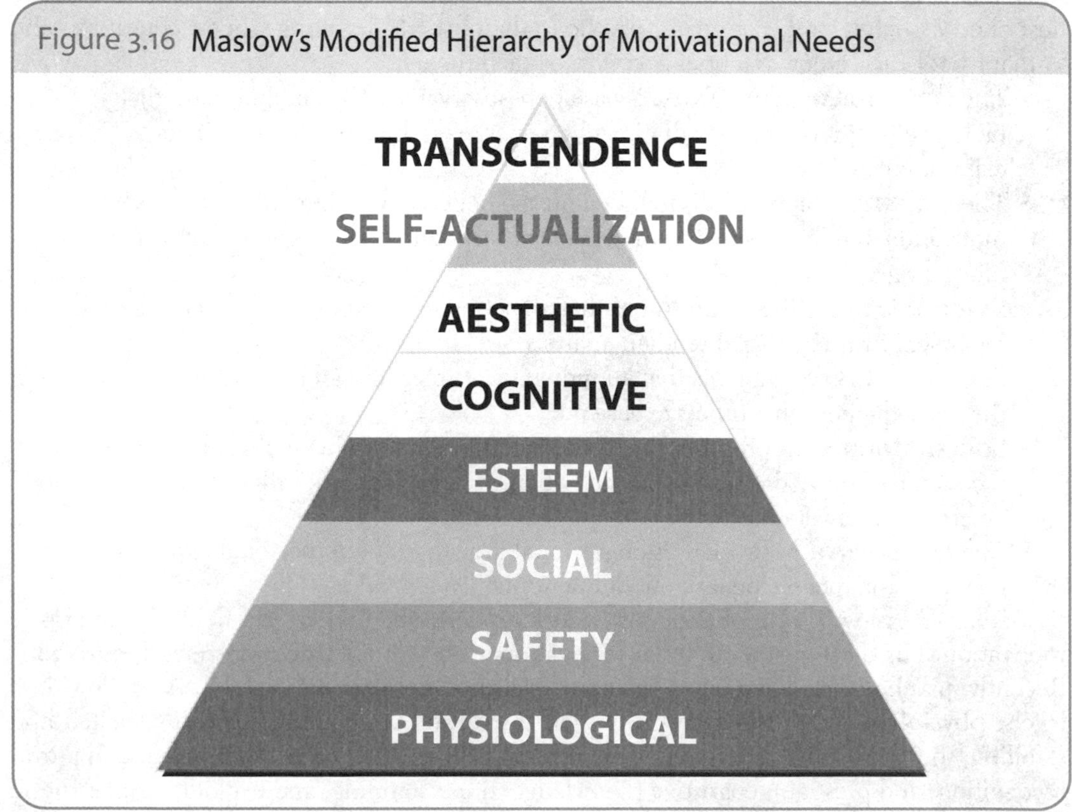

Self-motivation is an attitude that takes time to develop and fully integrate into your life. It may take longer to master motivation in some areas of your life than in others. The clearer you are about your purposes, priorities, and goals, the easier and more natural it is to become motivated by the sheer act of attaining your goals.

Your history plays a major role in attitude development. Throughout your life, your environment and the people around you have influenced you to some degree. Your cumulative experiences and feelings impact your perception. For example, you may view a certain task as boring while someone else might find the same task exciting. One technique for altering your feelings about an activity (and thus making it easier to accomplish) is to remove any negative descriptive terms associated with it.

The principal factor in motivation is goals. Without goals, motivation has no direction. You can even create goals about motivation. Your mind is a powerful tool that is ready and waiting for you to utilize it more effectively. If your motivation is still blocked, do some clearing exercises or the Dissolving Problems exercise as described in this chapter.

> "Ability is what you're capable of doing. Motivation determines what you do. Attitude determines how well you do it.
>
> —Lou Holtz

Figure 3.17 10 Ways to Sabotage Motivation

- Refrain from having written goals.
- Set unattainable goals.
- Agree to take responsibility for goals or activities that you don't believe in.
- Set goals in such a way that they take a long time to accomplish without small successes along the way.
- Establish important goals that conflict with your values or other aspects of your life.
- Withhold rewards on big projects until they're fully completed.
- Refuse to acknowledge your successes.
- Maintain a negative attitude about yourself, your abilities, your goals, and your activities.
- Ignore your mental, physical, and emotional wellbeing.
- Listen to the skepticism of your friends, family, and colleagues.

Self-Assessment

You already have been doing a lot of business skill building, soul-searching, and clearing throughout the process of "working" this book. Now it's time to evaluate yourself to determine the skills you need to learn or enhance. Be honest.

- What are your strengths?
- What are your challenges?
- How do your challenges compare with your strengths?
- How do you intend to alleviate those challenges?
  (Use the planning tools from Chapter 2 to create measurable steps. Integrate those steps into your regular routines, use them as motivation, and you will see those challenges diminish over time.)

The following poster is a summation of the principles and techniques covered in this book. Post it in strategic places, such as your bathroom mirror or bulletin board. Refer to it often.

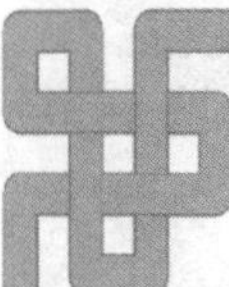
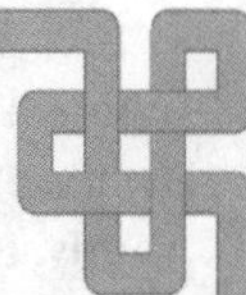

Be Your Own Best Manager

Believe in yourself!

Identify your values and operate from them.

Clarify your purpose, priorities, and goals.

Design and implement an effective business plan.

Create strategic plans of action.

Learn to work smarter—not harder.

Track important components.

Eliminate time wasters.

Plan your days.

Set a schedule and keep it.

Utilize proper body mechanics.

Respect your mind's and body's cycles.

Take a stretch break every 20 minutes.

Strengthen your business savvy.

Become proficient with your computer skills.

Be dressed for "work."

Get feedback from colleagues and experts.

Collect information: quotes, articles, statistics.

Keep your workspace organized.

Enhance your telephone skills.

Work from a client-centered approach.

Follow through with clients.

Market your business consistently.

Join at least 1 professional association.

Develop powerful networking abilities.

Keep accurate records.

Maintain healthy boundaries with clients and co-workers.

Keep up on the latest research findings.

Be a calculated risk-taker.

Be flexible.

Be willing to move on.

Make sure your needs are being met.

Exercise regularly.

Eat healthy foods.

Receive regular wellness treatments.

Create a support system.

Engage in group or peer supervision.

Take continuing education courses.

Enhance your communication skills.

Get out of the house/office EVERY DAY!!!

Have a life outside of work.

Schedule fun time that has nothing to do with your work.

Take responsibility for yourself.

Choose appropriate advisors.

Keep things in perspective.

For tasks you hate, delegate (or subcontract).

Balance your personal and professional life.

Maintain a good sense of humor.

Remember, we are human, we make mistakes.

Acknowledge your accomplishments every day.

Possess a positive mental attitude.

Do what you love, love what you do.

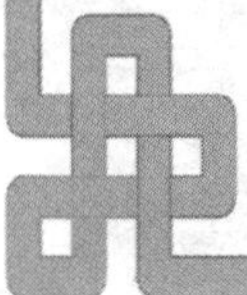
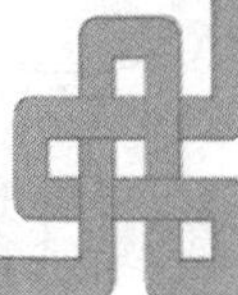

4
Boost Career Longevity

"If you ask me what is the single most important key to longevity,
I would have to say it is avoiding worry, stress, and tension.
And if you didn't ask me, I'd still have to say it."
—George Burns

Career Longevity Components
- Personality Characteristics
- Client Interactions
- Technical Capabilities
- Business Savvy
- Strong Client Base

Prevent Burnout
- Self-Care and Stress Management
- Scarcity Consciousness
- Sloppy Time Management
- Poor Boundaries
- Boredom Syndrome

Professional Development
- Continuing Education
- Research

Cultivate Your Support System
- Create a Safe Harbor with Supervision
- Find the Right Mentor
- How to Choose Advisors
- Mastermind Groups
- Join Online Discussion Forums

Key Terms

Advisor
Body Mechanics
Boredom Syndrome
Boundaries
Burnout
Career Longevity
Client Base
Client-Centered
Communication
Continuing Education
Continuing Education Provider
Ergonomics
Flexibility
Learning Environment
Mastermind Group
Mentor
Online Discussion Forums
Peer Support Group
Professional Development
Research Capacity
Research Literacy
Scarcity Consciousness
Scientific Method
Self-Care
Stress
Stress Management
Supervision
Support System
Time Management

According to career counselor Randall S. Hansen, Ph.D., "Studies indicate that the average worker will change careers—not just jobs—several times over the course of a lifetime."[1] But what if you're already in (or attending school for) your second or third career, and you want it to be your last? Or what if you're just beginning your career in this field and want to be in control of when—or if—you leave it someday?

Although there are no easy formulas that guarantee career longevity, steady efforts in the areas of professional development, positive attitude, communication skills, and self-renewal are a good way to plant seeds for success—and excel in your career day to day.

Career Longevity Components

The principal components of career longevity are personality characteristics, client interactions, technical capabilities, business savvy, and self-care. Most of the suggestions for longevity are the same for those who are self-employed as they are for those who work as employees.

See Chapter 12 for many **employment tips**.

The additional skills critical for employees to master are interpersonal communications with staff and management, and knowing how to adapt to various management styles. Most employers look for highly skilled practitioners who are positive and professional, flexible and adaptable, and who have an ability to put clients at ease. They want mature, team players with good people skills, and an ability to take initiative. They are also looking for employees with the wisdom to seek self-renewal, which enables a practitioner to function at his or her best and avoid burnout.

Personality Characteristics

Self-confidence Quiz
www.mindtools.com/pages/article/newTCS_84.htm

Successful practitioners are confident in their abilities, possess a positive mental attitude, maintain healthy boundaries, enjoy working with people, and are willing to take risks, such as speaking in public. They are willing to press through challenges and be uncomfortable for a while. They are determined and focused. They do what is necessary to ensure quality and success. They maintain consistency of quality.

Along with this determination is flexibility. Flexibility is crucial in the hands-on aspect of the work, as well as in business operations. For instance, there may be times when practitioners find themselves needing to change the type of work or treatment plan right in the middle of a session: perhaps a client isn't responding well to a particular technique; doesn't like what's being done; or it becomes apparent that the session needs to go in a different direction.

Flexibility is also needed to sail through the changes that occur in one's career. This includes adding modalities to one's repertoire and branching into other areas, such as education. Employees in particular need to be flexible, as they rarely have much control over their work environment.

> "If you think you can, you can. And if you think you can't, you're right.
> —Mary Kay Ash

The key personality characteristic is loving your work and appreciating people for who they are regardless of their physical condition. The work you do isn't limited to your technical abilities. Clients need to feel comfortable with you and know that you truly care for them.

Client Interactions

Practitioners who have been in the industry for a long time have a reverence for the inherent magnificence of the human body and spirit. They are compassionate and respect their clients regardless of their physical conditions or the particular reasons that they seek care. A highly judgmental person rarely lasts long in private practice, as clients sense subtle messages. Successful practitioners say that a client-centered approach is important, that it's crucial to stay present with clients, and to listen to what they're really saying. They customize each session to address clients' long-term goals and immediate concerns.

You can improve client relations by taking courses to enhance communication skills, learning effective intake interviewing skills, and creating treatment/session plans that encourage clients to take an active role in their own wellness.

§1

Technical Capabilities

Practitioners with staying power possess a high level of expertise and excel in what they do. They consider their initial schooling to be just the starting point, and they invest in regular continuing education. They stay current with the trends, read the new literature, attend seminars, and learn new techniques. While some long-time practitioners do well as generalists, most specialize in a particular technique, condition, or aspect of wellness care. Jean Shea, president and chief product formulator of BIOTONE, says that "over the course of your career, your marketplace will more than likely change, as will your professional interests. That's why learning throughout your career is essential."[2]

Note to students and new graduates: The first step to career longevity is to gain a solid base of experience to integrate what you've learned in school with hands-on practice in the field. Recognize that in the first few years of practice, it's vital to continue your education to expand your portfolio of skills and techniques. In fact, it's common to find successful wellness practitioners with several years of experience who have taken hundreds of hours of additional training. Continuing your professional education throughout your career opens many doors—to both personal fulfillment and professional growth. A commitment to lifelong learning provides a strong foundation for ongoing success.

Business Savvy

The more you make business a natural expression of who you are, the more successful you are.

The majority of people enter this field with limited business knowledge and many bear a negative attitude about business. Plenty of books, classes, marketing products, and online resources abound to assist practitioners in expanding their business knowledge. The savvy practitioner takes advantage of these tools.

Take every opportunity to learn all you can about effective communication. Successful professionals are those who have learned to communicate clearly and openly, and who have a knack for creating win-win solutions to everyday problems. They avoid defensive communication and focus on mature two-way communication grounded in respect for others. They make it a practice to listen with empathy and full attention. When others slip into gossip or criticizing a co-worker, boss, or competitor, they often bring up the bright side or positive qualities of the person.

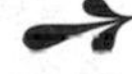

See Chapter 6, for more details on **communication**.

Learning to work smarter—not harder, is a chief tenet of success. Take the time to stay organized and keep excellent records. Look to the long term and consult with experts.

Strong Client Base

Keep in mind that the number one key to career longevity is a solid base of clients. After all, without them you don't have a practice. Exceptions do exist, such as when you work in a destination spa or resort where there's a continuous flow of new guests, or your work is of a particular approach or philosophy that advocates working with a client only once or twice.

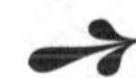

See Section 7 for **marketing tips.**

Doing what you love doesn't mean sitting in your office waiting for the phone to ring; it's about taking action to attract new clients and actually doing your work. If you don't have a full client load, either invest that free time in educating people about your work or donate your services (do what you love)—then the money will come.

Effective marketing in this field includes a mixture of promotion, advertising, community relations, and publicity—with the emphasis on promotion. The core of client retention is a solid customer-service plan. The best plans are founded upon making clients feel safe and welcome, finding effective ways to support clients' wellness and stress management efforts, and addressing any wellness needs.

Prevent Burnout

> "Realize that not all movement is progress. When stress and tension and chaos surround you, pause for a moment and relax. The best time to take a deep breath is when you don't have time for it.
>
> —Melchor Lim

Avoiding professional burnout can be challenging in today's fast-paced world. As a wellness practitioner, your personal wellbeing and balance is a major influence on your everyday effectiveness. Some common pitfalls that contribute to burnout are inadequate self-care and stress management, scarcity consciousness, sloppy time management, poor boundaries, and boredom syndrome. We explore each of these pitfalls and ways you can prevent burnout and thrive every day in your work.

Self-Care and Stress Management

Helping others is difficult if you neglect your own wellness. The signs of chronic stress include high blood pressure, digestive problems, sleep disorders, mood shifts, depression, anxiety, and decreases in mental acuity. It's so easy to forget about ourselves, yet as caregivers we must make certain we're also care-receivers. Developing a habit of self-renewal helps you stay energized and ensures you're at your professional best. To properly manage stress, your self-care routine should include most of the following:

- Take breaks, stretch, and do breathing exercises.
- Eat properly and stay hydrated.
- Carve out time for daily walking, yoga, or meditation.
- Exercise regularly.
- Enjoy time in nature.
- Take a little time to laugh and play each day.
- Enjoy your friends and family.
- Schedule fun outings.
- Participate in sports that relax and energize you.
- Make adjustments in your body mechanics and use proper equipment.
- Make time for a weekly touch therapy session.

Walk your talk: if you're a massage therapist, get weekly massages; if you're a nutritional consultant, eat healthy foods and take proper supplements; if you're an esthetician, get weekly facials; if you're a dentist, make sure your teeth are in great condition. How can you realistically expect clients to regularly incorporate your services into their lives if you aren't practicing what you preach?

Receiving wellness sessions from other practitioners not only benefits you, it's also a great way to build your knowledge of different techniques so you can make informed referrals for your clients. Even if you have a favorite practitioner, try out others. You may discover a technique or body of knowledge that is absolutely wonderful; you can then take the necessary steps to learn it and incorporate it into your practice. In addition, receiving these sessions on a regular basis can assist you in being more attuned to your clients' needs. How can you resist this wonderful opportunity to take care of yourself and grow professionally at the same time?

Regular exercise is essential for health and a feeling of wellbeing. If you're not already exercising, make this a habit by committing to at least 3, 20-minute exercise sessions each week. In about 6 weeks, you will feel much healthier and best of all your body becomes more efficient at processing oxygen—the magic key to enjoying more energy. Choosing types of exercise that you enjoy, or joining with others who have similar goals, boosts your success in this area of self-care.

Keeping balance in mind is the key to stress management. You need to keep things in perspective. Don't react to things that aren't your responsibility. Learn to deal with interruptions: internal and external. Learn to say "No."

Emotional burnout is a bit trickier. Attitude plays a critical role. You can avoid burnout by making time to meet with colleagues on a regular basis, attending conferences, varying the way you work, maintaining a strong personal support system, and enrolling in new classes to expand your knowledge and stay inspired.

§1

Develop a Self-Care Plan

Before you begin this activity, write a paragraph or two in your journal about your overall energy levels and how you feel (physically and mentally) about your weekly routine. Next, use the list above (or make up your own), and write down several self-care activities that you enjoy. Take a look at your weekly schedule. Pick times throughout your week that you can reasonably add an activity or two, and create a new weekly schedule. For the next 6 weeks, commit to the weekly schedule you have created.

Follow-Up: At the end of the 6 weeks, revisit your initial journal entry. How have your energy levels changed? How do you feel about the new weekly routine (physically and mentally)? Did you learn anything about yourself or about self-care over these 6 weeks?

Body Mechanics

The number one cause of physical burnout and injuries is poor body mechanics. Take the time to find out what works best for your body. For those of you who do hands-on work, invest in a high-quality table. Additionally, for those who do outcalls, be sure to purchase and use the accessories specially designed to help tote tables. If your work involves sitting with clients (e.g., nutritional consulting), then purchase an ergonomic chair. Set up your office in a manner that supports your posture and optimizes the physical demands of your work.

Purchase equipment and tools that enhance your own comfort, and invest in the proper training to use the equipment safely and effectively. Choose techniques and applications that are designed to reduce the wear and tear on your body (this would be a good use of your continuing education budget!). Career longevity depends on your ability to evaluate all avenues that can increase the effectiveness of your treatments while reducing your physical effort.

Scarcity Consciousness

Many people operate with a "go with the flow" philosophy in most areas of their lives, but when it comes to their business, their perspective often changes to one of scarcity. Poverty thinking burns you out faster than anything else.

I attended a party where a woman mentioned that although her 3-year-old practice was okay, she was considering getting a part-time job to help out. It wasn't as though she was just starting out and needed to transition into her career. If you figure that it takes approximately 3 hours of marketing to get a new client—why settle for a $10 an hour temporary job when you can spend these 3 hours to earn at least $60 instead of $40 (and that's if the client only comes in once). Her shortsightedness was staggering. This is a classic example of poverty thinking and scarcity consciousness at work.

> "Prosperity is a way of living and thinking, and not just money or things. Poverty is a way of living and thinking, and not just a lack of money or things
>
> —Eric Butterworth

Keeping a realistic frame of reference is crucial. Overcome this negative thinking by utilizing the tools covered in this chapter and reminding yourself of the value of your work and... Do the math!

Sloppy Time Management

See Chapter 3, pages 38-43 for more on **time management**.

Not paying enough attention to time management can also contribute significantly to burnout and imbalance. Practitioners invite burnout if they don't set appointments at accurate intervals, don't pace themselves well to accommodate breaks for clearing and centering, don't allow sufficient preparation time for clients, or don't schedule time just for themselves. A sloppy approach to time management prevents you from giving your best to your clients and creates a more stressful environment for yourself. In short, it makes sense to work smarter—not harder. (Are you noticing a theme here?)

Also, be sure to set aside time for planning and thinking—whether it's about your business agreements, goals, marketing, client relations, or evaluating what is working and what isn't. Think before you leap. Life is much more enjoyable and successful when one is coming from a proactive position than one of reaction.

Poor Boundaries

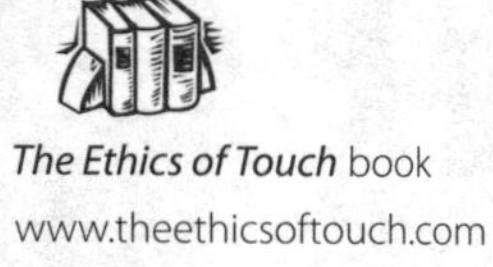
The Ethics of Touch book
www.theethicsoftouch.com

Alongside physical injury, the inability to effectively maintain and manage boundaries with clients, co-workers, and management is the leading cause of burnout for wellness practitioners. Boundaries help to protect the respect and dignity of each person. Resentment builds if you frequently allow your boundaries to be crossed. For instance, a client may repeatedly fail to respect your time by forgetting to cancel an appointment and refusing to pay for a missed session. Or you may encounter situations where others are prone to take advantage of your good nature or generosity. Set boundaries by learning to express your needs clearly and honestly so others know you expect to be treated with respect and dignity. Create policies and adhere to them. Work with a clinical supervisor or meet regularly with colleagues for peer supervision.

Boredom Syndrome

Practitioners who have been in business many years may find themselves falling prey to ennui. Sometimes a great rhythm turns into a deep rut. Here are some ideas to prevent this burnout:

- Diversify your practice.
- Alter your work environment.
- Join forces with other wellness providers.
- Start a whole new business.
- Take a sabbatical.
- Learn new skills.
- Volunteer your services.
- Revamp your business plan.

> “There's only one corner of the universe you can be certain of improving, and that's your own self.
> —Aldous Huxley

Keep in mind that any career has its ups and downs. The key is to recognize the difference between a natural phase and a downward spiral. Step back and objectively (as possible) evaluate the situation. Determine why you're encountering boredom and what might work best to remedy it. After you've assessed the situation and brainstormed possible solutions, discuss the issue with an advisor. Getting feedback from a trusted advisor can often shed new light on a challenging situation.

Professional Development

Learning is a lifelong process. Those who refrain from engaging their brains tend to lose their creative edge. While some people naturally gravitate toward continuous learning, others gravitate toward a comfort zone of familiar experiences. Some prefer informal to formal learning scenarios. Professional growth can take many shapes, from taking workshops or webinars, to reading books, to participating in professional associations. It may also involve activities such as public speaking, publishing articles in trade journals, or participating in research projects. Taking the time to develop a support system of like-minded professionals, as explored in the next section, can also be a powerful catalyst to professional growth.

While it's easy to say that professional development is a worthwhile endeavor, making it happen isn't always so easy. Scheduling time off from work or attending weekend courses can be logistically challenging. It can also be cost-prohibitive at times for those on an already stretched budget. However, career experts agree that if you want to reach your full career potential, carving out time and a budget for continued professional development is a must.

See Chapter 5, page 80 for information on **professional associations**.

Continuing Education

Although most everyone would agree that continuing education is valuable, performance anxiety or unpleasant childhood memories of academic pressures can act as big detractors. Even with the best of intentions to grow professionally, continuing education classes can easily slip to the bottom of one's to-do list. To help you overcome these hurdles, we will now explore various options for continuing education.

Continuing education courses range from 1 hour to hundreds of hours. You learn the basics in school, however, the true integration and honing of your skills comes with practice and years of working with clients. You keep the learning process active (and thus your professional and personal growth) by taking continuing education courses—either a series of short, specific classes or a long-term, advanced training program.

> "If you fill your mind with coins from your purse, your mind will fill your purse with coins.
> —Benjamin Franklin

Choose courses for the right reasons. Practitioners often save their pennies so they can take some new modality or product information workshop, desperate in the hope that this will bring them more clients or more security in their business. They take classes believing "This will be the magic formula to make me successful." If they don't market themselves well now, it's unlikely that additional training is the panacea. Unless a workshop includes a segment on how to market your new skills, it isn't likely to support your goal of creating more business.

Furthering your knowledge base is important, but don't confuse your ability to be good at your one-on-one work with the ability to market yourself well. They are different skills. If you need to learn more about marketing, take a marketing course. If you want to expand your technical repertoire, attend a modality or product knowledge training. Do each for the right reason.

Requirements

Many people are required to take continuing education to keep their certification or licensure current. Check with your certifying or licensing bodies to find out their parameters: the number of hours required annually; whether all (or a certain percentage) of the classes must be given by approved providers; the scope of topics that can be taken and which topics aren't allowed; the minimum or maximum number of hours that can be allotted to certain subjects (e.g., half of the hours must be hands-on, only up to one-third of the hours can be practice management); the method of learning allowed (some certifying bodies allow a limited number of hours for reading books or writing articles, others disallow distance learning for certain types of courses); and specific course requirements (e.g., 6 hours of ethics every 4 years, CPR recertification every 5 years).

> "I am convinced that it's of primordial importance to learn more every year than the year before. After all, what is education but a process by which a person begins to learn how to learn?
> —Peter Ustinov

When you know the requirements, you can carefully plan your continuing education far enough in advance to schedule the time and money for the courses you really want to take. Too many times practitioners wait until the last minute to fulfill their continuing education requirements for license renewal, and then they get stuck taking a course or workshop that happens to be offered at this specific time but doesn't even interest them. Plan ahead!

Exploring Educational Goals and Interests

What are your goals for continuing your education? Make a list of continuing education topics that interest you. Next to each topic, include at least 1 thing you want to get out of a course on that topic. Now do some research on providers that offer courses in your topics of interest. Keep a list of courses and providers in your journal, so when you're ready to sign-up for a course, you can follow your own interests.

How do you like to learn? Do you like to watch or read, and then practice on your own? Do you like to learn in a group or community? Do you like to have personal, reinforced instruction? Think about learning environments that you really enjoy and keep that information in your journal as well.

Sources

Many individuals, companies, and organizations provide continuing education courses on a wide range of topics. Check out advertisements in trade journals, magazines, newspapers, and newsletters; contact your professional association for a list of providers; request catalogs from schools as well as local community colleges, universities, and adult education programs; peruse local specialty publications; and surf the Internet (start your search with key terms such as training, continuing education, home-study, correspondence, schools, seminars, workshops, or the specific topic you're interested in exploring).

CE Requirements

Massage

integrativehealthcare.org/massage/state-list-massage-ceu-resources.html

Acupuncture

www.nccaom.org/wp-content/uploads/pdf/PDA/PDA%20Handbook.pdf

CE Sources

www.findce.com
www.worldwidelearn.com
www.afmte.org/ce-course-directory/

Learning Environments

The good news is that the manner in which you continue your learning isn't limited to a traditional school environment: you can read books; take distance-learning courses (e.g., correspondence, home-study, online); attend workshops; participate in self-exploration classes which benefit you directly and assist you in working with clients (e.g., movement, breathwork, communication skills); and go to conferences. Even continuing education courses offered by schools are usually administered quite differently than those in diploma programs.

If the environment isn't suited to your learning preferences, you can still do it, but it will most likely be more difficult, take longer, and the results won't be as clear. Some people learn best by reading or viewing a DVD and then processing the information on their own at their own pace. Distance-learning courses can be highly effective for these people. Keep in mind that these courses also vary widely: some provide reading materials while others include audio or video components. Assessments vary by course and can include multiple choice exams, written essays, and documented case studies.

Others learn better in a classroom or workshop environment. Teaching styles vary greatly when continuing education is done "live" (e.g., workshops, classes, conferences) and the leader's style might not be best for you. Some people prefer highly structured classes; others like a loose format. Some people want to hear only what the "expert" has to say and resent class discussions. Some people enjoy group activities; others would rather work on their own. Some people do just fine in a class with hundreds of people; others withdraw. Some people want a hands-on approach, others would rather watch a video. Once you've identified your preferred learning environment, you can assemble a list of questions to ask potential CE providers to get the best course for you.

§1

Figure 4.1 Questions for Colleagues about a CE Provider

- How easy was it to contact the provider about the course?
- What did you like the most about the course?
- What did you like the least about the course?
- What was the instructor's teaching style?
- Were the course materials beneficial and of high quality?
- On a scale of 1-10, how would you rate the overall value of this course?
- Did you learn what you expected to learn?
- Were agreements kept?
- Were you given a certificate upon completion?
- Do you think this was the best way to learn this subject? Why? Why not?
- What is the likelihood of you taking another course from this company?
- How often do you use what you learned in your daily practice?

Evaluating Continuing Education Providers

The depth, breadth, and overall quality of continuing education courses vary greatly. Do proper research before enrolling in any course. The key aspect is the credibility of the company and the individual facilitating the course. The following steps guide you in ascertaining credibility:

Review Marketing Materials

- Do the materials project a professional image?
- Are the courses clearly defined with specific objectives?
- Are the testimonials believable and are they from real people (not a vague reference such as "J.R. from Dallas")?
- Does the company offer a satisfaction guarantee or quality assurance?

Investigate Business History

- How long has the company (or individual) been in business?
- How many classes have been given?
- How many people have taken courses?
- What are the qualifications of the person leading the classes (or the developer of a distance-learning course)?
- What are the professional affiliations held?
- Has the company or individual received any awards?
- Does the company or individual have credentialing status (e.g., an approved NCBTMB provider)?

Obtain References

- Get feedback from others who have taken courses by this provider. The CE provider might furnish you with names and contact information of past participants. Be aware the referrals are slightly biased (those lists are usually comprised of happy customers).
- Talk with your colleagues and members of online newsgroups.

Research

The various disciplines that comprise the wellness professions have fascinating and diverse origins, and the unique public face of each discipline often depends heavily on these histories. Consumers vary in how they perceive these histories, and often it's these perceptions that lead them to choose one type of wellness care over another. There exists today, however, a method that levels the playing field and provides every technique an equal opportunity to prove its worth to today's savvy consumers. That method is research.

In recent years, a growing body of research in the holistic wellness field has paved the way for wider acceptance of modalities such as acupuncture, yoga, and massage therapy by both the mainstream medical community and by the general public. By providing practitioners with access to high-relevance information, research provides solid science to document the effectiveness of treatment.

Massage Research Tools

massagetherapyfoundation.org/research-tools

Locate Research Articles

www.massagemag.com/research-studies
www.biomedcentral.com
www.univadis.com
www.ncbi.nlm.nih.gov/pubmed
www.acupunctureresearch.org

In addition to what we know through our experience and clinical judgment, and through what our clients teach us about their experience, research can promote the wellbeing of our clients, our profession, and ourselves. It does so by facilitating the development of evidence-informed practice, by providing more democratic access to high-quality information, and by giving us a common language we can use to communicate with other wellness practitioners. Finally, it can inspire us to think outside of the box, and to ask more and better questions of our profession and ourselves.

Continued research that is rigorous, focused, and of high quality will inform training programs, direct treatments, and—most importantly—guide the choices of consumers who want to know what issues a technique is good for, what it does, and why it's worth paying for. The bottom line is clear: research is essential to the long-term commercial success of the wellness professions. If you're serious about maintaining a stable and long-term career in the wellness field, study the current research, integrate research findings into your practice and marketing, and determine what role you can play in the conduction of research.

The Scientific Method

The scientific method of research requires results to be repeatable, observable, and measurable. The steps consist of observing a sequence of action, measuring the data, and making a testable prediction about that sequence.

As an example of the scientific method used in research, a study by Ferrell-Torry and Glick focused on massage therapy treatments for patients with cancer pain. Results showed that massage lowered blood pressure in that patient group.[3] Another study by Olney applied the same treatment plan in a different group of patients with high blood pressure (hypertension).[4] This study found the same result: massage lowered high blood pressure.

In its simplest form, the scientific method consists of the following steps:

- Observe something that occurs (in our example above for the group of cancer patients, blood pressure was lowered).
- Create a hypothesis about what you observed. Ferrell-Torry and Glick hypothesize that massage lowers blood pressure in cancer patients.
- Use that hypothesis to make a prediction about what will occur. Olney predicted that since massage has been observed to lower blood pressure in other groups of patients, it would also lower blood pressure in people living with hypertension.
- Set up an experiment to see if that prediction is accurate. Olney tested the effects of 10 back massages, (lasting 10 minutes apiece, carried out 3 times a week), on the blood pressure of patients diagnosed with hypertension.
- Decide whether the experiment confirmed the hypothesis or contradicted it. Olney concluded that there was a significant reduction in the blood pressure of the people who received the massages; therefore there was evidence that massage is a treatment that could be considered for hypertension patients.

Research Literacy

Research literacy refers to an ability to find, read, evaluate, and apply relevant findings that may be useful in your wellness practice. At first, the idea of reading research articles may be intimidating, but remember that you don't need to analyze every detail of the article in tremendous depth. Read as carefully as you can and look for the high points: what was the research question the author tested, how was it tested, did that research question hold up when it was tested, and were there enough subjects tested to make the findings relevant? That is the heart of the article; the rest is details.

Knowing how to sift gems of information and insight from research is a learned ability that comes with practice. You may want to organize a group that meets monthly to discuss research articles and information useful in day-to-day practice. This is a great way to ensure you keep up with latest developments, as well as to network with like-minded professionals. Plus it can significantly enhance your skills as a practitioner.

You can find various kinds of articles, such as reviews, essays, and research summaries in scientific journals, trade magazines, and online. The structure of most research papers and articles mirrors the scientific method, so the more you read the more you will be familiar with the format.

Research Literacy Practice

Search peer-reviewed journals for 3 research studies that address the type of work you do on a condition that interests you. Evaluate the methods and results of each study. Determine whether the study findings support your specific work with this condition. Determine if you will adjust your session planning regarding this condition based on any new information you have learned. Note any difficulties you had in finding multiple research studies for your chosen condition. If so, what do you think that means in terms of the state of research on your type of work regarding this condition? What level of importance do you give research in your treatment planning?

Research Capacity

Research capacity refers to the ability to carry out research. Ruth Werner, past president of the Massage Therapy Foundation, says that the best way to become involved in research is to start by writing a case report. That is, start with exploring what happens between one client who has some goals, and one practitioner. The wellness professions need more well-written case reports. Werner calls it "citizen science." Writing good case reports can open doors to getting involved in larger studies. If you live near a university, you can check whether it's carrying out research in your field. If not, you can develop a research idea and approach potential funders in your community to carry it out. The funders will look closely at whether you have the skills and experience to carry out what you propose to do. Building a strong team of professionals who have solid experience in research design and implementation plays a key role in the success of such a proposal.

The **Massage Therapy Foundation** offers grants for various research projects

massagetherapyfoundation.org/grants-and-contests

Cultivate Your Support System

Professional growth includes developing relationships with other professionals in your field. Keeping up with standards, trends, and relevant research is easier and more fun when you join organizations of individuals who share your enthusiasm for learning.

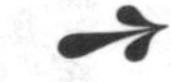

See Chapter 5, page 80 for more on **professional affiliations**.

Professional associations, online communities, and support groups provide forums for accessing other professional development activities such as continuing education and research. They can also provide up-to-date news and information on topics affecting your career and your profession.

A strong support system can greatly impact your career. Get advice and coaching from people who have essentially traveled the path you're on, as well as others who have greater expertise than you in specific areas concerning career growth and business development.

The major support system categories are supervision, peer support groups, mentors, advisors, mastermind groups, and online discussion forums. It's ideal to have more than one category in place, although finding a mentor may be the most difficult. Your support system may be comprised mainly of people you know who care about you and want to see you succeed. Then again, some, if not all, may be paid advisors. The nice aspect of paid advisors is that terminating the relationship is easy.

Create a Safe Harbor with Supervision

> "Experience is a good teacher, but her fees are very high.
> —W.R. Inge

Supervision has long been the primary professional training model for mental health clinicians. More recently, other wellness professionals have begun to recognize and use this forum to teach students. Supervision can take place on a one-on-one basis or in a group. It consists of the practitioner meeting regularly with another professional (or several) to discuss client treatments and professional issues in a structured way.

Les Kertay, Ph.D., states,[5]

> *If you're interested in doing work that has emotional and spiritual impact on your clients, then the most powerful way of dealing with the questions involved is to utilize ongoing professional supervision. Supervision isn't about being told how to do your job, rather it's a place to process your clients' work and your experiences of being with them.*

Supervision creates a shame-free setting for self-care, support, and nurturance. It is the right place to receive appreciation for the good and useful work a practitioner is doing. Participating in supervision helps you to maintain an ethical practice and avoid burnout by assisting you with the following:

- Diffuse intense feelings that arise in the therapeutic relationship.
- Resolve complex interpersonal dilemmas.
- Establish and manage boundaries.
- Recognize and manage transference and countertransference.
- Learn from your experiences.
- Progress in expertise.
- Ensure excellent client care.
- Enhance communication skills.
- Create balance.

Professional Supervision

Professional (also referred to as clinical) supervision provides an opportunity to discuss with a more experienced, psychologically savvy practitioner (usually one with mental health training) how to best help a client while promoting increased self-observation and awareness.

Rather than offering advice and telling the practitioner what to do, a good supervisor helps the practitioner to explore what's happening internally, define where the appropriate boundary is for the practitioner and the client, and determine what action might correct the situation. In general, these techniques, which draw on and validate the practitioner's problem-solving skills, lead to a more effective and empowering resolution. In a group setting, the supervisor often invites other members to help navigate a colleague toward the core issue underlying the problem.

How To Find A Supervisor

Psychotherapy disciplines have the longest tradition of providing clinical supervision and, thus, psychotherapists are fruitful sources. Psychiatrists, nurses, social workers, psychologists, and counselors are likely to be experienced supervisors. Personal recommendations by a colleague or a valued teacher are also fine ways to secure names of potential supervisors. If a referral by a colleague or instructor is difficult to obtain, it's possible to contact state or national professional organizations to obtain names of professionals in good standing.

A skillful supervisor is like a guide in unfamiliar territory, enhancing understanding and helping direct the practitioner toward constructive solutions. A supervisor often helps by asking a variety of questions about what is needed and what the practitioner was thinking and feeling when she encountered the problematic situation. In appropriate situations, advice can be offered about how to best assist a client. The most meaningful aspect of supervision, however, is the opportunity to explore and work through a problem.

Start a Peer Support Group

It's often useful to have the support of a small group of practitioners who are doing the same kind of work. This broadens the base of learning and creates an additional support system for each member. If the practitioner is in a group situation where she can learn from others' experiences, it's possible to master the fundamentals of practice through witnessing others' learning and not relying exclusively upon her own professional trial and error. Hearing the fears and doubts of other practitioners who are feeling challenged by unusual client situations can help practitioners feel less isolated and alone.

Peer support groups are valuable for practitioners at any phase of professional life. Beginning practitioners may find it beneficial to engage in both individual supervision and peer support. Mid- and late-career practitioners often participate regularly in peer groups and seek individual consultations as required. Each practitioner designs a network of support that suits the demands and needs of his practice, phase of professional development, and personality.

Peer support groups have easily identifiable advantages and some potential disadvantages. The strengths, limitations, and success of peer groups rest with the composition of the individual members and the clarity of the peer group contract. Peer support decreases professional isolation, increases professional support and networking, normalizes the stress and strain of professional life, and offers multiple perspectives on any concern or problem. Peer support has the added benefit of being free of charge, intellectually stimulating, and fun.

A brief, start-up consultation with a clinical supervisor or group specialist is helpful to define and establish the contract and framework for a successful peer support group. When successful, peer support groups far exceeds other forms of supervision and continuing education for individualized learning, intimacy, support, pleasure, and a sense of belonging that anchors professional work. Many peer groups opt to have a clinical supervisor moderate their meetings on a regular basis, such as quarterly or twice a year. It may also be appropriate to meet with this supervisor individually when additional support is needed.

Find the Right Mentor

A business or professional mentor is an individual, usually older and more experienced, who helps and guides another individual's career development. The benefits of finding the right mentor are many. A good mentor can be an invaluable career asset and greatly enhance your potential for success. One of the most valuable things a mentor can do is to help you take an honest look at yourself and identify areas where work is needed to achieve your goals. This guidance isn't done for financial gain yet can be personally rewarding for both parties. Most often people choose mentors who are in the same or related field. This person serves as a trusted confidante and the mentoring relationship usually lasts a long time—throughout a phase or throughout life.

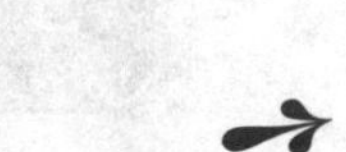

See Chapter 5, pages 85-88 for **social responsibility**.

People become mentors as a way of giving back to their community and to society at large. They may also do it to develop their skills as a teacher, manager, or consultant. An effective mentoring relationship also works in both directions. A critical aspect of mentoring is to make certain that both parties are getting something out of the deal. It cannot just be a one-sided relationship; there must be give and take. Both parties must understand the benefits and demands that are going to be experienced in this process.

Sometimes a mentor can be found through a professional or trade organization. Also, contact your alma mater to find out if it has a mentoring program in place. Another option that is similar to mentoring, and can ultimately lead into a true mentoring relationship, is to intern or apprentice with a highly regarded practitioner.

"Mentor: Someone whose hindsight can become your foresight.

—Unknown

In most instances, the best place to look for a mentor is right in front of you—perhaps someone from work or in your professional circle who you admire and respect. You might also know someone who doesn't do the same type of work as you but is an expert in the field. These are the types of individuals to approach first to ask if they would consider being your mentor.

How to Choose Advisors

Every business has management, marketing, legal, and accounting aspects. It is important to know trustworthy people for advice, particularly in areas where you lack knowledge, interest, or skill. Selecting the most appropriate advisors directly affects the success of your business. Before making any major decisions, discuss them with at least one other person—regardless of your expertise in the area. All too often, the tendency is to do it all on your own and it's almost impossible to be truly objective, especially with something as significant as your business or career. Your primary advisors are your lawyer, accountant, banker, and business consultant or coach.

Government organizations that **match people with mentors**

www.sba.gov/tools/local-assistance/sbdc

www.score.org

Reliable, affordable, and trustworthy counsel is crucial to your business health. Pick the members of your advisory team before you NEED them. Don't wait for an emergency when you may not have ample time to find an appropriate advisor to assist with the situation at hand. Begin to build your relationships now (particularly with a banker) so you can establish your credibility and develop rapport.

The process for selecting advisors begins by getting personal recommendations from friends and colleagues. In addition to the names, get specific information about them. Find out why they recommend these advisors and what types of dealings they have had with them. Whatever you do, don't stop at this point. You must also make your own assessments. The first thing is to trust your intuition. If you don't feel comfortable with a particular advisor—keep looking. Even if you feel good about the person, do further research. She may be an excellent advisor, yet not appropriate for you.

Check into the potential advisor's credentials and competency. If she has the required expertise and experience, the next phase is to discover if you're compatible. Find out the type of clientele she advises, particularly if she has clients in your profession.

Interview potential advisors (make certain this initial consultation is free of charge). See if your personalities and styles mesh. This is someone you're going to work with for a long time. You must share a similar philosophy and manner in which you like to get things done.

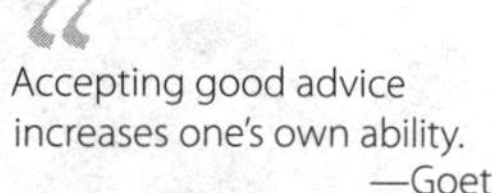

"Accepting good advice increases one's own ability.

—Goethe

Assess your level of confidence and trust in this person—professionally and personally. How well you communicate with each other is one of the most critical factors in choosing an advisor. For example, this person may be totally qualified, works with many others in your profession, has an impeccable character, and shares many of the same beliefs as you; yet it seems as though whenever you talk, you're speaking in 2 different languages. You have to decide if it's worth the time (and money) it takes to work through the communication barriers to have this person be your advisor.

Finally, determine if this person desires to have you as a client. A good advisor demonstrates a sense of commitment to you and your business and is readily available to answer questions.

Mastermind Groups

Joining a Mastermind group is a good way to strengthen your support system and widen your circle of professional acquaintances. Being involved in a Mastermind group is akin to having a volunteer board of directors that gives you guidance and support, and shares their proven success strategies. And the only cost to you is that you give back the same. The concept of Mastermind groups was coined by Napoleon Hill in his book *Think & Grow Rich.*[6] Hill defines Mastermind groups as the coordination of knowledge and effort in a spirit of harmony between two or more people for the attainment of a definite purpose. Members of Mastermind groups serve as a confidential sounding board—they listen to business concerns and ideas are shared, analyzed, and honed. The strength of this type of group is that the members are committed to supporting each other. This synergy fosters amazing creativity and results.

How They Work

Mastermind groups usually consist of 6-8 people, but no more than 10. The members are professionals with varied backgrounds, experiences, and areas of expertise. They meet on a regular basis (weekly, monthly, or quarterly) to brainstorm with each other, give and receive feedback, bestow their secrets for success, set goals, and share their successes as well as challenges. As an added benefit, members often provide business leads and client referrals.

Responsibilities are shared by all members. Each person takes a turn at hosting a meeting. The host sets the agenda, coordinates schedules, handles the logistics (e.g., room setup, refreshments), and facilitates the meeting.

If you cannot find an opening in an existing group, start your own Mastermind group. Be selective on who you invite to participate, and set up meeting rules to respect each participant's time.

Join Online Discussion Forums

Online discussion forums are a great place to get additional help. Professional forums and social media sites like Facebook and LinkedIn can provide timely support for specific situations. Because someone in the group is usually online, you can often get immediate answers to your questions. Protect client privacy and confidentiality by exercising caution when posting questions or comments in any online forum.

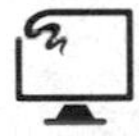

Online Forums

www.massageprofessionals.com
www.chiroweb.com
acupuncturetoday.com/forums

§2
Intentional Excellence

In Section 2 of *Business Mastery*, the theme of intentional excellence takes center stage. Intentional excellence requires unflinching honesty and courage, and it results from making your integrity central to whatever you do. It's the result of consistent and conscious effort made visible in the behaviors, interactions, and relationships you establish within your practice.

Chapter 5 focuses on measures of excellence that are different from markers of success like client numbers and bank balances. We start with a look at professional ethics, which exist not to catch people in wrongdoing, but to guide practitioners toward greatness, and present guidelines for recognizing ethical dilemmas and resolving them. This discussion flows naturally into the key role that a professional image plays in building a successful practice. The last two topics of the chapter consider how goodwill and social responsibility bring excellence into your practice—as you share your talents, time, and resources to support the causes closest to your heart.

Chapter 6 discusses why good communication skills are essential in business and highlights ways to fine-tune key skills, such as active listening and reflective feedback. It looks at the power of first impressions and rapport building, as well as several common barriers to effective communication. It includes useful tips on how to handle the inevitable conflicts and difficult situations that are part of professional life. This chapter also offers practical insights into how to conduct effective client interviews. Excellent recordkeeping is another aspect of good communication, so we discuss SOAP and Wellness formats for documenting client sessions and charting progress. You will also find a wealth of practical tips and resources for developing excellent communication skills and using technology appropriately.

5
Conscious Practice

"Life is an echo. What you send out comes back. What you sow, you reap. What you give, you get. What you see in others, exists in you."

—Zig Ziglar

Ethics
- Key Interpersonal Ethics Concerns
- Key Business Ethics Concerns
- Resolving Ethical Dilemmas
- Codes of Ethics

Professionalism
- Professional Affiliations
- Professional Credentials
- Image

Goodwill
- Public Recognition

Social Responsibility
- Profiles
- Steps You Can Take Now

Key Terms

Ambiance
Bigotry
Boundaries
Certification
Client Records
Codes of Ethics
Compassion
Competence
Confidence
Confidentiality
Dual Relationships
Empathy
Ethical Decision-Making Model
Ethical Dilemma
Ethics
Goodwill
Guarantee
HIPAA
Honesty
Image
Integrity
Laws
Licensure
Morals
Power Differential
Pro Bono
Professional Affiliations
Professional Credentials
Professionalism
Purchasing Power
Registration
Regulations
Reputation
Respect
Responsibility
Scope of Practice
Self-Accountability
Self-Esteem
Six Step Resolution Model
Social Responsibility
Title Protection
Values

A conscious practice is one in which you take the steps to make certain your outward impressions match your intentions. The information in this chapter helps you to develop a professional image and provides tools for handling ethical dilemmas. It also supports you in generating goodwill, recognizing your unique connection to your community, and determining your desired level of social responsibility.

Ethics

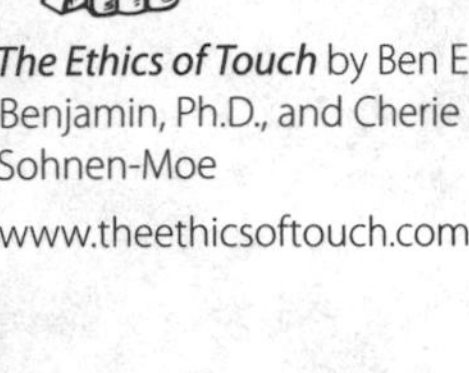

The Ethics of Touch by Ben E. Benjamin, Ph.D., and Cherie Sohnen-Moe

www.theethicsoftouch.com

Ethics have been debated by philosophers great and small for millennia. While there are several aspects of human behavior that are clearly good or bad, it's extremely difficult to agree upon what is good and bad—so much depends on the situation. Ethics can be defined as: a system or code of morals and conduct of a person or group; the discipline dealing with what is good and bad or right and wrong. The book, *The Power of Ethical Management* by Norman Vincent Peale and Kenneth Blanchard, relates ethical behavior to self-esteem: people who feel good about themselves withstand outside pressure and do what is right rather than what is expedient, popular, or lucrative.[1]

Ethics are different from morals and laws. Morals relate to character. Laws are codified rules of conduct that are based on ethical or moral principles. Laws often set the minimum standard necessary to protect the public's welfare, while ethics epitomize the ideal standards embraced by a profession.

Ethical behavior involves striving to bring the highest values into one's work and aspiring to do one's best in all interactions. It means doing the right thing for the right reason with the right attitude. The cornerstone of ethics is self-accountability. When you have a well-developed sense of self-accountability, you're honest with yourself and fully responsible for what you say and do at all times. You have the ability to look beyond the immediate moment to consider all the consequences and know if you're willing to accept them. In general, typical business ethics cover adhering to prevailing laws, upholding the dignity of the profession, being service-oriented, staying committed to quality, and demonstrating loyalty to staff.

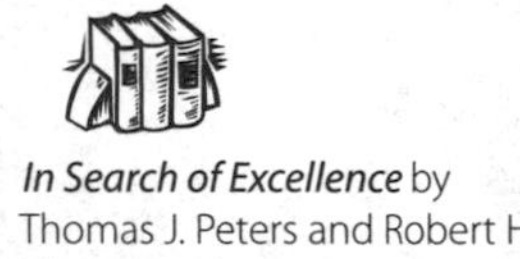

In Search of Excellence by Thomas J. Peters and Robert H. Waterman Jr.

Tom Peters offers a practical definition of ethics:[2]

> *High ethical standards—business or otherwise—are, above all, about treating people decently. To me (as a person, business person and business owner) that means respect for a person's privacy, dignity, opinions and natural desire to grow; and people's respect for (and by) co-workers.*

We're continually faced with ethical concerns. Most of them are easily reconciled, though occasionally we encounter a major conflict. Examples of common ethical dilemmas in the wellness professions are:

- Practicing beyond your scope
- Breaking confidentiality
- Sexual misconduct
- Misrepresentation of educational status
- Financial impropriety
- Exploiting the power differential
- Misleading claims of curative abilities
- Improper dual relationships
- Bigotry
- Dishonesty
- Inappropriate advertising
- Violation of state/city laws or regulations
- Boundary crossings and violations

Key Interpersonal Ethics Concerns

The attainment of wholeness requires one to stake one's whole being. Nothing less will do; there can be no easier conditions, no substitutes, no compromises.

—C.J. Jung

§2

As stated previously, the most common ethical dilemmas wellness practitioners experience involve personal boundaries, power differential, confidentiality, and dual relationships. Following are examples of these types of situations that may require careful consideration.

Boundaries: In relationships, a boundary is a limit that separates one person from another. It protects the integrity of each person. A boundary can be as tangible as the skin that surrounds our body or as ethereal as an attitude. The primary problem in defining boundaries is that in most instances they're intangible. Understanding boundaries is crucial to creating an ethical practice and building professional relationships. You can improve the therapeutic relationship and avoid any inadvertent slips into unethical behavior by increasing your awareness of your own and your clients' boundaries.

Power Differential: It's difficult to understand the therapeutic relationship between client and practitioner without comprehending the dynamics of power in a therapeutic relationship. There is a natural power differential in many relationships: between parent and child; between teacher and student; between employer and employee; and, of course, between wellness practitioner and client. A parent, teacher, employer, or wellness practitioner has the more powerful position. They are the authority figures whose actions, by virtue of their role, directly affect the wellbeing of the other.

The power differential is inherent in any therapeutic relationship. There is an implicit acknowledgment that the practitioner has more knowledge in this area than the client. In the wellness field, the power differential is amplified by the physical aspects of practice. The client takes a position—usually lying or sitting—which allows the practitioner access to his body. The practitioner positions herself within the client's physical space, often leaning over the client. Furthermore, in many professions, the client is partially or fully unclothed. Finally, as the practitioner makes physical contact with the client's body, the client's physical safety is literally in the practitioner's hands. For these reasons, the practitioner must take more responsibility than the client in creating a balanced relationship, however unequal the power differential may be.

Confidentiality: Confidentiality is the cornerstone of every positive and powerful therapeutic relationship. Confidentiality can be defined as the client's guarantee that what occurs in the therapeutic setting remains private and protected. First and foremost, the issue of confidentiality concerns the client's rights to privacy and safety. These rights belong equally to every client you see regardless of age, status, or relationship to you or another client. These same rights apply to whenever you share a client's information with others, whether written or verbal.

Most professionals are clear about what constitutes a major confidentiality breach, such as sharing personal information about a client with a third party. However, subtle situations may occur where it can be easy to cross boundaries if one is not vigilant, such as public recognition. Clients shouldn't be acknowledged in public unless they recognize and greet the professional first. To do so puts clients in a position of having it revealed that they were seeking professional services that they may want kept private. Social media posts and comments should be considered "public" as well, with the same confidential care exercised anywhere online. If you work with celebrities or public figures and you think you might want to let others know (e.g., including a statement on a flyer such as, "Some of my clients include [insert celebrity's name]."), it's wise to get permission—preferably in writing.

See Chapter 19, pages 264-266 for more information on **confidentiality and HIPAA regulations.**

Occasions when it's appropriate to break confidentiality include: when there's a clear and imminent danger to the client or another individual; a client discloses an intention to commit a crime; suspected abuse or neglect of a child, an elderly person, or an incapacitated individual; or a court subpoena for a client's records. A confidentiality agreement that notes these situations can be a crucial tool for communicating to a client these exceptions to standard confidentiality practices.

Dual Relationships: The term dual relationships describes the overlapping of professional and social roles and interactions between two people. Human beings naturally develop multiple relationships in various arenas—among family, friends, neighbors, employees, employers, professional peers, clients, students, and teachers. People often fit into more than just one of those categories, and certain individuals play a mixture of roles. The classic depiction of a dual relationship is when two persons who interact professionally develop other roles of social interaction.

For example, you and a working colleague discover a mutual interest in tennis and begin to play together, or you and your teacher develop a longstanding friendship. Dual relationships also develop in the other direction, from the social to the professional realm: you and your sister decide to go into business together; or a social acquaintance or a friend seeks your professional services. In small towns or rural communities, dual relationships are even more common because of the limited numbers of people and choices for professional services.

Figure 5.1 Key Ethical Concerns

Interpersonal	Business
• Boundaries	• Finances
• Power Differential	• Product Sales
• Confidentiality	• Client Records
• Dual Relationships	• Legal Issues
	• Insurance Issues
	• Referrals
	• Taxes

Key Business Ethics Concerns

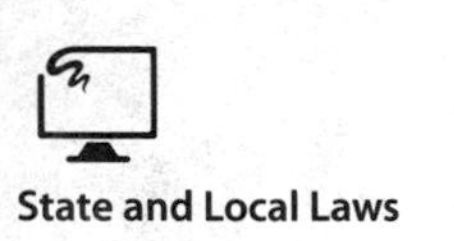
State and Local Laws
smallbusiness.findlaw.com

Whether you're a business owner or employee of a spa, group practice, or medical clinic, you may encounter situations that require you to apply sound ethical judgment. Following are highlights of business situations involving ethical issues. The nuts and bolts of these topics are covered in depth in other chapters.

Finances: In the realm of financial transactions, ethical issues can arise relating to gift certificates, fee structures, and tips. There have been reported instances of practitioners deliberately setting gift certificate expiration dates or redemption policies that result in a high percentage of unredeemed certificates. On the other hand, ethical practitioners often place a reminder call to a gift certificate holder one month prior to the expiration date, or return funds to the gift certificate purchaser if a certificate is not redeemed within the allotted time. Another area of ethical concern involves scenarios in which a practitioner charges a higher fee to clients who pay by insurance versus clients who pay by cash. Lack of income tax reporting of tips from sessions is also an area of ethical concern.

See Chapter 21 for more information on **product sales**.

Product Sales: At times, unethical practices such as pushy sales techniques or hype can characterize product sales in wellness settings. Fortunately, this is the exception rather than the rule. Ethical product sales involve providing clients with easy access to high-quality products that enrich their wellbeing. As a wellness practitioner, clients depend on you to provide them with sound information and guidance in the realm of product sales. Thus, it's essential to know your products well and convey the proper use, benefits, and possible side effects or contraindications of each product.

Client Records: Keeping accurate records is paramount. Also, confidentiality must be maintained in a therapeutic relationship to promote an atmosphere of safety. Although confidential recordkeeping has always been a cornerstone of ethical practice, government scrutiny of this issue has added extra weight to compliance—via the Health Insurance Portability and Accountability Act (HIPPA). These regulations were enacted to ensure compliance with high ethical standards of confidentiality, and define what healthcare providers must do to protect the confidentiality of client information and recordkeeping.

See Chapter 19, pages 264-266 for more information on **HIPAA regulations.**

Legal Issues: A practitioner must comply with all legal requirements whose aspects include: complying with local, state, and federal laws; maintaining appropriate insurance coverage; slander and libel; negotiating and complying with contracts; civil lawsuits; and employees. Sometimes a practitioner may feel confusion about what is legal and what seems the right thing to do. Practitioners may feel forced to find legal loopholes to justify their choices. These dilemmas require thoughtful choices.

§2

Insurance Issues: Insurance coverage for complementary healthcare treatments is an evolving issue. Careful attention and recordkeeping can maximize the benefits for both clients and practitioners. For instance, a client's eligibility for medical insurance reimbursement may be limited to "authorized treatment." According to standard insurance definitions, treatment is warranted until a condition is corrected or maximum improvement is made. By identifying guidelines for delineating treatment versus wellness care, you can ethically apply those standards to the insurance issue: who pays for care? However, there is often a fine line between the two, especially if the condition is chronic. Ethical decision-making can require careful thought and attention to treatment documentation.

See Chapter 19, pages 267-273 for details on **insurance reimbursement**.

Referrals: Thanking people for referrals seems straightforward, yet such a simple gesture can be easily misconstrued. The key is the nature of the business relationship. It can become an ethical issue when a person in a power differential relationship makes a recommendation to a client and the practitioner receives financial remuneration for the referral. Might the concept of a referral fee come to outweigh the client's need for the best possible objective referral? Accepting payment for referrals clouds that ability and puts the practitioner's ethics in a compromising position. In all cases, this creates a conflict of interest.

See Chapter 25, pages 388-393 for Information on **building professional alliances**.

Taxes: Taxation is a topic fraught with emotional charge. Many people resent the amount of money they pay in taxes (or how that money is spent) and use this anger to justify shady business practices. The two most common actions are concealing income (mainly cash payments and barter) and exaggerating expenses. An ethical practitioner keeps precise records, declares all income received, refrains from inflating expenses, and accurately files governmental reports.

See Chapter 20, pages 294-300 for details on **taxes**.

Resolving Ethical Dilemmas

An ethical dilemma occurs when two or more principles are in conflict and, regardless of your choice, something of value is compromised. At such times, you may find that you have several viable options, each with merit, and you aren't clear as to the most appropriate choice. You may also find yourself in a position whereby your values are in conflict. To resolve an ethical dilemma, follow this 6-part process.

1. **Identify the problem**. This is the point at which you would gather as much relevant information as possible to determine whether it's truly an ethical problem.
2. **Identify the potential issues involved**. List and describe the critical issues. Evaluate the rights, responsibilities, and welfare of those affected by the decision. Ascertain the potential dangers to the practitioner, client, and the profession.
3. **Review your profession's code of ethics and relevant laws**. Determine if this issue violates either the letter or the spirit of applicable laws, regulations, or professional codes. Check if your policies or procedures address this issue.

4. **Evaluate potential courses of action.** Brainstorm lots of ideas. Usually the first few options are based upon your personal values or an emotional response to the issue. Identify the benefits, drawbacks, and outcomes of various decisions. Identify your motivations and stake in the outcome. Consider the consequences of inaction and contemplate how you will feel about yourself when all is done.
5. **Obtain consultation.** Engage in self-reflection and consider how society and members of your community might view these actions. Determine the impact it could have on your profession and justify a course of action based on sound reasoning which you can test in a consultation with a colleague.
6. **Determine the best course of action.** Map out the best way to resolve the problem. Who should be contacted first if multiple parties are involved? Do you need outside support? Do you need to talk to a supervisor? Should anyone else know about the problem?

Figure 5.2 Steps to Resolve Ethical Dilemmas

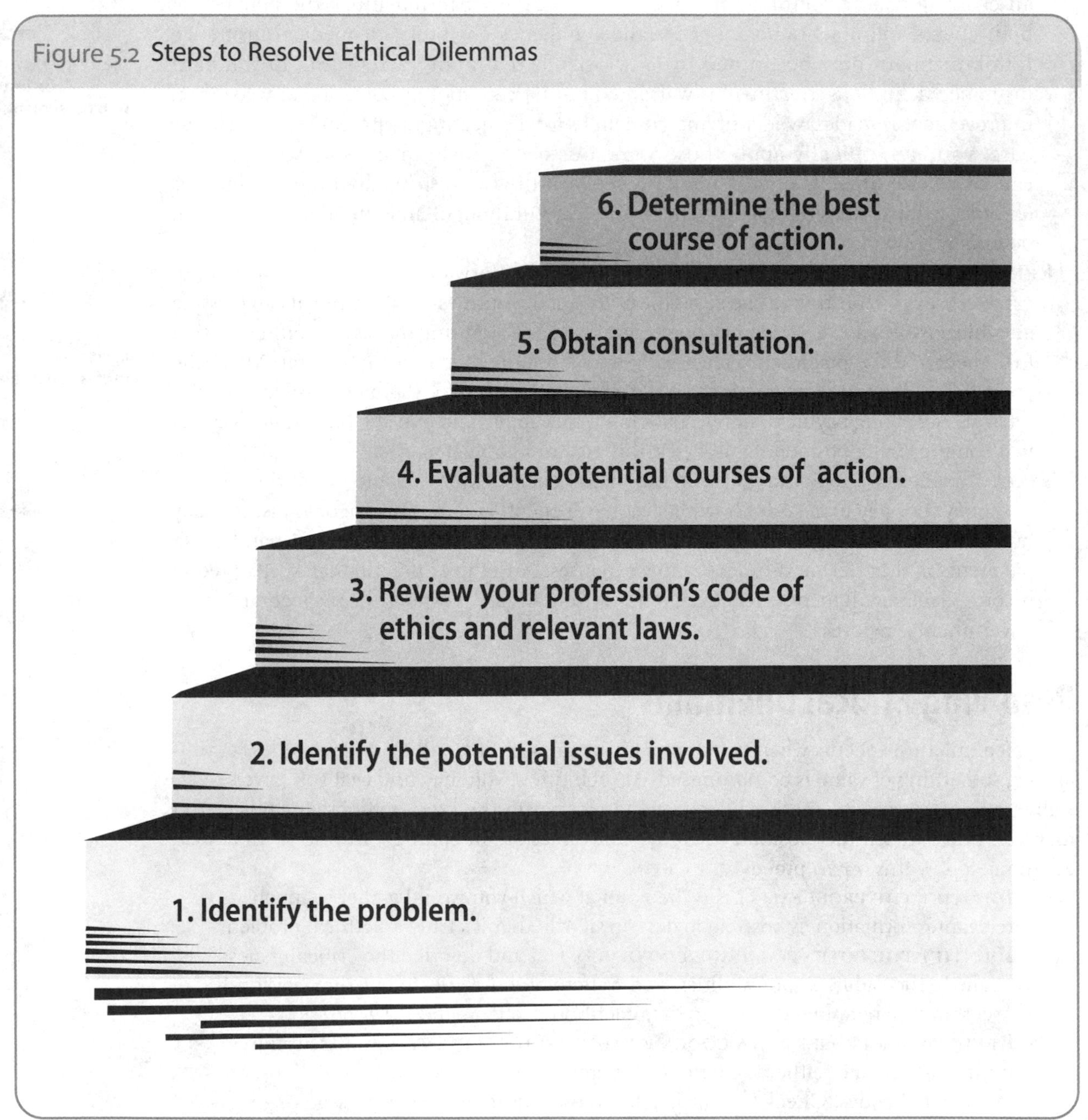
6. Determine the best course of action.
5. Obtain consultation.
4. Evaluate potential courses of action.
3. Review your profession's code of ethics and relevant laws.
2. Identify the potential issues involved.
1. Identify the problem.

Let's analyze a scenario using the 6-step resolution model:

On Monday your session with Sally was very intense. She was experiencing significant pain in her legs and lower back. During the session she also released a lot of emotions and briefly spoke about her personal issues. Sally's partner, Terry, shows up for his weekly treatment on Tuesday afternoon. He mentions that Sally was exhausted and a bit withdrawn after her session. He jokingly makes a comment about how powerful it must have been and asks you what happened.

1. **Identify the problem**: This is a common occurrence when working with clients who know each other. They often ask how the other person is doing or how the session went. This is usually done out of genuine concern and not a need for gossip. Yet even just saying, "Oh, it was a good session" is inappropriate and may feel awkward. You determine this is an ethical problem.
2. **Identify the potential issues involved.** By telling Terry about Sally's session, you would be committing a breach of confidentiality. Yet you believe that it would be helpful to Sally if Terry was aware of what occurred. The potential hazards of sharing this information with Terry are: Sally may become upset with you and decide not to return; you may lose your credibility with both Terry and Sally; this action could interfere with Sally's healing process; and you may lose potential clients due to the bad-will generated by this incident.
3. **Review your profession's code of ethics and relevant laws.** While you're unable to find any legal specifications, your professional Code of Ethics states that you must maintain client confidentiality.
4. **Evaluate potential courses of action.** You have several options. First you need to decide what to say to Terry. You can shrug your shoulders and say, "Well, I guess it was rather intense," and then continue your session. Or you can say, "I highly value my commitment to client confidentiality. It would be best if you ask Sally directly about her session." You determine if you should pursue this any further at all (remind Terry to talk to Sally, or recommend to Sally that she talk with Terry), depending upon how Terry responded to your reply about the session and your sense of the benefits resulting from Sally sharing the information with Terry.
5. **Obtain consultation.** You talk with several colleagues and get a mixed response. Some think that it isn't really a problem since the clients are partners. Other colleagues are adamant about it being a breach of confidentiality.
6. **Determine the best course of action.** You decide not to breach confidentiality by disclosing nothing about Sally's session. You choose to restate your confidentiality policy to both Terry and Sally and encourage them to share their experiences with each other.

Points to Ponder

What if you responded to Terry with something like, "Yes, it was a great session," and then you realized afterward that you had indeed broken confidentiality? What are some options for rectifying that situation?

The challenge is that many times we are faced with these types of dilemmas and we don't have the luxury of walking away and choosing a best course of action. For illustration purposes, we worked through all 6 steps in the previous scenario, yet if this happened in real life, the practitioner would have needed to choose a response immediately. Prepare yourself in advance so that you know where you stand and you can gracefully address dilemmas when they arise.

Develop Ethical Dilemma Responses

Make a list of potential ethical dilemmas that would require an immediate response. Use the Six Step Resolution Process to develop a plan of action on how you will handle each one. Script your potential responses and practice them until you feel comfortable and confident. Understand that the "human factor" will come into play, so they may not go exactly as you have planned.

BMW

See the ***Business Mastery Workbook*** for an expanded activity.

https://sohnen-moe.com/bm5-workbook-request/

Codes of Ethics

Codes of ethics are conduct guidelines and are often created to address issues that don't exist as specific laws. While individuals may have developed their own personal codes of ethics, codes that relate to business practices are most commonly set by professional organizations. These codes serve to do the following:

- Inform practitioners of appropriate ethical norms and behavior.
- Supply direction for challenging situations.
- Encourage practitioners to provide excellent service.
- Protect clients.
- Provide a means for enforcing desired professional behavior.

Most codes of ethics are broad and vague, partly due to the contextual nature of "right" and "wrong." Research, consultation, and self-exploration are usually required to determine what is appropriate and ethical. Among the components of most wellness providers' codes of ethics are: a statement of basic concerns (e.g., honesty, integrity, respect, compassion, making a difference); standards of service; a description of how the treatment or session is delivered (condition, place); when the treatments are given and by whom; the quality of materials used; and service guarantees.

Ideally, the wellness community would develop a general code of ethics that all wellness professionals endorse with provisos for specific fields. Such a document would serve as a tool to educate the public about the basic conduct and level of professionalism they can expect from any wellness provider. Once this code of ethics is adopted, we also face other exciting challenges, such as: deciding how to implement it; determining the consequences of breaches; resolving the manner of enforcement; and educating the public. This calls for much introspection and dialogue within the wellness community (see Figure 5.3).

Code of Ethics vs. Values

Find the Code of Ethics for your profession. Go back to your values list from Chapter 1 and compare and contrast the two. Are there specifications in the Code of Ethics that don't match your values? If so, how might you adjust your values to match more closely with the code? What would you do if there was a major conflict between your values and the Code of Ethics?

Figure 5.3 Sample Code of Ethics

We, as wellness providers, have the responsibility to guide our actions to serve the best interests of the client. As members of a wellness profession, we realize this responsibility can only be upheld by maintaining the highest degree of personal and professional integrity. We make the commitment to provide personalized care and knowledgeable techniques, in a clean, comfortable atmosphere, thereby ensuring the client's safety and wellbeing.

Therefore, I agree to do the following:

1. Maintain a professional appearance and demeanor by keeping good hygiene and wearing attire that is appropriate for the client setting.
2. Respect all clients regardless of their age, gender, race, national origin, sexual orientation, religion, socioeconomic status, body type, political affiliation, state of health, and personal habits.
3. Demonstrate respect by honoring a client's process, being present, listening, asking only pertinent questions, keeping my agreements, being on time, draping properly, and maintaining professionalism.
4. Maintain confidentiality of information concerning clients, and refrain from discussing client care details except under appropriate circumstances or as required by law.
5. Provide a safe, comfortable, clean environment that is stocked with quality equipment and supplies.
6. Perform only those services for which I'm qualified and (physically and emotionally) capable, and refer to appropriate specialists when work is not within my scope of practice or not in the client's best interest.
7. Be honest in all marketing endeavors.
8. Customize my treatments to meet the client's needs.
9. Charge a fair price for my services and offer a sliding scale when appropriate.
10. Keep accurate records and review charts before each session.
11. Educate clients by providing them with feedback and resources.
12. Make return and follow-up calls when appropriate and in a timely manner.
13. Post my credentials and policies.
14. Undergo peer review bi-annually.
15. Never engage in any sexual activity with clients.
16. Refrain from the use of any mind-altering substances before or during sessions.
17. Stay current with information and techniques by reading, receiving wellness treatments regularly, and taking at least 1 workshop per year.
18. Continue membership in at least 1 professional association.
19. Adhere to city, county, state, national, and international requirements.
20. Educate the public about my services and benefits through activities such as: giving presentations, workshops, and demonstrations; holding open houses; and writing articles.

Professionalism

Professionalism stems from your attitudes and is manifested through the image you portray, your technical skill level, your communication abilities, and your business practices. The term professionalism also relates to ethical behavior. High standards of action with clients result in both ethical and professional behavior.

No matter how many hours you work, this is your profession. There is a major distinction between part time and spare time. You may have other facets to your career besides being a wellness practitioner, but you must be clear about the roles each facet plays and be committed to excellence in each one. Quantity does not equate to quality. You're a wellness professional, and you're a business person—even if you only work 3 hours a week. The more you treat your practice as a business, the more professional you appear and the more successful you become. Sometimes this can be difficult, particularly if you don't have a modicum of technical business experience. Your attitudes toward yourself and your business are communicated directly and indirectly to your clients, colleagues, and potential clients. You need to respect yourself and your abilities.

Professionalism isn't measured by how many clients you see or how much money you earn but rather by who you are, your attitudes, and how you treat others. The basis for true professionalism lies in integrity. *Webster's Dictionary* defines integrity as "the quality or state of being complete; unbroken condition; wholeness; honesty; and sincerity."[3] Someone may talk, walk, and appear the part, but if that person doesn't come from a base of integrity, the facade wears thin quickly. If you don't treat your clients with the utmost respect, you won't have many clients. Integrity is often considered an important thing to have—people have integrity if they're ethical, can keep confidences, and keep their word. But there is more to it than that.

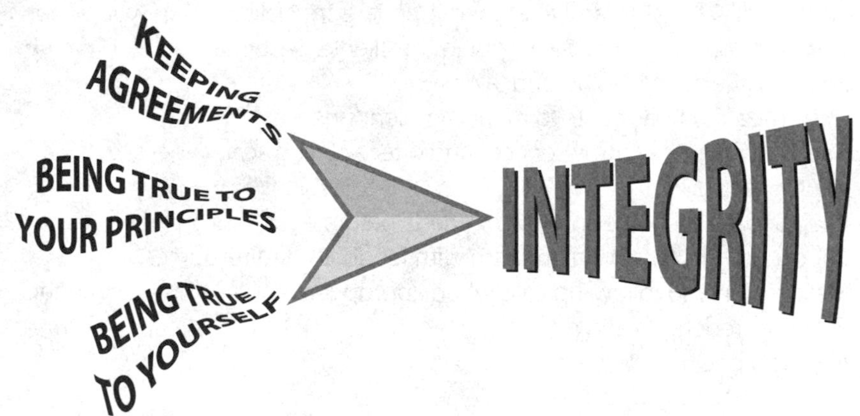

Integrity can be divided into three major levels: the first level is keeping your agreements; the second is being true to your principles; and the third level is being true to yourself. It's rare to find practitioners who put on an air of professionalism without the integrity behind it. More often, they love what they do and are genuinely concerned about the wellbeing of their clients. Nevertheless, some neglect to develop a professional demeanor.

Professional Affiliations

Professional Associations Directory

sohnen-moe.com/resources/professional.php

Professional affiliations are an important part of the business world and the development of a professional image, in addition to the educational, social, and networking benefits. Join at least 2 organizations: 1 that specifically relates to your profession and 1 that supports your visibility in your community.

Numerous associations exist for wellness professions, ranging from modality-specific associations to more general health and wellbeing organizations. An excellent source for these groups is the *Encyclopedia of Associations* (at your library or at www.gale.cengage.com). Look under the "Health and Medical" section for thousands of listings of specialized, auxiliary, and local branches of associations. You can also find online links to many associations.Membership in a professional association makes a statement of your commitment to your career field.

Involvement in business organizations also demonstrates belief in yourself as a professional. Many groups exist on a national level. Locate them by referring to the "Business" section of the *Encyclopedia of Associations*. Locally, groups, such as the Chamber of Commerce and business support groups, can be found by talking with other business owners, researching online, and checking local calendars of events.

Professional Credentials

Credentials establish professionalism to the public. The four regulatory methods of credentials are known as Licensure, Certification, Registration, and Title Protection. Each method has its particular requirements and provisions.

Licensure: requires practitioners to obtain a license to perform their services; unlicensed persons who practice break the law. This form of regulation is the most restrictive and provides the greatest level of public protection. Some municipalities require a business or occupational license in addition to your license to practice your trade. Legal names and professional titles cited in the law are numerous and varied. License titles are not necessarily the same as professional certification titles.

Certification: from a governmental view is a voluntary option which offers the use of vocational titles to distinguish professional services from adult entertainment. Other certification documents that you can post show that you have passed specific professional tests, such as those from the National Certification Board for Therapeutic Massage and Bodywork (NCBTMB) or The National Certification Commission for Acupuncture and Oriental Medicine (NCCAOM).

Registration: is the means by which a government agency keeps track of practitioners by informational recordkeeping. In Canada and some states in the United States, practitioners must be registered to legally use their professional title.

Title Protection: does not require practitioners to register or notify the state. Anyone may engage in the particular practice, but only those who satisfy the prescribed requirements may use the specific title.

Professional Associations

Massage
www.amtamassage.org
www.abmp.com
www.crmta.ca

Acupuncture
www.aaaomonline.org

Asian Bodywork
www.aobta.org

Chiropractic
www.acatoday.org

Yoga
www.yogaalliance.org

Fitness
www.ideafit.com
www.netafit.org
www.aapte.org

Image

The image you portray influences how people react to you. Your public image is determined by the way you present yourself, your office, your business practices, and the manner in which you treat your clients. How you look, act, and treat people influences if they will become your clients and how regularly they will return. Your level of integrity, professionalism, and style determine how you are perceived. Taking the time to project a professional image is always worth the investment. It isn't necessary to have a huge budget either—just creativity.

I'm not advocating being someone other than yourself; I'm suggesting you take the time to make certain your "outward" image supports your vision of success. The next sections provide guidelines to bolster your image and reputation. Most of the guidelines don't involve any financial outlay. The desired result is that your image is professional, and it's vital that you don't lose yourself in this process. Who you are is what makes you good at what you do. It distinguishes you from the others. Keep your style and personality intact.

Exude Confidence, Competence, and Compassion

- Dress stylishly yet neatly, and keep jewelry to a minimum: your attire isn't meant to be a distraction.
- Keep good personal hygiene. Don't wear heavy perfume or cologne due to chemical sensitivities. Make certain that your clothes, person, equipment, and linens are free from the smell of smoke if you are a smoker.
- Keep your technical skills excellent and current: don't pretend to be an expert where you're not.
- Be punctual and prepared: make your clients feel important and respected.
- Know how to introduce yourself and others: it can be very embarrassing if you stumble over your own tongue.
- Get involved in your community: become active in civic, social, and political groups.

Generate a Comfortable, Professional Ambiance

- Be aware of the noise level and make any necessary adjustments: mute the phone and soundproof thin walls.
- Keep the interior clean, particularly the bathroom.
- Make sure that the building and address is visible from the street: this may mean investing in signage.
- Maintain the area outside your office: this may include landscaping.
- Keep the temperature comfortable for the client: if you don't have easy access to the temperature control, put a portable heater and fan in the room.
- Create a sense of privacy: you may have to be very inventive.
- Make certain that all equipment and furniture is comfortable and sturdy: you don't want a table to squeak and groan with every movement or to collapse under a client!
- Provide closet space or a shelf (at the very least, a hook) for your clients' belongings: most people don't like to throw their possessions in a corner.
- Keep supplies stocked and handy: you don't want your clients searching for a tissue while they're sneezing.
- Post your business license, policies, certifications, association memberships, continuing education certificates, and awards in a conspicuous place: these items represent the time and effort you've invested in your career.
- Have your business cards and literature available: make it easy for your clients to take what they need to help promote your business.

Treat Clients with Respect

- Be empathetic and understanding: keep in mind that not everyone shares your particular beliefs about health, wellbeing, religion, or politics.
- Greet your clients appropriately: some people may not be up to a hug, while others may welcome it.
- Keep what happens during a session confidential: this can be tricky when your clients know each other and ask about the other's appointment. Be noncommittal and recommend they speak to the person directly. Even a casual remark can damage your trust factor.
- Remember that you're here to serve your clients: it isn't their job to counsel you during their sessions.
- Observe your clients' likes and dislikes: make the effort to do those "extra little things."
- Answer your phone professionally: you don't have to be overly formal, but remember you're a business. If you don't have a receptionist, consider hiring a reliable appointment service or offer online scheduling. They can significantly increase your bookings.

- Return calls within 24 hours: you never know the influence and connections that a potential client may have; promptness is always appreciated.
- Answer emails as you would phone calls, within 24 hours. Even if it's a nonessential matter, respond with a "thank you for your email" type of response and information on when they can expect to hear from you next.
- Answer important mail within 4 days and nonessential mail within 2 weeks: don't wait until you have the time to write a brilliant letter. Keep a supply of postcards handy. This way you can quickly acknowledge correspondence without worrying about having to fill up the page.
- Send newspaper clippings, articles, and items of interest to clients and colleagues: this lets people know that you're thinking about them and are genuinely concerned.
- Acknowledge in writing any item or gift sent to you: thanking people over the phone is okay, but people usually keep cards for several days. Every time they look at your card, it reinforces their feelings of goodwill.
- Send thank-you notes for referrals: it's vital to show your appreciation. Thank-you notes are good for building goodwill and expressing sincere appreciation for your client's confidence in you.
- Use caution with social media. Only post appropriate content and photos. Respond to clients messages promptly.
- Set clear boundaries: don't let your personal life interfere with business.
- Return borrowed property promptly and in good condition: never borrow anything that you cannot replace should you damage or lose it.
- Never repeat a rumor that could hurt someone's reputation: it's wise to stay neutral. Gossip never reflects well on any of the parties.
- Keep accurate client files: review them before you see each client. Don't rely on your memory for all the details of your last session.

§2

See Chapter 27, pages 438-443 for details on **social media**.

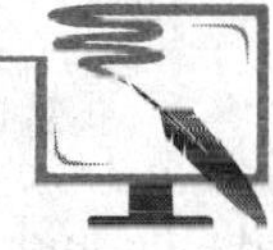

Clarify Professionalism

Characteristics of a Professional

Think about someone you regard as being very professional and answer these questions:

- What is this person's occupation?
- What is this person's philosophy of life?
- How does this person feel about her/his career?
- What does this person look like?
- Where is this person's place of business? What does the business look like from the outside? Can you easily see the office from the street? Is parking easily accessible? What does the office look like?
- How does this person greet you?
- What does this person say and do?
- How do you feel when you're with this person?

Personal Inventory

- Describe yourself in terms of professionalism.
- Describe how you imagine others see you in terms of professionalism.
- List any changes you would like to make to demonstrate your professionalism.

Enhance Your Professionalism

- How closely does the personal description from your inventory match the professional's characteristics you described above?
- What additional actions do you want to take to enhance your professionalism?

Goodwill

> You cannot do a kindness too soon, for you will never know how soon it will be too late.
> —Ralph Waldo Emerson

Goodwill is an integral component for success in any service industry, and especially so in the wellness field. Goodwill is benevolence, friendly disposition, cheerful consent, willingness, and readiness. In the business world, goodwill is the commercial advantage of any professional practice due to its established popularity, reputation, patronage, advertising, and location, over and above its tangible assets. In other words, goodwill is an abstract impression, the "positive feelings" you inspire in others. It's based upon the supposition that you're doing the best you can and are fair and ethical in your dealings and behavior. It implies warmth, congeniality, and trust.

Take a moment to think about the businesses and people that you respect. Why do you hold them in such regard? What have they done to encourage these feelings of goodwill? How have they demonstrated their concern? Your responses are the key to understanding the concept of goodwill. It's essential to cultivate alliances.

> A candle loses nothing of its light by lighting another candle.
> — James Keller

In his book, *Give and Take: A Revolutionary Approach to Success*, researcher Adam Grant explores the roles (of what he terms *giver, matcher,* and *taker*) preferences play in success. As you can guess, his research revealed that givers end up at the bottom of the success ladder. If that's true, then why the emphasis on cultivating goodwill? Well, because as Grant's research also revealed, givers also end up at the top (while "takers and matchers are more likely to land in the middle"). There are the selfless givers that we usually think of, who tend to get walked on in their various interactions and eventually burn out. But there are also "otherish" givers, those who care about the interests of others, but also focus on their own interests. Grant says that this type of giver "reverses the popular plan of succeeding first and giving back later, raising the possibility that those who give first are often best positioned for success later."[4] This plan illustrates how the largest benefit of your professionalism just may be goodwill.

Public Recognition

Many branches of the wellness field (particularly "alternative" ones) have substantial distances to cover before they achieve the recognition they deserve from the general public and the health industry. A major part of this guarded acceptance stems from a lack of standardization. The general public doesn't know what to expect. The variety of educational levels, styles, modalities, philosophies, and fee structures are as diverse as those who practice them.

> You can't build a reputation on what you are going to do.
> — Henry Ford

To gain further headway for recognition, it's imperative to enhance the public image of your specific industry—that is, promote more goodwill.

The wellness field tends to rely on attraction (e.g., word-of-mouth, reputation, client referrals) rather than traditional methods of promotion. The downside is that word-of-mouth often revolves around "who" you know more than "what" you know. And, even then, it isn't enough to just know the "right" people. You need to nurture those associations to obtain their support. You must have good people skills. For example, you could be the most brilliant practitioner in your area, yet if you don't promote goodwill with your clients, centers of influence, colleagues, and the community, you still may not do well financially. One of the most essential habits to develop is prompt and gracious acknowledgment of all of the people who support you. A little recognition goes a long way!

It takes time, thought, creativity, and some money to foster goodwill. Being good at what you do is only one aspect of it. Make certain that your actions reflect that you're proud of your profession and are sincerely concerned about people's wellbeing.

You can't buy goodwill, particularly if it's an attempt to repair a bad reputation (although corporations spend millions of dollars attempting to do just that). You can bolster the general public's opinion of you and your profession by donating your services and knowledge to charitable organizations and events—especially if you get media coverage.

Finding out the "whys and hows" of community involvement and goodwill helps you to choose activities for your own business involvement, discover organizations that align with your mission and values, and decide which events to support.

New Traditions in Business
— edited by John Renesch

§2

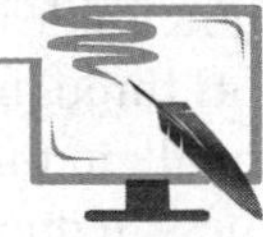

Generating Goodwill

Think of a professional or a business that elicits warmth, congeniality, and trust. What do they do in your community that generates these feelings of goodwill? Contact this person or business and ask them the following questions:

1. How long have you been in business?
2. How long has your business been giving back to the community?
3. Why do you participate in community events and activities?
4. How does your community involvement support your business activities?

Social Responsibility

Social responsibility is twofold. It holds that a business has a responsibility to refrain from unethical behavior that may bring harm to the community, its people, or the environment. It also recognizes that a business has a responsibility to give back to society to help solve social problems through means such as grants, in-kind donations, community outreach, and employee volunteer programs.

In short, socially responsible companies operate in environmentally friendly ways, invest in the communities they serve, and focus on ways to improve working conditions for employees. A growing number of companies recognize that social responsibility isn't just good business or a public relations gimmick—it's simply the right thing to do.

The goodwill and heightened visibility generated by being a socially responsible business can greatly impact your success.

As an individual and business owner, you can make a difference socially, economically, environmentally, and politically. Running your practice from a place of compassion, integrity, and personal values creates a sense of empowerment and fulfillment. Many businesses are learning how to be profitable and heed their social missions. As the concept of "quality of life" evolves, time and freedom become the dominant concerns (although financial security is clearly important). In addition, companies are becoming more ecologically aware, reducing the number of consumables, choosing "environment-friendly" products, and instituting recycling programs.

As growing numbers of small and large businesses incorporate values that reflect social responsibility into their everyday practices, political pressure comes to bear upon governments to create policies and laws along the same lines. As a result of the changes in business philosophy, new operating procedures are often developed. Purchasing products and services is no longer based only on price and quality. Companies that embrace the philosophy of social responsibility often offer discounts to businesses that belong to like-minded political, professional, social, or networking organizations.

Many companies demonstrate the feasibility of being financially successful while doing good in the community, treating their employees well, and providing excellent customer service. In addition, company support of volunteerism and tithing is on the rise. Many individuals and companies are donating their time, money, and expertise to their favorite charities. Also, groups of individuals are joining together to form organizations expressly committed to responding to emergency conditions.

Profiles

Good360
good360.org

Good360 (formerly Gifts In Kind International) is a wonderful example of social responsibility at work. Driven by a mission of providing an effective conduit for the donation of products and services from the private sector to the charitable sector, Good360 is a leader in product philanthropy. It provides valuable resources to thousands of nonprofits through its network of corporate and association partners. Large corporations, as well as small and mid-sized companies, benefit by supporting the communities where they do business, reducing inventory and warehousing expenses, and qualifying for a tax deduction. Forbes magazine consistently ranks Good360 as one of the top 10 most efficient charities.

Ben & Jerry's
benandjerrysfoundation.org

Ben & Jerry's premium ice cream and frozen yogurt manufacturing company believes in what they call "Caring Capitalism": a business that makes top-quality, all-natural products; is a force for social change; and is financially successful. Co-founder Ben Cohen once said, "Business has a responsibility to give back to the community." Thus, the company's social mission is to improve the quality of life of a broad community—local, national, and international. Ben & Jerry's product donations support the work of a wide range of nonprofit organizations across the country and the company sponsors a variety of community service projects and individual volunteer efforts. In addition, some of the company's profits go directly to the Ben & Jerry's Foundation, which makes grants to grassroots organizations around the country that address social and environmental problems.

TOMS: One for One
www.toms.com

TOMS Shoes is a recent example of what is referred to as social enterprise. TOMS is in business to help improve people's lives, they just happen to do it with shoes. TOMS promises "with every product you purchase, TOMS will help a person in need. One for One.®" TOMS started with shoes, providing a free pair of shoes for every pair sold. They now sell eyewear and coffee, helping to provide sight and fresh water to people in need, and other products that support their mission.

Team Children
www.teamchildren.com

Team Children is a prime example of how great movements spring from small individual actions. Robert Toporek, a Rolfing practitioner in Philadelphia, had a mission to make a positive impact on the children who live in the "Badlands," one of the worst neighborhoods in Philadelphia. In 1993, he founded a children's project now known as Team Children. Every summer since then, he recruits volunteers to go to these neighborhoods weekly to offer Rolfing structural integration, massage, music, books, and computers. Since that time, he has collected, repaired, and distributed more than 11,000 computers. Toporek has discovered that this is another way to relieve stress in these economically challenged families.

A unique community effort created a **Massage Emergency Response Team** in California after the Loma Prieta earthquake struck in October 1989. People at the National Holistic Institute (NHI) masterminded the logistics and got involved to help heal the community—8,000 massages were given by 300 massage therapists. It has evolved since then to become the AMTA Massage Emergency Response Team AMTA-MERT), now organized by individual state chapters. There are eligibility requirements to join—although being a member of the American Massage Therapy Association is not mandatory—and members all receive standardized training in providing massage at an emergency response scene.

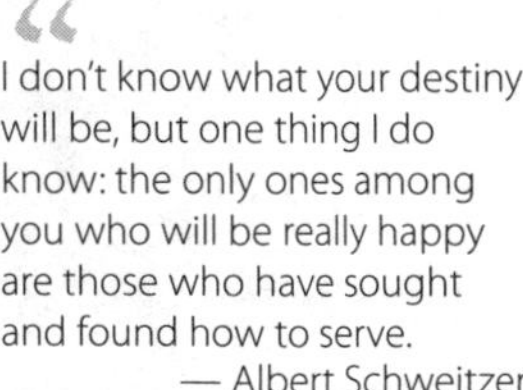

> I don't know what your destiny will be, but one thing I do know: the only ones among you who will be really happy are those who have sought and found how to serve.
> — Albert Schweitzer

Steps You Can Take Now

The five major ways to make a difference are to act responsibly, volunteer, fund projects, use your purchasing power, and be respectful.

Act Responsibly

Acting responsibly requires that you be aware of your environment. In addition to embracing the slogan, "Reduce, Reuse, Recycle, and buy Recycled," become knowledgeable about the world and expand your horizons: read your industry trade journals, national magazines, and community publications, to stay up on events where you can make a difference. In your waiting room, post brochures, flyers, and announcements on these events and ways your clients can make a difference too.

Be an advocate: vote; write letters and place phone calls to politicians about issues that concern you; join a progressive campaigning group like Friends of the Earth or Amnesty International.

You aren't limited to contributing your specific vocational services. You can stuff envelopes, organize events, and even build homes.

Volunteer

Donate your time and expertise to your favorite charities: join an industry group such as the AMTA-MERT or Acupuncturists Without Borders; do community service work with organizations such as Habitat for Humanity or the Literacy Foundation; donate blood; be a mentor for a child; pick a population of people who can't afford your services and "adopt" them; form a local community group; volunteer to walk a dog at your local animal shelter (there's often not enough staff to take animals for walks and you get to be a virtual pet owner—no muss, no fuss); give presentations in public schools (e.g., career day, health education week); take part in special events such as Make A Difference Day; and sponsor an activity such as "Adopt a Highway."

§2

Volunteer

www.foe.org
www.amnesty.org
www.amtamassage.org
www.acuwithoutborders.org
www.handsforheroes.net
www.integrativetouch.org
www.hearttouch.org

Fund Projects

In addition to donating money to worthwhile causes, you can grant scholarships and help coordinate fundraising activities. You can donate your services as prizes or raise money by sponsoring an event such as a "massage-a-thon." You can designate a charity and donate a day's revenues or run a promotion such as for every specified dollar amount (e.g., \$50) that a client donates to your favorite charity, he gets a free treatment (such as a half-hour session or an adjunct service).

One of the most common ways to fund causes is through tithing. Tithing is contributing a set amount (usually 10%) of time or money to charitable causes. This is a convenient and effective way to give back to your community. People often associate tithing with religion, but that's only one option. Some popular forms of tithing include donating a specific amount of profits to an organization, doing pro bono work (providing services free of charge), and offering a sliding fee scale.

Random Acts of Kindness by Conari Press

Figure 5.5 Make A Difference Day

This annual day of doing good was created by USA WEEKEND in partnership with the Points of Light Foundation. It was started more than 20 years ago. Held on the fourth Saturday in October, Make A Difference Day is the largest annual national day of helping others. Projects can be personal (e.g., helping an elderly relative with their chores), neighborly (e.g., organizing a neighborhood beautification day), or major productions such as refurbishing a children's recreational center.

Join in with millions of volunteers as they contribute to millions of others. The organizers request that if you currently volunteer regularly, make an extra effort in your volunteer activity. If you need more than 1 day for your project, still do a significant part of your volunteering on the fourth Saturday. If you can't participate on Saturday for religious reasons, do your project Friday or Sunday. Contact the organizers so they can include your volunteer activities as part of the DAYtaBANK. www.makeadifferenceday.com

"When strangers start acting like neighbors, communities are reinvigorated.
— Ralph Nader

> “The greatest pleasure I know is to do a good action by stealth, and to have it found out by accident.
> —Charles Lamb

Use Your Purchasing Power

Let your voice be heard through your acquisitions. Purchase ecologically sound products (e.g., natural fiber linens), use environmentally friendly detergent for linens and clothes, and print your promotional materials on recycled stock. Invest wisely. Actively support businesses that are aligned with your values and boycott companies that oppose them.

Be Respectful

Respect is the foundation of a socially responsible business: respecting yourself, the environment, and your clients. Caregivers enter this field because they want to be of service. In her article, "The Value of Sharing Your Values," Michelle Blake tells us, "I tended to think my professional and volunteer work inhabited separate universes. In truth, by keeping them sequestered, I was missing opportunities to deepen my client relationships." Sharing values with clients "can benefit both clients and practitioners in profound and unexpected ways."[5] Clients are looking for practitioners with whom they share similar values. Be true to your beliefs, and express them in ways that respect differing viewpoints. While it isn't appropriate to foist your beliefs on your clients, you can encourage them to explore alternatives. Better yet, make sure your marketing attracts clients with similar beliefs. Not only do people like to participate in meaningful ways, they are often discerning about where they spend their money. They are much more likely to choose those businesses with shared values.

Identify Companies You Love

Make a list of companies that you love and utilize your purchasing power to support. Beside each company, list the reasons why you feel good about shopping with them. Note how many of them support your political and/or social views, and how many of them are on the list "just because." Conduct research to find companies that align with your values to replace the "just because" businesses.

6

Therapeutic Communications

"The single biggest problem with communication is the illusion that it has taken place."

—George Bernard Shaw

Communication Fundamentals
- First Impressions
- Building Rapport
- Keys to Excellent Communication

Listening Skills
- Active Listening
- Reflective Feedback
- Body Language

Communication Barriers
- Upset Clients and Difficult Situations
- Emotional Triggers

Documenting Client Sessions
- Client Forms

Client Interviews
- Timing
- Artful Phrasing
- Interview Stages
- Client Compliance
- Client Education
- Hone Your Interviewing Skills

The Client Technology Connection
- Machines vs. Humans
- Phone Etiquette
- Email and Text Etiquette
- Screening Clients

Declining and Dismissing Clients
- Declining a Potential New Client
- Dismissing a Current Client

Key Terms

Active Listening
Body Language
Client Compliance
Client Education
Client Interview
Closed-ended Questions
Closure Stage
Communication
Contraindications
Countertransference
Demeanor
Dissonance
Documentation
Empathy
Etiquette
Exploration Stage
Exit Interview
Feedback
HIPAA
Indications
Informed Consent
Initiation Stage
Insurance Reimbursement
Intake Form
Intake Interview
Listening
Malpractice
Malpractice Insurance
Noise
Non-verbal Cues
Open-ended Question
Planning Stage
Policy
Presence
Protocol
Rapport
Recordkeeping
Referral
Reflective Feedback
SOAP Charting
Therapeutic Relationship
Transference
Trauma
Treatment Plan
Trigger
Wellness Notes

Good communication is the foundation of healthy relationships and thriving practices. In fact, one of the common threads of highly successful practitioners is effective communication skills. Advanced technical skills and business savvy are simply not enough. Without good communication skills, the growth of your business is likely to lag.

Taking the time and effort to enhance your communication skills will serve you well. Like any skill, achieving a degree of mastery takes practice—and in this case, a willingness to take a fresh look at your communication style and behaviors.

Communication Fundamentals

> "Seek first to understand, then to be understood.
> —Steven Covey

Communication skills are also known as "people skills," because, at its best, communicating involves connecting with people in positive and productive ways. This is done through speaking, writing, vocal tone, and body language. As you enhance your skills in this area, you can expect to increase productivity, reduce stress, and improve teamwork. You can also build stronger client relationships and minimize the potential for misunderstandings with colleagues, co-workers, and clients. However, the greatest benefit manifests in clients who feel at ease and experience high levels of satisfaction with your work.

Good communication is a two-way process that involves an exchange of ideas, emotions, and attitudes. The ultimate goal of communication is to elicit some type of action. The communication skills necessary in effective therapeutic relationships are the ability to establish rapport, listen to answers, utilize communication technology, be patient, make astute observations, elicit information, ask open-ended questions, gain cooperation, conduct excellent interviews, ask for input, assert boundaries, use active listening techniques, and show genuine concern.

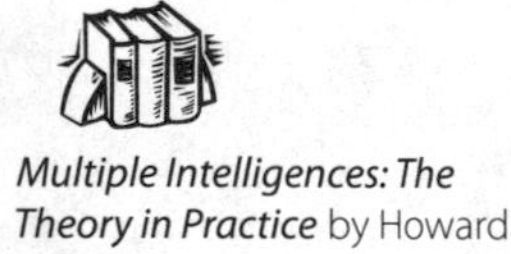

Multiple Intelligences: The Theory in Practice by Howard Gardner

Understanding people and personality types is a good start to developing good communication skills. You can improve your everyday interactions by leaps and bounds by developing an awareness of how different personality types view the world and the preferred communication style of each. Sometimes effective communication requires you to adjust your communication style, and it can feel a bit unnatural at first. But, with basic knowledge and steady practice, you can quickly gain proficiency.

First Impressions

First impressions are powerful—and often irreversible. Your first interaction with a person sets the tone for future communication. Did you know that you have between 4 and 20 seconds to make that vital first impression?[1, 2] The elements of a first impression include characteristics such as your appearance, facial expressions, body language, what you say, what's not said, your ability to gain rapport, your energy level, and the actual message. A vast amount of information is exchanged, and many judgments are formed at lightning speed.

Personality Inventories

www.nlp.com

www.surfaquarium.com/MI/inventory.htm

www.personalityexplorer.com

www.nipreston.com/publications/excerpts/personalitytypes.pdf

Sometimes practitioners unknowingly alienate new and potential clients because they don't present themselves positively and professionally. To avoid this potential pitfall, take some time to think about how you present yourself and your work in that vital first meeting. When you're thoroughly prepared and aren't worrying about how to introduce yourself and what to say, it's easier to focus on being with your clients and listening fully to them.

Avoid prejudging yourself or your clients, as this prejudice can substantially alter your first impression. Focus on building rapport and keeping an open mind. Your confidence in yourself and your abilities increases the comfort your clients experience.

Building Rapport

Rapport is the bond that develops between you and clients; it's based on mutual trust and accord. After you've made a good first impression, rapport can be the single most important factor in whether a client sees you once or becomes a long-term client. Rapport develops by being open and demonstrating genuine concern. Some techniques for developing rapport are to correctly pronounce clients' names, use clients' names frequently, smile, shake hands, maintain good eye contact, allow ample time for clients to talk, speak with enthusiasm and conviction, be punctual, listen, and ask a light, personal question about the client's family, hobby, or job. You demonstrate care and concern by using language that validates your clients' thoughts, feelings, and experiences, and by maintaining confidentiality. You demonstrate respect by not offering unsolicited advice and acting like you know what's better for clients than they do. Most of all, you build rapport and encourage returning visits by not shaming your clients with judgmental comments on how they take care of themselves.

See Chapter 25, pages 386-397 for details on developing a **self-introduction**.

§2

Figure 6.1 Tips on How NOT to Create Rapport

- Arrive late.
- Use invalidating language.
- Don't give the client your full attention.
- Eat or chew gum.
- Avoid eye contact.
- Talk about yourself a lot.
- Gossip.
- Be messy.
- Disregard ambient noise.
- Shame clients into coming back.
- Give unsolicited advice.
- Act like you know what's best.
- Be judgmental.

"You can handle people more successfully by enlisting their feelings than by convincing their reason.
—Paul P. Parker

It All Begins with You

An excellent strategy for building rapport as well as enhancing understanding and impact is to begin as many sentences as possible with the word "you." This technique is also referred to as an embedded command. When you say "you," people pay attention because what you say relates to them. Incorporate expressions such as: "You are," "you have," "you will notice," "you will discover," "you will find," "you will receive," "you will experience," "you will see," "you will smell," "you will touch," and "you will feel." It's also very effective to use the client's first name in place of "you," when appropriate. If you say a client's name too often, it may seem forced or ingenuine. So, be selective, and when appropriate, personalize the statement.

Keys to Excellent Communication

The principle concept to remember about communication is that people act and react to fulfill needs. When you better understand their needs, you can create a better strategy for improving communication. Start by taking into consideration the person's natural tendencies and capacities. For example, if someone prefers to see things in writing, don't expect him to be very responsive to verbal communication, without also giving him something to read. If you're talking to someone who doesn't speak English well, avoid using polysyllabic words, rapid speech, and colloquialisms. Also, be considerate of the other person's mental, physical, and emotional state, particularly if he is under a lot of stress. Attempt to communicate on an equal level; don't act superior or inferior. And pay attention to your emotions. It's difficult to have clear communication when you're coming from a reactionary position, so focus on the facts.

Enhance Communication
www.cnvc.org
www.savicommunications.com
www.healingfromthecore.com

Be aware of how much the other person knows about you. If someone fully respects your expertise, it isn't necessary to take the time to build up your credibility. If she doesn't know you,

you need to take the time to build rapport and trust. Introduce yourself and your credentials, explain everything fully, and be honest. Practice good timing by appropriately pacing your questions and leaving ample time for answers. And listen carefully.

Figure 6.2 10 Keys for Excellent Communication

1. Understand the other person's needs.
2. Take into consideration natural tendencies and capacities.
3. Be considerate.
4. Communicate on an equal level.
5. Be honest.
6. Know the other person's opinion of you.
7. Have good timing.
8. Separate your emotions from the facts.
9. Ask questions.
10. Listen. Listen. Listen.

Listening Skills

Although more than half of all communication time is spent listening, very few of us have received training in the most effective ways to listen. In fact, by the time we reach adulthood, many of us have become highly skilled at tuning out messages—either from well meaning but overly critical parents or teachers, or from the constant bombardment of media advertisements.

> "The most basic and powerful way to connect to another person is to listen. Just listen. Perhaps the most important thing we ever give each other is our attention.... A loving silence often has far more power to heal and to connect than the most well-intentioned words.
>
> —Rachel Naomi Remen

Listening goes beyond hearing. Hearing is simply the physiological process by which the brain registers information received through the ears. Listening involves taking the time to understand and interpret heard information. Listening means giving the speaker your full attention.

Effective listening skills affect clients in positive and powerful ways. They can help a client to feel at ease. They can also help defuse difficult or awkward situations when you may encounter an emotionally upset client. Being heard can profoundly help a client to relax and heal. After feeling truly heard, a client may breathe deeper, sleep better, and feel less tension in his body—and this doesn't even have anything to do with the actual treatment.

One of the most common mistakes in both personal and professional communications is to give unsolicited advice or turn the focus back to yourself when someone expresses a concern or frustration. By jumping in with a solution or inserting your experiences into the conversation, the person you're talking with won't feel heard. In a professional setting, you also risk traversing into territory better handled by a psychotherapist. However, with training and experience you can learn to manage the fine line between being supportive and moving into the territory of a psychotherapist.

To help enhance your listening skills, we explore how you can use the communication techniques of active listening and reflective feedback to ensure your clients feel truly heard.

People Skills: How to Assert Yourself, Listen to Others and Resolve Conflicts by Robert Bolton

Active Listening

Active listening involves giving your full attention to the speaker. Oftentimes, that can mean listening for the feelings behind words, facial expressions, or gestures. Words convey only part of the message. To completely comprehend what a speaker is saying, a listener needs to understand what the message means to the speaker. That entails understanding what's said from within the speaker's frame of reference. It also requires a willingness to set aside wandering thoughts to stay focused on the speaker's message.

An active listener conveys interest with nonverbal communication, such as open body language and steady eye contact, and avoids distractions such as fiddling with a pen. The active listener also pays close attention to a client's verbal and nonverbal communication. The old saying, "Walk a mile in my shoes," captures the essence of active listening.

Figure 6.3 Tips for Active Listening

- Maintain steady eye contact.
- Hold your body in an open position: face the speaker and lean slightly into the conversation.
- Be active: nod your head, nonverbally acknowledge what is being said.
- Use body language and tone to reflect the intent of what's being said.
- Ask questions to clarify or get more information when necessary.
- Pay attention to what is being said as well as what isn't being said.
- Check in with the speaker about nonverbal cues.
- Avoid distractions: turn off phone, place "Do Not Disturb" or "Session in Progress" sign on the door.

§2

Reflective Feedback

Reflective feedback is one of the most effective techniques for enhancing communication. This involves briefly restating the feelings, concerns, or content of what the speaker has said. An active listener that uses reflective feedback first allows a speaker to relate her story without interrupting, and then responds by asking further questions or rephrasing what was heard. Don't merely parrot back what someone has said. This can be counterproductive. Instead, find the core of the message and reflect that succinctly and in your own words. Use tone and intention to convey what was heard and check to see if what you heard is accurate. For example, a client claims to be experiencing pain in her right shoulder. An active listener would explore that pain with the following: "Tell me a bit more about the pain." "How does this pain inhibit your activities?" "What I hear you saying is that the pain…."

> "Listen long enough and the person will generally come up with an adequate solution.
> —Mary Kay Ash

Marshall Rosenberg, founder and educational director of the Center for Nonviolent Communication, says this about reflective feedback: "If we have accurately received the party's message, our paraphrasing will confirm this for them. If, on the other hand our paraphrase is incorrect, the speaker has an opportunity to correct us. Another advantage of our choosing to reflect a message back to the other party is that it offers them time to reflect on what they've said and an opportunity to delve deeper into themselves."[3]

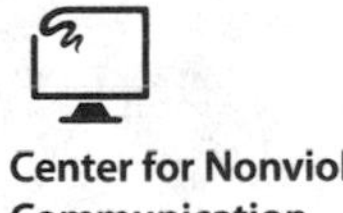

Center for Nonviolent Communication

www.cnvc.org

Rosenberg suggests practicing reflective feedback through asking questions, such as, "What you're saying is that you've been having bad headaches since you were rear-ended last week?" Or, "It sounds like you're feeling really frustrated that other treatments you received have not significantly decreased your pain level?" Reflecting in the form of a question gives the client the opportunity to tell you if you've heard him correctly and add any additional information he may want to convey.

Validate the speaker's feelings and experiences, regardless of what you think about them. Also, refrain from expressing any judgments or personal opinions. This can be more difficult than you may think. Simple agreement or disagreement with the content of the information can be judgmental, or judgment can be more direct as in the following example: A client is very distraught because her teenage son was caught drinking last night, and you say something like, "Wow, I hear how upset you are when your son behaves stupidly!"

> "Judge a person by their questions, rather than their answers.
> —Voltaire

Figure 6.4 **Tips for Reflective Feedback**

- Be aware that reflective feedback requires total presence: people see, hear, and feel when you're paying attention to what they say.
- Paraphrase instead of repeating what you heard word for word; only reflect back what is essential.
- Set aside your own feelings and opinions.
- Validate the speaker's feelings and experiences, regardless of whether you agree with him.
- Avoid comments that express judgment.
- Use a question format to reflect back the essence of a person's concern.
- Give ample time for the speaker to complete her thoughts; don't interrupt.

Body Language

For touch practitioners, listening involves more than hearing, we must also pay attention to body language. Non-verbal cues are often the only signal we get that our client may have additional needs. Even when you use active listening and reflective feedback skills, responding to body language can make communicating more difficult. You can't simply provide a reflection when there is no verbal content to reflect. Also, we often make mistakes when reading body language, particularly if we aren't careful to understand the context of the message or we filter the message through our own personal and cultural biases.

Figure 6.5 **Tips for Responding to Nonverbal Cues**

- Use direct observations like, "I noticed you were holding your breath when I pressed down on your shoulder."
- Use third-person statements when addressing sensitive boundary issues. For example, "Some clients disrobe completely, while others choose to leave on certain items, like underwear."
- Explain choices or alternatives. As in the above example, you might add, "Either way is fine. I can work on any area through your clothes, or avoid certain areas altogether. The choice is yours."
- Express openness to client input, "Please let me know if anything changes throughout your treatment, if you would like an area worked or avoided, or if there is anything else I can do to help you be more comfortable."

Even outside of the treatment room, remember to use body language to your advantage, leaving a positive impression with everyone you meet. When you shake hands and display confidence, you put others at ease and continue building rapport.

Communication Barriers

Words are imprecise vehicles of communication. The 500 most frequently used words in the English language have 12,078 separate and distinct meanings in The Oxford English Dictionary.[4] On average, that's 24 meanings per word! People have to guess at what is meant by a word—usually from the context in which it's used. Often they're right; sometimes they aren't.

The biggest problem with language is that the meaning of words is in people, not in dictionaries. Each of us projects our own meanings onto the words we say and hear. The tone and accompanying body language are often more significant than the actual words. Ambiguous comments like, "You have an interesting style of dress;" sarcastic comments like, "Oh sure, she's a really nice person;" and redundant comments that are repeated over and over, tend to interfere with the transfer of information. This type of interference is called noise.[4] If you've ever seen someone expressing irritation or anger while smiling at the same time, you probably experienced this feeling of dissonance. Likewise, if someone apologizes to you with a smirk on his face and an arrogant tone, you'll experience a mixed message that causes you to doubt his sincerity. When you're aware of this unnecessary noise in conversations, you can help reduce it by shifting your focus from what you say to how you say it, and make better choices in your words and voice tone.

Communication can also break down at the listener's end. Researchers have found that people listen 4-5 times faster than people speak.[5] The listener has spare time in which to become bored and may mentally drift off to other thoughts. Also, without even realizing it, the listener may miss important elements of the message. Furthermore, we all listen through filters that screen out some messages and distort others. Our concerns, needs, moods, roles, prejudices, and other factors color what we hear. The possibility for error increases when the speaker, the listener, or both, experience strong feelings about the message.

The good news is that you can overcome communication barriers by applying a few basic skills and insights such as:

- Active listening
- Awareness of varied personality and communication styles
- Clarity when expressing a personal need or request
- Giving critical feedback in a positive and constructive manner
- Appropriately expressing feelings, such as anger and frustration
- Managing boundaries effectively
- Understanding how negative communications and dysfunctional patterns get in the way of good communication
- Expressing appropriate empathy

§2

"Honor is the capacity to confer respect to another individual. We become honorable when our capacities for respect are expressed and strengthened. The term respect comes from the Latin word respicere, which means "the willingness to look again."

—Angeles Arrien

The Ethics of Touch by Ben E. Benjamin, Ph.D., and Cherie Sohnen Moe

Upset Clients and Difficult Situations

Although most of us would rather avoid upset clients and difficult situations, they're an inescapable part of professional life. In the realm of customer service, the focus isn't whether clients are right or wrong. The optimal goal is to ensure that clients feel that their concerns have been truly heard and addressed in an appropriate manner.

For instance, you may encounter a situation in which a client is having an "off" day and a simple misunderstanding can quickly gather speed. The client's emotions can start whirling, and you may find yourself in the center of a storm. Realize that in some cases, no matter what you say or do, you're perceived as "wrong" by the client. Staying centered, using active listening and reflective feedback techniques, and responding with clarity may be the best you can do. The least helpful thing you can say is, "There's no reason to be so upset."

You may then need to brainstorm with the client to arrive at a solution agreeable to both parties. However, if a client is irrational, it's best to distance yourself from the client by saying

"Everything that irritates us about others can lead us to an understanding of ourselves.

—Carl Jung

that although the client may have a valid concern, you need time to think about what has been said and would prefer to respond later. You may then want to consult with a supervisor or trusted peer to explore effective ways to deal with the situation. In the worst case scenarios, you may need to involve a manager or another on-site peer to help defuse the situation. If you as a practitioner made a mistake, did something inappropriate, or inadvertently crossed a boundary, an acknowledgment and an apology would be the appropriate response in the next meeting. If a client's concerns are valid, the practitioner should take steps to correct the problem and communicate that to the client.

Always document issues in the client's file.

If a client has misinterpreted information or actions, it often works well to discuss the matter with the client at the next meeting. Sometimes a cooling off period may allow the incident to be discussed more easily. You can acknowledge how your actions could have been misunderstood and work to bring clarity to the situation.

Figure 6.6 Tips for Effective Communication in Difficult Situations

- Carefully listen to the person's concern and the emotion behind the words.
- Avoid reacting by venting back at the person with anger or frustration of your own. Though it may be difficult, do everything you can to hold your tongue. Focus on staying centered.
- Acknowledge and reflect the person's concern and feelings. For example, "It sounds like you're really frustrated right now. If I understand correctly…."
- Don't pacify. Don't over-apologize. Upset people respond much better to a genuine apology that comes from strength not weakness.
- Focus on core issues and solutions. Don't get sidetracked by unimportant details.

Emotional Triggers

If you're a wellness practitioner who specializes in hands-on bodywork, you're probably aware of how this modality can sometimes elicit emotional reactions—such as crying, anxiety, or anger. Your response in these emotionally charged situations can profoundly impact the positive impact of the bodywork and the long-term therapeutic relationship with your client. Thus, learning how to handle these delicate situations skillfully is essential.

If you work with clients with known trauma, confirm that they're also seeing a psychotherapist.

Prior to beginning a session, practitioners should discuss with a client how bodywork can sometimes trigger strong emotions, and explain that emotional releases sometimes occur and are a natural part of the healing process. This type of conversation accomplishes two things. First, it paves the way for a client to feel safe and at ease if emotions should arise. Secondly, it frames the experience in a matter-of-fact and positive way.

When working with clients who have experienced trauma, sometimes touching a particular area can trigger an emotional response associated with a past occurrence. If this occurs, the client might want to share with the practitioner. Allowing expression is usually acceptable, but encouraging it, asking questions, or interpreting it often exceeds the practitioner's scope of practice. During an emotional release, keep the client focused on the present moment. You can suggest that the client breathe into the area, relax, and perhaps open her eyes. If the client appears in great distress, ask the client if she would like to stop the session. If the client prefers to continue the session and asks you to work on the trigger area, you must proceed carefully. Keep in mind that there is a significant difference between assisting a client in letting go of a memory or feeling that has surfaced, and promoting an emotional reaction or release. The latter is usually inappropriate.

Whenever a client has an intense emotional release during a session, it's wise to call the next day to check in.

Be aware of how easy it can be for a practitioner to get drawn into inappropriate responses to a client's strong emotions. Checking in with the client is appropriate, but it's best to refrain from asking questions that probe into the cause of emotional releases. Examples of some inappropriate questions are: "Do you know why you felt sad when I touched your leg?" "Were you thinking of someone in particular when you began to feel angry?" "Do I remind you of someone from your past?" Avoid playing the role of an armchair psychiatrist. Emotional release is a gray area where professional boundaries are easily crossed.

Unless you have specialized communication skills, knowledge, and training in working with clients' strong emotions, it's best to defuse the situation and change the focus of the session with a statement such as, "This seems to be an area in your body where a strong experience is being held. Should I move to a different area?" The practitioner may then take the opportunity to explain that emotional experiences are often held in the body and mention that counseling or therapy can be beneficial in processing the emotional issues that come up in bodywork.

There's an art of knowing how to let clients have their feelings without requiring them to stop crying or express their feelings. Most times, the practitioner doesn't need to do anything except be open and available and keep working. Overreacting to an emotional release can stop the client from feeling safe. If you encounter a situation in which you feel overwhelmed by a client's strong emotions, consider calling a timeout, leaving the room, or stopping the session. All are appropriate responses that respect your professional boundaries. You can say something like, "I think it's best to give you a few minutes to let this integrate. I'm going to step right outside the door. Let me know when you would like to continue."

Documenting Client Sessions

The documentation of client sessions—also known as charting—is a vital activity in all wellness practices, regardless of whether the files are for recordkeeping or for insurance billing purposes. Documentation provides historical perspective, protects you in case of legal actions, demonstrates professionalism, and verifies progress. It also enables wellness practitioners to clearly communicate with each other about a client's treatment plan. Note that insurance companies won't honor your malpractice coverage if you fail to keep accurate, detailed records.

Some practitioners have clients sign contracts and waivers, and request they fill out evaluation forms after each session.

Client files serve three major purposes. The first is recordkeeping, including proper documentation to support Internal Revenue Service filings. When you're in a service industry, the only way you can document your "work" is to create and maintain client files. The rudimentary information to include in each file is the client's name, address, phone number, session dates, and amounts paid. Second, up-to-date files document a client's needs and progress, which help you to develop the most effective treatment sessions. In group practices, client files provide continuity in treatment planning and provide the primary means for practitioners to share information about a client. Third, client files provide documentation necessary for insurance reimbursement. Many insurance companies don't pay for maintenance care. "Reasonable and necessary" is the term used to validate a treatment modality. Thus, if a wellness provider can show proof of an injury or condition (reasonable) and substantiate the success of treatment (e.g., a decrease in symptoms), the care is considered curative (necessary), not palliative.

In the book, *Hands Heal*, Diana Thompson says, "Ideally, serving our patients is the ultimate motivation for documentation. We document to gather and record information that ensures safe treatment and effective care, educates the patient, and clearly states the treatment results so that the patient acknowledges the benefits of the treatment."[6] Essentially, we document because it's in the best interest of our clients. The added benefits are toward the interests and protections of our own business.

See Chapter 19, pages 264-266 for more information on **HIPAA and confidentiality**.

In addition to client files, it's recommended that you have a sign-in sheet at the front desk or on a clipboard if you're providing services at a public event. This form is for your protection—it verifies the client did see you. Keep this sheet simple and don't risk breaching confidentiality by requesting personal information such as "reason for visit."

Client file and charting procedures vary depending upon the working environment. For instance, due to tight time frames at spas, charting isn't always required of practitioners. Some spas use a general intake form that a guest completes upon arrival. Due to the strict HIPAA laws, information is then passed on to the practitioner on a need-to-know basis.

Figure 6.7 Basic Charting Tips

- Review a client's file immediately before you meet with him. This helps refresh your memory and focus on the client's unique needs.
- Make concise and complete notes after each session. Include anything unexpected that may have happened, techniques you want to focus on next time, client education activities, and any other pertinent information.
- Be cautious of labeling or diagnosing clients in a manner that could reflect negatively upon them. For example, if a client says, "I've been feeling low energy and moody lately," it would be appropriate to reflect the client's words as: "Client states he has been feeling…" rather than saying, "client is depressed." You never know when a client's files could be subpoenaed.
- Pay close attention to confidentiality. Although files need to contain accurate and thorough information, session records should only include information directly related to sessions.
- Focus on facts; avoid analysis or judgments.
- Avoid using abbreviations or symbols not specifically defined by your employer, group practice, or standard industry practices.
- In some medical and healthcare environments you may need to chart electronically. In these cases, it may be helpful to brush up on your technology skills to maintain a high level of productivity in charting.
- Don't change or delete information once it's in a chart. If you realize an error was made, attach an addendum to the document or note the error (perhaps draw a thin line through it), initial it, and date it.

Client Forms

See Chapter 26, page 419 for more on **welcome kits**.

Various client file formats have been developed over the years. You may want to use "ready-made" forms, adapt them, or create customized forms. Every client should fill out an intake form, a health information form (sometimes the two are combined), a client policy form, and an informed consent form. Some practitioners provide these forms on their websites or email them to clients prior to their first session. Additional forms to be filled out depend on the nature of the work being done and if the client's sessions are covered by insurance. Here is a list of common forms:

- Client Policies (including fee structure)
- Health Information Sheet
- Health History
- Client Intake Form
- Financial Agreement (for insurance)
- Pain Questionnaires
- Informed Consent Form
- Injury Information Form
- Health Report
- Session Charting Forms
- Client Treatment Plan
- Medical Records Release Form

Once you have collected this information from a client, you must get the client's permission to share it with any other healthcare provider. Be sure to get this permission in writing.

Intake Forms

The fundamental facts to include on your client intake forms are: the client's name; address; phone numbers; email address; medical history; chief complaints; current medication; and reason(s) for using your services.

Some practitioners incorporate a disclaimer on their intake forms. For example, many massage therapists include a clear statement that massage is nonsexual. Other wellness practitioners state that their type of therapy isn't a substitute for medical examination or diagnosis, and recommend that clients see a physician for any physical ailments they may have.

You must decide what purpose your client files are going to serve and choose appropriate forms. As you and your needs change, so do the forms you use. For example, in addition to the general health information intake forms, you may want to have clients sign an acknowledgement of your fees and policies, fill out pain questionnaires, or complete billing information forms for insurance reimbursement.

§2

Session Forms

The two primary standardized formats for documenting what occurred in sessions are known as SOAP notes (Subjective, Objective, Assessment, Plan) and Wellness notes. SOAP notes are generally used for charting specific conditions, treatment plans, progress, and outcomes. Wellness notes are used in the many cases where clients may not have a specific issue, are in good health, and are seeking care for relaxation and overall wellness purposes.

The SOAP charting format (see Figure 6.8), was initially used to document physical therapy sessions, and has been adapted and used widely by many wellness practitioners. Variations of this charting system are part of the curriculum in many clinically oriented programs, and are easily adapted to other similar charting formats, such as the CARE (Condition, Action, Response, Evaluation) format. The SOAP categories include:

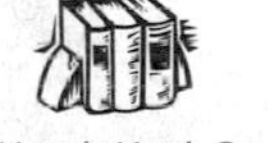

Hands Heal: Communication, Documentation, and Insurance Billing for Manual Therapists by Diana Thompson

Subjective: A description of symptoms and conditions as described by the client or a referring primary healthcare provider. Quotation marks are used to denote a client's own words. Key words are symptoms, location, intensity, duration, frequency, and onset. These notes reflect a client's perception of his condition.

Objective: An account of your observations and immediate results of the treatments you administer. This includes what the practitioner saw, felt, and did.

Assessment: A record of the changes in a client's condition as a result of treatment. How the treatment worked, what changes (positive or negative) occurred, and functional goals and outcomes based on activities of daily living.

Plan: A list of recommended actions and client preferences.

SOAP charting is now easier than ever, with online programs that allow practitioners to chart with a tablet or smartphone. When choosing an online SOAP notes program, ensure that it follows HIPAA confidentiality guidelines, and that your notes are secure and dated for accuracy. If your handwriting is rough, electronic charting can be an easy and legible option.

Printable Forms

www.sohnen-moe.com/products/tools/#product-client-forms

Many types of wellness care or spa-type settings don't lend themselves well to the healthcare model with a focus on treatment goals. In these settings, simply jotting down a few sentences about the treatment and client preferences on a Wellness chart can be more appropriate and achievable than a complete SOAP chart. Simple Wellness chart categories include:

Treatment (Tx): Details on the treatment provided, such as the techniques and modalities used, the area where applied, and the length of the session.

Comments (C): Additional information, such as personal preferences, variations from the routine, and client progress.

What format you use largely depends on your work setting and your personal preferences. No matter which you choose, sign and date every treatment chart, and observe all confidentiality laws that apply to your practice.

Figure 6.8 **Client Session SOAP Chart**

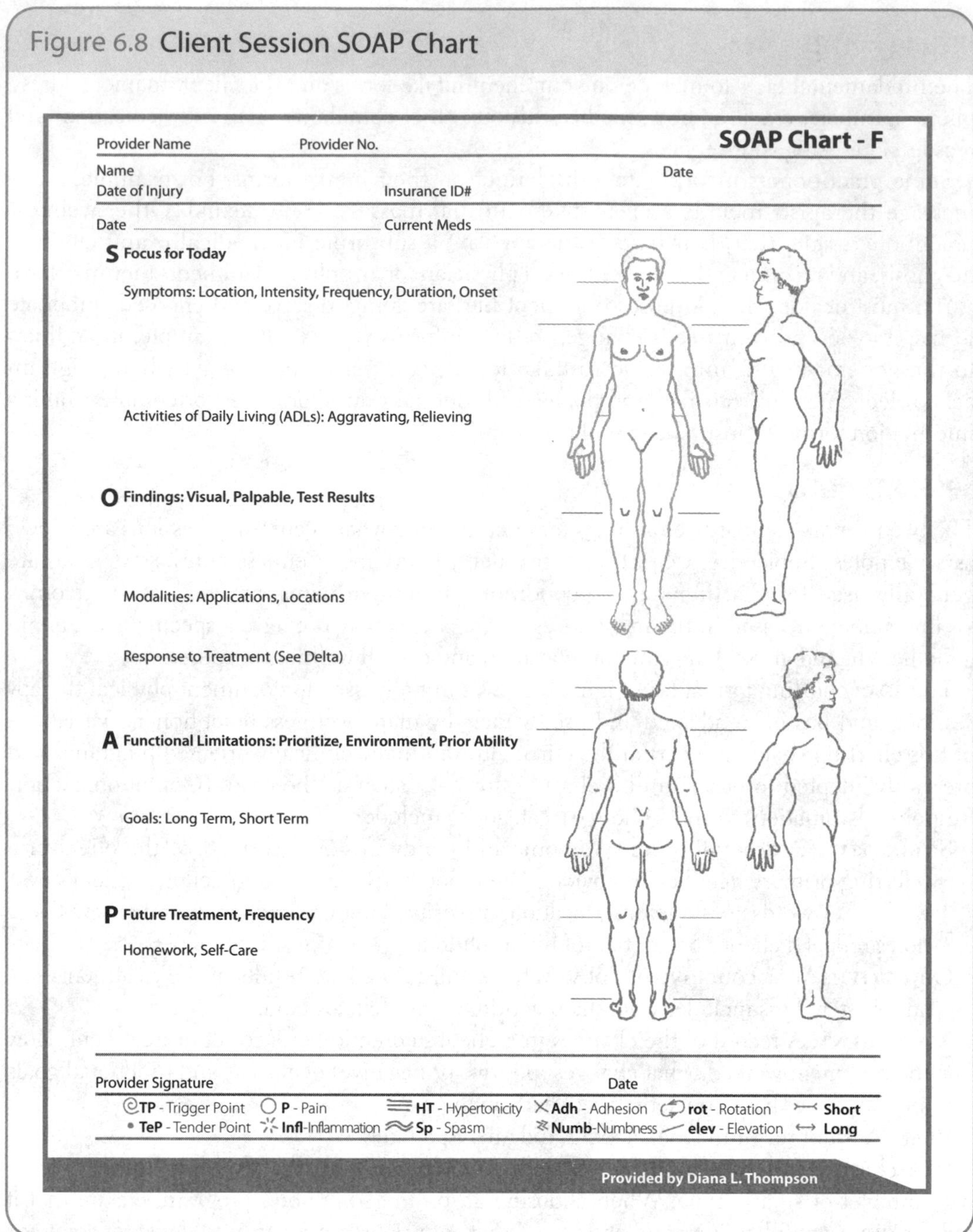

SOAP Chart - F
Provider Name
Provider No.
Name
Date
Date of Injury
Insurance ID#
Date
Current Meds
S Focus for Today
Symptoms: Location, Intensity, Frequency, Duration, Onset
Activities of Daily Living (ADLs): Aggravating, Relieving
O Findings: Visual, Palpable, Test Results
Modalities: Applications, Locations
Response to Treatment (See Delta)
A Functional Limitations: Prioritize, Environment, Prior Ability
Goals: Long Term, Short Term
P Future Treatment, Frequency
Homework, Self-Care
Provider Signature
Date
TP - Trigger Point
P - Pain
HT - Hypertonicity
Adh - Adhesion
rot - Rotation
Short
TeP - Tender Point
Infl-Inflammation
Sp - Spasm
Numb-Numbness
elev - Elevation
Long
Provided by Diana L. Thompson

Client Interviews

Interviews play a key role in creating lasting, healthy relationships between practitioners and clients. Information is gathered, rapport is built, trust is developed, and ideas are shared. Ideally, they occur at regular intervals. The most extensive one is the initial intake interview. It sets the tone for your working relationship. An effective intake interview can take from 20 to 60 minutes and requires good communication skills, especially the ability to listen. An intake interview isn't simply about obtaining a client history; it's an opportunity to explain procedures, clarify boundaries, determine the course of treatment, and educate clients. It's also a time to build a climate of trust by listening carefully to a client's concerns and questions.

Figure 6.9 **Sample Interview Checklist**

- ❑ Review File
- ❑ Greet Client
- ❑ Give Client a Tour of the Premises
- ❑ Fill Out Intake Forms
- ❑ Review Policies
- ❑ Discuss Overall Goals
- ❑ Preview Session Procedure
- ❑ Perform Assessment
- ❑ Provide Treatment
- ❑ Develop a Treatment Plan
- ❑ Summarize Session
- ❑ Assign Homework
- ❑ Suggest Referrals
- ❑ Make Product Recommendations
- ❑ Schedule Next Session

§2

Timing

Unless you carefully allot your time with clients, interviews can be rushed and less than effective. Conducting a thorough intake interview is time well spent. Consider that it takes approximately 6 times more money and 3 times more effort to get a new client than to keep one you already have. So, an extra half-hour is a minor investment on your part.

Allow ample time for your clients to fill out forms and ask questions. Keep in mind that your clients may not have the awareness or the vocabulary to accurately describe their conditions and goals. Your ability to ask pertinent questions and draw out useful information can make a big difference in the treatment results. A well-planned and thorough intake interview ensures the most effective experience for a client. Whether you allot 3 minutes or 30 minutes for an intake interview, help your client feel safe and comfortable, and gather key insights about your client's condition. With time and practice, you become highly skilled at both tasks.

> "Drawing on my fine command of the English language, I said nothing.
>
> —Robert Benchley

Figure 6.10 **Tips for Keeping the Interview on Track**

- Inform your clients about what they can expect to experience on their first visit. For instance, "Today we're going to go over your health history questionnaire and identify your concerns. I'm gathering all of this information to get a clear picture of your specific needs. All of this is important for me to create the best possible course for you."
- Explain how you plan to allot time. For instance, "We will spend about 20 minutes discussing concerns and health history, and the treatment on the first visit will be 45 minutes. After that, sessions will usually last 50 minutes."
- If a client starts to ramble, kindly redirect him to the topic at hand and assure him you want to allow as much time as possible for his session.
- In a spa setting, it can be challenging to complete a thorough intake interview in the time allotted. Key questions to ask include: Any major health challenges or accidents in the last 6 months? Are you currently under medical care or taking medication for any condition? How is your body feeling today? Any specific areas of focus or concern? (Keep in mind that you can also get more information on preferences as you're working.)

Artful Phrasing

> "Of one thing I am certain, the body is not the measure of healing, peace is the measure.
> —George Melton

Deftness at artful phrasing and asking clients open-ended questions is a skill that's honed over time. It involves forethought and lots of practice. Open-ended questions facilitate therapeutic communication as they encourage clients to express their thoughts and feelings. Open-ended questions usually begin with how, what, when, or could. For example, "What would you like to achieve in today's session?" These types of questions also help the client to feel like an active partner in the treatment process. In contrast, closed-ended questions are limited in scope, as the answer is usually a simple "yes" or "no."

One of the most frequently asked questions in an intake interview is whether the client has experienced this type of treatment; for instance, "Have you ever been hypnotized before?" Two problems are inherent in this question. First of all, the scope of hypnotherapy isn't clear. A client could have listened to self-hypnosis tapes but never visited a professional hypnotherapist. Secondly, the question only calls for a one-word answer. A better series of questions would be as follows: "What is your experience with hypnotherapy?" "How often have you received hypnotherapy sessions?" "When was your last hypnotherapy session?"

Figure 6.11 **Open- and Closed-Ended Questions**

Open-Ended Questions
- How do you react to stress?
- What types of wellness activities and treatments have you done?
- What would you like me to focus on in this session?
- How are you feeling today?
- What are your concerns?
- What products would you like to take home today?

Closed-Ended Questions
- Do you experience a lot of stress?
- Have you ever experienced this type of treatment before?
- Shall we focus on your headaches today?
- Are you feeling better today?
- Do you have any concerns?
- Would you like to take home any products today?

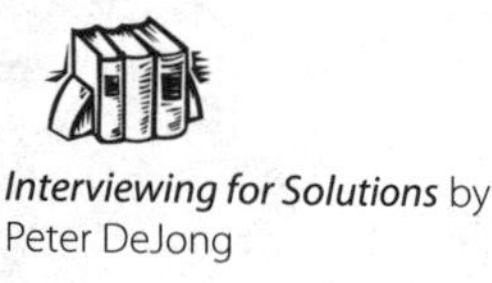

Interviewing for Solutions by Peter DeJong

Another useful practice is to incorporate phrases such as "how much?" "how long?" and "what is the level of intensity?" into your questioning routine. Let's say you're a shiatsu practitioner working with a client and you sense that the pressure may be a bit too much. If you ask, "Is this pressure okay?" the response will most likely be "yes" or "I guess so" (possibly with gritted teeth). Yet, if you ask your client to rate the pressure on a pain scale (after agreeing upon what the numbers mean), you get a much more accurate response. Even asking a question with a short answer like, "Do you prefer more or less pressure?" empowers the client to take responsibility for getting the desired pressure level.

You can use other questions to express concern for your client's comfort and wellbeing. Consider the following example that frequently occurs during a session: You sense your client is getting a bit chilly. Instead of asking, "Are you cold?" or "Would you like a blanket?" ask "Would you like a blanket on your feet and legs, or would you prefer to be fully covered with a blanket?" This type of question gives the client options and shows careful forethought on your part.

Use clear and simple language when talking with clients and avoid medical jargon and technical terms that may be unfamiliar to someone outside of your industry. The following interview questions (see Figure 6.12) help you understand your clients' needs. As each wellness modality is unique, you also need to ask questions specific to the type of work you do.

"I think the one lesson I have learned is that there is no substitute for paying attention.
— Diane Sawyer

§2

Figure 6.12 Client Interview Questions

- How are you feeling today?
- Tell me about your physical or emotional condition.
- How long have you been experiencing this condition?
- When was the onset of this condition?
- What is the intensity and frequency of this condition?
- What causes you stress?
- What activities aggravate this condition?
- What actions relieve or reduce the discomfort of this condition?
- What are your long-term wellness goals?
- What do you want to achieve in today's session?
- What kind of mobility assistance might you need from me?
- What is your experience with [your profession here]? What were the results (if applicable)?
- Are you currently under medical or therapeutic treatment? If so, for what condition and what medications or supplements are you taking?
- What products have you used to address this condition?
- What questions and concerns do you have about my services?
- What are your expectations about my profession or me?
- What can I do to make this session effective and enjoyable?

Interview Stages

Client interviews consist of four major stages—initiation, exploration, planning, and closure. You move from introductions and establishing rapport, to gathering specifics on the client's condition, to engaging the client in planning the first and subsequent treatments, to a timely and comfortable closure. Help ensure a smooth and effective intake interview process by keeping the essential interview elements (see Figure 6.13) in mind as you navigate the stages.

The first time you work with a client, the interview process is usually more extensive than in subsequent sessions. You can retain the quality of your interviews, even though the time spent is reduced, by making sure you include all 4 stages each time you see a client.

Figure 6.13 Top 10 Essential Interview Elements

1. Actively listen.
2. Reflect what you've heard.
3. Ask for clarification.
4. Take notes.
5. Make assessments.
6. Describe your treatments.
7. Answer questions.
8. Obtain client consent.
9. Engage client in planning.
10. Plan treatment(s).

Initiation Stage

The initiation stage of an initial interview is the one in which you introduce yourself, establish rapport, discuss the client's general issues and expectations, describe what you can do, review your policies, and explain procedures. Knowing what clients expect improves treatment results and client satisfaction. The initiation stage of subsequent sessions involves actions to continue building rapport, such as greeting each client appropriately and engaging in light chitchat.

Exploration Stage

> "It is what we think we know already that often prevents us from learning.
> —Claude Bernard

The exploration stage encompasses reviewing a client's history, performing a physical assessment, and determining the treatment course of the specific session. The flow of the exploration stage varies depending upon the actual type of service you provide and your environment. Ideally, in your initial session, you would review the client's intake forms, clarify any vague responses, get a sense of the client's general wellbeing goals and specific goals for receiving treatments, administer some type of assessment, determine the course of action and techniques to use for the current session, and obtain the client's informed consent (i.e., you have sufficiently discussed goals and treatment options for the session, and the client has agreed to go forward with the planning stage, including the actual treatment).

The exploration stage of subsequent sessions encompasses reviewing the client's files, discussing any changes that may have occurred between sessions, documenting observations, setting treatment goals, and determining the course of the specific session.

Planning Stage

Planning is the stage that the practitioner and client create together. Long-range treatment plans are the key to having clients who receive treatments on a regular basis. Treatment plans are blueprints to follow while working with any specific client. Long-range treatment plans also serve as a reminder for the client to take responsibility for his goals.

> "Some patients, though conscious that their condition is perilous, recover their health simply through their contentment with the goodness of the physician.
> —Hippocrates

The first time you see a client, you do much of the planning before the hands-on portion of the session, yet you will most likely need to update it after the hands-on portion. Ultimately, the plan is based upon all the information gathered in the initiation and exploration stages of the interview, as well as the session. It may seem awkward to break up the interview with a treatment, but it's the only way you can accurately develop a long-range treatment plan. It's usually difficult to accurately evaluate a client's condition until you've given a treatment. Also, during the session, clients often discover unsuspected problems or remember previous physical or psychological trauma. This information can be crucial in designing the treatment plan.

Some items to include in the plan are: the client's short-term and long-range wellness goals; indications and contraindications; treatment frequency; specific modalities to be used; homework; and possible referrals to other wellness providers. Create a vision with your clients so they can experience themselves having attained their goals. This makes the treatment more powerful and inspires clients to take an active role in their wellbeing (e.g., do homework assignments, use products). This can also elicit secondary goals.

The tricky part to designing a long-range treatment plan is setting realistic goals. Many people don't know enough about themselves or your services to gauge the potential outcomes. Begin by discussing general goals and letting them know which conditions can be successfully addressed by your services. Create short-term goals (for individual sessions and the next few treatments) and long-term goals related to the overall wellness picture your client has in mind. The difficulty is that unless you're a primary care provider, you can't prescribe—but you can describe. Make sure you're clear about the proven benefits of your work (that's where familiarity with research helps), so you can safely make those statements. It's best to let your clients determine the treatment frequency. You can provide them guidelines such as: "Other clients with similar goals obtained their desired results by coming in twice per week for 2-3 weeks, then once per week for 3 months, and tapering off to a minimum of twice monthly." or

"If I had a condition like this, I would...." A statement I often used in my massage practice was, "I recommend massage as often as you can afford physically, timewise, and financially."

The planning process for subsequent sessions includes updating the long-term treatment plan and making notes for activities and modalities to incorporate into the next session.

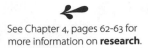

See Chapter 4, pages 62-63 for more information on **research**.

It can also be helpful to encourage clients to listen to their bodies to determine how often to schedule wellness treatments. Oftentimes, this can vary due to life circumstances and stress levels. Clients that listen to their bodies may schedule sessions every few days or once a month depending on their comfort level and needs.

Update long-range treatment plans after each visit. Make notes for subsequent sessions, taking into account any changes in your client's lifestyle and treatment results (e.g., what worked and didn't, the areas or modalities you didn't cover, what you want to include next time). All too often, practitioners omit this stage, particularly with clients who have been receiving regular treatments or clients who are very educated about and involved in their own wellness. Keep in mind, most people want objective evidence that they're reaching their wellness goals. I know I appreciate it when a practitioner looks at a chart and tells me the specific changes and progress I've made since the last session and where I'm at in relation to my long-term goals.

Closure Stage

Closure is the final interview stage, often referred to as the "exit interview." This can be done fairly quickly with the first session since you've spent a significant amount of time designing the treatment plan. Give a very brief overview of what took place, highlight some of the client's major goals, make any needed adjustments in the long-term plan, assign homework, give the client an opportunity to ask questions, make any necessary referrals, and schedule the next appointment. Allow clients to connect how they are feeling after the session to the the work that was done by asking a few follow-up questions about their impression of the session and how they feel now.

Closure tends to take longer in subsequent sessions than with the first visit. After the treatment, review the session with your client (this doesn't need to be lengthy and can be informal). Summarize what you did, address issues that might have surfaced, and answer any questions. Briefly review the client's long-term goals and make any appropriate recommendations and homework assignments. Finally, ask when she would like to schedule the following session.

> "Every person who ends up buying into your idea does so by changing it into his idea (even if it still looks a lot like your idea).
>
> —Tom Peters

Client Compliance

Many practitioners complain about a lack of client compliance (e.g., clients don't do their homework, make no lifestyle changes, don't use appropriate products, fail to return for follow-up sessions). Although you can't force someone to comply with your recommendations, your communication skills can increase the odds.

First of all, recognize the factors that prevent full compliance: lack of discipline, time restraints, insufficient funds or insurance coverage, social pressures, beliefs, and other obligations. Explain why it's in their best interest to adhere to your recommendations, clarify the instructions, and discuss ways to overcome barriers. Have clients repeat instructions or perform exercises or stretches to be sure they understand them. Give them printed reference material to take home. The most critical aspect is gaining your clients' concordance about their treatment plans and assignments.

Even using good communications, a client may still choose not to comply. Don't reprimand or treat the client differently because of non-compliance, as it will negatively affect your rapport, and it's ultimately up to the client. Continue to make your recommendations for achievement of the client's long-term goals in a positive, non-judgmental manner.

Client Education

Everyone in the wellness field is an educator. Client education occurs in two ways: you support the body's learning of how to optimally respond to states of relaxation and repair; and you increase your clients' general awareness of body function and self-care. Some practitioners offer added measures to help broaden their clients' knowledge by: describing what they're doing and why; demonstrating stretches and self-care techniques; showing videos; describing how a product works; sharing information on related wellness topics; providing educational materials; and assigning homework.

Educating clients so that they can better understand the cause of their pain or health condition, and methods to alleviate it, empowers them to take more responsibility for their wellness. They become active partners instead of passive recipients of treatments. A side benefit is that as clients learn new ways to enjoy greater wellness, they're more likely to share this information and recommend your treatment services to friends and family.

Client Education Handouts

www.sohnen-moe.com/products/tools/#product-client-handouts

When providing client education, the more methods of delivery you use, the better chance the client will absorb and retain the information. For example, when you're demonstrating a stretching technique, it works well to discuss the stretch verbally, perform a demonstration, provide a take-away handout, and inquire if there are any questions. You should then ask the client to demonstrate the stretching technique so you can observe and offer any helpful feedback.

By taking time for questions, you ensure that the client has grasped the information, and by asking the client to demonstrate the stretching technique, you provide an opportunity for body-based or kinesthetic learning. The handout serves to reinforce and support the client's at-home learning in a visual manner.

Hone Your Interviewing Skills

Interviewing skills take time and practice to develop. The best way to sharpen your skills in this area is to role-play several intake interviews. Other techniques to improve communication skills are to read books, take seminars, post reminders to yourself about areas you wish to improve (e.g., ask open-ended questions, don't interrupt, suspend judgments), and ask for feedback from clients. Excellent communication skills evolve from a lifelong process of observation, study, and experimentation. Have fun!

Interview Simulation

Get together with 2 other colleagues. Allot at least 3 hours for this activity. Run through an intake interview (without doing the treatment or session consultation). One person is the practitioner, one portrays a client, and the third person is the observer. As you practice, focus on asking open-ended questions and listening carefully to the client to obtain useful information.

At the conclusion, the observer reports on what she noticed in terms of the overall flow, the client's apparent comfort level, types of questions asked, body language, and what did and didn't work. The client shares his reactions to the interview, and then the practitioner discusses what she experienced. Run the simulation 3 times so that each person gets to play every part. After all 3 rounds are completed, reflect upon the following: Which role did you find most difficult? In which role did you feel most like yourself? How can you use this information to help clients feel most comfortable during the interview process? The final step is to create an action plan for incorporating any desired changes.

The Client Technology Connection

Next to your occupational abilities, technology can be the most important tool in your business—or it can be an obstacle. This section covers techniques for improving your effectiveness when communicating with your clients via phone, text, and email, and dealing with inappropriate calls and messages. In addition to allocating financial resources for appropriate equipment, be sure to invest the time to improve your communication effectiveness with these technologies.

§2

Machines vs. Humans

Since many practitioners are in sole practice and don't have a receptionist, they rely on voicemail, text, and email to exchange messages with clients and potential clients. These technologies serve a good purpose but are generally not well suited for this field. Even people who are comfortable with technology, appreciate it for things like scheduling, but still want a personal touch for questions that aren't easily answered via text or website FAQs. Most people prefer talking to another human being with their questions, particularly if they aren't current clients.

Another significant drawback relates to scheduling. For example, imagine that you're working with a client and the phone rings. Someone wants to schedule an appointment right away. You have the next hour open, but by the time you're finished with the current client and listen to your messages, it's too late for the other person to come into the office. A prospective client may have called the next available practitioner while you were busy. If you had an appointment service or an online scheduler, that person could have scheduled an appointment and been in your office by the time you were done with your current client. An appointment service is similar to an answering service, plus they book clients.

Wellness Practitioners Answering Service

www.myreceptionist.com

Appointment services are usually well worth the money! All it takes is 1-3 sessions to pay for this service, which could easily be done by attracting just 1 new regular client. Of course, you're best off researching the different services. After you've chosen one, explain the work you do to the receptionists, furnish them with brochures, and then give them a complimentary session. The receptionists can help turn an inquiry into a client.

You may also want to explore setting up an online scheduling system. These systems work much like a self-serve appointment service. Plus, they are affordable, easy to work with, and clients often appreciate the added flexibility that comes with scheduling appointments at their convenience. Everyone benefits from less time spent in "phone or email tag."

Phone Etiquette

If your files are computerized, you can create a new client account and directly input the information while you're on the phone.

Every time you answer the telephone, you create an impression. The question remains what that impression will be. Within the first few seconds of a conversation you convey how you feel about yourself, your practice, and the caller. Just because the caller can't see you doesn't mean that she can't sense the attitudes you convey through the tone of your voice and the words you use. So, dress as if the caller could see you, get feedback from others, notice how others handle themselves on the phone, practice and role-play, vary your "script," and follow the telephone guidelines below. Utilize the telephone wisely to build your practice. Keep in mind that every time you answer the phone you have the opportunity to gain or lose a client. Your emotional state gets conveyed and possibly misconstrued, so don't answer the phone if you're busy, distracted, or upset.

Without visual cues, it can be quite difficult to determine the intent of someone's statement. For example, a caller might possess a sardonic sense of humor, and you could be offended by a remark that would have been humorous with visual cues. We can't eliminate the inherent communication problems associated with telephones, but we can reduce distractors and increase rapport by incorporating the following techniques:

Be prepared. You don't want to keep callers waiting while you search for supplies or information. Store needed provisions (e.g., paper, pen, appointment book) within reach and be knowledgeable about your practice.

Inspire interest. You must know how to eloquently describe in 30 seconds or less the offerings of your practice, your policies, and the type of work each practitioner does. The caller may be a potential client, so you need to immediately inspire interest.

Answer promptly. Plan to answer the phone promptly: after 2 rings, but before 5 rings. By picking up right at the first ring, you may give the impression that you've nothing else to do but sit idly by the phone. Also, most people don't expect someone to pick up the phone right away, so it throws them off balance. If you wait too long to answer the phone, the effect is usually negative. The caller gets impatient or anxious that voicemail is about to pick up...then you answer in person.

Courtesy first. Greet the caller courteously. Your tone sets the stage for the whole conversation. Before you pick up the phone, be sure to smile. It sounds hokey, but smiling makes a difference in your vocal quality as well as your attitude. You never know who is on the other end of the line (unless you recognize the number on your Caller ID).

For instance, I was at home writing an article on telephone communications and it was late on a Saturday afternoon. I had received 6 or 7 unsolicited sales calls in less than an hour. Lo and behold! The phone rang again and I must admit I wasn't my most "professional" self when I answered the call. After all, it was a weekend and this was my personal line. Well, it was a school owner wanting to schedule me for a seminar. He thought he called my business number. I recovered the conversation (after all, I wasn't rude—just not at my best), but it took a little while to change the tone.

See the ***Business Mastery Workbook*** for a **New Client Checklist.**

https://sohnen-moe.com/bm5-workbook-request/

Identify yourself. Never assume your voice will be recognized. Also, ask to be of service. When you answer the telephone, your greeting might be like this: "Good morning. Thank you for calling The Northwest Health Center. This is Nancy. How can we assist you?"

Be clear. Speak in a clear and friendly manner. Personalize the conversation whenever possible by using the caller's name. Listen, give feedback, and mirror language patterns.

Avoid distractors. One of the most important techniques for improving telephone communications is to keep down background noises: don't drink beverages, eat food, or chew gum while on the phone. Also, if you listen to music or watch television, be sure that the volume controls are close to the telephone: turn off the sound before you answer a call. If you work out of your home and children or animals are present, you need to create a sound-proof environment around the phone. Your credibility as a professional can be adversely affected if your dog barks or children holler while you're talking with a potential client.

Avoid the hold option. Most people dislike being put on hold, so avoid it whenever possible. If you must put someone on hold, follow these guidelines:

- Get the caller's name before asking to "please hold." When you return to the caller, address the caller by name.
- Be specific about how long you expect to be on the other line. If it goes longer, check back in to let the caller know she is not forgotten. Even 30 seconds can seem like a lifetime when you're in telephone limbo.
- Always ask if the person would prefer to be called back.
- Give the first caller preference.

Follow through. Keep any promises you make to your callers. This is why it's imperative to take notes. Return all calls within 24 hours unless other arrangements have been made.

Focus on services. An effective response to a potential client who asks for prices immediately is, "Before I can answer that, please tell me what you're needing." You must understand clients' needs so that you can clearly guide them.

Figure 6.14 **Telephone Tips**

- Be prepared
- Inspire interest
- Answer promptly
- Be courteous and smile
- Identify yourself and offer to be of service
- Speak clearly
- Avoid distractors
- Avoid putting people on hold
- Take notes and follow through
- Focus on service

§2

Email and Text Etiquette

Clients often find it very convenient to use email or texting for questions and appointment requests. Unfortunately, this can also complicate communications because a large percentage of communication impact is nonverbal.

Before you choose to send an email, ask yourself: "Is email appropriate for this correspondence?" Email can be a great option if you're making announcements, passing on information or online links, and sending newsletters. A phone conversation is the best option if you need to resolve a conflict, you're upset or frustrated, you want to express feelings about something, you need to ask follow-up questions or negotiate, or you need to give information that may upset the other person. Follow these guidelines if you do choose to send email:

- Use simple, straightforward sentences, with familiar words.
- Use active, rather than passive language. For example, "Our new location opens Sunday." rather than "Our new location will be opening Sunday."
- Use positive language. For example, if you want to remind someone of something, say "remember to…", instead of "don't forget to…."

If you choose to respond to text messages, only do so to answer quick, simple questions. Call them back if it's anything more complicated. Always get permission before initiating a text message conversation (it's helpful to include communication preferences on your intake form).

Screening Clients

During an initial conversation with a potential client, you have an opportunity to gather essential information that can save a lot of time and trouble down the road. By efficiently answering questions and sharing information about your services, you can quickly build rapport and inspire interest in making an appointment. Conduct a preliminary interview to find out the reason for calling and the expectations. This assists you in determining if you're the appropriate provider for the caller (sometimes ending relationships with clients you don't want can be harder than obtaining new clients). If you're unable to talk with the potential client initially (e.g., you have a client in the next few minutes or someone else took the call), place a personal confirmation call as soon as possible. Your screening checklist might look something like this:

- What's your name?
- How did you hear about me?
- What motivated you to call me? (Stress, pain, injury, illness? Ask follow-up questions related to the response, like "Did you seek medical attention?")
- What type of treatment are you looking for?
- Has this type of treatment been successful for you in the past?
- What are your expectations for this treatment?

- Will the session be charged to an individual or a business?
- Will anyone else be attending the session with you (e.g., spouse, children)?
- What is your phone number (home, business, or cell) in case I need to reschedule?

Some people are naturally at ease talking on the telephone while others feel less comfortable. If someone else answers your phone, consider developing scripts so that they know how you want callers to be treated, the information you want to obtain and give, the image you desire to portray, and policies for handling specific issues. Topics to cover include: prospective clients; cancellations; rescheduling; follow-up visits; disgruntled clients; fees; setting an appointment for a minor; scope of services; clients with special needs (e.g., people with disabilities); insurance reimbursement; and clients who want to speak directly with you. Rehearse the scripts and role-play scenarios.

Telephone Scripts

Design a questionnaire to ensure you obtain the information desired, disseminate your client requirements (e.g., prices, scope of services, cancellation policy), and determine if a client has special needs (e.g., assistance getting in and out of a wheelchair). Role-play your new scripts with a colleague or friend.

Reflection: Did you keep the script and the question and answer period to a reasonable length for a phone conversation? Are there any more efficient ways to disseminate the necessary information while remaining thorough?

Inappropriate Calls

Receiving inappropriate calls can be a source of immense discomfort. Unfortunately, many practitioners—particularly massage therapists—still get calls from people who are ill-informed about the nature and scope of wellness services. Sometimes people are indirect about wanting sexual services. You can often determine inappropriate callers by their tone of voice, awkward periods of silence, calls placed late at night, and if they request late-night appointments. A common tip-off for massage therapists is when a caller requests "full-body massage."

When someone calls requesting sexual services, you have two choices: you can get upset and hang up the phone, or you can use it as an opportunity to educate the caller. Too many practitioners take these calls as a personal affront.

If you receive this type of call, it works well to stay centered in your professionalism. If people want sexual services, that's their prerogative, but they don't have the right to expect it from you or any other wellness provider. Tell them that isn't what you do, give a brief description of the services you do provide, and let them know that a legitimate practitioner does not perform that kind of work. You might also say something along these lines: "Because prostitution is not legal in most states, and prostitutes need some way to let others know how to reach them, they tend to put advertisements under massage or touch therapy. This is changing as the general public becomes more aware of the therapeutic practice of massage. If you would like further information about the therapeutic benefits of massage, I'd be happy to speak with you about it or you can visit my website."

This gives the caller the opportunity to learn more about massage or gracefully remove themselves from the conversation. Remember, these callers are human beings. Just because they want something you don't offer doesn't mean they might not want a legitimate massage in the future or don't have friends who want a professional massage. Besides, these are the people we really need to educate. They are the ones perpetuating the myths about massage and the entire healing arts field. You can transform a potentially negative experience into a positive one by responding professionally and keeping perspective.

Declining and Dismissing Clients

There are several reasons why you may need to decline a potential new client, or dismiss a current client. In either case, you want to do so in an appropriate and professional way, to maintain a positive image for your practice.

§2

Declining a Potential New Client

If you have built your practice successfully, there is always the possibility of having a full practice. If your appointment book is filled with established clients, make sure you have a list of practitioners ready for referrals. You might say, "Currently all my appointment slots are filled with established clients. May I recommend some nearby practitioners who do similar work?" Another reason to decline is when, after you have conducted a preliminary interview, you determine that the client has needs beyond your specialty or scope of practice. In this case, you should refer them to an appropriate specialist or to their primary care practitioner for further evaluation.

The most delicate reason to decline a potential new client is when you experience countertransference. If you find yourself feeling a great attraction or repulsion, a sensation of intense dislike, or a vague lack of affinity, you should ask yourself, "can I give this client clear, caring, compassionate attention in the course of a treatment?" If your honest answer is no, you must refer the client elsewhere. To do this gently, in a neutral and positive way, you might say, "I don't believe my skills are developed enough to give you the standard of care you deserve. Let me offer you the names of practitioners with more experience in this area." Or simply, "I think my ability to help you is limited. I would like to refer you to a more experienced practitioner who can give you better care."

Dismissing a Current Client

No matter how hard you try, sometimes you just need to say goodbye. If after a course of treatments, you determine that the client is not benefiting, you may decide to end the therapeutic relationship and offer referral elsewhere. This is where your charting can come in handy in your communications. As you track the client's progress, you and the client can determine that the treatments have not moved her toward her wellness goals, and together you may decide to terminate treatment.

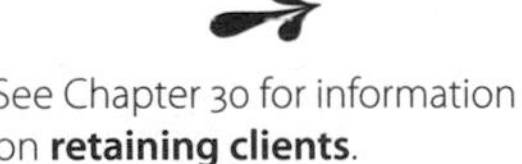
See Chapter 30 for information on **retaining clients**.

Like with declining a new client, if you experience discomfort or countertransference, or your client is experiencing transference, you may need to dismiss the client. For example, if the client becomes overly dependent, suffers from some emotional disorder that threatens you, asks you for help outside of your scope of practice, or you're unable to set workable boundaries, you may need to refer him to another practitioner, or to psychotherapy if aggression or infatuation is present. In these cases, consulting with a supervisor or peer can be very helpful in determining the best course of action. If you decide to terminate treatment, you might say, "I've become aware that something you're asking for in our sessions (e.g., emotional support, memory processing) is outside my expertise. I believe we've reached the limits of how much I can help you. I want the best for you as you continue your healing process, therefore, I'd like to offer the names of some excellent practitioners who offer a more suitable type of therapy."

The best reason to dismiss a client is when the therapeutic goals have been reached. This is the happy circumstance in which your work was effective and you finish what you can do for your client. At this time you can terminate treatment, or help the client set new goals if she chooses. You might say, "Congratulations, the problem you came to me with has been resolved. I've enjoyed having you as a client and if you wish to continue sessions with other goals in mind, I would be happy to work with you."

Figure 6.15 Declining and Dismissing Clients

Reasons to Decline a New Client	Reasons to Dismiss a Current Client
• Practice is Full	• Discomfort
• Inability to Help	• Lack of Results
• Countertransference	• Transference/Countertransference
	• Completion

§3 Exploring Career Paths

Section 3 of *Business Mastery* provides an insider's look into career opportunities in the wellness field. This section provides an overview of wellness career trends, and information to help you determine if working as an employee or being self-employed is the best option for you. You'll also gain valuable insights into different work environments so that you can approach your career choices with credibility and confidence.

Chapter 7 starts with a statistical review of complementary and alternative healthcare usage and then follows up with an overview of the trends in wellness careers. It discusses why career focus is essential and the steps involved in clarifying that focus. The topics of employment, self-employment, and independent contractor status are explored, including the pros and cons of each choice. The chapter wraps up with an activity to assist you in defining your ideal career.

Chapter 8 provides you with insights into working in spas and salons, whether you are an employee or an independent contractor. It highlights what you can expect to find in these environments, such as the corporate culture, training requirements, scheduling concerns, and seniority issues. It also includes success tips for each of the most common types of spas.

Primary healthcare settings offer a variety of CAM services on both an inpatient and outpatient basis. This translates into a growing number of career placement opportunities. **Chapter 9** focuses on what to expect when working in primary healthcare settings and provides suggestions to enhance your experience in this environment.

Chapter 10 explores the advantages and disadvantages of group practices. It examines the key aspects of this option and includes overall tips for success in group practice. The chapter then identifies specific concerns and success strategies for working in a wellness center or a specialty center.

The majority of practitioners work at least part time as sole proprietors. **Chapter 11** takes an in-depth look at the challenges and opportunities with private practice options, such as working in a home office, commercial office space, primary care provider's office, fitness center, or on an outcall basis.

7
Career Tracks

"There is no passion to be found in playing small, in settling for a life that is less than you are capable of living."
—Nelson Mandela

Wellness Career Trends

Why Career Focus Is Essential
- Multi-Discipline Options

Employee vs. Independent Contractor vs. Self-Employed
- Employment
- Independent Contractor Status
- Self-Employment
- Your Ideal Career

Key Terms

Ambiance
Autonomy
Boundary
Compensation
Complementary and Alternative Medicine (CAM)
Corporate Culture
Employee
Image
Independent Contractor
Interpersonal Skills
Mismanagement
Multi-Disciplines
Policies
Preventive Wellness
Procedures
Professionalism
Self-Employed
Self-Evaluation
Sexual Misconduct
Stress Management
Teamwork
Undercapitalization

Employment in the complementary and alternative medicine (CAM) fields has risen significantly over the more than 2 decades since the first edition of this book has been in print. According to the most recent report on CAM survey data released by the National Center for Health Statistics (NCHS), more than 33% of U.S. adults are using some form of CAM.[1] According to the NCHS, the breakdown of CAM usage is as follows:[2]

"Trends in the Use of Complementary Health Approaches Among Adults"

www.cdc.gov/nchs/data/nhsr/nhsr079.pdf

Massage Therapy Fact Sheet & Press Releases

https://www.amtamassage.org/publications/massage-industry-fact-sheet/

- 17.7% took nonvitamin, nonmineral, natural products
- 10.9% did deep breathing exercises
- 10.1% practiced yoga, tai chi, and qi gong
- 8.4% had chiropractic or osteopathic manipulation
- 8.0% meditated
- 6.9% received massage
- 3.0% used special diets
- 2.2% received homeopathic treatment
- 2.1% practiced progressive relaxation
- 1.7% used guided imagery
- 1.5% had acupuncture

Additionally, adults in the U.S. spend more than $33.9 billion annually in out-of-pocket expenses for the products and services of professional CAM healthcare providers which include chiropractic, acupuncture, and massage/bodywork practitioners.[3]

A recent Associated Bodywork & Massage Professionals (ABMP) report is even more optimistic stating that 16% of U.S. adults visited a massage therapist in the previous year (22% of women, 10% of men), and 37% of adults have received a professional massage at some time in their life. Further, the U.S. spa industry is closing in on $13 billion per year.[4]

Practice location statistics are more readily available for massage therapists than for other wellness practitioners, so those are included here. According to the 2015 Massage Profession Research Report[5], the breakdown of where consumers received massage is:

Contact your professional associations for current industry trends and statistics.

- 21% Spa
- 13% Chain
- 12% Massage Therapist's Office
- 10% Chiropractor's Office
- 9% Other
- 8% Hotel, Resort, Cruise
- 8% Home
- 5% Salon
- 3% Medical Clinic
- 2% Massage School Clinic
- 2% Alternative Therapy Clinic
- 1% Workplace
- 1% Healthclub
- 1% Physical Therapist's Office
- 1% Don't Know

Wellness Career Trends

In view of these statistics, the career outlook for wellness practitioners is bright. The expanding career opportunities are due to a constellation of factors: a widening interest in stress management and preventive wellness; the public's disillusionment with the high cost of traditional medical care and prescriptions (plus the negative side-effects of those medications); and a fast-growing population of baby boomers (age 55 and over) looking for ways to cope with the physical challenges and stress associated with aging.

Most wellness practitioners love what they do. How could one not love a career where you can help people reduce stress, improve their health, get in touch with themselves, and feel better so quickly? What is not so often mentioned is the high percentage of graduates who fail to become successful in their careers. Although the causes are many, most failures are rooted in a lack of business savvy.

At first glance, it may seem that acquiring advanced technical skills and a high degree of expertise are sure ways to success. However, this is only one part of the equation. Other key factors for success are business acumen and strong interpersonal skills. Without this solid foundation, your career and technical skills cannot flourish.

Fundamental interpersonal skills include: creating rapport and building relationships; developing a soothing and inspiring manner with clients; setting appropriate personal and professional boundaries; and creating a safe space for clients. Developing awareness of, and adhering to, high standards of professionalism are crucial, as these skills serve you well whether you run your own business or work for someone else.

Figure 7.1 provides a brief overview of career paths for wellness practitioners. Keep in mind that the specific venues listed under Employee and Self-Employed can overlap.

In the next sections, we explore some effective ways to sharpen your career focus and look at the advantages and disadvantages of self-employment versus working for someone else. The more information and insights you have into possible career paths, the better prepared you are to make choices best suited to your unique personality and overall goals.

Figure 7.1 **The Wide World of Holistic Wellness**

Full-/Part-time Employee

Spas

- Day Spa
- Dental Spa
- Destination Spa
- Resort Spa
- Luxury Hotel Spa
- Cruise Ship Spa
- Medical Spa

Holistic Healthcare Clinic or Wellness Center

Specialty Clinic/Center

- Single Modality Clinic (e.g., all Acupuncture, all Massage Therapy)

Hospital or Medical Clinic

- Medical Center
- Orthopedic Physician's Office
- Physical Therapy Clinic
- Rehabilitation Center
- Sports Medicine Clinic

Self-Employed

Private Practice

- Home Office
- Private Office in a Professional Building
- Room in Another's Practice (e.g., Chiropractor's Office)*
- On-site/Outcalls
- Fitness Center/Gym/Health Club*
- Corporate Wellness Program
- Day Spa*
- Dental Spa*
- Hospital
- Hospice
- Personal Practitioner for a Celebrity or Professional Athlete
- Salon*

Group Practice

- Holistic Healthcare Clinic or Wellness Center*
- Medical Clinic*

*Possible Independent Contractor Situations

Why Career Focus Is Essential

Career focus is essential to long-term success. In addition to choosing an overall field, it's crucial to clarify the specific career focus parameters. Douglas Helmer, Ph.D., author of *The Massage Therapy Career Focus Workbook*,[6] says that if you ask an aspiring somatic practitioner what she wants to "do," she'll usually give you her job title. For example, "I'm training to be a massage therapist," or, "I'm learning to be an acupuncturist." Probe any deeper and these same aspiring wellness providers are often stuck for an answer. If you ask them where they want to work, you'll often get, "I don't know." Ask who they want to treat and the response is usually, "I'm not sure." Ask them if they want to be an employee or work on their own, and you'll most likely hear, "I haven't decided." Finally, ask if they think not knowing the answers

"Your work is to discover your work and then with all your heart to give yourself to it.
—Buddha

> It is the commonest of mistakes to consider that the limit of our power of perception is also the limit of all there is to perceive.
> —C.W. Leadbeater

to these questions is a problem, and most reply, "It's not a problem, and there's lots of time to figure that out after graduation." Unfortunately, there simply isn't "lots of time" to make these vital career decisions. Practitioners who arrive at graduation day without a crystal clear vision of some basic parameters that define a preferred career are likely to land up in the "Did Not Stay in the Profession After Two Years" column.

Helmer also points out that the career focus parameters can be as simple as knowing the answers to the journalist's 5 W's and 1 H: Who? What? When? Where? Why? How? Looking for an easy way to sharpen your career focus? Take a few minutes to reflect upon the questions in Figure 7.2.

Figure 7.2 The 5 W's and 1 H

Who

Who do you want to work with? or, Who (i.e., what type of client) do you want to work on? Young people? Elderly people? Athletic people?

What

What do you want to provide to your clients? What kind of treatment? What kind of outcome do you desire? What kind of environment will you provide?

When

When do you want to work? Strictly 9-5? Do you want your weekends free? Do you have a preference or are you flexible?

Where

Where do you want to work? Are you looking for a spa/resort setting? Clinical? On-site?

Why

Why do you want to work in a certain area or focus? Is it to communicate more effectively? Do you want to build your referral network? Is your main goal to help people?

How

How do you want to care for your clients? How will you approach your clients? Will you approach the whole client or their specific condition? Will you actively work with them so they learn to care for themselves, or passively so they'll depend on you for future treatments?

Multi-Discipline Options

Many wellness practitioners combine several professional roles to create a unique, blended career. For instance, personal trainers are seeking massage therapy credentials, skin care technicians are getting yoga teacher certifications, and chiropractors are becoming movement therapists. Holding more than one credential in related disciplines allows you to add additional income streams and employment opportunities, expand potential target markets and referrals, and experience a more varied and fulfilling work life. However, it can be challenging to balance your various roles along with your personal commitments. Also, it's wise to hone your first profession before adding additional ones. Choosing a multi-discipline career requires a commitment to self-discipline. Consider the following questions to explore whether or not a blended career is right for you.

In her article "The Benefits of a Blended Career,"[7] Heidi Smith Luedtke says you should ask yourself these questions if you're considering a multi-discipline career:

- What do I wish I could spend more time doing?
- What interests have I put on the back burner?
- What do I have to offer that I'm not currently offering my clients?
- How could I increase my impact?
- What else do my clients want from me?
- How could I be more authentically me?
- How much risk am I comfortable taking?
- What will I scale back (or give up) to allow a new role to flourish?
- Do I need formal training for this role?
- How will this new role fit with my current career?

If the thought of having a different schedule throughout the week sounds exciting, maybe adding another credential is right for you. On the contrary, if you get anxiety just thinking about it, you may want to keep a single discipline focus.

§3

Employee vs. Independent Contractor vs. Self-Employed

The two primary career tracks are to work for a company or be self-employed. Within those paths are a number of possibilities. Some people kick-start their careers by working at a spa or clinic, others take part-time jobs to augment their private practices, some choose a private practice right away, and there are those who prefer to only work for others.

See Chapters 12–14 for specific details on **successful employment strategies**.

If you're "hired" by a company as an Independent Contractor, the reality is that you're self-employed. Be aware that you might be treated more like an employee (without benefits), and that might not fit in with your personality.

Another consideration is the amount of time you want to work. Some people want to work full time while others choose to permanently work in their field on a part-time basis (they either have another career, are raising a family, or want to pursue other interests).

Employment

See Chapter 11 for information on **setting up a private practice**.

Working as an employee provides many potential benefits such as the following: the possibility of walking into a full practice with little marketing; providing a larger scope of services for your clients' wellbeing; starting out with a ready-made professional image; reduced paperwork (there's usually an office manager); the ability to focus on hands-on work; access to better and more varied equipment and supplies; excellent built-in referral base; laundry service; and an office staff that does the scheduling, places confirmation calls, and handles financial transactions. Employers are responsible for all facility liability, overhead costs, marketing, financial management, and business operations.

By agreeing to accept employment, an individual enters a world where commitment, loyalty, cooperation, and obligation play important roles. Hopefully the business earns these from its employees through its own ethical behavior; nevertheless, these qualities, on the part of the employees, aren't optional. The employees' commitment, loyalty, cooperation, and obligation remains with their clients and the services they provide.

Employers also must act responsibly. In *The Ethics of Touch*, the chapter on The Team Approach talks about how "a business should take a protective role towards its employees. Laws and regulations provide this ethical framework, which is ideally completed through policies and procedures that demonstrate the business' respect for its employees and defense of their individual rights. Important areas where these attitudes must and should be expressed are in practices of fairness and diversity, safety, security, and integrity."[8]

Think about yourself. Do you enjoy working as part of a team? Do you enjoy focusing primarily on client wellbeing? Do you prefer the convenience of an office support staff and less paperwork? Do you like the idea of someone else handling marketing and business logistics? Do you like working within an established structure? Working in these settings also requires conforming to a set image, policies, and procedures. You might need to alter your style and scope of practice to align with the company's vision and schedule. Success as an employee requires you to understand the rationale behind the policies and procedures set by the employer. These guidelines protect clients, the company, and the practitioners.

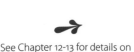

See Chapter 12-13 for details on **résumés** and **job interviews**.

Figure 7.3 highlights the pros and cons of working for an employer. It may provide some new insights as you consider your career path.

Figure 7.3 **Employment Pros and Cons**

Pros of Working for an Employer

- Possibility of walking into a full practice with little marketing
- Providing a larger scope of services for your clients' wellbeing
- Starting out with a ready-made professional image
- Being part of a team with clear and established boundaries
- Reduced paperwork (there is usually an office manager)
- Ability to focus on hands-on work
- Access to better and more varied equipment and supplies
- Additional training on specific techniques
- Excellent built-in referral base
- Office staff that does scheduling, places confirmation calls, and handles financial transactions
- Discounts on services and products
- Use of the facilities
- Benefits (e.g., health insurance, paid vacations, paid sick days, pension plans, profit sharing, continuing education reimbursement)

Cons of Working for an Employer

- Lack of control over the scheduling
- Rarely get to choose your clients
- Possibly needing to alter your treatments in terms of style, modalities, and length
- Conforming to a set image, policies, and procedures
- There is no guarantee your shifts will be filled
- Potential to get booked for a specific service even if it isn't clear that you're proficient in that technique or if contraindications are present
- Return clients are rare in some settings, such as destination spas and resorts, leaving little chance to mark progress or make lasting connections
- Possibly required to perform other services when not doing your primary service

Corporate Culture and Image

Many practitioners enjoy the team environment of working as an employee—that is, if the corporate culture of the business promotes a positive attitude, discourages gossip, and expects a high degree of professionalism and respect for co-workers and clients. The most enlightened business owners aspire to build businesses in which both clients and employees thrive. The best managers recognize that clients perceive subtle undercurrents of disharmony, and will aim to create a sense of community among team members and good working relationships with employees.

When it comes to image, you can expect to encounter a clear list of do's and don'ts. Ambiance and image are often key elements of a business brand and corporate identity, requiring employees conform to policies about image and personal appearance. For instance, some workplaces may require employees not to have visible tattoos or excessive piercings. Some require practitioners to conform to a dress code or wear a designated uniform.

Policies and Procedures

Employees are expected to follow company policies and procedures, provide the services outlined in their job description, and are held accountable for professional behavior and job performance. For instance, many employers have stringent hygiene policies, such as long hair pulled back, no facial hair, and no perfume. The personalities, styles, and philosophies of the various wellness professionals must blend or conflict can arise over working conditions and what's best for the client. When you start your new job, take the time to review policy and procedure manuals. Clarify any ambiguous policies. Ascertain what's expected of you when you're not directly working with clients (e.g., paperwork, clerical duties, assisting the other practitioners, marketing, cleaning chores, providing treatments for staff).

Compensation

Employees can be paid an annual salary, an hourly wage, or an hourly wage plus commission. Regardless of the wage terms, the total hours worked divided by the wages received must always equal at least the minimum wages. At the end of the year, the employer must provide employees Form W-2: Wage and Tax Statement.

See Chapter 20, page 297 for a list of **employer's tax forms**.

Some businesses base salaries and preferential scheduling on seniority. It's important to take this into account when you're new. As in most careers, it may take some time for your income to grow to its full potential. Compensation varies greatly among the type of business and its geographic location. Other possible compensations include gratuities, commission on product sales, increases based on rebookings, and benefits. Employee benefits can include health insurance coverage, paid time off and sick days, pension plans, profit sharing, tuition reimbursement for continuing education, discounted services, and use of facilities.

The policies on tipping can also vary greatly. For instance, some spas don't allow tips to simplify logistics for clients. Others allow tips but have moved to a cashless system that enables a guest to note a tip on a credit card receipt or hotel folio. Other work settings, such as medical spas and primary healthcare facilities, should offer higher base wages, as gratuities aren't common in those environments.

Keep track of what payments are due to you as mistakes can happen (usually due to incorrectly inputting a fee or a tip into the system). Find out ahead of time how such mistakes are rectified: Do you receive an immediate payout or is the amount added to your next pay period?

Sexual Misconduct

In most cases when you work as an employee in a business setting, you don't have to worry about sexual misconduct from clients—it rarely happens, and, if it does, assistance is nearby. More common are reports of subtle inappropriate behaviors, such as suggestive comments, offensive jokes, or inappropriate touching. In these cases, terminating a session may be the appropriate response. Simply state you're uncomfortable with continuing the session, or excuse yourself from the session by saying you don't feel well.

In short, be aware of the potential for problems in this area and use your best judgment and diplomacy to deal effectively with difficult or awkward situations. Don't hesitate to end a session immediately if a client's behavior is inappropriate, and report problems or concerns to management as soon as possible. Professional ethics dictate that you refrain from talking about a client's inappropriate behavior with anyone other than management.

Teamwork

As in many business environments, politics can sometimes get in the way of equitably resolving scheduling issues or work conditions. Make an effort to express your views in a balanced way, and then release your expectations. Accept that some things are beyond your control.

Help with clients' needs that might not technically be "your job." Teamwork is paramount in settings where clients receive multiple services. Time is a very important consideration so as not to throw everyone off of their schedules. For instance, if a practitioner is running behind schedule, jump in and help (e.g., reset the room, escort the client to the next station) whenever possible.

Take courses to enhance your communication skills with co-workers. Learn and practice conscious detachment. For example, make an effort not to take anything personally, especially when a client is difficult.

Employment Status

When exploring job openings, evaluate the advantages and disadvantages of joining a company as an independent contractor versus an employee. Sometimes you may work first as an independent contractor, then negotiate a change to employee status. Or you may be offered a position as an employee after the manager has had a chance to observe your skills and success in building a solid base of clients. Be prepared to discuss compensation by researching industry trade journals to get insights into salary structures.

Please note that some business owners classify practitioners as independent contractors to simplify paperwork and avoid the tax implications and other liabilities associated with an employer/employee relationship. The penalties can be quite high if the government determines that the company misclassified employees.

Independent Contractor Status

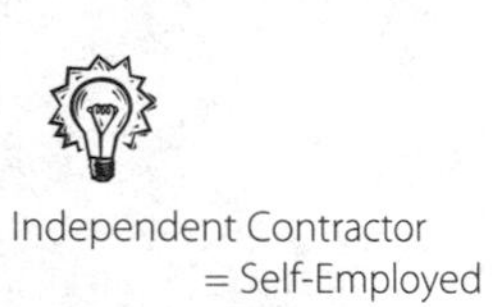

Independent Contractor = Self-Employed

Oftentimes, private practitioners pursue short-term or long-term independent contractor arrangements as an effective way to supplement their income. In these settings, you're technically a separate business operating within another business: you generally rent office space on a flat rate or percentage basis of the income you generate. Independent contractors typically pay the business a percentage of the client service fee charged in exchange for the space and shared operational services such as the receptionist. Other times, practitioners work as an independent contractor for special events, such as providing chair massage at a business convention or providing acupuncture to the members of a film crew that are in town for a week.

Some practitioners even work as independent contractors for several companies and rarely see clients in their own offices. These opportunities provide a degree of variety that appeal to many.

See Chapter 15, page 200 for **sole proprietorship regulations**.

Keep in mind that as an independent contractor, the hiring business isn't obligated to pay a minimum wage, guarantee any income, or withhold any taxes. In general, independent contractors only receive income from actual sessions provided, they must pay all taxes, and receive a specific tax form (1099-MISC: Miscellaneous Income) from the contracting business at the end of the year.

If you're thinking about working as an independent contractor for one or more companies, remember that while it means you operate as a business owner (sole proprietor), you may be treated more like an employee without the employee benefits. In these settings, however, your start-up business tasks are fewer in number and complexity than practitioners who establish a private or group practice.

See Chapter 22, pages 325-327 for more details on **independent contractor status**.

If you're an independent contractor and also operate a private practice, define parameters for working with the "company's" clients in your private practice setting. In general, it's unethical to seek out clients for a private practice from the pool of clients at your workplace, unless you have an explicit agreement with the hiring company that allows it. Consult with a business coach, attorney, or financial advisor before finalizing and signing an independent contractor agreement. The time and money you invest in consultation more than repays you by avoiding lost time, disappointment, and potential legal problems resulting from conflicts.

The three main categories that the IRS uses to assess the degree of control and independence are behavioral, financial, and the type of relationship. To determine whether you qualify for independent contractor status, you would be able to affirm:

- I control what I do and how I do it.
- I determine how I'm paid, how my expenses are paid, and the tools I use.
- I provide myself with any benefits available.

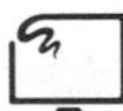

IRS form for determining worker status

irs.gov/pub/irs-pdf/fss8.pdf

According to the Internal Revenue Service, "an individual is an independent contractor if the payer has the right to control or direct only the result of the work and not what will be done and how it will be done."[9]

In some instances an independent contractor might subcontract work to others. For example, a film company contracts with a massage therapist to provide massage and other wellness care for the cast and crew during a movie shoot. The massage therapist would "hire" additional practitioners as independent contractors to provide any additional needed services.

Self-Employment

Most wellness practitioners choose to be self-employed at some point in their careers. These sole proprietors work in private practice settings, either out of home offices or business offices. These businesses may also include outcall services. Practitioners often work in multiple environments. For example, a practitioner might see clients 3 days a week from a home office, go to several clients' homes each week, provide employee wellness at a corporation twice a month, and work from another wellness provider's office 1 day per week.

Unfortunately, not everyone is well suited for this type of enterprise. It takes a certain personality type to be truly successful in one's own business. Successful business owners are inventive and follow through with their plans. They respect money. They possess considerable expertise in their particular career field and have broad experience in several others. They have very good verbal and written communication skills and are usually considered very personable. They are positive thinkers, determined, self-disciplined, service oriented, and persistent—they don't quit!

Think about yourself. Do you possess these qualities? In most instances (unless, for example, you have a partner with a lot of business acumen), it's not enough just to have talent, you need to manage the business. Many small businesses that don't succeed are examples of this problem—talent without proper business skills.

See Section 6 for specifics on the actual **running of a business**.

According to the U.S. Small Business Administration (SBA), two-thirds of new companies survive at least 2 years and about half continue for at least 5 years—instead of the more often cited (but inaccurate) statistics that claim that 1 out of 5 (20%) businesses are successful after 5 years.[10]

Though the odds are improving, these statistics can be cause for concern. The two major reasons for failure are mismanagement and undercapitalization. Mismanagement is generally a result of poor planning, not realistically evaluating strengths and weaknesses, failing to anticipate obstacles, improper budgeting, and lacking the necessary business skills. Undercapitalization is not having enough start-up capital or needing to take draw (salary) before the business is firmly established.

"Do economic or industry factors affect business survival?"

www.sba.gov/sites/default/files/Business-Survival.pdf

Take a few moments to review the chart that highlights the pros and cons of self-employment (Figure 7.4). This career path presents some unique challenges. The chart may help you realistically assess if you have what it takes to run a business.

Figure 7.4 Self-Employment Pros and Cons

Pros of Self-Employment
- Ability to choose your target markets
- Control over standards and scope of practice
- Freedom to determine your image
- Control of the client screening procedures
- Potential for unlimited income
- Opportunity for creativity
- Flexible schedule
- Independence
- Be your own boss
- Tax write-offs
- Increased potential to contribute to others

Cons of Self-Employment
- Potential loneliness and isolation
- Long hours: work with clients, marketing, and management
- Taking all the risks
- Responsibility for getting and retaining clients
- Potential cash flow problems
- Initial funding of the business
- Safety risks increase if you work alone or provide on-site services
- Possibility of needing to delay financial expenditures such as expensive equipment
- Responsibility for administrative and logistical activities
- The only "employment benefits" are the ones you pay for yourself
- No true paid vacations, holidays, or sick days
- Responsibility for making certain everything is done

Autonomy

Although you may enjoy the freedom of private practice, a potential drawback is a sense of professional isolation. Private practice can be a stark contrast to educational programs which offer plenty of opportunities to share professional opinions and insights with colleagues. Nonetheless, some practitioners thrive in a private practice setting. Others find they must actively work to minimize isolation. Some good ways to do this are to establish a support system of colleagues and advisors, join a networking group, attend industry conferences as your time and budget allow, and trade tasks with a colleague (e.g., you balance her checkbook and she helps you develop your marketing plan). These are all great ways to make new friends, generate leads, and find business opportunities.

> "The only way to do great work is to love what you do.
> —Steve Jobs

You may also experience days when the endless array of business tasks seem to take on mammoth proportions. As the appointment scheduler, bookkeeper, business manager, marketing director, and wellness provider, you're responsible for making sure everything gets done. You may choose to hire someone to handle some of these business tasks, such as bookkeeping, so that you can focus on working with clients. This makes good business sense and frees you up to do more of what you love. For instance, if you pay someone $12 per hour for 10 hours a week ($120) and that frees you up to do 8 more sessions at $50 each ($400), you'll net $280.

A mistake many practitioners make when they are new is to work whenever clients want. This can lead to burnout. Make a schedule that works for you, includes ample breaks, and allots time to take care of yourself. Take off at least 1 day per week and 2 days in a row when possible. Include cancellation and no-show policies on your client forms and review them with clients. This assists your time management, as well.

Safety

Safety is a standard concern for any business owner, but even more so for a self-employed wellness practitioner. Take a vigilant approach to personal safety. For instance, first-time clients can present potential trouble spots, as it's difficult to know much about their character or background, so use a screening protocol for new clients. In most cases you can quickly and aptly sense unbalanced individuals, an unsafe neighborhood, or other safety concerns, and remove yourself from the situation with haste or end a session, if need be. However, operating this "inner radar" at top efficiency requires that you first develop an awareness of potential personal harm and take it seriously.

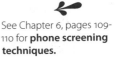

See Chapter 6, pages 109-110 for **phone screening techniques.**

Fortunately, safety incidents are rare in private practices. From a safety standpoint, it's best to only work hours when someone else is in the building (or your home). In addition, lock your treatment door or main office so uninvited people can't wander in, make sure outdoor lighting is adequate, and call a friend before (in hearing range of the client) and after sessions. The old saying, "An ounce of prevention is worth a pound of cure," certainly applies here. Don't hesitate to end a session immediately if you feel unsafe.

§3

Planning

Take the time to write a business plan that includes a vision statement and maps out best-case and worst-case financial scenarios. Focus special attention on your marketing plan and allot ample time each week for marketing tasks.

See Chapter 17 for details on **business plans**.

Finances

When you're the only source of revenue in your business, you must carefully manage your cash flow. If you're just starting out, it can help ease financial pressures if you work part time at another job until you can build a strong client base. You need to plan for items such as professional association fees, licenses and permits, tax payments, supplies and equipment purchases, insurance premiums, and marketing expenses. Help launch your business on solid footing by meeting with a financial advisor or referring to a business self-help book to map out an effective system for estimating monthly operating expenses and revenues, and making quarterly tax payments. Learn about tax deductions and set up an easy-to-use recordkeeping system to save time and headaches at tax time. Track where your time and money go so you can monitor results and change course if needed.

See Chapter 20 for more information on **financial management**.

Insurance

Insurance policies are necessities and should be a priority. Make sure your malpractice and liability insurance covers you wherever you practice. Research health and disability insurance options to find the best value and coverage. Ask colleagues for their recommendations. Verify that your auto insurance covers lost income if you're in an accident, as this typically isn't a standard coverage feature.

See Chapter 15, page 207 for more information on **insurance coverage**.

Benefits

The only "employment benefits" you receive are the ones you pay for yourself (which kind of defeats the whole concept of "perks"). As a self-employed practitioner, there are no true paid vacations, holidays, or sick days. Some practitioners find it helpful to open a savings account to set aside cash resources as "self pay" for vacations and days off.

Self-Employment Checklist

Under each question, check the answer that says what you feel or comes closest to it. Be honest with yourself!

Are you a self-starter?

- ❑ I do things on my own, nobody has to tell me to get going.
- ❑ If someone gets me started, I keep going all right.
- ❑ I don't prefer to put myself out until I have to.

How do you feel about other people?

- ❑ I like people. I can get along with just about everybody.
- ❑ I have plenty of friends—I don't need anyone else.
- ❑ Most people irritate me.

What type of work do you prefer?

- ❑ I prefer a balance of hands-on and mental work.
- ❑ I prefer to focus primarily on client wellbeing and hands-on work.
- ❑ I prefer to do the least amount of work possible.

Can you lead others?

- ❑ I can get most people to go along when I start something.
- ❑ I can give the orders if someone tells me what we should do.
- ❑ I let someone else get things moving. Then, I go along if I feel like it.

Can you take responsibility?

- ❑ I like to take charge of things and see them through.
- ❑ I'll take over if I have to, but I'd rather let someone else be responsible.
- ❑ There's always some eager beaver around wanting to show how smart he is. I say let him.

How good an organizer are you?

- ❑ I like to have a plan before I start. I'm usually the one to get things lined up when the group wants to do something.
- ❑ I do all right unless things get too confused. Then I quit.
- ❑ I get all set and then something comes along and presents too many problems. So I just take things as they come.

How good a worker are you?

- ❑ I can keep going as long as I need to. I don't mind working hard for something I want.
- ❑ I'll work hard for a while, but when I've had enough, that's it!
- ❑ I can't see that hard work gets you anywhere.

Can you make decisions?

- ❑ I can make up my mind in a hurry if I have to. It usually turns out okay, too.
- ❑ I can if I have plenty of time. If I have to make up my mind fast, I think later I should have decided the other way.
- ❑ I don't like to be the one who has to decide things.

Can people trust what you say?

- ❑ You bet they can. I don't say things I don't mean.
- ❑ I try to be on the level most of the time, but sometimes I just say what is easiest.
- ❑ Why bother if the other person doesn't know the difference?

Can you stick with it?

- ❑ If I make up my mind to do something, I don't let anything stop me.
- ❑ I usually finish what I start—if it goes well.
- ❑ If it doesn't go my way right away, I tend to quit.

How good is your health?

- ❑ I never run down.
- ❑ I have enough energy for most things I want to do.
- ❑ I run out of energy sooner than most of my friends do.

Suggestion: This checklist is also in the online workbook.

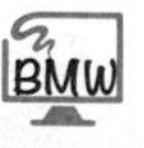

The Business Mastery Workbook

https://sohnen-moe.com/bm5-workbook-request/

Self-Employment Checklist Scoring Key

After completing the Self-Employment Checklist, count the checks you made beside the answers to each question. How many checks are beside the first answer? The second answer? The third answer? If most of your checks are beside the first answer, you probably have what it takes to run a business. If not, you're likely to have more trouble than you can handle by yourself. Find a partner who is strong on the points in which you experience challenges. If many checks are beside the third answer, not even a good partner could shore you up.

Self-Evaluation

Without a boss or supervisor to provide feedback or performance evaluations, a self-employed practitioner lacks valuable input to identify the adjustments and improvements that are necessary for planning and growth. Therefore, you need to get feedback from clients, colleagues, and advisors. Send a service evaluation form to all clients seen in the past 6 months. Email them an online survey tool or mail a printed form. If using a printed form, ensure anonymity, provide space for general comments, and include a stamped, self-addressed envelope to encourage participation.

§3

"Create Surveys, Get Answers"
www.surveymonkey.com

Offer a free treatment to a colleague whose skills you admire, in return for a frank assessment of your skills. Meet with well-respected sole practitioners to compare and assess the effectiveness of current practice policies and procedures. Consult a trusted accountant, or consider updating (or replacing) practice management software, to provide a complete picture of the financial health of your practice. Finally, use the results of these efforts to strategize how your business can best flourish, and to pinpoint resources (e.g., experts, services) that can assist in that process.

Self-Employment Assessment

- Are you willing to take the risks in being self-employed?
- Do you know how much credit you can get from your suppliers?
- Do you know where you're going to get your start-up funding?
- Have you talked to a banker about your plans?
- If you need/want a partner with money or skills that you don't have, do you know someone who is qualified and appropriate?
- Have you talked to a lawyer about your business?
- Does your family support your plan to be in business?
- Could you net more money working for someone else?

Self-Employment Reflection

Reflect on your Self-Employment Checklist and the Self-Employment Assessment. Were you surprised by anything? Did your responses and scores measure up to your initial ideas about your future? What are some of the action steps you can take?

Your Ideal Career

At this point you still may be uncertain about being self-employed or working for someone else. The next activity assists you in discerning what you really want in your career. After completing this activity, the subsequent chapters illuminate the key aspects of a variety of practice settings.

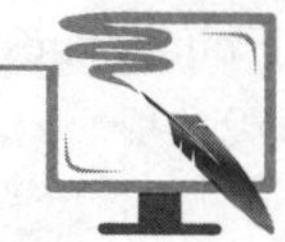

Your Ideal Career Elements

1. Where do you want to practice? What city, state, or country?
2. Do you want to travel as part of your career?
   ❑ Yes ❑ No ❑ Maybe If yes, where?
3. How many hours per week do you want to work? Doing what specifically? (In addition to client interaction, include the other business-related activities such as marketing, bookkeeping, networking, and planning.)
4. What type of work location do you want? Do you want to have a private office or work at a medical facility? Do you want an office in your home? Would you rather just do outcalls? Or would you prefer a combination of the above?
5. What type(s) of people do you want to have as clients?
6. Which professions could provide referrals to your business?
7. For which professions can you be a good source of referrals?
8. What benefits do you want your business (or employer) to offer (e.g., health insurance, paid vacations, retirement fund)?
9. Do you want to work as an employee or run your own business?

If you plan to be self-employed, answer the following questions:

10. Do you want to have multiple locations?
    ❑ Yes ❑ No ❑ Maybe If yes, where?
11. Do you want any associates?
    ❑ Yes ❑ No ❑ Maybe How many? What would they do?
12. What type of business atmosphere do you want?
13. How much do you want the net business profit to be annually? $
14. How much money do you want for your salary/draw after taxes? $
15. Describe your ideal office/location in detail including external features, the style of decorations, equipment, and ambiance.

If you plan to work for someone else, answer the following questions:

16. What is the lowest fee or percentage you will accept?
17. List at least 5 places or people for whom you'd like to work.
18. Describe the ideal business agreement. What would you like your employer to offer? What are you willing to provide?

Follow-up: After you have completed this activity, refer back to the Life Planning activity in Chapter 2 and update your career goals.

8

An Insider's Look at Spa and Salon Settings

"The biggest mistake that you can make is to believe that you are working for somebody else. Job security is gone. The driving force of a career must come from the individual. Remember: Jobs are owned by the company, you own your career!"

— Earl Nightingale

What to Expect
- Key Aspects of Spa Settings

Day Spas and Salons

Cruise Ship Spas

Destination, Resort, and Luxury Hotel Spas
- Resort and Luxury Hotel Spas
- Destination Spas

Medical and Dental Spas

Key Terms

Ambiance
Boundaries
Confidentiality
Contraindications
Corporate Culture
Cruise Ship Spa
Day Spa
Dental Spa
Destination Spa
Dual Relationships
Luxury Hotel Spa
Medical Spa
Resort Spa
Salon
Scope of Practice
Seniority
Spa
Treatment Space

In an era in which consumers are looking for ways to slow down, rejuvenate, and connect with like-minded individuals, spa visits have become a desirable lifestyle experience. According to the International Spa Association (ISPA), more than 20,000 spas were operating in the United States by the end of 2013, with nearly 350,000 employees, accommodating 164 million visits.[1] These figures are expected to continue their upward trend, indicating an increasing need for wellness practitioners in spa settings.

The growth of the spa industry is evidenced by the popularity of franchise businesses in the wellness fields. The following wellness franchises were listed in Entrepreneur Magazine's top 100 fastest growing companies from the 2015 Franchise 500® list.[2]

- Planet Fitness (fitness club)
- Anytime Fitness (fitness center)
- Massage Envy Spa
- The Joint (chiropractic services)
- Orangetheory Fitness (personal training)
- Hand and Stone Massage and Facial Spa
- Elements Massage

Spas range in image from holistic wellness centers to posh pampering resorts. It's commonplace to find wellness practitioners, such as acupuncturists, massage therapists, nutritional consultants, estheticians, energy workers, and other somatic practitioners, in all of these settings. Today the wide world of spas includes day spas, resort and hotel spas, destination spas, cruise ship spas, and medical and dental spas.

What to Expect

As the spa market continues to flourish, so do employment opportunities for wellness practitioners. New practitioners can gain valuable experience by working in a spa. In addition to building expertise through client feedback, you have the opportunity to learn proper etiquette, interact with clients in a professional manner and, in many cases, expand your skills through in-house trainings and tuition reimbursement programs. There are even advancement options for those who aspire to move beyond the treatment room. Team leader, assistant spa manager, spa director, and even spa owner are all possibilities for the business-minded and extremely motivated practitioner.

> "Diamonds are only lumps of coal that stuck to their jobs.
> —B.C. Forbes

Although the majority of spas hire practitioners as employees, some day spas and dental spas prefer to establish independent contractor relationships with practitioners, where the practitioners run their own businesses underneath the umbrella of the spa.

All spas share common characteristics, and the overall working environment can be similar. After we acquaint you with the big picture view of spas, we provide insights into the different types of spas.

As in any business, spas have rules, expectations, and guidelines that exist to ensure profitability. By appreciating the business side of spa work, you pave the way to success. Interview several wellness practitioners who work in specific spa environments that interest you to gain more insights into the pros and cons of those working environments.

Once you've identified a spa that most interests you, do some research before contacting them for an interview. Collect brochures or website information about the spa and its mission. Learn about its history, its clients, its spa treatments, and its unique qualities compared to competitors. During the interview, ask the right questions to find out if this particular spa is a good fit for you, such as:

- What is the spa's vision?
- How long is a shift?
- What other spa services are employees required to perform?
- What are the expectations regarding retail sales?

- What type of orientation and training program do you provide?
- How much time is allotted between clients?
- What kind of employee turnover do you have?
- Is there a strong team environment?
- Does the spa value open communication and employee feedback?
- What is the required dress code?
- How are practitioners compensated?
- Is there a continuing education allowance?
- How does seniority affect booking and compensation?

Figure 8.1 Wide World of Spas

Type of Spa	Clientele
Day Spa	Clients seek wellness, rejuvenation, beautifying, relaxing, or pampering experiences that last for several hours or the entire day.
Resort Spa or Luxury Hotel Spa	Vacation or business travelers seek beautifying, relaxing, stress-reducing, or pampering experiences.
Destination Spa	Clients seek to make healthy lifestyle changes, enhance their wellbeing, or rejuvenate from the stresses of a high pressure career. Destination spa settings often offer the widest variety of wellness services under one roof.
Cruise Ship Spa	Passengers seek beautifying, relaxing, or pampering experiences for several hours or an entire day.
Medical or Dental Spa	Clients who enjoy the convenience of spa-like services as an adjunct to their medical or dental visits. Clients undergoing surgical procedures may seek therapeutic spa services to enhance the healing process, promote relaxation, and support skin beautification. Services may include massage, craniosacral therapy, acupuncture, reflexology, professional skin care, manicures, and pedicures.

Boost your chances of getting hired and increase your compensation rate by obtaining certification or advanced training in spa specialty therapies such as aromatherapy, reflexology, body wraps, or energy work. A benefit of working in spas is that they often pay to train you in these modalities. Take advantage of opportunities to expand your knowledge base and skill portfolio by attending in-house training programs. Learning adjunct treatments can help prevent burnout and reduce repetitive stress injuries.

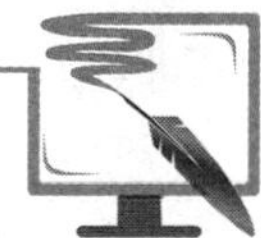

Identify Spa Modalities

Research the various modalities that are offered at spas. Make a list and note the service in which you are both trained and experienced in giving. Next, highlight the modalities you don't know well, but interest you, and include taking those trainings into your goals. Also, note any modalities that you know, but need to hone your skills, and find some willing folks on whom you can practice.

While most of the major ethical concerns of working in a spa are similar to those in any type of practice, the spa environment contributes additional twists. The areas of greatest concern are: establishing appropriate boundaries; working outside the scope of practice; not having a detailed intake form to identify a client's health issues; and breaches of confidentiality.

The Ethics of Touch[3] suggests these ethical guidelines for Spa Employees:

- Know the goals, mission, and standards of the spa.
- Conform to corporate image and represent unity to clients.
- Utilize established means of communications with management, especially treatments you're willing to do and training you're willing to undertake.
- Know your scope of practice and contraindications to treatments.
- Maintain professional standards and client confidentiality at all times.
- Avoid dual relationships with management, peers, and clients.
- Participate in marketing and product sales, when required.

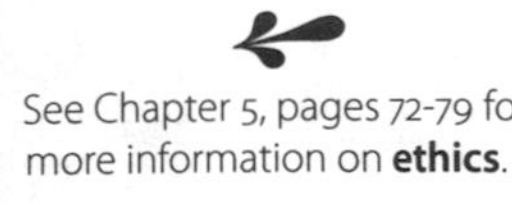

See Chapter 5, pages 72-79 for more information on **ethics**.

Key Aspects of Spa Settings

The following are some of the key aspects to consider when working in any type of spa: corporate culture, training, scheduling, treatment space, expanded responsibilities, confidentiality, contraindications, scope of practice, seniority, and boundaries.

Corporate Culture

Follow the spa's hands-on protocols regarding how clients are to be treated (e.g., greeting, draping, the session sequence). Be aware that most spa visitors are called guests, not clients, but for consistency in this book, we refer to them as clients. Consistency is paramount to spas. They want to make sure that clients receive the same service from all practitioners. Most spas, particularly destination spas, are team environments. Be a team player. Learn which spa treatments complement what you do to create the most effective and integrated experience for the guest.

Training

While some spas provide comprehensive training programs, others provide minimal or no training (also known as "sink or swim"). When interviewing for a spa job, ask about orientation and training programs. If you ascertain in advance that the training program is skimpy and you still decide to take the job, adjust your expectations accordingly so you can better weather the first weeks of your new job.

Training issues are not limited to orientation. Problematic situations can arise when a spa expects a practitioner to teach proprietary treatment modalities to other practitioners, even though this may break the professional agreement between the treatment owner and the practitioner. In contrast, highly ethical spas hire professional trainers to facilitate workshops on products, treatments, and other types of continuing education, which may include topics such as sexual harassment and nonviolent communication.

Scheduling

The most challenging aspect of spa or salon work often relates to scheduling. Before accepting employment, determine if the scheduling policies allow you to work at a comfortable pace that accommodates your special modalities and style of working. Some spas may require 5-7 client sessions per shift. Others may require a hectic pace of 10-12 sessions per shift, sometimes without breaks between 50-minute sessions. Some progressive spas actually book a full 15 minutes between sessions.

Clarify scheduling practices prior to accepting employment so you can clearly understand what's expected. Learn how to do a session in the allotted time (usually 50 minutes for the treatment and 10 minutes turnaround time) without appearing rushed. Many spas require weekend and evening shifts, while others require working on holidays. If you work as an independent contractor, you might not have to adhere to these rules. If you just rent space in the facility, then you can set your own pace.

Expect and plan for slow seasons or open times between client appointments. If you aren't expected to perform other spa-related job duties during these times, bring reading materials, catch up on correspondence, listen to relaxation music, or enjoy some simple yoga stretches.

Spas often offer a wide variety of services. Be aware of how your service is currently marketed. Keep track of your bookings. Communicate regularly with the staff to learn about marketing plans and ask how you may assist (possibly unpaid) in promoting your service.

Treatment Space

In most cases, the room you work in constantly changes. This can be from day to day or even session to session. It can be a challenge to focus when the room isn't yours (e.g., it lacks your personality, layout may not be what you prefer). Additionally, the treatment room may not be adequately sized or insulated, and the equipment may vary from room to room. It can require some adaptability to adjust to these working conditions.

Expanded Responsibilities

Some spas ask employee practitioners to expand their skills and perform other spa treatments, such as hydrotherapy, seaweed body wraps, and paraffin treatments, when not providing their primary service. Overcome any phobia you have for selling products and other spa services. Most spas expect practitioners to generate from 5-20% of their total sales in home-care products or supplies (and up to 50% for estheticians).

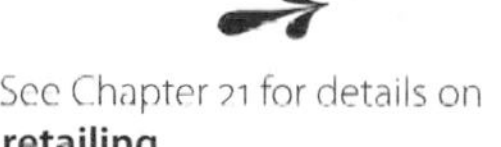

See Chapter 21 for details on **retailing**.

In addition, some facilities expect practitioners to assist wherever they're needed, from greeting clients to cleaning. These expectations may be present even when practitioners are not paid for non-client interactions. Ask questions in the interview about such spa policies so you can know what to expect if you're hired.

Confidentiality

Confidentiality issues can sometimes occur in a spa setting—either due to the physical environment (a lack of private space) or less than professional behavior on the part of staff. Management's role is to clearly communicate and oversee professional standards and behavior. According to standard confidentiality guidelines applicable to wellness practitioners, any information shared between client and practitioner during a session or related to a session remains private (e.g., client names, details of treatment, information shared by clients during a session are not discussed by the practitioner with anyone else). If you work at a high-end spa or wellness center, management expects strict adherence to confidentiality policies. Many celebrities, or other high-profile individuals, count on a spa and its employees to "go the extra mile" to protect their privacy.

Contraindications

You may sometimes encounter situations in which you have a concern about working with certain clients when contraindications are present such as: clients who take certain medications; those with suspicious skin conditions; clients with uncontrolled high blood pressure; those who request work you feel is inappropriate; and clients arriving under the influence of drugs or alcohol.

Because it's essential to accommodate clients with medical conditions, industry best practices dictate that a spa provide an intake form that includes health history, and allot proper time for any needed discussion between practitioner and client. If you find that an intake form is missing in your work environment, design an appropriate intake form and diplomatically raise the issue to management with the solution in hand. An intake form protects you, the client, and the long-term reputation of the spa where you work.

Design a Simple Intake Form

Pretend you work in a spa that doesn't have an intake form. Create a simple intake form that addresses the contraindications for your services. Next, make a list of the most important reasons you could present to your employer for utilizing such a form.

> "There is no respect for others without humility in one's self.
> —Henri Amiel

Develop good recordkeeping habits to ensure client files are complete and current. This helps you track client progress and be aware of potential contraindications, and it also provides a useful reference point for each session. Clients appreciate this type of thorough and professional attention to their unique needs.

Scope of Practice

Sometimes a client asks for a service that is outside of your skill set. For instance, a receptionist may book a specific service even if it isn't clear that the practitioner on duty is proficient in that technique. If the service is within your scope of practice, but not within your current skill set, commit to learning additional services offered at the spa.

Seniority

Seniority works a bit differently at every spa, and it can affect both your salary and volume of client bookings. Like many other aspects of employment, it's a good idea to learn about seniority policies before you accept a job—rather than be surprised after you join the spa.

This can mean that during every hour that calls are accepted for appointments, the person with the most seniority gets booked first, then the next person and so on. The next hour, the process starts all over again. Thus, practitioners with high seniority may be fully booked for the day and you may have no clients for that day. Obviously, this system is less than desirable for a new practitioner. Nonetheless, if you decide to work at such a spa in spite of this initial drawback, factor this in and budget accordingly until you can move up in seniority.

Fortunately, many spas use a more balanced seniority system, such as a rotation system that favors seniority yet makes an effort to even out the bookings.

Although the seniority system can be frustrating to new practitioners, you can increase your chances of getting more client bookings by being trained in as many modalities as possible that the spa offers. The wider range of skills you offer, the better chance you will be needed in any given time slot. Many spas also have a tiered pay system that takes into account your years of experience plus the modalities you offer. Also, spas may pay you a different rate for different treatments, such as a higher rate for more physically demanding or labor-intensive treatments.

Boundaries

Understanding boundaries is crucial to creating an ethical practice, building professional relationships, and succeeding in a spa environment. By increasing awareness of client boundaries (as well as our own), we can improve the therapeutic relationship and avoid inadvertent slips into unethical behavior. Unfortunately, boundaries are often blurred in a spa environment, given that people can play a variety of roles. Some spas have strict rules about boundaries and dual relationships, particularly regarding guests and practitioners.

Figure 8.2 Success Tips for Working in All Spa Environments

- Know the rules, expectations, and guidelines of the business.
- Review policy and procedure manuals, clarify any ambiguous policies.
- Follow the spa's hands-on protocols regarding how clients are to be treated.
- Communicate regularly with the staff.
- Be a team player.
- Make an effort to express your views, and then release your expectations.
- Learn and practice conscious detachment.
- Be aware of how your service is currently marketed, ask how you may assist.
- Keep track of your bookings.
- Develop good record keeping habits.
- Attend in-house training programs.
- Overcome any phobia you have for selling products and services.
- Adapt to changes in treatment rooms and working conditions.
- Be prepared to work long shifts with few breaks.
- Learn how to do multiple sessions without appearing rushed.
- Practice good body mechanics and stretch regularly to avoid injuries.
- Expect and plan for slow seasons or open times between appointments.
- Recognize what the spa does for you and appreciate the benefits.

Day Spas and Salons

Day spas account for almost 80% of all spas in the U.S.[4] The ISPA defines a day spa as: "an establishment that provides beautifying, relaxing or pampering experiences that can last an hour or may take a whole day."[5] Many day spas embrace the true origin of the meaning of spa, "taking the waters," and focus on wellness and rejuvenation. The phrase, "taking the waters" refers to drinking or bathing in the famed, mineral-rich waters of Bath, England.[6] A day spa can be a stand-alone business venue or connected to a luxury hotel, resort, health retreat, cruise ship, or department store.

See Chapter 7, pages 123-127 for information about **being self-employed**.

The ambiance in day spas can range from spare and simple to elegant and opulent. Whatever the means, whatever the style, all day spas aim to create a haven of tranquility and rejuvenation for clients. Working in these surroundings is pleasant. Spa clients are usually easygoing and generous in expressing their appreciation. Staff is usually available to handle marketing, scheduling, confirmation calls, and financial transactions. A potential downside of this environment is that you might be responsible for generating most of your client base.

Some day spas promote themselves to the masses, while others target niche markets, such as upscale clients, aging baby boomers, moms and babies, or young professionals. In recent years, a new breed of discount spas and spa chains have emerged that offer high-quality services at affordable prices. Another growing market niche is "men-only" spas. Men now compose more than 47% of all U.S. spa-goers.[7] As the day spa market continues to flourish, so do employment opportunities for wellness practitioners.

Salons, which many classify as a close cousin to day spas, range from bustling turnstiles to tranquil escapes from everyday stress. Although most day spas hire wellness practitioners as employees, opportunities may arise to work as an independent contractor in this type of setting. Salons customarily rent rooms to practitioners and rarely have more than 3 wellness providers (usually somatic practitioners and estheticians).

Salons provide you with a built-in clientele of people who need your services—the other employees!

In certain salons or day spas, you're assigned a permanent treatment room, and you can personalize the decor to some extent. In most cases, you share the treatment room with other practitioners. A potential drawback is that some treatment rooms are located in close proximity to other salon activities and lack room-specific temperature control units. Some aren't well-insulated from sounds and odors. Ideally, arrange the treatment room so it isn't adjacent to hair designer stations (to avoid the intrusive noise of hair dryers) or where harsh chemicals are used.

Be prepared to include all of the supplies and equipment in your operating budget if you're an independent contractor. Most salons require you to provide those items, particularly linens, lubricants, treatment chairs, or massage tables.

Day Spa Association
dayspaassociation.com
Spa Finder
www.spafinder.com
Salon Employment
www.salonemployment.com

In this setting, you must actively and consistently market your services through brochures, special introductory offers, gift certificate programs, or other means. In general, body therapies and other wellness services are of primary interest to day spa visitors. In contrast, building a successful wellness practice in a salon may require considerably more time and effort. If you work in a salon, place your business cards and brochures on display at the reception desk. Create good signage. Have the front desk place your brochure in the bags when clients purchase products. Make sure that everyone who works at the salon experiences your services. Be visible. Give free demonstrations of your products or services to clients waiting for other services. Offer referral incentives. Hold educational meetings for your co-workers: explain the benefits of your work; give demonstrations; and show them tips for self-care.

Figure 8.3 Specific Success Tips for Working in Day Spas and Salons

- **Build long-term relationships**. It can be very rewarding to track a client's progress over time and tailor ongoing sessions to support a client's health and wellness goals.
- **Follow-up**. If you haven't seen a client for awhile, place a follow-up call to ask how she is, and invite her to visit the spa again.
- **Keep detailed records**. Be sure to indicate which clients are locals. Review locals' files monthly and follow up as appropriate.
- **Adapt your treatment space**. Ideally, have your room be in an area that is isolated from sounds and smells.
- **Market yourself appropriately and abundantly**. Invest time in developing a client retention plan in addition to attracting new clients.

Cruise Ship Spas

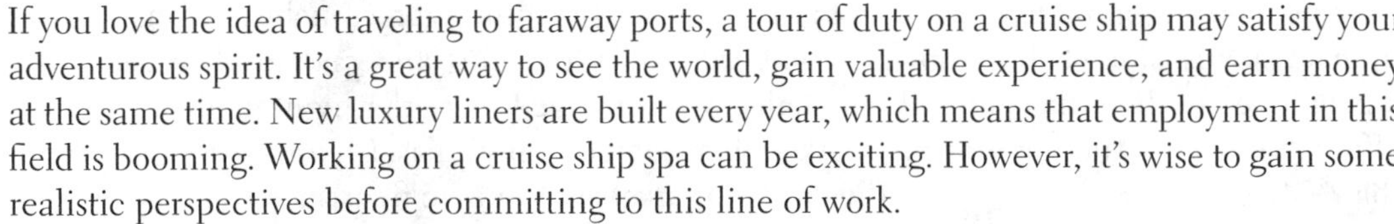

Cruise Jobs
www.theonboardspa.com
www.indeed.com
www.cruiseshipjob.com

If you love the idea of traveling to faraway ports, a tour of duty on a cruise ship may satisfy your adventurous spirit. It's a great way to see the world, gain valuable experience, and earn money at the same time. New luxury liners are built every year, which means that employment in this field is booming. Working on a cruise ship spa can be exciting. However, it's wise to gain some realistic perspectives before committing to this line of work.

The positive aspects of working in this setting are: the opportunity to get lots of experience under your belt (especially attractive to new practitioners); a major change of pace from wherever you are now; the opportunity to meet and make friends with crew members from all over the world; the ability to save some money if you budget wisely; and plenty of travel to exotic destinations. During off-time, you're free to do anything you like, just like a passenger, which includes going into port when the ship docks.

The potential downside is that life on a cruise ship can be trying at times. A cruise ship spa can be very different from working at a land-based spa. A 12-hour workday is standard aboard ship. The number of sessions you're expected to give per day is higher than other working environments. You could easily do 10 or more treatments per day, although some days you may only do 4 to 6 sessions. Wellness practitioners often administer a variety of spa treatments outside their specialty and are expected to comfortably and successfully sell beauty and wellness products. You're likely to have other guest-care responsibilities, as well as logistical chores, such as doing laundry or helping out in another department.

Generally, you get one and a half days off per week. It can require patience and determination to ride out rough seas and cramped living quarters. In many cases, you may share quarters with 1-3 strangers. It's common to encounter very little personal privacy. In some cases, you may find a lack of healthy food in the crew cafeteria. Lastly, you're away from home for long periods of time.

Although training programs vary, depending on the cruise line, often many luxury cruise lines offer corporate training and orientation programs that span from 2-8 weeks. Recruits learn about the essentials of customer service, the realities of working on cruises, and how to become skilled in specialized treatment offerings.

§3

The employment process typically begins with wellness practitioners signing an employment contract for anywhere from 4-9 months, and living on a ship with room and board and laundry services provided. Prior experience working on a cruise ship isn't necessary. An upbeat attitude, high energy, flexibility, and the ability to sell wellness products are a plus. Compensation varies widely depending on season and ship. A good portion of your income may depend on product sales. Benefits may include medical insurance and reduced-price vacations for family and friends.

Beware of fictitious companies on the Internet that pretend to be legitimate agencies for employment on cruise ships. You should not pay a fee for a list of current job openings or to submit your résumé to a cruise ship company. Also, don't fall for a "no-risk guarantee" of employment from a website that requires you to pay a fee. There is no such thing as a guarantee of employment.

"Champions keep playing until they get it right.

—Billie Jean King

Figure 8.4 Specific Success Tips for Working in Cruise Ship Spas

- **Expect demanding work conditions**. Treatment rooms can be cramped, and long hours are the norm.
- **Have an upbeat attitude, high energy, and be flexible**. As an employee on a cruise ship, you must be "on" nearly 24 hours a day. For all that time, you're expected to represent your company to the public, which means that you must always show a sunny personality.
- **Be in excellent physical and emotional condition**. Stamina, good boundaries, an open heart, and an open mind may be essential to survival.

Destination, Resort, and Luxury Hotel Spas

Destination spas, resort spas, and luxury hotel spas share commonalities. These establishments cater to an affluent clientele with high expectations of customer service from both management and practitioners. Surroundings are elegant, the ambiance is tranquil. The equipment tends to be first-rate and products are high quality. Unfortunately, little opportunity exists to build repeat business on a long-term basis, although guests often develop an appreciation for a highly skilled practitioner and schedule several visits during their stay. Practitioners are usually fully booked unless their service is uncommon or it's a slow season.

Resort and Luxury Hotel Spas

Resort and luxury hotel spas are very similar. Working at a resort spa in the Bahamas, Hawaii, or the Caribbean is a great way to meet new friends and enjoy an island lifestyle. Whether you prefer ocean, mountain, or desert resorts, a variety of spa jobs are located in these settings. You may also like some perks of the job—employees often get discounts on spa services so they can rest and rejuvenate at their leisure.

Working at a luxury hotel spa in an urban area can be very similar to working at a day spa. The pace is usually brisk and the surroundings are pleasant. Most clients are vacationers or business travelers in town for a short visit. At some luxury hotel spas, people from the local community enjoy visiting the spa and partaking of its services. These clients often forge long-term customer relationships with favorite practitioners.

A potential advantage of working in this type of a spa environment is career longevity. Because practitioners are often expected to perform a variety of spa treatments, this reduces the likelihood of repetitive stress syndrome, as some types of treatments are less taxing on the body than others. For instance, a day can be divided into 70% massage sessions and 25% treatments like salt glows and body wraps. The rest of the time is spent in escorting clients to treatment rooms and completing paperwork.

Spa work at resort and luxury hotel spas can be demanding for all types of practitioners, but especially for massage therapists. In general, the turnover rate is quite high, however, this is not always the case, as some practitioners have found an enjoyable career niche working at resort and luxury hotel spas on a long-term basis. A lot depends on finding the right scheduling situation, with the right team and the right compensation.

Destination Spas

A destination spa is an upscale health retreat dedicated solely to guests who come for weeklong or weekend spa programs. These types of spas are often located in the mountains or near the ocean where guests can enjoy the peace and beauty of nature while experiencing every amenity imaginable. Guests usually visit these spas to enhance their health, make lifestyle changes, or rejuvenate from the stresses of a high-pressure career. Clients include executives, celebrities, professional athletes, health-conscious families, aging baby boomers, and just about anyone interested in enhanced wellbeing.

If you work at a destination spa, developing a client base becomes more a matter of retaining a "guest" and that guest's friends. As some long-time practitioners working in these settings have observed, guests often tell their friends if they find an exceptionally good practitioner. Often these guests and their friends return year after year, and request the same practitioner. Word-of-mouth is a powerful force in building clientele, particularly when a client experiences a deeply relaxing session, gets relief from a troubling pain syndrome, or learns from a nutritionist how simple modification can make a profound change in her life.

Figure 8.5 Specific Success Tips for Working in Destination, Resort, or Luxury Hotel Spas

- **Time your application to arrive prior to the beginning of the busy season**. You may have a better chance of getting interviewed.
- **Polish your customer service skills**. Clients expect to be catered to and demand exceptional customer service.
- **Develop advanced training and a wide portfolio of skills**. Reduce the repetitive nature of busy schedules by offering a variety of session options.
- **Build stamina**. Practitioners may perform from 8 to 10 one-hour sessions each day. The pace can be demanding, especially during the busy season at resorts.

Medical and Dental Spas

The phenomenon of medical spas started in the mid-1990s and has continued to thrive as holistic approaches to health and beauty have gained in popularity. Most medical spas are owned and managed by dermatologists or board-certified plastic surgeons. Medical spas cater to the luxury market, offering a menu of cosmetic surgery procedures, holistic health services, and skin rejuvenation treatments. The services may range from massage therapy, acupuncture, aromatherapy, and facials, to modern laser therapies, injections, and plastic surgery procedures such as facelifts. It's generally acknowledged that medical patients who schedule concurrent holistic health treatments often heal faster, feel less pain, and have a decreased medication dependency after surgery. Most medical spas have high professional standards and seek practitioners who are highly educated and skilled in using appropriate medical terminology.

In recent years, massage therapy has solidified its presence in traditional health care due to validated outcome measures (i.e., proven results). Massage is generally recognized as one of the key therapeutic interventions that support effective pain management.

You're likely to find a trickling waterfall or soothing candles in your dentist's office too. According to an American Dental Association survey[8], a growing number of dentists say spa-like amenities and services persuade patients to make and keep appointments and help them stay relaxed during dental procedures. Spa services such as massage, facials, manicures, pedicures, reflexology, acupuncture, and craniosacral therapy are welcome amenities to time-pressed dental customers—or to customers that dread visits to the dentist.

Spa services offered by doctors and dentists vary widely depending on the demographics and preferences of customers. Some offer full-service massage therapy within their office setting, while others find that 10-minute chair massages, facials, and manicures are more popular. Although some doctors and dentists don't refer to their offices as spas, they pamper loyal customers and attract new ones by offering practical and relaxing spa-style comforts. A busy medical or dental spa might hire a practitioner as an employee, while others hire them as independent contractors.

With the right doctor or dentist, it's possible to gain many referrals and build a loyal following fairly quickly. Most offices who offer wellness services do so because they believe in them and want happy patients. This element of support boosts your chance of success.

Figure 8.6 Specific Success Tips for Working in Medical and Dental Spas

- **Do your own market research**. Search the internet for information about medical and dental spas throughout the country for insights into operations and how they market themselves.
- **Educate yourself**. Gain credibility by becoming familiar with medical terminology and recordkeeping specific to medical and surgical procedures.
- **Be flexible**. Medical settings often require adaptability and flexibility due to unexpected scheduling twists or changes to patient conditions.

9
An Insider's Look at Primary Healthcare Settings

"What is the recipe for successful achievement?
To my mind there are just four essential ingredients:
Choose a career you love, give it the best there is in you,
seize your opportunities, and be a member of the team."
— Benjamin F. Fairless

What to Expect
- Key Aspects of Primary Healthcare Settings

Hospitals and Hospice

Medical Clinics

Key Terms

Acupuncture
Care Coordination
Case Management
Case Manager
Chiropractic
Complementary and Alternative Medicine (CAM)
Health Insurance Portability and Accountability Act (HIPAA)
Hospice
Hospital
Massage Therapy
Medical Clinic
Midwifery
Multidisciplinary Team
Naturopathic Medicine
Osteopathy
Primary Care Provider (PCP)
Primary Health Care

In response to the public's growing interest in Complementary and Alternative Medicine (CAM) therapies, an increasing number of hospitals are establishing adjunct clinics for services such as chiropractic, massage therapy, and acupuncture. Others hospitals integrate CAM programs directly into their operating environments.

Primary healthcare settings may include hospitals or clinics, such as a rehabilitation center, medical center, sports medicine clinic, physical therapy clinic, or an orthopedic physician's office.

What to Expect

Working in a medical setting requires the integration of the CAM therapy into a multidisciplinary team as a key member, where the wellness practitioners work in tandem with medical doctors or physical therapists. In a hospital setting, you may become a part of the medical team treating trauma patients, amputees, cancer survivors, or burn survivors. You may be treating a client prior to surgery to enhance relaxation and reduce stress. Treatments may be on an inpatient or outpatient basis.

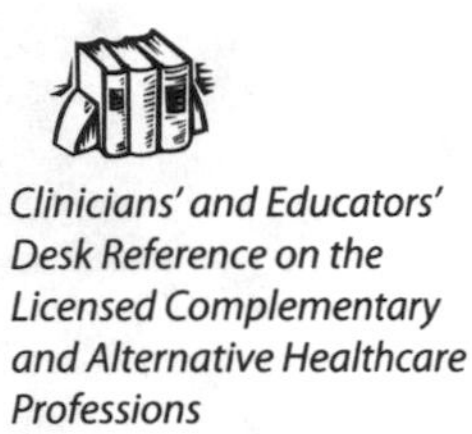

Clinicians' and Educators' Desk Reference on the Licensed Complementary and Alternative Healthcare Professions

Determine what type of medical practice or specialty attracts you. Learn about it and the types of clients it helps. Interview several wellness practitioners who work in specific primary healthcare settings that interest you to gain more insights into the pros and cons of those working environments. Ascertain the specific skill set needed to be successful in this environment. For example, somatic practitioners are much more employable if they also are trained in lymphatic drainage, myofascial release, aquatic massage, and scar massage. Most practitioners discover that they need to alter their treatments or scope of practice in a clinic setting. The time you spend with clients and the actual work you do may be determined by the lead primary care provider (PCP). You may be directed very specifically on what to do, how to do it, and the time allotted.

One of the advantages of working in a medical setting is the opportunity to develop ongoing relationships with clients and observe outcomes of care over time. It can be very rewarding to see a client endure and triumph during a difficult healing journey. However, in some cases, you may see a client for only a limited number of treatments. As the settings vary, it's important to understand what's expected of you in any medical environment.

The Academic Consortium for Complementary and Alternative Health Care (ACCAHC) is a collaboration of academics from 5 disciplines (chiropractic, naturopathic medicine, massage therapy, acupuncture and Oriental medicine, and direct-entry midwifery). In 2010 they published the *Competencies for Optimal Practices in Integrated Environments*.[1] This document outlines the essential skills for all healthcare practitioners interested in practice opportunities in interdisciplinary, inpatient, and outpatient environments.

Key Aspects of Primary Healthcare Settings

The following are some key considerations when working in any type of primary healthcare setting: administration; additional training; care coordination and case management; and research opportunities.

Administration

Developing an awareness of the various organizational structures and chains of command typical in these settings is critical to success. Practitioners who work in a medical setting or clinic are expected to participate in various activities in addition to direct client treatment, such as completing various medical reports, participating in team meetings, and documenting daily workload. Working agreements may be negotiated as an employee or independent contractor, usually either by on-site appointments or contracted hours. If you're a private practitioner, allot ample time to market your services to attract new clients and obtain referrals from physicians.

No matter your classification, you're expected to conform to the organization's structure the same as any employee.

Additional Training

A high degree of knowledge and skill is vital to effectively and safely treat clients with medical conditions. You need to have excellent clinical skills, such as assessment, clear identification of short- and long-term treatment plans, and techniques appropriate to specific conditions. In addition, specific protocols, procedures, documentation, and medical language are used by clinicians and physicians in hospital and clinic settings. Fluency in these practices and terminology is required to participate as an inclusive member of the healthcare team.

Broaden your employment possibilities by learning a variety of techniques for assorted medical conditions. Seek to understand the benefits of treatment for each medical condition, as well as conditions for which a CAM procedure is contraindicated. For instance, a client with cancer requires a different approach than a client that is scheduling a session for relaxation prior to surgery.

§3

Care Coordination and Case Management

Some hospitals or clinics have designated case managers whose exclusive role is to coordinate care and services among providers. The purpose of case management is to help clients more effectively reach positive health outcomes. Wellness practitioners need to understand the case management processes of assessment, planning, implementation, coordination, and evaluation, which takes superior critical thinking, communication, and collaborative skills.

In the U.S., changes in health insurance laws and the Affordable Care Act, may allow your client to bill her insurance for your services, along with services from the other practitioners involved in the case. Knowledge of insurance billing procedures, as well as HIPAA compliance, should be integral with your care coordination training.

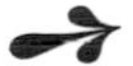

See Chapter 19, pages 264-273 for more information on **HIPAA compliance and insurance reimbursement**.

Research Opportunities

To ensure the ongoing success of CAM programs, most hospitals and clinics develop practices that incorporate standard outcome measures, such as the McGill Pain Rating, Vancouver Burn Scar Index, Goniometry (for measuring range of motion), or the Arizona Integrative Outcomes Scale. These measuring tools enable practitioners to identify the therapeutic outcomes and benefits to clients in a language shared by all healthcare professionals. Evidence documenting a program's effectiveness is key in the long-term viability of CAM programs. As wellness research continues to evolve, you may have the opportunity to contribute to research studies or be asked to share periodic research findings with physicians and administrators.

After you gain some solid experience working in medical settings, consider volunteering. Many cities have formed organizations that offer free wellness care to hospital patients, especially those with AIDS and people in hospice care.

Figure 9.1 Overall Success Tips for Working in a Primary Healthcare Setting

- **Interview several wellness practitioners**. Talk with practitioners who work in a hospital or clinic to gain insights into these environments.
- **Educate yourself**. Gain credibility by being well versed in medical terminology and recordkeeping specific to different types of medical practices.
- **Know the limitations.** Familiarize yourself with current contraindications for medical conditions.
- **Learn proper documentation**. Know how to conduct research and how to measure therapeutic outcomes. Medical settings often rely on funding from agencies that require this type of documentation.
- **Be flexible**. Medical settings often require adaptability and flexibility due to unexpected scheduling twists or changes in client conditions.

Hospitals and Hospice

Many wellness practitioners work in hospital or hospice settings, either as employees, independent contractors, or volunteers. The clinical considerations in these environments can vary greatly from the environments with which many such professionals are familiar. Adherence to HIPAA is more strictly enforced, as access to sensitive and detailed medical and health history information is greater. It's also typical to be working as part of a team made up of a variety of other professionals like physicians, nurses, and occupational, physical, or respiratory therapists; all working together within an established plan of care for each patient.[2]

See Chapter 5, page 87 for more on **volunteering**.

Practitioners may treat patients with many conditions not seen in non-hospital settings, such as trauma patients, amputees, cancer survivors, burn victims, patients preparing for or recovering from surgeries, and patients preparing to die. An excellent working knowledge of medical terminology and contraindications for medical conditions is essential to communicate concerns to the medical team. Document patient sessions carefully. A record of a wellness session is usually placed in a patient file for reference by other team members, such as the patient care coordinator or primary care provider.

In some hospitals, wellness practitioners are fully integrated as paid employees working within a funded program with full access to medical records. In other cases, practitioners are permitted only to work with ostensibly healthy staff members, often as part of a wellness program or a hospital's attempt to provide self-care options for clinicians.

Many practitioners find working in a hospice program rewarding and fulfilling. In medieval times, the word "hospice" referred to a way station where travelers were cared for and refreshed. Today, hospice programs combine advanced medical technology with compassionate care, enabling individuals with terminal or incurable health conditions to live as fully and comfortably as possible, in familiar surroundings, in the company of family and friends.

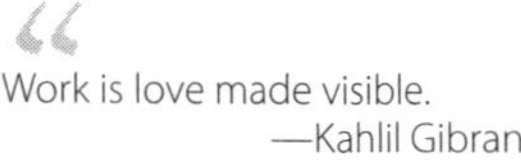

Work is love made visible.
—Kahlil Gibran

Those who apply to a hospice program are usually required to have an opinion from a medical professional that their disease is likely to lead to death in 6 months or less. Although some hospice programs are part of medical centers, the majority of hospice programs offer in-home care and support. People of all ages are admitted to hospice programs. In this setting, you may very well work with patients from 3 to 93 years old.

In hospice settings, practitioners generally work on a part-time basis. If not volunteering, practitioners usually work as independent contractors who receive a flat rate fee that doesn't include travel time to patients' homes. Once a referral is made through the hospice program, a practitioner often continues visits on a weekly or bimonthly basis. Practitioners should request a clear working directive from the medical team, patient, and family regarding how to approach the work with each patient.

Hospice work can be emotionally demanding. Honestly evaluate your readiness to undertake such work. You must be able to maintain equilibrium in the presence of the patient and family. It's wise to have some outlet, such as supervisory or peer support, to help manage your emotional responses to intense session work.

Figure 9.2 Specific Success Tips for Working in a Hospital or Hospice

- **Ensure you have access** to medical history, care plannings, and impressions recorded by other members of patient care teams.
- **Ask to be included in hospital-wide notifications**, trainings, updates, and Grand Rounds.
- **Offer to provide "in-service" trainings** to the clinicians about the benefits and appropriateness of your services.
- **Connect with the Employee Health Office** to ensure that you have all immunizations and protections in place.
- **Prepare yourself mentally**. Working with seriously ill or dying patients can be emotionally taxing. Many practitioners prefer part-time work of this nature.
- **Establish a support system with hospital or hospice-based colleagues**. Many considerations in these settings are unlike those in private practice or other outpatient settings.

§3

Medical Clinics

Medical clinics are like hospitals in the sense that both are staffed by professionals who can assess, diagnose, and treat patients. The main differences between clinics and hospitals are in terms of scope. A clinic may be headed by a single practicing physician (PCP) while a hospital has a complex leadership hierarchy. Clinics have limited hours while hospitals run 24 hours a day. Clinics work on an outpatient basis while hospitals have inpatient wards. When a clinic sees a patient who has suffered a severe trauma, or whose condition has worsened beyond the ability to be cared for by the patient herself or in the home, then the clinic refers the patient to a hospital.[3]

Clinics manage patients' wellness care and supervise home treatment regimens for chronic conditions. The clinic specialty is determined by the combined skills of its staff and the purpose of its practice. A general outpatient clinic may have primary care physicians in several practice areas that provide the main health care for a community. Specialized clinics include rehabilitation centers, physical therapy clinics, sports medicine clinics, orthopedic physician's offices, and immunologist practices. Many somatic practitioners work in these types of clinic environments in tandem with medical doctors or physical therapists.

When joining a medical clinic, consider the following: the possibility of needing to alter your style and scope of practice to suit the clinic's visions, policies, and procedures; and the issue of being hired as an independent contractor versus employee.

To avoid future complications, be sure the clinic attracts the kind of clients with whom you want to work, provides opportunities for you to use your favorite modalities, and allows you to work at the pace and in the style with which you're comfortable. Many practitioners discover they need to alter their treatments in a clinic setting. The time you spend with clients and the actual work you do may be determined by the lead care physician. As in hospital settings, you could be told what to do, how to do it, when to do it, and the time allowed to work. You may even experience a sense of detachment from the client because someone else usually handles the greeting, scheduling, payment, paperwork, and, sometimes even, the follow-up.

On the positive side, freedom from administrative tasks provides you with more hands-on time with your clients. In addition, your clients benefit from your association with the clinic because the setting provides access to managed care and possibly to state-of-the-art equipment that you, otherwise, might not afford.

Figure 9.3 **Specific Success Tips for Working in a Medical Clinic**

- **Ensure you have access** to medical history, care plannings, and impressions recorded by other members of patient care teams.
- **Adhere to clinic policies** for dress code, finances, logistics, practitioner/practitioner interactions, client/practitioner interactions, and marketing.
- **Build long-term relationships**. It can be very rewarding to track a client's progress over time and tailor ongoing sessions to support the client's and healthcare team's overall goals.
- **Keep detailed records**. Be sure to follow the clinic's guidelines for charting, and follow up as appropriate.
- **Accept direction from medical personnel**. You must be willing to defer to the primary care provider (supervising physician or nurse) for critical care decision, and sometimes minor decisions as well.

10

An Insider's Look at Group Practice Settings

"Your profession is not what brings home your paycheck. Your profession is what you were put on earth to do with such passion and such intensity that it becomes spiritual in calling"

— Vincent Van Gogh

What to Expect

- Key Aspects of Group Practice Settings

Wellness Centers

Specialty Centers

Key Terms

Associate
Associations
Business Plan
Ethical Dilemma
Goals
Group Practice Settings
Holistic Healthcare Clinics
Image
Legal Status
Marketing
Medical Clinics
Office Logistics
Policy and Procedure Manual
Self-Assessment
Specialty Clinics
Values
Wellness Centers

Working for yourself can be rewarding, yet working by yourself can also be lonely. Joining an environment with other professionals can be a great way to add collaboration and camaraderie to your practice.

Many wellness practitioners join forces with other healthcare providers to create associations, group practices, and partnerships, potentially sharing some overhead expenses. It's also becoming more commonplace to hire practitioners as employees in these settings. The other professionals in these environments may be practitioners of your same discipline, or they may practice various other complementary therapies. You may share facilities, equipment, or staffing. You may promote yourself independently, market as a group, or share clients as assigned by an employer.

What to Expect

These alliances can be quite beneficial for the practitioners as well as for their clients. The benefits of a group practice are numerous. Many practitioners enjoy the camaraderie and creative synergy that happens when two or more professionals work together on case management or everyday brainstorming. In addition, group practice often provides a variety of wellness services under one roof, which can attract new clients and lead to greater income potential. If you're joining an established practice, the other benefits include access to a ready-made professional image and extensive office resources (e.g., staff to handle scheduling, greet clients, manage financial transactions), along with an increased sense of personal safety when dealing with problematic clients.

Group practice offers added flexibility when you're ill or want to take a vacation, as you can make arrangements with other staff to provide services for your clients during these times. Group practice can also be highly cost-effective. You often encounter reduced overhead and greater buying power via volume discounts on supplies and holistic healthcare products for resale. Lastly, it can be more fun and rewarding to share space with others in a team environment—providing the team works in harmony and shares professional values.

If you're interested in joining or establishing a group practice, the primary settings are holistic healthcare clinics, wellness centers, specialty clinics, or medical clinics. Typically, holistic healthcare clinics and wellness centers offer a variety of services, such as chiropractic, acupuncture, massage therapy, yoga, movement therapy, nutritional counseling, and aromatherapy. In contrast, specialty clinics focus on a single specialty, such as chiropractic, acupuncture, or massage therapy.

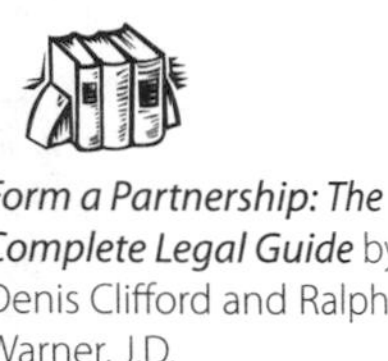

Form a Partnership: The Complete Legal Guide by Denis Clifford and Ralph Warner, J.D.

Group practices differ from medical clinics and hospitals in the services they offer and the purposes of the practice. In wellness settings, clients are primarily interested in preventive care, stress management, relief from everyday aches and pains, or support for various health challenges. Practitioners focus on identifying imbalances in the body, assisting clients in achieving their wellness goals, and educating and guiding clients about preventive measures they can practice at home.[1] A sub-category of group practices are specialty centers that focus on one of these modalities.

Some aspects of clinic or wellness center work require careful consideration if you join the group as an independent contractor. Finances tend to be complex, especially in view of the need to maintain fairness in shared expenses, client scheduling, and revenues from product sales. Clear, written agreements with other group practitioners are vital to avoid entanglements and misunderstandings. From a cash flow standpoint, keep in mind that if you're dealing with insurance reimbursement, you may not receive payment for months after you've done the work. Track your operating expenses and continuing education events so you can confidently raise your prices periodically to account for cost factors and your growing skill level. It is also usually easier to get insurance reimbursement if one of the practitioners is already a recognized primary care provider.

Unfortunately, too many people develop these alliances or take jobs in companies without creating a proper structure to clarify expectations and guide interactions, consequently, creating an environment where ethical dilemmas arise.

Group Practice Case Study

Steve, a chiropractor, decides to share an already established office with chiropractor, Terry. The office is situated in a prime location, and Steve has been feeling rather isolated in his practice. He has known Terry for several years and respects her work. Steve asks Terry to create an association agreement, but Terry refuses and acts offended. This red flag should have immediately sent Steve running in the opposite direction. Steve decides to proceed anyway. After all, they're both caring, responsible adults, and he feels confident they could work out any problems.

Things go fairly well for several years. Terry starts getting involved in accounts that take her outside of the office, so she brings in another chiropractor, Stacy, to work with clients in her treatment room. This is done without consulting Steve. Now there are 3 people sharing the total space, yet Steve is still paying half of the expenses. Resentment brews. Then Steve discovers something that sends him over the edge: Several times clients had called to book sessions with him when he wasn't in the office. Stacy talked with the clients and instead of trying to figure out another time when they could schedule with Steve, she booked the appointments for herself.

He could not resolve these issues, and no guidelines had been set for how to deal with unresolved conflicts. So Steve gives notice. He wants to leave as soon as possible but agrees to stay for several months. Meanwhile, things go from bad to worse. He feels uncomfortable in his own office. He realizes that communication is difficult, so when the time nears for him to leave, he submits a written, 30-day notice. The next day, Steve goes to work only to discover that the locks to the office had been changed. Ultimately, the situation gets resolved, but not without unnecessary grief and anger (as well as the intervention of an attorney).

Points to Ponder

Was Terry's behavior unreasonable? Was Stacy's behavior unethical? Think about other options that Steve could have pursued? What could he have done differently?

§3

Key Aspects of Group Practice Settings

You can avoid the pitfalls described above and garner the benefits of working with others by paying careful attention to some nuts and bolts of business start-up, such as the following: scheduling time for self-assessment; performing careful interviews with potential associates; clarifying roles, goals, and expectations; evaluating legal status options; defining image and marketing goals; creating a game plan for product sales; setting up financial operations; defining office logistics; and establishing scheduling procedures for clients. Although holistic healthcare clinics, wellness centers, specialty clinics, and medical clinics have unique aspects, they all share common operating and marketing challenges—and potential pitfalls. This section explores a range of aspects which can help you find a group practice setting that best matches your talents and interests.

Self-Assessment

The first phase in choosing a group practice is clarifying your reasons for wanting to share your business (or space) with another person, or for wanting to join an established practice. For instance, are you doing this because you want to or is it mainly stemming from financial considerations? Assess your temperament to determine if it's appropriate for you to have another person involved in your business. Think about how you want to share your space and how much control you need to exert. If you're uncomfortable when things aren't done in a specific manner, it may become difficult for you to share an office, let alone be in partnership or work as an employee.

If you decide to go ahead with the idea, you need to be clear about the desired relationship with your potential associate/partner/employer. Do you want others to play an active role in your business, or would you rather just have someone to share ideas and expenses? Consider that it might be beneficial to affiliate with someone who does something totally different from you. On the other hand, you may prefer someone who does similar work as you.

Interviews

After you've clarified your reasons for wanting to work in a group practice and have envisioned the qualities of the people with whom you want to work, it's time to conduct interviews. This process is helpful whether you're thinking of joining a practice or bringing someone into yours. Your closest friends or colleagues may not be the wisest choices when looking for a business partner. Invest the time required to do this well; after all, this is someone you may be seeing every day. Share with each other your goals and concerns. Some of the questions to consider are: How long do you intend to stay in this location? What kind of work schedule do you prefer to keep? What type of atmosphere do you want? Who do you want as clients? Do you want to be an employee? Do you ultimately want additional associates or employees? Do you plan on incorporating other services or products?

> "It's not hard to make decisions when you know what your values are.
>
> —Roy Disney

Look for the commonalities and possible areas of conflict. Do the different practitioners' types of services or individual businesses complement each other? Are your fee structures similar? Also, get to know each other's communication style and see if your personalities are compatible. Everyone has their own personality and way of doing things, and these styles don't always mesh well in a business setting. For example, if you prefer a methodical approach to business and your partner tends to work best under pressure or in chaos—you may be in for a tempestuous association.

Make certain the types of therapy offered aren't in conflict. For example, a massage therapist who works with elderly clients and does a lot of quiet guided meditations would not co-exist well with a counselor who does Primal Scream Therapy (which can get very noisy).

Common Values

Investigate whether your presence in the group practice would be a good fit. Ask about the types of clients who are seen at the group practice. Gain a clear understanding of target markets, conditions addressed, and health philosophies. Ask to meet other team members prior to accepting employment or joining as an associate. A brief team meeting or one-on-one meetings gives valuable insight into whether this setting and team is a fit for you. Do you share similar values and views? Do you sense that team members are dedicated to excellent client service?

Roles, Goals, and Expectations

After you decide to join or form a group practice, the next step is to delineate—in writing—your roles and expectations. List all of the things that are important to each of you in running the business. Also, clarify what is expected of all group members when not directly working with clients (e.g., paperwork, janitorial chores, clerical duties, assisting the other practitioners, providing treatments for staff, marketing). Whether you get paid for these activities depends upon your employment status.

Be certain to agree upon the image you wish to portray. Nothing is quite as frustrating as sharing space with others who don't hold similar visions or standards.

For those who are associates in a group practice, create a dissolution (or buy-out) agreement in addition to writing your shared vision, goals, roles, and expectations. Who knows what the future holds? People's goals change or major life-altering circumstances happen. Make sure that all parties have a realistic means to ethically and amicably part ways. If you decide to become partners (and not just associates), I highly recommend you design a full business plan before the partnership is official. The process of developing your business plan compels you to evaluate your strengths and weaknesses, clarify your financial arrangements, delineate your roles, determine legal responsibilities, and refine your business vision. Also, memories aren't always accurate; you can avoid many misunderstandings by referring to a written agreement.

Include a section on image in your written agreement. Cover items such as the following: the way clients are greeted; practitioners' attire; the physical layout and esthetic of the office; and acceptable refreshments, music, and noise levels.

Although communications and time spent together vary, it's crucial to clarify your desired levels of interaction. It takes time, energy, and concern to maintain decent relationships. Holding weekly or bi-weekly office meetings can be a good way to keep everyone up to date about business matters and talk about concerns or new ideas.

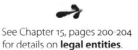

See Chapter 11 for more on **private practice**.

Peer Support

A key advantage to working in a group practice is peer support and supervision. A group setting easily supports a team approach to client wellness, from the opportunity to ask another practitioner's opinion about a treatment scenario to discussing integrated care plans for clients whom you share in common. Working in a group practice even part time can help a practitioner feel a sense of community and support often lacking in private practice.

Legal Status

Most group practices are associations, not partnerships: the practitioners get together to share resources and expenses while keeping separate business identities. A partnership is two or more people contributing assets to a jointly-owned business and sharing in the profits or losses (although not necessarily equally). To be considered a partnership, you don't need to use the term "partner" or have a written partnership agreement. The operative phrase is "jointly owned." In many states, if you're perceived to be a partnership, you could be held liable for something your associate does. Legalese aside, your reputation could be on the line if anyone else within your group does something unprofessional. Avoid any misconceptions about association status by posting a sign in the office reception area that states that each person in the office operates her business separately.

See Chapter 15, pages 200-204 for details on **legal entities**.

Finances

Financial obligations can be a major source of entanglement in an association. Typically, one person is required to assume responsibility for each major account (e.g., rent, utilities, telephone). If you commingle too many funds, you're in essence creating a partnership.

Avoid misunderstandings by drawing up a contract that outlines each person's financial obligations, and how profits are to be distributed. Next, agree upon an operating budget and perform financial projections. You may want to involve a financial advisor in the planning process or simply have the advisor review any financial contracts or plans before finalizing them. Be cautious when jointly making major purchases, unless you're indeed partners.

Product Sales

Product sales are a great diversification method and profits from them can defray overhead expenses. The three biggest problems are: choosing the product lines, determining who is responsible for overseeing sales, and calculating who gets what profit—particularly when a client sees more than one practitioner in the group setting. If your business is a partnership, the funds can be commingled. If you're an employee, the financial terms should be detailed in your employment contract. If you're part of an association, consider one of the following models for handling the logistics of product sales:

Option 1 — Individual Profit Centers

- Designate a weekly or monthly order date. Combine practitioners' product order lists and place 1 order.

- Each practitioner pays for his portion of the order.
- Each practitioner receives requested product quantities and sells products separately.
- Each individual collects payment for product sales and retains the profit.

See Chapter 21 for details on **retailing**.

Option 2 — Distributed Profits

- The group assigns one practitioner to manage product sales. Tasks include tracking inventory, stocking products, placing orders, handling payment through the manager's individual account (this assumes an office assistant handles payment processing tasks).
- The product manager is compensated for her time in managing product sales.
- Remaining profits are applied to lower shared overhead expenses (e.g., rent, linen service, telephone, internet, marketing).

Marketing

Many marketing activities and expenses can be shared, even when group practices are associations and not partnerships. Actually, this is one of the strongest benefits to being in a group practice. The combined energy, expertise, and financial resources can provide diversity and afford you the opportunity to experiment with avenues that were previously unaffordable or infeasible.

Determine what percentage of marketing is handled jointly. Next, develop a joint marketing plan that defines goals, target dates, and a budget. Before placing any long-term advertising, such as a radio or television ad, create a payment agreement to cover the possibility of an associate leaving.

Office Logistics

Office logistics encompass the day-to-day activities in running a business, such as preparing the office for clients, stocking supplies, cleaning, and coordinating repairs. Most people in group practices develop a task list, designate who is responsible for what tasks, and agree upon weekly or monthly schedules. Also, agree upon how expenses are handled for ongoing items, such as fresh flowers or other office decor.

See Chapter 18, pages 242-252 for more information about developing **policies and procedures**.

Although few people thrill at the thought of writing a policy and procedure manual, it's an essential tool to smoothly operate a business. It simply documents how the group has agreed to run the business—what policies apply to what situations and how office procedures work. It doesn't have to be elaborate. It just needs to state the facts simply and clearly so everyone knows what to expect. Topics can run the gamut from ethics, to how to answer the phone, to what is considered to be a clean kitchen (e.g., dirty dishes belong in the dishwasher, not the sink). It can be helpful to all parties to clearly define what consequences apply when there's a serious or repeated violation of policy or procedure. This is especially paramount if you hire employees because establishing grounds for termination is essential from a legal standpoint.

Scheduling Clients

In most group practices, each individual is responsible for booking his own clients (although you might share the cost of a receptionist). This gets fuzzy when the group practice consists of people who provide the same services and clients come in from shared marketing activities (particularly a media ad or website). You can avoid many misunderstandings and resentments by creating a new client scheduling policy. For instance, simply make a list of all the practitioners and place a check next to each one's name every time she gets a new client. In general, it's best to match the first caller with the first practitioner on the list and then proceed down the list. This isn't always possible when a client wants an appointment at a certain time (or desires a specific approach) and the only person available is the one who received the last referral. But by referring to the list, whoever answers the phone knows that practitioner B gets first choice of the next new client.

Figure 10.1 Overall Success Tips for Working in a Group Practice

- **Interview practitioners** who work in a group practice to gain insights into this type of work. (If you're a student, do this while you're in school.)
- **Clarify your reasons** for entering into, or developing, a group practice.
- **Make a list of essential qualities** you want in the people who make up the group practice.
- **Review the group's written materials**: mission, policies, and promotional materials.
- **Develop a detailed agreement** that defines roles and expectations.
- **Develop a long-term business plan** and a professional code of ethics.
- **Negotiate practice boundaries**. Also, be sure to define parameters for working with clients outside of the group setting.
- **Clarify what is expected** of all group members when not directly working with clients.
- **Include each practitioner's name on the office lease**. If that isn't an option, create a separate written agreement that all members sign.
- **Budget accordingly**. Be prepared to do cash flow forecasting, particularly if you receive deferred insurance payments.
- **Create a written telephone script** for greeting callers.
- **Coordinate office decor**, as first impressions do count.
- **Create a group action plan** for product sales, including goals and a budget.
- **Schedule time** for a marketing review each week.

§3

Wellness Centers

Many wellness practitioners enjoy being part of a clinic with clear and established professional boundaries. This setting also offers opportunities for professional development through mentoring or tuition reimbursement programs.

As with medical settings, wellness centers also provide opportunities for case management. When a team of highly skilled wellness practitioners works together to create optimal support for a client, positive results can be greatly amplified. This requires open communication, consistent cooperation, shared values among practitioners, and carving out time throughout the day or week for informal or formal team meetings.

An ethical dilemma that can occur relates to working part time in a wellness center while maintaining a small home-based practice. Following is an example:

Conflict of Interest Scenario

A clinic client has received his total insurance-covered sessions for the current year, yet is still in need of further treatment. The rate for Tracy's services at the clinic is substantially higher than her home-based practice. The client has somehow discovered this and has requested private sessions. Tracy wants to support her client, but doesn't want to cause problems at the center. She informs the client that she can only see him at the center.

Points to Ponder

What other options could Tracy have pursued? What are the potential consequences of each option? What would you do?

As a practitioner, you have a responsibility to the client's treatment plan. As a professional, you have a responsibility to your employer/associates and ethical business conduct. When you negotiate your employment contract or independent contractor relationship with a clinic, clarify how this type of situation would be handled. By setting up guidelines, these types of issues can be avoided or at least resolved with minimal conflict.

Figure 10.2 Specific Success Tips for Working in a Wellness Center

- **Educate yourself**. If you work in a chiropractic or acupuncture clinic, you need a firm grasp of clinical terminology and protocol, and skill at insurance charting.
- **Make full use of the group benefits**. Enjoy what is provided for you, such as scheduling services, laundry, and marketing.
- **Honor the Chain of Command**. Follow the center's protocol regarding how new clients are handled, charting requirements, and cross-referral protocols.
- **Identify your strengths**. Give each member of the practice a demonstration or a handout describing how your services can complement their services.

Specialty Centers

Specialty centers are businesses that specialize in one type of wellness service, such as acupuncture, massage, or chiropractic care, and often at a discount. They range from a group of like-minded practitioners joining forces to nationwide franchises that encourage clients to become members and get discounted treatments. The average price for a treatment even for non-members is usually slightly less than the going rate in the area.

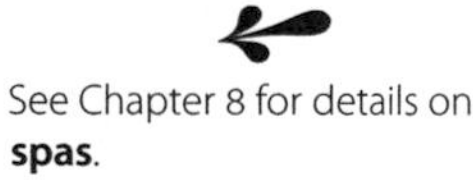

See Chapter 8 for details on **spas**.

There are many advantages to working in this type of setting. It's a great way for new practitioners to gain valuable experience and often receive free continuing education as an employment benefit. Practitioners who are in transition or who have recently relocated can kick-start their practice by working in this setting. Also there's the advantage of walking into a situation in which everything is provided: you just show up to do the work. The disadvantages are that often the pay is low as the fees being charged are low, and clients tend to be more loyal to the business than to the individual practitioners.

Figure 10.3 Specific Success Tips for Working in a Specialty Center

- **Make full use of the group benefits**. If you're an employee, enjoy what is provided for you, such as scheduling services, laundry, marketing, and CE opportunities.
- **Differentiate yourself.** There can be a lot of competition between practitioners when you all do the same thing. Go the extra mile with clients so your work stands out. Improve bookings by incorporating small touches such as aromatherapy or hot towels during the session.
- **Learn to sell products**. Increase your income by using retail products in your sessions. If a client enjoys the product, you can tell him how to purchase it for home use.

11
An Insider's Look at Private Practice Settings

"Think not of yourself as the architect of your career but as the sculptor. Expect to have to do a lot of hard hammering and chiseling and scraping and polishing."
—BC Forbes

What to Expect

Commercial Office Space

Home Office

Primary Care Provider's Office

Fitness Centers and Health Clubs

Practitioner for a Celebrity or Athlete

Corporate Wellness Programs

On-Site and Outcall Settings

Key Terms

Commercial Office Space
Corporate Wellness Programs
Fitness Center
Health Club
Home Office
On-Site
Primary Care Provider (PCP)
Private Practice
Professionalism
Return on Investment (ROI)
Safety
Zoning

As a small business owner, you need to develop a solid base of business knowledge and understand the advantages and disadvantages of various practice settings. To help you establish your ideal business, this chapter looks at career options such as private practice in a home office, business setting, or on an outcall basis.

Figure 11.1 Private Practice Settings

- Commercial Office Space
- Home Office
- Room in Another's Practice (e.g., chiropractor's office)
- On-site or Outcall Settings
- Corporate Wellness Program
- Salon, Day Spa, or Dental Spa
- Fitness Center, Gym, or Health Club
- Hospice
- Personal Practitioner for a Celebrity or Professional Athlete

What to Expect

"I have found enthusiasm for work to be the most priceless ingredient in any recipe for success.
—Samuel Goldwyn

The main reason people start a private practice is control. They can choose when they work, how they work, and with whom they work. A private practice provides freedom and flexibility. You choose the attire, clients, environment, music, lighting, ambiance, creativity, modalities, fees, and scheduling. You can essentially do anything you want as long as it's legal, ethical, and moral. Besides the overall start-up tasks and the general practice management activities covered later in this chapter, a sole practitioner must contend with some aspects unique to this working environment. We briefly review these aspects and offer tips on how to effectively manage them. Please refer to Chapter 7 for the key considerations of self-employment that exist (e.g., autonomy, safety, planning, finances, insurance, benefits) regardless of the specific private practice environment.

Figure 11.2 Success Tips for Private Practice

- Find mentors and trusted advisors with whom you can consult.
- Network! Attend at least 1 networking event each month.
- Hire someone to handle time-consuming business tasks.
- Take safety precautions. Don't hesitate to end a session immediately if you encounter inappropriate comments or behavior.
- Keep good records in an easy-to-use system that works.
- Allot ample time each week to focus on marketing tasks.
- Create a reserve account for purchasing high-ticket items.
- Develop clear policies.
- Schedule efficiently.
- Make lifelong learning a priority.

The following sections contain brief overviews on the most common practice settings for people in private practice. Each setting has its advantages and disadvantages. As you review these options, keep in mind that you may choose to work in multiple settings. Flexibility is essential when your business operates in multiple settings, as your expectations, behavior, attire, and client interactions may need to change depending on the environment. This can be an added benefit to being in private practice, because making those subtle alterations in behavior and attitude can be fun!

Commercial Office Space

Choosing an office space is a very important decision. Having a private office space in a professional building gives you the freedom to decorate the office according to your taste (although some restrictions could be placed by the landlord). It also conveys professionalism.

The building in which your office is located impacts the atmosphere you wish to create. Your room (or office suite) doesn't exist independently of its surroundings. Your clients are affected by the totality, including the lobby, restroom facilities, parking area, adjacent businesses, and even the building itself. Most people want their offices close to home, yet that choice can be disadvantageous. Your clients' needs should come first. The most important questions to ask are, "Will your clients want to come here?" and "Is the parking convenient?"

§3

You can also add to your revenue by maximizing the usage of your square footage. Consider renting your office space to other practitioners on an hourly or daily basis. If you only work a limited number of days per week, perhaps sublet those other days to another practitioner. Make sure your lease allows these options.

See Chapter 16, pages 220-225 for details on **office design** and **leasing**.

Figure 11.3 Specific Success Tips for Commercial Office Space

- Choose an office space that reflects your image.
- Find a space that your target markets can easily access.
- Make sure the other businesses in the building are compatible with your practice.
- Review the lease with an attorney before signing it.
- Introduce yourself to the neighboring businesses and do cooperative marketing.
- Set up a safety protocol for when you're alone in the office.

Home Office

A large number of practitioners have home offices as their main business site. Some practitioners with commercial office space still see some clients at home. A home office yields many advantages: it's usually more economical to run than a commercial office; you can take a tax deduction; you can more easily accomplish household tasks (e.g., do laundry between sessions); you can spend more time with your family; and there's no commute.

The flip side is that some people aren't productive at home. They are too easily distracted and lack discipline. Other problems arise from family members not respecting their boundaries. Plus, zoning restrictions often restrict or prohibit home businesses. Commercial office space conveys an image of professionalism that is rarely found in a home office, no matter how nice it is. However, this perception is changing as more people in diverse professions work from home.

The main things to consider in conveying professionalism are privacy, sounds, cleanliness, and environment. First of all, make sure there's a separate workspace in your home. Ideally, this room would have a private entrance from the main house. The next best option would be to have a separate room. If you must meet with clients in the main living quarters, do your best to set up a private area. Room screens work well for this.

Sounds are a major concern. Make sure you silence your telephone(s). Pick a quiet area to answer phone calls from potential clients. I highly recommend a separate business telephone line, especially if you have children. You always want your business line to be answered in a professional manner.

Consider adding a **Permitted Incidental Occupancies** endorsement to your homeowners policy that deletes the liability exclusions for business activities conducted on the residence premises and modifies the business personal property special limit.

Also, figure out a way to let others who may come to the door know that you cannot be interrupted. Be aware of ambient sounds, such as children playing. A major problem could arise when family members are in your home during a session. Set clear boundaries and rules with family members. Make sure they're quiet and never disturb you during a session. Pets aren't always cooperative in honoring the silence rule. Extra steps may need to be taken to ensure quiet.

Cleanliness is imperative to your professional image. Pets can present a potential problem, because no matter how well you vacuum, dander is always present if they're allowed in the session area. Also take into consideration that many people are allergic to animals. Any area in your home that your clients may see needs to be kept clean and tidy.

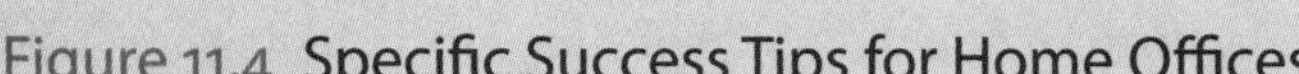

Figure 11.4 Specific Success Tips for Home Offices

- Ideally, create a separate entrance and waiting area.
- Soundproof the room as much as possible to block outside ambient noise.
- Keep personal items (e.g., photos, trinkets) to a minimum.
- Set office hours.
- Create written boundaries with household members.
- Keep your family members and pets out of the office space.

Primary Care Provider's Office

Another practice option is renting a room in the office of a primary care provider (PCP), such as a chiropractor, medical doctor, naturopath, osteopath, or a physical therapist. These situations range from sharing a room to having the room to yourself. The fee structure also varies. You can either pay a flat rate for the room or pay per session. Payment based on sessions provides a safety net for new practitioners, since they only pay when they see clients.

As with all practice settings, this has advantages and disadvantages. On the positive side, you may have a good source for new clientele from referrals. On the negative side, you may rarely get referrals. Some PCPs simply have other practitioners there to lower their costs and look good, while others do it because they believe in what you do and want to have alternatives available to their patients.

Other pluses can include sharing marketing expenses, a sense of community, and possible shared reception or office help. As an independent contractor or renter, you usually supply all materials used in your work. Before you agree to work in the office, make sure you know how the PCP plans to interact with you and how referrals and marketing are handled. If you pay a rental fee per session, negotiate a maximum of how much you will pay per week or month.

Have a good marketing plan to make your services known to current patients. Place your business cards and brochures on display at the reception desk and create good signage.

Make sure that everyone who works at the office experiences your services. Hold educational meetings for your co-workers to explain the benefits of your work, give demonstrations, and show them tips for self-care. Give free demonstrations of your products or services to patients waiting for other services.

Figure 11.5 Specific Success Tips for Working in a Primary Care Provider's Office

- Negotiate a clear agreement regarding your role, marketing, scheduling, and the use of office staff.
- Determine what to expect as far as referrals from the PCP.
- Familiarize yourself with contraindications for medical conditions and medical terminology.
- Keep good client records.
- Market yourself appropriately and abundantly.

§3

Fitness Centers and Health Clubs

Working at a fitness center, gym, or health club requires you to tailor services to your client's health concerns and interests. Many highly motivated career professionals and aging baby boomers have taken the initiative to develop a personal wellness program at local fitness centers, and enjoy the convenience of scheduling massage therapy, bodywork, yoga classes, or nutrition consulting under the same roof. This provides ample opportunities for practitioners who prefer to work in fitness settings.

Building a practice at a fitness center, gym, or health club setting can be a good way to gain valuable experience if you're a new practitioner—or if you're an experienced practitioner who likes working with the type of health-conscious clientele common to these settings. You may particularly enjoy this type of work if you're interested in sports injuries, or if you like working with athletes or other clients who are looking for effective ways to manage chronic pain or health conditions. It can be fun and rewarding to work with regular clients and witness progress in their efforts to reduce stress, heal from injuries, and enjoy good health. Utilize a comprehensive intake form, so you can become aware of and accommodate a client's medical conditions or contraindications.

> "The talent of success is nothing more than doing what you can do, well.
> —Henry W. Longfellow

Like the salon environment, you need to market yourself. Place your business cards and brochures on display at the reception desk. Create good signage. Education is the key to building a practice in this environment. Offer free demonstrations and classes. Offer special "welcome" marketing programs (e.g., $10 discount coupons for the first visit, gift certificate promotions) to help build your business. Make sure that anyone who interacts with members experiences your services. Educate staff on how your service helps clients meet their health and fitness goals. Using the facilities yourself can be an informal way to network and market your services, plus get a good workout!

Figure 11.6 Specific Success Tips for Fitness Centers and Health Clubs

- Market yourself appropriately and abundantly.
- Network with other wellness practitioners in your area who work in similar settings.
- Take classes and exercise at the facility.
- Make sure that everyone who works at the facility experiences your services.

Practitioner for a Celebrity or Athlete

Sometimes working at a fitness center or health club can lead to a job as a personal practitioner for a celebrity or athlete. These clients may be patrons of the establishment and, after getting to know your skills and abilities firsthand, they may offer you a job traveling with them on concert tours, movie sets, or during the game season.

> "Nothing great was ever achieved without enthusiasm.
> —Ralph Waldo Emerson

On the other hand, you may hear of these types of career opportunities through personal or professional contacts. In most cases, you work as an independent contractor, although occasionally you may be offered employment. As in any working environment, it's important to assess the advantages and disadvantages, and take a realistic look at what the job involves. Although these types of jobs can be glamorous, they're often physically demanding and require a great deal of flexibility in terms of scheduling and adapting to travel and lifestyle issues.

Work with a legal advisor to review the terms of your independent contractor agreement (or employment contract). Clarify what is reasonable in terms of scheduling (e.g., minimum and maximum number of treatment sessions per day and per week, time off, the time limit after which you would not be available). Maybe you don't mind working at 2 a.m., but maybe you do. Will you be paid a weekly salary or compensated by the number of hours worked? Determine if there is a bonus for working beyond the standard number of hours each week. If you will be traveling, clarify how expenses for air travel, lodging, meals, and incidentals such as laundry will be handled. Will you have an allowance for these expenses? Will all charges be handled directly by your client?

If you work for a client who is on tour, you may be on the road for 6-8 months. Think about how you will handle the logistics of maintaining a home base while you travel or what storage solutions may work for you. Are you willing to adapt to your client's preferences in terms of restaurants and hotels? Clarify expectations around the times when you will not be providing wellness services. For instance, are you expected to run errands or handle other chores? Good communication skills and boundaries help create a professional working relationship that balances your needs with the needs of your client.

Figure 11.7 Specific Success Tips for Working with a Celebrity or Athlete

- Attain legal advice to carefully review the terms of your agreement.
- Document how travel expenses will be handled.
- Outline the logistics of leaving home for an extended period of time.
- Consider lifestyle issues.
- Maintain excellent boundaries.

Corporate Wellness Programs

The return on investment in corporate wellness programs is no longer in dispute. For every 1 dollar that employers spend on wellness programs, they save 3 dollars in healthcare expenses.[1] Faced with steadily rising healthcare costs, most large employers are expanding workplace wellness initiatives. This helps to create a healthy, happy, and productive workforce—and a healthier bottom line.

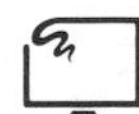

The Wellness Council of America

www.welcoa.org

Recognized benefits of employee wellness programs include reduced absenteeism, reduced number of sick days, an overall reduction in healthcare and workers compensation costs, and increased productivity. An article titled *Massage Is In Business*[2] reported that of the "100 Best for Working Mothers" companies mentioned, 77% offered massage therapy to their employees.

Corporate wellness programs may include on-site seated massage, table massage, acupressure, chiropractic care, fitness classes, smoking cessation, nutritional consulting, meditation, and yoga classes. These services usually take place in a designated area in the company's building, a company gym, or through a sponsored program at a health club.

§3

The expansion in corporate wellness programs bodes well for wellness practitioners. Many companies offer flex benefits which allow employees to apply eligible dollars to wellness services and classes. You may also find opportunities working within wellness programs at upscale retirement communities. Hospitals may offer wellness programs for staff to help reduce stress and enhance health.

In the majority of cases, wellness practitioners work as independent contractors. Some practitioners consider corporate wellness programs as an adjunct to their main practice and offer an adjusted type of treatment in this setting. This could be a good way to grow some extra income and make contact with prospective clients for their private practices. For instance, massage therapists could consider offering corporate on-site chair massage as a complement to their table massage private practice.

Contact local businesses, hospitals, colleges, and universities about wellness programs for employees and staff. Send the contact person a letter with articles about other companies that offer such services. Follow up with a phone call to request a meeting to introduce your service and its benefits. Offer to give a demonstration of your services during your introductory meeting. Employee participation is higher if the company pays for on-site wellness care versus if the employer pays only partial costs. Negotiate this from a win-win standpoint. The more employees who participate, the healthier they become, which ultimately translates into lower employer healthcare costs. Also, suggest that the company pay you by the hour rather than by the session. This takes into account the transition time between clients; otherwise you will be on-site and unpaid for this time.

Figure 11.8 Specific Success Tips for Corporate Wellness Programs

- Get to know other wellness professionals in your area and network.
- Contact local businesses about wellness programs for employees.
- Demonstrate the ROI (return on investment) benefits for employers.
- Offer wellness presentations to businesses and their employees.
- Negotiate with employers to pay all or part of the costs.

On-Site and Outcall Settings

Outcall Companies

https://www.zeel.com
www.soothe.com

Mobile practices have become very popular. Many wellness practitioners prefer to go to a client's home or office. The major advantage is very low overhead for the practitioner—no rent to pay! Clients also love the convenience of receiving services at their home or work.

The disadvantages include lugging around heavy equipment and driving a lot. You may spend more time with clients when you're in their home setting up and breaking down (which doesn't happen when there is another client waiting in your office). Good boundaries can help to avoid spending too much time at the client's premises. One idea is to schedule a business or personal appointment within an hour after the expected completion of the session. Whenever possible, group clients who are located close to each other to be seen on the same day. Allow enough time to get to your next client in heavy traffic. Keep in mind that there can be many distractions you cannot easily control, so try to set up your session area in a peaceful space away from telephones, kids, and other distractions.

Safety can be an issue if you're unfamiliar with the client and the environment. Avoid problematic situations with first time outcall clients by clarifying the scope of services you offer. Avoid booking appointments in unfamiliar neighborhoods at night. Be cautious with late-night appointments for new clients, unless it's through a hotel or agency you trust to carefully screen clients. As a safety practice, call a friend (while the client is nearby) and tell him that you will call him after your session.

New technologies are providing additional avenues for private practitioners who wish to provide outcall services. You may choose to become part of a business that finds and screens clients for you.

Figure 11.9 Specific Success Tips for On-Site and Outcall Settings

- Keep safety concerns foremost.
- Set up your session area in a comfortable space.
- Set good boundaries and schedule wisely.
- Set a price that takes into consideration driving, setup, and breakdown times.
- Give a discount for more than 1 client per location.

§4 Navigate Your Way to the Perfect Job

Section 4 of *Business Mastery* provides information on how to find and keep a job. Even if you plan on being an independent practitioner, you never know when you might want to work as an employee, even if it's just on a temporary or part-time basis.

Chapter 12 covers the fundamental aspects of employment. The chapter begins with a section on career success secrets and then describes how to find potential employers, research companies, and hone your interviewing skills.

Successful job seekers assemble an employment kit with all of the items needed to help procure an interview and get hired. **Chapter 13** reviews the key items to put in that kit and focuses on how to write a top-notch résumé and accompanying cover letter.

Chapter 14 reviews how to effectively navigate employment contracts, and, when the time is right, to renegotiate terms (e.g., a raise, booking seniority, benefits, advancement). The chapter concludes by covering ways to excel in a performance review.

12
Employment Fundamentals

"To find a career to which you are adapted by nature, and then to work hard at it, is about as near to a formula for success and happiness as the world provides."
— Mark Sullivan

Career Success Secrets
- Traits of Successful Employees

Research Potential Employers
- Informational Interviews

Contact Potential Employers

Polish Your Interviewing Skills
- Tough Questions

Key Terms

Appreciation
Communication Skills
Compensation Package
Differential Advantage
Flexibility
Image
Informational Interviews
Integrity
Loyalty
Mission Statement
Positive Attitude
Professionalism
Reputation
Respect
Solution-oriented
Target Market
Time Management

How do you make sure your talent and hard work get noticed, appreciated, and rewarded by your employer? How do you create the best chance of a promising career path? First, embrace the traits of successful employees at the beginning of this chapter. Then, make it your aim to land a job with an employer—either a company or an individual—that values happy employees and a positive work environment. Besides making it more enjoyable to go to work each day, it's simply good business.

Career Success Secrets

An international study showed that companies with positive employee attitudes are more profitable.[1] As a result, these employers are also more likely to recognize and reward talented and dedicated employees accordingly.

Oftentimes, gauging whether an employer offers a positive work atmosphere starts with first impressions. How are you greeted when you arrive for an interview? How are you treated on the phone when being contacted about scheduling an interview? Are the people you talked with engaged with their job, or are they in zombie mode, barely there?

> "Choose a job you love, and you will never have to work a day in your life.
> —Confucius

When you arrived for the interview, did you sense positive and upbeat energy and a sincere interest in providing the best customer experience, or ho-hum energy and a focus on quantity versus quality? Did you observe professionalism versus an overly informal approach to business? Did you sense a strong team environment? Although there are times when first impressions aren't always representative of a company or individual's business persona, more often than not they're a good indicator of what's to come.

It's crucial to research the company and its mission, and what you can expect in terms of hours, clients, and salary range. These are the measurable and tangible elements of your job search. Just as important are the "vibes" you get when you interact with people in the company. Observe carefully, consult your research, and talk with trusted advisors—then follow your instincts.

Keep in mind that sometimes when you're first starting out, finding the ideal employer may not happen right away. However, in time, the right door will open for you as you build your skills and expertise, and keep a clear focus on finding your ideal employer.

Traits of Successful Employees

Highly successful employees share these common traits and career success secrets. Keep these traits in mind as you prepare to find your ideal employment situation in the following sections.

Professionalism. Professionalism includes appropriate dress, good hygiene, good boundaries, excellent time management, integrity, flexibility, and loyalty. Flexibility means conforming to a company's routine, adapting your treatments to the company's preferences, ability to move from room to room, etc. Loyalty means making the company's priorities your priorities; acting as if the company was your own. (Not surprisingly, professionalism issues are reported by employers as the most common barriers to practitioner success.)

Respect. Respect for others means honoring clients, co-workers, and managers as unique individuals. Although others may have different outlooks or ideas, it means treating others as you would like to be treated.

Respect can manifest in social courtesies such as greeting co-workers pleasantly each morning. Or it can mean holding back an angry or unkind remark during a difficult conversation. It can also mean coming in to work on time or even a little early. Respect also includes going out of your way to pitch in when others need help, and, if you share a room, making sure you leave that room clean and appropriately stocked for the next practitioner. Whatever shape it takes, respect requires a conscious effort to honor both the terms of your employment and your team members' needs to be treated in a positive and kind manner.

Appreciation. To appreciate is to acknowledge the positive effort, unique talent, or personality characteristics of co-workers and employers. It creates a sense of teamwork and inspires people to be their best.

Solution-oriented. An employee who can identify creative solutions to problems, or find new ways at looking at old problems, stands out from the crowd. If you see difficult situations and difficult people as opportunities to put your creativity to work and learn new skills, you're sure to shine. Most companies highly value and reward this type of employee.

Communication skills. Great communicators are good listeners. They know how to communicate with clarity and genuine respect for others. They take every opportunity to hone their skills through practice, continuing education, and study.

Positive attitude. Simply put, attitude is everything. A positive attitude is like a magnet. It attracts good people and fortunate circumstances. It ensures that you excel in your career. An interesting labor statistic is that approximately 70% of those fired are let go because they cannot get along with other people.[2] Keeping a positive mindset isn't always easy, but it's always worth it. When challenges loom large, a good sense of humor can work wonders to help revive a positive attitude.

> "There are few, if any, jobs in which ability alone is sufficient. Needed, also, are loyalty, sincerity, enthusiasm and team play.
>
> —William B. Given, Jr.

Research Potential Employers

Once you have determined what type of setting is the best fit for your skills and personality, the next step is to research potential employers. Look through the Help Wanted sections in trade journals and online job posting sites. Check with local schools to find out if they have any job postings or job fair events coming up. Contact school alumni to see if they have any openings in their practices. If you're unable to get a list, then perhaps you can write a "Position Wanted" post in alumni social media groups. Check your professional association's website for job postings, and if none exist, you can often find contact information for practitioners in the area where you wish to practice. Also, consider posting your résumé on professional online bulletin boards.

If you're still in school, you can jump-start your career by having a job lined up before you graduate. Most students are so overwhelmed with all the tasks necessary to complete their education that they don't start their job search until after graduation. Take advantage of this to get your name higher on the "potential employee" list. One of the personality traits employers highly value is initiative. Contacting potential employers while you're still in school demonstrates foresight and strong initiative.

Create a list of potential employers. Gather the information in Figure 12.1 for each potential employer, so you can compare your options. Note the addresses, phone numbers, email addresses, and the names and titles of the people who have hiring authority. Meanwhile network, network, network. Talk to people, let them know you're available. Ask for leads. Remember, quite often, it's who you know that gets you the job (or at least an interview).

Job Search Websites

www.hcareers.com
www.hospitalityonline.com
www.jobvertise.com
www.salonemployment.com
www.americanspa.com
www.allhospitaljobs.com
www.fitnessjobs.com
www.wellnessjobs.com
globalhospitality.com/spa

Informational Interviews

Informational interviews are a good way to gain insights into different work environments and the people who work in each. They're also a way to make valuable contacts; people may remember you when there is a job opening down the road. Before you start the formal interview process with employers, meet with several practitioners and managers who work in the type of settings you're targeting in your job search. Most people are willing to schedule a half hour to share insights and guide you in your research. Figure 12.2 lists some sample questions to ask during an informational interview.

Figure 12.1 Potential Employer Checklist

- ❑ Company Name
- ❑ Address
- ❑ Phone
- ❑ Fax
- ❑ Website
- ❑ Email
- ❑ Owner/Manager/Director
- ❑ Years in Business
- ❑ Years in Present Location
- ❑ Other Locations
- ❑ Types of Wellness Services Offered
- ❑ Types of Products Sold
- ❑ Number of Practitioners Currently Employed
- ❑ Desired Number of Practitioners
- ❑ Target Markets
- ❑ Mission Statement
- ❑ Image and Standing
- ❑ Differential Advantage
- ❑ Reputation
- ❑ Organizational Structure
- ❑ Major Competitors
- ❑ Type of Employment Status
- ❑ Compensation Package (wage range, insurance, vacation pay)
- ❑ Job Description (include expectations of what you're to do when not performing hands-on work)
- ❑ Unique Skills or Attributes You Can Bring to this Business

See Chapter 24, page 358 for information on the **differential advantage**.

Figure 12.2 Informational Interview Questions

- What are some attributes of practitioners who have been the most successful in this environment?
- Is there a strong team environment?
- What do you think is the most challenging part of this work environment?
- What do you like best about working here?
- How would you describe communication between management and staff? Are there regular staff meetings?
- Because so much depends on seniority, how did you endure the slow days in the beginning when you were not scheduled for many treatment sessions?
- What advice do you have for doing the best job possible and developing a career in this type of setting?
- What advice do you have for adjusting to this environment and management (e.g., rules, personalities)?
- How does the hiring process work (e.g., are there several rounds of interviews or just one)?
- **If you're a student, ask:** What do you suggest I do while in school to increase my odds of getting hired by this company?

Conduct Informational Interviews

Set up at least 2 interviews with managers and practitioners who work in a setting that you're considering. Ask them the questions from Figure 12.2. Afterward, compare the answers. Did you get any conflicting responses? What were the most helpful suggestions you received? What information do you still want to know and how can you discover that information? How did this activity influence your desire to work in that type of setting?

See Chapter 25, pages 383-385 for more specifics on **networking**.

Contact Potential Employers

Sometimes it's possible to make an initial contact by phone. In other cases, you may need to send your résumé and cover letter by mail, email, or personal delivery. When calling about a job opportunity, ask to talk to the manager that makes hiring decisions. If you're fortunate enough to connect directly to that person, be prepared to express your interest in employment opportunities and ask how the interview process works. Answer any questions concisely and completely. If you gauge that you've established rapport and there is mutual interest, ask about scheduling an interview.

If the hiring manager is unavailable when you call, make a note of the person's name and title, and confirm the correct spelling. Then send a résumé with a cover letter to the attention of the manager. Although some job openings are filled through online applications or résumés, it's a good idea to send a paper résumé and letter. It shows you're willing to take some extra time and effort in your employment search.

If you haven't received a response within 5 days of the potential manager having received your letter, call to follow up. Continue to place follow-up calls weekly. Sometimes endurance pays off. If you keep yourself so visible that a manager is aware that you really want to work for her company, you may get the job out of sheer persistence.

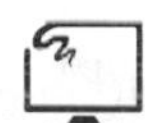

Find **Alternative Health Jobs**
alternativehealthjobs.com

Polish Your Interviewing Skills

The key to a successful interview is preparation (see Figure 12.3). Review your research. Be ready with answers to questions that an interviewer is likely to ask (see Figure 12.4 for sample questions). To get comfortable with talking about your skills and experience, and what you're looking for in a job, practice interviewing with a friend. Work on polishing your answers to possible interview questions and asking meaningful questions about the job. Focus on concise phrasing and conveying a positive attitude. Keep in mind that the best communicators are also the best listeners. You must be confident, and most important of all, you must be prepared.

Figure 12.3 Interview Tips

- Dress appropriately and be well groomed.
- Be enthusiastic, confident, and polite.
- Bring an appointment book or an electronic calendar.
- Bring 2 copies of the appropriate materials from your Employment Kit.
- Bring a printed sheet with at least 3 references.
- Be on time.
- Be prepared.
- Be well poised, centered, and relaxed.
- Maintain good eye contact.
- Use positive wording and listen carefully.
- Control the interview without monopolizing the conversation.
- Look for closing signals.
- Have a list of unique skills, education, or attributes you can bring to this business.
- Know your strengths and weaknesses and how you plan to compensate for those weaknesses.
- Be prepared to discuss each item on your résumé or job application.
- Have at least 3 questions that you can ask the interviewer.
- Prepare a response to the inevitable interview question, "Tell me about yourself."
- Know what sets you apart from the other candidates.
- Avoid discussing salary and benefits in the first interview.
- Thank the interviewer when done.
- Send a thank-you card to everyone with whom you've spoken.

See Chapter 13 for details on the **employment kit**.

Tough Questions

During the interview you're talking up your strengths and experience and how you're a good fit for the job. You can also expect an interviewer to ask you some tough questions. For example: "What are your weaknesses?" Think carefully about your response. Whatever weakness you choose, it shouldn't be a true liability. Turn a weakness into a strength. A good example: "I have a tendency to be a perfectionist, but I also work to keep a sense of balance about this." This conveys that you're conscientious and interested in self-improvement.

"How to Answer Interview Questions"

careerconfidential.com/how-to-answer-interview-questions-top-50.php

Another tough question an interviewer may throw at you is: "Why should I hire you?" This is often asked toward the end of the meeting. Some possible responses are, "Based on our meeting, I believe you're looking for… based on my experience and training [elaborate], I know that this would be a good fit for my skills and abilities." Another sample answer is: "Based on our meeting, it sounds like you're looking for a highly skilled, flexible person with initiative and an ability to put clients at ease—someone who is dedicated to doing their professional best each day. My experience tells me that I'm a good fit for the job…[elaborate]. Also, I like the company and admire its success. It seems there is a good team environment here and I value that." In short, communicate why you're a good match for the position. (See Figure 12.4 for common interview questions.)

Note: Taking interview notes can come in handy for follow-up after the interview, but it isn't wise to refer to them during the actual interview. In the article, "Taking Notes in the Job Interview," Andrew Klappholz states. "The point is to appear competent, and a great way to do that is to appear as if you know what you're doing. Relying on notes, however subtle, demonstrates the opposite message: I have no idea what I'm doing here and can't even remember what I'm supposed to say. The possible downside consequences are so much greater than any possible upside."[3]

Figure 12.4 Common Questions Employers Ask

Work History

Of all your jobs, which one was the most rewarding, and why?
Of all your jobs, which one was the least helpful to you and why?
What will your references say about you?
What accomplishments bring you the most pride?
What do you like best and least about your profession?

School History

Why did you choose this field?
How did you pick the school you attended?
What were your favorite courses? Why?

Ability & Personality

What would make you successful in this job?
How do you cope when work is very demanding?
What experiences have you had dealing with the public?
How would you describe your personality using 10 words or less?
What 3 words would your friends/colleagues use to describe you?
How do you motivate yourself?
What was the most difficult situation you've ever been in?
Has there ever been a time when you changed your schedule to accommodate work? What was the situation? How did you respond when asked?
What are the situations when you won't bend or give in?
Do you have a goal-setting system to determine priorities and get them completed?

Manageability

How do managers get you to do your best work?
What would the perfect relationship between a manager and employee look like?
Describe the best and worst managers you ever had.
How can a manager reward you for doing a good job?

Communication

What was the most difficult communication situation you've dealt with?
How do you deal with people when there is a disagreement?
Have you ever had a time when you turned an unhappy customer into a happy one?
What type of people do you get along with best?
How do you work with people you don't like?
Describe a time when you had to make an immediate decision that you may not have had the authority to make. Why and how did you make the decision?
What kinds of decisions do you not like to make?

Team Building

What is your strategy in working with a group to accomplish a goal?
What are some of the things co-workers do that irritate you?

Job Suitability

What is the most important thing you do in your job?
What do you think a typical day would be like here?
Describe your perfect job.
What does success mean to you?
What types of clients do you like to work with?
In what area could you expect to make the biggest impact?
Why should I consider you for the job?

Future

How will this job help you reach your personal and professional goals?
How long do you plan on staying with this company?
What are your plans for future education?

§4

Polish Your Answers to Interview Questions

Schedule an hour or so to review the questions in Figure 12.4 and jot down your answers. Then spend some time with a friend who will give you tips on how to polish your answers. You need to articulate your strengths. Use concrete examples and stories to emphasize how your skills and abilities are a fit for the job. Know the company's mission and explain why you want to work for the company. Be yourself, prepare clear and concise answers to potential interview questions, and remember to relax.

Take Charge of the Interview

Instill confidence in your potential employer by asking several thoughtful questions. Use the information that you gathered about the employer during your research phase to illustrate how your skill set is a good fit. Several people with equally good qualifications could be interviewing for this position, and your knowledge of the employer's mission, goals, and business philosophy can go a long way to demonstrate your interest and work ethic. At some point in the beginning of the interview, ask the interviewer to describe the skill set that he or she is looking for in the position. This information helps you determine what education and experience you'll highlight in the interview.

> "Your chances of success in any undertaking can always be measured by your belief in yourself.
>
> —Robert Collier

Toward the end of the interview, you may be asked, "Do you have any questions for me?" This is your chance to shine. Here are some sample questions you can pose:

- What was it about this company that made you want to work here?
- What does this company value the most?
- What is the most important thing I can do to help within the first 2 months of my employment?
- When senior practitioners leave the company, why do they leave and where do they usually go?
- What do you see as my strongest assets and possible weaknesses?
- Do you have any concerns about me fulfilling the responsibilities of this position?

13
The Employment Kit

"The closest most people come to perfection is when they fill out a job application."
—Don L. Griffith

Write an Inspiring Résumé
- Résumé Formats

Cover Letters

Targeted Inquiry Letters

Key Terms

Career Objective
Chronological Résumé
Combination Résumé
Cover Letter
Employment Kit
Functional Résumé
Inquiry Letter
References
Résumé

A complete and up-to-date employment kit can save you time and unnecessary stress when preparing to apply and interview for an employment position. Remember, each potential employer may be inspired by something different on your résumé, so do your homework and customize a cover letter and résumé for each specific employer.

To simplify this process, create several résumé, cover letter, and inquiry letter templates. Keep those templates in an "Employment Kit" folder on your computer. Also create a list of references so it's available when the employer requests it. Check your own references periodically to ensure you have the correct contact information. Keep your credentials, proof of insurance, and any other advanced training documents in this same folder for easy access.

In addition to the "Employment Kit" folder on your computer, print the most current version of each document on premium stationery paper, and keep them in a master hard-copy folder.

Figure 13.1 Employment Kit Checklist

- ❑ Résumé
- ❑ Cover Letter
- ❑ Targeted Inquiry Letter
- ❑ Reference List
- ❑ Proof of Licensure/Certification (if applicable)
- ❑ Proof of Liability/Malpractice Insurance (if applicable)
- ❑ Copies of advanced and specialized training documents
- ❑ Background check (if applicable)
- ❑ HIPAA compliance certificates (if working in a primary healthcare facility)
- ❑ A sheet that documents the benefits of your type of work in specific settings or with specific conditions (include research citations)
- ❑ Copies of any referenced research studies

Write an Inspiring Résumé

A résumé is a tool with one specific goal: to inspire a potential employer to interview you. A résumé that clearly highlights your professional training and experience, and that conveys an understanding of an employer's mission, is the one most likely to lead to an interview. To create an effective résumé you need to learn about the company's history, mission, needs, and problems. Determine the ways in which your skills and experience can contribute to the company's success and emphasize these points. Finally, find the name and title of the person in charge of hiring (which isn't always the personnel administrator).

Résumé Magic, 4th Ed: Trade Secrets of a Professional Résumé Writer by Susan B. Whitcomb

The three major types of résumés are chronological, functional, and a combination of both. The chronological résumé is used when you want to emphasize a good work history that's directly related to your desired job. The functional résumé is used when you want to emphasize your talents, abilities, and potential—not your work history. In most instances, new practitioners use more of a functional résumé to highlight new skills and qualifications. Some employers find the functional résumé confusing, without some record of work history. In that case, you may choose to use a combination résumé to highlight your skills and qualifications (functional), as well as your stellar work history and dependability (chronological).

A résumé is a useful tool for promotion, even if you own your own business. If nothing else, the process of developing your résumé clarifies your strengths and reinforces your self-esteem.

In today's electronic world, it's essential to have a digital copy of your résumé at the ready, in addition to printed copies. Many job listings and potential employers request that you send a résumé via email. One option is to simply copy your résumé information from the word processing application you created it in, and paste it directly into an email. This option, however, is the least attractive way to present yourself, as you will likely lose all the formatting that exists in the original document. A better option is to attach your original document to an introductory email. The downside of this option is that your recipient may not be able to open the document if they don't have the application in which you created it. Even if they do have the correct application, if they don't have the fonts you used, the document may still not appear as your intended. Appearance is crucial at this introductory stage, so I recommend saving your résumé as a PDF file. All businesses have the ability to open a PDF file, and the file will retain the formatting you select, appearing to the receiver just as you intend. When you're at the actual face-to-face interview, you should also submit a copy of your résumé printed on premium paper.

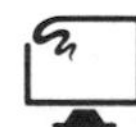

Résumé Resources

www.careersteering.com
https://rockportinstitute.com/resources/how-to-write-a-masterpiece-of-a-resume/
www.careerdoctor.org

Figure 13.2 **Résumé Checklist**

- ❑ Does the résumé focus on why the employer should hire you over your competitors?
- ❑ Is the résumé targeted to the employer rather than a one-size-fits-all document?
- ❑ Have you included a concisely stated career objective?
- ❑ Does the résumé clearly describe your training, experience, and accomplishments?
- ❑ Does the résumé have a visually pleasing, polished presentation? For example:
  - ❑ Are margins even on all sides?
  - ❑ Are design elements like spacing and font size consistent throughout the document?
  - ❑ Is the résumé free of spelling errors and grammatical errors?
  - ❑ Is there a good balance of white space and words? Does the résumé look overcrowded with words, or is it too skimpy and vague?
- ❑ Does the résumé include sentences that begin with action words, such as, prepared, developed, monitored, maintained, and presented?
- ❑ Does the résumé include appropriate industry terminology?
- ❑ Have you included experience or personality traits that address the top skills that employers want?
- ❑ Have you asked friends or colleagues to proof it for accuracy and to share feedback?

Résumé Formats

The following chart highlights the elements of chronological, functional, and combination résumés. Also included are sample résumés for wellness practitioners. (See Figures 13.3, 13.4, 13.5, and 13.6.)

Figure 13.3 **Résumé Format Comparison**

	Chronological Highlights Work History and Experience	Functional Highlights Talents, Abilities, and Potential	Combination Highlights Talents, Abilities, and Work Experience
Heading	**Name, address, and contact information at the top of the page.**		
Objective or Professional Profile	This is optional, especially if you address it in your cover letter. If you do use an objective résumé, make it very specific and concise. State what you can contribute to the organization. Objectives can help focus résumés when you have an eclectic background or you are embarking on a new career. It can also be a place to state your healing or therapeutic intentions: a sentence, statement, or paragraph, that communicates your desired goals and effects of your work.		
Work Experience ---- Function or Specialty Focus	Start with your present or most recent job. It isn't necessary to give the month and day, just the year. List your employer, job title, and a brief description of your duties. Emphasize your major accomplishments and abilities. You don't have to list each position change within a company. Next, list your other jobs in reverse chronological order.	List your strongest abilities or accomplishments in 4 or 5 separate paragraphs—put them in order of relevance to desired job. Have a major headline for each paragraph. If you have a strong work history, it can be by position (e.g., Staff Management). If you have limited work history and are relying on your education, list by modality (e.g., Sports Massage, Hydrotherapy), specialty populations (e.g., Seniors, Post-Operative), or related skills such as Organizational Skills.	List your job experience chronologically, but categorize the descriptions by sets of skills (e.g., practical hands-on skills, leadership skills, communications skills).
Education	Include the name of the school, year graduated (optional), degree(s), certification(s), and any honors. If your education is within the past 3 years, it should be the first thing listed after the heading, otherwise put it at the bottom.		
Personal	[This is optional.] Include information you feel is valuable toward getting you the job (e.g., relevant volunteer positions, community involvement, memberships, awards, other personal achievements).		

Figure 13.4 Sample Chronological Résumé

Nikki Mountain, LMT
4141 Winding Way, Tucson, AZ 85750
520-555-5555 • nikkimountain@example.com

Professional Profile

Highly skilled massage therapist with more than 10 years experience in a wide range of healing modalities. I am seeking to join an active wellness center. The ideal setting would include practitioners who value open communication, high ethical standards, and dedication to providing high-quality client care. My goal is to provide bodywork that honors the body, mind, and heart of each client, combining my skills in Swedish massage, deep tissue massage, aquatic massage, energy work, Chi Nei Tsang, and nonviolent communication.

Work Experience

Moving Spirit Massage Therapy, Tucson, AZ
Sole Proprietor 2010 - Present.

Highly skilled in combining various healing modalities, such as Swedish massage, craniosacral therapy, deep tissue massage, energy work, and Chi Nei Tsang.
Responsible for managing business tasks, including scheduling, bookkeeping, marketing, and publishing monthly newsletter for clients.
Maintained a diverse practice, including many long-term clients of five years or more.

Wellness Institute, Tucson, AZ
Massage School Coordinator. 2017 - 2020

Coordinated and managed multiple aspects of massage therapy education program, including curriculum development, course planning, scheduling and faculty relations.
Maintained database of all student records.
Developed and presented study skills training for students.
Coordinated professional development programs for faculty.

Healing Arts Spa, Tucson, AZ
Assistant Manager. 2014 - 2016

Responsible for working with marketing consultant to develop new logo, promotional brochures, and business cards.
Maintained appointment books and confirmed client appointments.
Responsible for tracking product inventory and ordering products for resale.
Coordinated laundry service to ensure smooth operation.
Developed weekly schedules for spa practitioners; helped to troubleshoot last-minute schedule conflicts.

Education

Mountain Institute Holistic Health, Tucson, AZ
Completed 750-hour Therapeutic Massage Program, 2010
Arizona Licensed Massage Therapist, 2010
Reiki I and II with Susan Wright, 2012-2013
Chi Nei Tsang I with John Sterling, 2016
Craniosacral Therapy with Mary Suntree, 2017 and 2019

§4

Figure 13.5 Sample Functional Résumé

David Waters
2001 N. Pine Road, San Francisco, CA 94995
415-555-5555 • dwaters@example.com

Objective

To establish an acupuncture practice working with clients who seek a safe and natural way to get well and enjoy vibrant health. My goal is to join a group practice at a holistic health center with other practitioners, such as physical therapists, chiropractors, bodyworkers, naturopathic physicians, and medical doctors.

Specialty Focus

Areas of special interest include pediatrics, pre- and post-surgery support, and eye diseases. Received a letter of commendation from the faculty for demonstrating highly effective diagnostic assessment and acupuncture treatment skills during my senior internship.

Education

California College of Traditional Chinese Medicine, Master of Science in Health Science, Oriental Medicine Program (O.M.D.), San Francisco, CA. 2019.

Curriculum and training focused on history and philosophy of Chinese medicine, diagnostic assessment, acupuncture needling techniques, Chinese herbology, tongue and pulse diagnosis, adjunct treatments such as moxibustion, case studies, ethics, and practice management.

California Licensed Acupuncturist, 2020

Clinic Practice, Internship, and Experience

California College of Traditional Chinese Medicine curriculum and internship practice focuses on blending the holistic approach of ancient Chinese acupuncture and herbology with modern healthcare. The program closely aligned with current O.M.D. training in China. Clinical practice and internship included:

Assistantship (60 hours). Assisted acupuncturists in treatment procedures such as moxibustion and cupping, and withdrew needles from the patient.

Junior Internship (240 hours). Provided acupuncture treatments to patients under close supervision and performed diagnoses with guidance from a clinical instructor.

Senior Internship (270 hours). Diagnosed and treated acupuncture clinic clients with minimal supervision.

As an adjunct to the clinical training component of the program, I annually attended two grand rounds conducted by California College of Traditional Chinese Medicine faculty. During these sessions, faculty presented interesting or difficult cases and demonstrated appropriate treatment.

San Rafael College of Acupuncture provides acupuncture treatments to the community. Prior to studying acupuncture as a clinician, I managed the clinic business:

Business Manager. Managed student acupuncture clinic. Responsible for patient scheduling, bookkeeping, ordering clinic supplies, coordinating laundry services, and maintaining student practitioner attendance records.

Figure 13.6 Sample Combination Résumé

Jean Forrester, LMT
1212 Green Grass Drive
Boulder, CO 80301
303-555-5555
jeanforrester@example.com

OBJECTIVE

Highly skilled massage therapist and manager seeking a leadership position in an active wellness center. My goal is to collaborate with a team of client-centered individuals to provide successful training and management to benefit the center.

RELEVANT WORK EXPERIENCE

Boulder Wellness Center, Boulder, CO, Clinic Coordinator. 2017 - 2021

Managerial/Communication Skills

Planned and taught treatment protocol to new practitioners.
Assisted and advised practitioners about their employee performance.
Rated as an excellent manager by practitioners for three consecutive years.

Organizational Skills

Planned, organized, and implemented treatment schedules within company guidelines.
Updated and maintained company website.

Recruiting/Mentoring Skills

Actively recruited prospective employees.
Provided career advice to practitioners.

Healing Spirit Spa, Boulder, CO, Massage Therapist. 2011 - 2016

Technical Skills

Provided appropriate client-centered treatments for center clients.
Assisted new practitioners with protocol and treatment planning.
Maintained a diverse repeat clientele, including many clients of five years.

EDUCATION

Snow Mountain Institute, Denver, CO

Completed 1000-hour Therapeutic Massage Program, 2010

LICENSES/AFFILIATIONS

Colorado Licensed Massage Therapist, 2010
American Wellness Practitioners Association Member since 2010

§4

Cover Letters

Your cover letter is an integral part of your employment packet; it complements your résumé and inspires the recipient to read further. A cover letter is where you build rapport. Keep your tone friendly and use terminology that's appropriate to your field. The best cover letters clearly communicate your understanding of an employer's needs, and convey your professionalism and personality.

Writing a good letter can be a challenge. Experienced writers often write, rewrite, edit, and edit some more. Plan to do the same. Don't expect to complete your letter in one sitting. Write the first draft, then come back later to edit. Find the hot topics, concerns, trends, and buzzwords by researching trade journals, websites, newsletters, and consumer publications targeted for your particular industry.

> "Perseverance is failing nineteen times and succeeding the twentieth.
> —Julie Andrews

Cover letters typically consist of three sections: an opening, body, and close. The opening establishes rapport and communicates your interest. The body conveys how your skills and experience meet the needs of the potential employer, and highlights unique aspects of your professional experience. The closing thanks the reader and suggests the next step, such as a telephone call or interview. Print your cover letter on stationery that matches your résumé, and keep the letter length to 1 page. Some career experts suggest sending your letter and résumé in a 9 x 12 inch envelope because it's bigger than the average mail item, and the presentation of your letter is a bit crisper.

Figure 13.7 Résumé Cover Letter Tips

- Employers hire humans, not robots. Beyond your professional experience, they like to get a sense of your personality and interpersonal skills.
- Use conversational language in your cover letter, and avoid copying sample letters word for word. Find your own voice. Include brief insights into your career experiences or why you chose your career path, and why you chose to apply to this particular company.
- Sample phrases:
  - Some of my most rewarding work has centered on...
  - I am passionate about...
  - I love my profession—the satisfaction that comes from...
- Avoid overly formal language and refrain from starting the cover letter with a sentence such as, "Enclosed please find a copy of my résumé..." Instead use: "I am writing to express interest..."
- Briefly highlight relevant experience; avoid repeating information verbatim from your résumé.
- If you've recently graduated from an educational program, reference your intern experience or include brief testimonials from those who have experienced your work in a student clinic or other apprenticeships.
- If applicable, mention a referral source. For example, "Jane Doe mentioned you were looking for an experienced nutritional consultant to join your clinic."
- The best cover letters focus on how you can meet an employer's needs, and convey unique aspects of your training and professional experience.

Figure 13.8 Sample Cover Letter

Nikki Mountain, LMT
4141 Winding Way, Tucson, AZ 85750
520-555-5555 • nikkimountain@example.com

July 10, 2021

Ms. Susan Sample, Center Manager
Desert Wellness Center
1234 East First Street
Tucson, AZ 85750

Dear Ms. Sample:

You recently advertised an opening for a highly skilled, licensed massage therapist at the Desert Wellness Center. My cousin and several of her friends are clients at your center. They speak highly of the quality care they receive and how comfortable they feel.

Given my 10 years' experience in this field, unique skill set, and dedication to high-quality client care, I would make a great addition to your team.

During my years in private practice, I greatly enjoyed seeing how regular massage sessions helped long- term clients weather stress and navigate through health challenges with greater ease than they thought possible.

I enjoy working with a diverse clientele. I am in excellent health and can easily work with a large number of clients each week.

I would appreciate the opportunity to personally convey what I might contribute as a member of your center. Thank you for your time and consideration.

Sincerely,

Nikki Mountain

Nikki Mountain

Enclosure

*Note: This cover letter style matches the résumé style in Figure 13.4.

§4

Targeted Inquiry Letters

Another type of job search tool is a targeted inquiry letter. This type of letter is appropriate when you've a identified a company where you would like to work, but the company isn't currently hiring. It's particularly valuable when you want to focus on your abilities—regardless of whether you've had much experience or training. In this case, you aren't targeting a job opening. You're introducing yourself and your unique talents, and proclaiming your interest in a future job opening. You must determine the type of job you want and specify it up front with a title, and possibly include a short description if the title doesn't fully convey the job description.

Marketing Communications Kit for Massage Therapists
by Sohnen-Moe Associates
sohnen-moe.com/prodinfo/mck01.php

As with a cover letter, the first thing to do is develop rapport. Then identify the type of job you want (e.g., spa coordinator, massage therapist, esthetician, yoga instructor, staff counselor), and give a concise, dynamic summary of your experience, capabilities, and achievements that relate to the targeted job.

Include specific work history and education, but keep the focus on what you have to offer, including any unique training or internship experiences. Close the letter by suggesting a time to get together. Print your letter on stationery that matches your résumé (in case you send one in the future), and keep the letter length to 1 page.

Assemble Your Employment Kit

1. Assemble your kit that includes the documents listed in Figure 13.1.
2. List the additional skills or experiences that would improve your employability.
3. Identify the steps to take to attain those additional qualifications.

Did you have any difficulty finding any of those documents? How can you better organize these files so that you can easily access them whenever an employment opportunity arises?

14
Terms of Employment

"There is no security in life, only opportunity."
—Mark Twain

Key Terms

Advancement
Benefits
Business Advisor
Cost of Living Adjustment
Employment Agreement
Employment Benefits
Legal Advisor
Negotiate
Performance Review
Raise
Salary
Wages

Applying, interviewing, and landing the job are just the first few steps in creating long-term employment for yourself. Negotiating the initial terms of employment happens during the hiring process, yet you will find additional opportunities to renegotiate those initial terms over the course of your employment.

Negotiating Initial Terms

See Chapter 7, page 122 for more information on being an **independent contractor**.

See Chapter 22, pages 328-329 for a **sample employment agreement**.

The initial terms of your employment may be explained in an employment contract. The old saying, "The devil is in the details," certainly applies. Although it may seem a cumbersome task at first glance, the time you take to carefully review a proposed employment contract can save many headaches down the road. Many practitioners have a legal or business advisor review a contract prior to signing it. Before meeting with an advisor, make a list of points that you would like to clarify, or where you would like to add new information to the contract. In some cases, you may want to negotiate terms that you perceive are more equitable. Often, you can clarify any questions in a brief conversation with your potential employer. A careful and thorough review of your contract is smart business.

Many employers don't create written employment agreements (although it's a good idea), they only rely on the employment application and the requisite government forms. Figure 14.2 shows examples of what you might find in an employment agreement. I recommend you use it in your negotiations when no contract exists.

Renegotiating Terms

At some point in your career, you will need to renegotiate your employment terms. In those situations, excellent performance on the job is your biggest ally. The three major areas for renegotiation are scheduling, money, and advancement.

Scheduling

How your time is scheduled is important. Your employer controls that schedule while you are on the job. If you have been a loyal, hard working employee that consistently meets the expectations of your employer, you may be in a good position to propose schedule options. Maybe you would like to work on specific days of the week. Or maybe you would like to alter the number of sessions you perform or the types of treatments you provide, per shift. These are excellent requests to make during a performance review meeting that is going well.

One request that might be a challenge (because business owners often budget based on the number of sessions per practitioner), is the idea of having more time between sessions for set-up and self-care. If your time between sessions is extremely short, you should discuss this with your employer even if you think nothing will change. Explain your challenges and offer solutions. You may be surprised at the creative options that exist.

Figure 14.1 Potential Schedule-Related Requests

- Specific Days of the Week
- Number of Sessions per Shift
- Types of Treatments per Shift
- Number of Hours per Shift
- Time between Sessions
- Vacation/Time Off

Figure 14.2 **Employment Agreement Checklist**

Employee Responsibilities

- ❑ Provide services within the scope of licensure
- ❑ Maintain appropriate certification and licensure (including all costs thereof)
- ❑ Maintain malpractice insurance
- ❑ Dress in a style consistent with the Employer's image and as stated in the Employee Manual
- ❑ Maintain client records in the manner prescribed by employer and applicable state laws
- ❑ Assist with other office duties as directed, when not engaged in treatments (e.g., assisting other practitioners with clients, performing clerical duties, cleaning, organizing the clinic)

Employer Responsibilities

- ❑ Provide a safe, clean environment, furnished with [chair or settee, stool, hydraulic table, hydrotherapy equipment, storage area]
- ❑ Provide receptionist services, appointment scheduling, insurance billing, and marketing
- ❑ Provide all necessary supplies and materials used in the performance of services (e.g., oils, lotions, linens, music)
- ❑ Pay all required local, state, and federal withholding, Social Security and Medicare taxes
- ❑ Provide Workers' Compensation and Unemployment Insurance
- ❑ Maintain insurance coverage for liability, fire, and theft

Fees, Terms of Payment, and Fringe Benefits

- ❑ Compensation (e.g., per hour, per treatment, additional services)
- ❑ Payroll schedule
- ❑ Health insurance, vacation time, pension plan, employee discounts, CE reimbursement

Other Possible Provisions

- ❑ Employee has the right to perform services for others during the term of employment, however such services are not to be performed on Employer's premises.
- ❑ Employee shall not solicit or provide services to the Employer's clients for private practice while employed or for 6 months after termination of employment, except as noted.
- ❑ All Employee's non-clinic marketing materials that include any information about Employer, must be approved in advance.
- ❑ Upon termination of employment, Employer and Employee shall discuss which clients, under what conditions, and with what compensation, Employee may maintain continuity of service.
- ❑ All client records shall remain the property of the Employer.

Asking for a Raise

Asking for a raise can be an excruciatingly painful process—or may flow as smoothly as a river running downstream. Your comfort level in talking or thinking about money hinges a great deal on two factors: your attitude toward money and feelings about your self-worth. Money is simply a medium of exchange for products, services, and ideas. Ask yourself these questions:

- What is your attitude toward money?
- Do you view money skills like any other skill—requiring education and practice to achieve optimal results?
- Do you manage money matters by default and let this part of your life operate on autopilot?
- Do you set financial goals?

The Money Class by Suze Orman

Developing a healthy attitude toward money can take time and effort, and this doesn't happen overnight. It requires developing basic knowledge about money matters and then practicing what you've learned. There are plenty of good books and magazines that can help you build your money skills and confidence.

A strong sense of self-esteem is vital to discuss or evaluate your compensation package with ease and confidence. Self-esteem is a feeling—how you feel about yourself. It isn't based on what you look like, how much money you have, or your position in the business world. If all your accomplishments, looks, and material goods were taken away, how would you feel about yourself? Do you believe in yourself and your ability to be your best and overcome obstacles? Who you are goes beyond the externals. Simply stated, self-esteem is how you feel about who you are and plays a major role in your negotiations.

See Chapter 20, pages 280-281 to further explore the **concept of money**..

How Much Do I Request?

The two most common wage adjustments are for performance and cost-of-living. Performance increases are based on excellent performance (e.g., the percentage that your efficiency has improved, client satisfaction ratings, going beyond your basic job description duties), the standards and averages of the industry, and the local going rate for your type of service. So, if you are already making $26 per hour, you may not get a raise if no one else in your city is getting more than $20 per hour for the same service (even if you are the best employee the company has ever had).

To find out if you are in a negotiable salary range, you need to know your industry's average for employees and your local job market. Find statistics on your industry's average by contacting the Bureau of Labor Statistics or professional associations who generate statistics based on practitioner surveys. Local chapters may also have specific information on your local area. If you are unable to find statistics, take a look at the employment listings for your area to see the number of job openings in your field and what those positions offer.

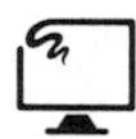

Wages by Area and Occupation

www.bls.gov/bls/blswage.htm

Consumer Price Index

www.bls.gov/cpi

Massage Industry Statistics

www.amtamassage.org/infocenter/economic_industry-fact-sheet.html

Another strategy is to ask the employer to consider raising the price of your services. That increase could even be set at a rate that would cover your raise and provide the company with a small net revenue increase.

Cost-of-living raises are more common for full-time employees than they are for part-time and contract workers in the service industry. This may change as more employers begin viewing wellness practitioners as healthcare workers rather than service providers. Cost-of-living raises can vary significantly by locale, and, in the U.S., are usually based on the Consumer Price Index that is calculated by the Bureau of Labor Statistics.[1] Inflation and deflation affect this index, and so companies may give cost-of-living adjustments of 4% one year, but nothing the next. For example, the Social Security Administration cost-of-living adjustment for 2014 was 1.7%.[2] If your employer isn't prepared to offer you a performance increase, you might negotiate for a cost-of-living adjustment. Before you negotiate, research the average cost-of-living adjustments for your area.

Figure 14.3 Tips for Determining Appropriate Raise Amount

- Gather Industry Statistics
- Research Average Cost-of-Living Adjustments for Your Area
- Identify Your Employer's Expectations
- Evaluate Your Own Performance

Advancement

Another option for your future is the possibility for advancement. If you have aspirations to manage or own your own operation someday, you may ask this question of potential employers, "what are the possibilities for advancement?" Large companies with many departments or locations usually offer many opportunities. However, if it's a small company with only a few employees, you may not have that option. Find out if your company has advanced practitioner positions, treatment specialists, lead practitioners, department heads, spa managers, and so on. If any of those positions interest you, you should add these desires to your performance review negotiations.

Figure 14.4 Potential Advancement-Related Requests

- New Job Title
- New Position
- Additional Responsibilities
- Product Development
- Leadership or Mentor Role
- Community Outreach Opportunities

Rate Your Performance

When negotiating with your employer, keep in mind that who you are as a person doesn't necessarily correlate with your value to an employer or client. You may be dedicated, outgoing, and honest, yet you still may not live up to external performance standards. The better you can distinguish "you" from your actions, the easier it becomes for you to analyze your strengths and create a powerful negotiating base.

First of all, make sure that your services are worth more than you now receive. Your desires and needs have nothing to do with your worth as an employee (see Figure 14.5 to help assess the worth of your services). Your skills may not be as valuable in the eyes of your company as you would like them to be. Don't worry if you aren't certain about being qualified to ask for more after answering the questions. Think about the areas you want to improve and set goals to improve your performance. Strengthen the areas that are weak. Take a seminar or read a book. Identify and follow through on whatever is necessary for you to grow and improve your skills. Keep track of your accomplishments. Regularly review your accomplishments and goals. Then when you feel more confident about your results, schedule a meeting with your manager to discuss a performance review.

> "My father taught me always to do more than you get paid for as an investment in your future.
>
> —Jim Rohn

Figure 14.5 Questions to Assess the Worth of Your Services

- Am I achieving my goals?
- Am I performing at my peak level in quality and quantity?
- How have I improved my business skills?
- How have I improved my technical skills and knowledge?
- Am I reliable and consistent?
- Do I get my work done on or before deadline?
- Are my clients achieving their desired treatment goals?
- How do I know that my clients are achieving goals?
- In what ways have I taken initiative?
- How have I contributed to the success of the company?
- Are my relationships with co-workers pleasant and productive?
- How have I improved my leadership abilities?
- In what ways have I given better/more service than I was paid to give?
- If I was my employer, would I be satisfied with my performance?

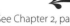

See Chapter 2, pages 12-20 for a review on **goal setting**.

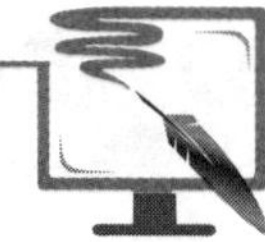

Analyze the Worth of Your Services

Write your responses to the questions in Figure 14.5. Were you able to give specific examples? What are your challenges? What can you do to improve your perceived worth?

Review Your Performance Record

Review your performance records. Many practitioners like to create a file to track accomplishments and training achieved during each year along with thank-you notes from happy clients. Note the times that you've exceeded expectations or achieved outstanding results under difficult circumstances. Compile a list of your accomplishments. Refer to the self-analysis questions in the previous activity. Whenever possible, include numbers. Be specific. Some examples are: "Clients are completing their treatment courses on or before projected date," "The number of clients on maintenance programs has increased by 40%," "My department's productivity increased 20%," "My promotion idea garnered us a $15,000 corporate contract," "Turnover rate has decreased by 50%," "Product sales increased by 42%," and "We were $5,000 under budget this year."

Also, include some of the less tangible results. For example, "Morale has improved," "Case management is more effective," and "I'm more organized." Actually, you could figure out how much money you were saving the company even with the intangible results by analyzing the amount of time saved and multiplying that by the average salary per minute. Unfortunately, many people either overlook or underestimate the financial value of time.

The Performance Review Meeting

One of the first steps to prepare for your performance review meeting is to look at the big picture. Have you ever been granted a schedule change? How many days off have you been given? How long has it been since you received a raise? Is your income comparable to your peers? Research industry salary surveys and economic indicators; look for articles in trade publications or association websites that provide facts and charts about salary trends. Be careful that you compare apples to apples when looking at this data. Sometimes these figures also include those in private practice. The ones in private practice may "earn" more income per client or hour, but are also responsible for expenses, such as office rent, supplies, and marketing. If data is available, research your company's history: how often has it given raises? What is the average percentage increase? What are some of the available perks or other benefits?

Carefully evaluate if your desire for special schedules or more money is based upon your needs or your performance. Assess your company's, supervisor's, and clients' standards for excellence and compare them with your standards. Make certain your perceived priorities are the same as theirs.

> "You miss 100 percent of the shots you don't take.
> — Wayne Gretzky

Mental Preparation

The next step in preparing for your review meeting is to imagine asking for an increase in compensation. Brainstorm the possible objections you might encounter and prepare responses to each one. Include "why" questions: Why don't you feel this job is worth $40,000 per year? Why don't you think I deserve $35 per hour? What do you think I need to do differently in the next 6 months to earn a performance increase? We would all hope the discussion wouldn't get to this point, but it's best to be fully prepared. This may seem like a lot of work, but, asking for more money is like selling—you're communicating the benefits of what you have to offer and asking for appropriate compensation for your talents and abilities.

Factor in Benefits

After evaluating yourself and following the suggested steps to prepare for a performance review, take stock of the employee benefits you already have. Sometimes employers may not be willing or able to give you more money, but they may increase benefits or accommodate some of your other requests. Alternatives to cash include: an expense account; a company car; stock options; profit sharing; pension and retirement plans; insurance; paid travel; vacations; use of corporate lodge or resort; professional association dues; educational expenses; memberships to health clubs; tickets to sporting events and theatrical productions; company discount on products or services, nursery and day care centers; and flexible working hours.

The Negotiation Presentation

This is when the fine art of negotiation comes in. Tailor your presentation to the manager's communication style and personality. Be grounded in your capabilities and accomplishments. Remember, timing is very critical. What is a good time for you may not be the right time for the other person. Although substance is important, style can play a big role in successful communication. Your attitude tremendously impacts negotiations. Before you ask for anything, practice your presentation with a friend. Listen to feedback. Visualize a win-win experience in your mind's eye. Imagine everyone getting what he or she wants. Have a positive mental attitude. You know you and your services are worthy of earning more, and you've prepared an excellent presentation. You're now ready to renegotiate!

§5 Business Fundamentals

Studies show that most business failures are due to improper management or undercapitalization, not because the owners were underskilled in the performance of their job duties. Section 5 of *Business Mastery* provides the necessary groundwork for a business to grow and prosper. It encourages you to take the time to master the basic business fundamentals so you can maximize your chance of success and avoid common pitfalls that plague many small business owners.

Chapter 15 looks at the critical elements involved in a business start-up. It covers how to assess the feasibility of your business idea, find start-up financing, determine the laws and regulations you must follow, choose a business name, and determine client fee structures. The chapter closes with exploring the option of buying a practice.

Choosing an appropriate business location can dramatically impact your success. **Chapter 16** covers the important elements to consider when looking for a location, how to negotiate a fair lease, and how to navigate zoning, insurance, and licensing regulations. It also explores how to design the interior office space. For practitioners on the move, the chapter closes by discussing how to manage the relocation of your practice, near or far.

Finally, **Chapter 17** provides detailed instructions for creating your business plan—an indispensable tool for mastering both short- and long-term success. The chapter details the major components of a business plan, including how to create a financial forecast to realistically assess the finances required to launch and maintain your business. We also include a guide of additional tips and useful resources to help you create a solid business plan.

15
Business Start-Up

"Many of life's failures are people who did not realize how close they were to success when they gave up."
—Thomas Edison

Initial Research
- Scope Out the Competition
- Meet People with Insider Information
- Determine the Business Feasibility
- Complete a Self-Assessment
- Assemble Your Business Advisors

Start-Up Financing

Legal Entity Status
- Sole Proprietorship
- Partnerships
- Corporations
- Limited Liability Companies (LLCs)

Business Name
- Domain Name

Laws and Regulations
- Professional Licenses and Requirements
- Business Licenses and Permits

Insurance Coverage

Setting Your Fees
- Sliding Fee Scales
- Prepaid Package Plans
- Raising Your Rates
- Value-Added Service

Buying a Practice
- Evaluate Your Reasons For Buying
- Determine the Fit
- Conduct a Preliminary Evaluation
- Assess the Business Premises
- Open Negotiations
- Final Stages
- Purchasing a Franchise

Key Terms

Bank Loan
Building Safety Permit
Business Feasibility
Business Interruption Insurance
Business License
C Corporation
Certificate of Occupancy
Competition
Corporation
Crowdfunding
Doing Business As (DBA)
Domain Name
Draw
Employer Identification Number (EIN)
Estimated Taxes
Fire and Theft Insurance
Franchise
General Liability Insurance
Grants
Insider Information
Lawsuit
Legal Entity
Liability Insurance
Limited Liability Company (LLC)
Logo
Malpractice Liability Insurance
Medical Health Insurance
Negotiations
Occupational License
Partnership
Partnership Insurance
Personal Disability Insurance
Personal Service Corporation (PSC)
Planning and Zoning Permits
Prepaid Package Plan
Professional Limited Liability Company (PLLC)
Regulations
S Corporation
SBA Loan
Sliding Fee Scale
Small Business Insurance
Sole Proprietorship
Supply and Demand
Trade Name
Trademark
Transaction Privilege Tax License
Value-Added Service
Workers' Compensation Insurance

As a new small business owner, you may be wondering where to start. You have a huge checklist of business start-up tasks and the energy, enthusiasm, and inspiration to match. Because knowledge is power, it makes sense to start with knowing your market—your clients, colleagues, and competition.

Initial Research

Determine the best way to set up your practice by researching your industry facets and local market. Begin by spending some time browsing through industry trade journals, magazines, and books related to your field. Attend professional association meetings and subscribe to their newsletters. Scope out the competition and meet with people who understand the wellness industry. This gives you a good sense of the competitive landscape and an appreciation for effective and lackluster marketing. Figure out if your specific practice model can flourish in your community. Follow that up by doing a self-assessment and identifying your needed business advisors.

Scope Out the Competition

See Chapter 24, pages 368-369 for details on **analyzing your competition**.

Find out the number of other businesses that are the same or similar to yours. Start by looking at listings and advertisements on the Internet, in specialty directories, and in local publications. Interview the owners of these businesses, ask them how they got started, the services they offer, what trends they see happening that will affect the success of this field, and then ask them for any advice. Most people like to talk about themselves, although some might not eagerly share this information. It helps if you can give them a name of someone who suggested that you contact them. If this isn't possible, find something about them that grabs your interest (check their website, brochure, or business card). Start off by telling the practitioner/owner what intrigues you about her business and then ask her if she would be willing to share some insights with you.

Figure 15.1 Questions to Ask When Interviewing Business Owners

- How long have you been in practice?
- What obstacles did you have to overcome?
- What are some of the smartest decisions you made in terms of business success?
- What are some poor decisions or mistakes that you made that I should avoid?
- What are the keys to long-term success in this industry?
- At what point in your career did you first feel successful?
- How much has your business model changed now from when you first started?
- What advice can you offer me about gaining the best results with a business support group?
- If you could do it all over again, what would you do differently?
- Students should also ask: What would you suggest I do while in school to prepare me for being in business?

After conducting an information interview, send a handwritten thank-you note to express your appreciation for that person's time and professional generosity. Also, ask that person if she would like to be a referral source if you have a client you cannot help or is beyond your experience.

Meet People with Insider Information

Another way to gain valuable business perspectives is to meet with professionals who provide services or supplies to your segment of the wellness industry. They can often shed light on trends and potential trouble spots for a new business owner. Schedule several informational interviews with sales representatives, product suppliers, equipment manufacturers, bankers, accountants, or consultants.

Research your potential markets. You may do an informal survey or hire a marketing consultant to do the research. Discuss the industry with other people who service your potential clients. Let's take athletes as a sample target market. The professions and companies that provide products and services to athletes include massage therapists, medical doctors, sports psychologists, chiropractors, trainers, sporting goods stores, nutritionists, equipment manufacturers, and hypnotherapists. These people may give you a broader view than someone who does your specific type of work.

See Chapter 24, pages 361-367 for details on identifying **target markets**.

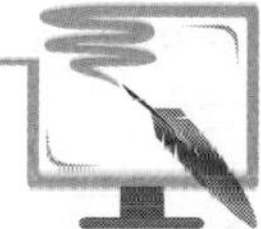

Gather Information in Your Area

1. Schedule an informational interview with a practitioner who does your kind of work. Use the questions from Figure 15.1 to gather information.
2. Schedule an informational interview with someone in a different profession, but who also services your same target market(s). Use appropriate questions from Figure 15.1 to gather information.
3. Compare your notes from each interview, noting similarities and differences of experience. Use this information when writing your operating and marketing plans.

§5

Determine the Business Feasibility

Ascertain the economic capacity of the community to support your business. You may find you need to expand your target markets or diversify your practice to increase your business viability. This information gathering process is also crucial when expanding or revamping a current business. "It's never too late to start over" is a common saying, although one not normally associated with business. You can start over regardless of how long you've been in practice. Although it can be more difficult to make changes after you're established, it's often worth the time and energy.

Supply and Demand

The old economics cliché states that business success is based upon supply and demand: find the demand then supply what's needed. This information is crucial for determining where you choose to practice and whom you target as clients. Look at the general demand for wellness care in your city and the specific need for your particular services. Figure 15.2 lists the types of information to gather and Figure 15.3 provides an example of how to calculate supply and demand.

2012 National Health Interview Survey

nccih.nih.gov/research/statistics/NHIS/2012

U.S. Department of Labor, Bureau of Labor Statistics

www.bls.gov/ooh

Figure 15.2 Evaluating Your Business Potential

Gather Income Statistics, Client Usage, and Trends
- U.S. Department of Labor
- Professional Associations
- Practitioners in Your Field
- Trade Journals
- State and Local Licensing Agencies
- Online Resources

Research Potential Markets
- People most likely to utilize your services
- People or conditions with whom you wish to work

Estimate Supply and Demand
- Calculate the numbers of potential clients
- Find out the average number of people receiving your type of work
- Determine the average number of sessions per client
- Ascertain the number of practitioners in your field in your city
- Project the average number of clients seen by current practitioners
- Divide the potential clients by the number of practitioners

Figure 15.3 Supply and Demand Example

Data Collected
- City Population = 100,000
- Current practitioners in your field = 100
- Average number of people receiving your type of work = 15%
- Average number of treatments per year that a client receives = 10

Calculations
- 100,000 x 15% = 15,000 people receiving your type of work
- 15,000 x 10 = 150,000 sessions per year
- 150,000 ÷ 100 = 1,500 sessions per practitioner per year
- 1,500 ÷ 48 weeks per year = 31.25 sessions per week*

*31 sessions per week is really too much for one practitioner (in this example), therefore, it's likely that this city can support a few additional practitioners.

Assess Supply and Demand

Gather supply and demand information for your services in the city where you wish to practice:

1. What is the population? (You can usually find this information on the city's official website.)
2. What percentage of the population receives your type of work? (You can usually find this information on professional association websites.)
3. What are the average number of sessions per client per year for your type of work? (Check professional association websites.)
4. What are the average number of sessions per practitioner per year for your type of work? (Check professional association websites.)
5. How many practitioners are there? (You can usually find this information on your state's Licensing Board website.)

Calculate how many additional practitioners the city can easily accommodate:

6. Number of people receiving your type of work. (Multiply **Number 1** by **Number 2**.)
7. Total number of sessions per year. (Multiply **Number 6** by **Number 3**.)
8. Number of practitioners the population needs. (Multiply **Number 7** by **Number 4**.)
9. Number of additional practitioners the city can accommodate. (Subtract **Number 5** from **Number 8**.)

Blank Supply and Demand Calculation Form

www.businessmastery.us/workbook.php

Complete a Self-Assessment

Now that you have a good picture of the business landscape, take a few minutes to answer the following questions. They will help you realistically assess your plans and pinpoint any actions needed to move you closer to your ideal practice.

§5

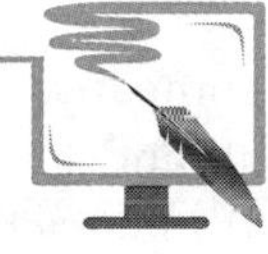

Self-Exploration Questionnaire

- How well does your educational and career experience fit this industry?
- How soon will you need advanced training to effectively grow your business?
- Have you interviewed colleagues and industry experts?
- Do you feel comfortable with the "business" aspects?
- Does this business provide sufficient opportunities?
- Are you aware of industry trends and regulations?
- Have you assessed your strengths and challenges?
- Do you have adequate financial resources to start your business?
- Is the time commitment compatible with the rest of your life?
- Are your friends and family supportive?
- Can you identify at least 2 target markets that will eagerly embrace your practice?
- Have you identified what makes your business unique and gives you a competitive edge?
- Do you have the personality and aptitude to market your services?
- Do you have a support system of colleagues and advisors?

See Chapter 24, page 358 for information on the **differential advantage**.

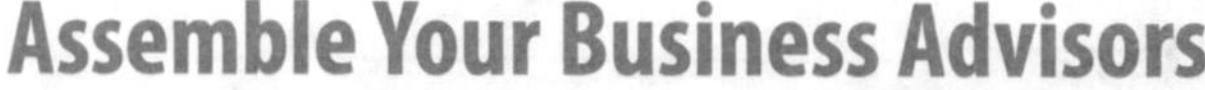

Assemble Your Business Advisors

Before you even get started "starting-up," seriously consider creating a personal group of advisors with whom you meet regularly for business advice. Your group may consist of a business coach, a bookkeeper or accountant, an attorney, an experienced practitioner/mentor, and a marketing specialist. Consulting professional advisors, like business attorneys who are experts in their field, is the best way to avoid potential issues and future problems.

See Chapter 4, pages 64-67 for details on **building a support team**.

Nina Kaufman, founder of The Legal Edge LLC, says these are the top 10 legal pitfalls to avoid:[1]

1. Not starting the business as a limited liability entity.
2. Not keeping proper corporate records.
3. Not having a written ownership agreement.
4. Doing business on a handshake.
5. Copying contracts from the Internet.
6. Having vague or inconsistent employee expectations.
7. Letting your proprietary and intellectual property go unprotected.
8. Giving unintended credit to customers.
9. Getting involved in litigation.
10. Not getting an experienced business attorney.

The most valuable of all capital is that invested in human beings.

—Alfred Marshall

The above pitfalls can be avoided by getting expert advice and keeping detailed records. Practice these skills now, while getting started, so they're habits by the time you're busy and successful.

Start-Up Financing

The costs of starting up and running a business can be daunting, which is why many people opt to work for others. According to the Small Business Administration (SBA), the median start-up cost for a solo business owner to just open the door is between $5,000 - $18,000.[2] The actual start-up costs depend on the scope of the business, the location and build-out costs, and the requisite equipment. Many wellness practices are fairly easy to set up, particularly since the initial costs tend to be minimal. In many instances, you can operate out of your home, rent space by the hour, or provide on-site work.

Small Business Administration

www.sba.gov

Service Corps Of Retired Executives

www.score.org

People often build their private practices slowly while working for another company. This is an acceptable route, as long as you develop an action plan for attracting clients and actively market your practice. Otherwise, you may find yourself with a permanent, part-time practice.

When determining start-up costs, include operating and personal living expenses for at least 6 months. Decide whether the costs are essential or optional. A realistic start-up budget should only include items that are necessary to start the business. Research similar businesses and seek advice from a realtor, accountant, and lawyer. Also contact your local SBA and SCORE offices.

Crowdfunding Info

www.entrepreneur.com/topic/crowdfunding

www.kickstarter.com
www.indiegogo.com
www.crowdfunder.com
www.gofundme.com

Be creative in obtaining services and supplies. Consider bartering and buying previously owned equipment and products. Your creativity, talent, and persistence are the qualities that help balance out the shortage of start-up resources.

Initial Expenses: Opening a business checking account; business telephone; equipment; first and last month's rent and security deposit; marketing materials (e.g., business cards, stationery, brochures); logo design; website design; opening promotion package (e.g., ads, direct mailers); decorations; office supplies; furniture; music system and CDs, iPod, MP3 player, or satellite stations.

Annual Expenses: Property insurance; business license; permits; liability insurance; professional association membership; continuing education; legal and accounting fees.

Common Monthly Expenses: Rent; utilities; telephone; bank fees; supplies; networking club dues; education; marketing; internet access; postage; repair and maintenance; business travel; inventory; business loan payments.

Financing your business (whether for start-up or expansion) can be frustrating. Even though a lot of venture capital is available, it's extremely difficult to procure investment money for a service business. Be extremely wary of any company that guarantees (for an up-front fee) to find you venture capital. There are a lot of scam operations. Check out the resource guides at your local SBA office to find reputable sources of funding.

A bank may be willing to give you a loan; the amount is usually based upon your assets. Applying for a loan (or venture investment) takes a lot of work: research, correspondence, proposals, refining your business plan—including financial statements and cash flow forecasts (they want to see numbers), and putting together an impressive presentation.

See Chapter 20, pages 287-288 for specific information on **business costs**.

Grants

www.successfulhandsgrants.com
www.grants.gov
www.foundationcenter.org
www.freegovmoney.us

www.sba.gov/content/find-grants

www.startupnation.com/articles/grants-to-start-a-business-hidden-trove-of-small-business-start-up-capital

Figure 15.4 Options for Financing a Practice

Personal Savings: Be conservative in your spending so you can build a start-up nest egg.

Personal Loans: If you own your home, you could take out a second mortgage or an equity loan. Some people use their credit cards (not usually advisable due to high interest rates). Another option is to cash out a retirement account (with the goal of returning those funds back into a retirement account).

Student Loans: If allowable, maximize the amount of your student loans and put the extra into savings.

Family & Friends Loans: Avoid potential discomfort and resentment by designing a loan contract that clearly delineates the terms and repayment schedule.

Private Investor Loans: Most private investors want to make a healthy return either in dollars or a percentage of the business. This route requires research, correspondence, proposals, and a refined business plan.

Bank Loans: The amount loaned is usually based upon your assets, and banks require a complete business plan.

SBA Loans: The SBA offers several types of funding, from guaranteeing up to 85% of a commercial bank loan to directly loaning money.

Grants: Many organizations provide grants to people who fall within the parameters of special interest groups, either as the business owner or the market you plan to serve. At a minimum, this route requires research and proposals.

Partnerships: This affiliation can vary from a "silent" partner (more of an investor) to someone who works alongside you to build your business.

Community Development Corporation (CDC) **Investors**: Local organizations that partner with government, business owners, and community leaders to provide economic assistance (e.g., loans, grants, consulting, subsidized office space). This is usually geared toward specific populations or the enhancement of a particular area of the city.

Crowdfunding: Internet sites that allow you to share your vision and business proposal, and collect contributions from a large number of people.

§5

Most small business owners finance their company with money from personal savings or through loans from friends and relatives. If you decide to borrow money from friends or family, treat them with the same consideration that you would give to a formal lending institution. Make an official presentation and submit a loan proposal and a business plan. Clearly delineate the terms of the loan and the repayment schedule. If you follow these guidelines and set your boundaries, it can be a rewarding experience—one in which everyone benefits personally and financially.

Legal Entity Status

Disclaimer!

This is **not a legal book**. The material in this chapter is provided to assist you in understanding basic legal concepts. Consult with appropriate legal advisors before deciding which structure best suits your needs.

The most common legal entity choices for your practice include sole proprietorship, partnership, corporation, and Limited Liability Company (LLC). The majority of new businesses open as sole proprietorships, mainly because this is the simplest, fastest, and least expensive structure. The decision to opt for a different structure is usually based on tax and liability considerations. Consult with an accountant or tax attorney, because each person's situation and needs are unique, tax laws frequently change, and requirements vary by locale. This section describes types of business structures and some of the advantages and disadvantages (see Figure 15.5 for a summary comparison chart).

Sole Proprietorship

If you don't incorporate, create a partnership, or form an LLC, your business is automatically considered a sole proprietorship. The Internal Revenue Service (IRS) usually allows a married couple to operate as a sole proprietorship. In all other cases in which two or more people co-own a business, they must choose an entity other than sole proprietorship.

The major disadvantages of sole proprietorship are having to be responsible for all business aspects, relative difficulty in obtaining financing, and unlimited liability. All business debts and liabilities are the personal responsibility of the owner. Damages from lawsuits brought against the business can be taken from your personal assets.

"Success seems to be largely a matter of hanging on after others have let go.
—William Feather

The main advantages of sole proprietorship are the ease of formation (minimal governmental regulation on how the business is operated), possession of profits, control of all decisions, and relatively simple financial recordkeeping.

The type of business license required for a sole proprietor who is a wellness provider varies from state to state. You may even need more than 1 license.

From a legal standpoint, as a sole proprietor, you and your business are one entity. You can't be treated as an employee of the business. You may withdraw money from your business, but it isn't considered a wage and can't be deducted as a business expense. Although you don't pay payroll taxes on "draw," you pay self-employment (SE) taxes and income taxes. The business doesn't file income tax returns or pay income taxes. In the United States, you file a Schedule C with your 1040 Form and pay personal income taxes on the profits.

Partnerships

A partnership is when two or more people contribute assets to carry on a jointly-owned business and share in the profits or losses. To be considered a partnership, you don't have to use the term "partners" or have a written partnership agreement or equally share ownership. The operative phrase is "jointly-owned."

A partnership is similar to a sole proprietorship in that governmental regulation is still fairly minimal. The financial recordkeeping is a bit more involved, although it's insignificant compared to a corporation. You must obtain a federal identification number (contact the IRS and request Form SS-4). Partnerships file a Schedule K-1 (Form 1065, partnership informational tax return), but the partnership itself pays no taxes. Each partner submits a copy of the K-1 to report his share of profits or losses on his individual tax return (Form 1040). You can be held personally responsible for debts and legal obligations incurred by the partnership, even for those made without your knowledge or consent. Incorporation, or forming a Limited Liability Company (LLC), is the best way to protect yourself against this kind of liability.

Having an associate or partner can be quite beneficial. It can help ease the loneliness of being self-employed, allow you to take time off, and add diversity of services and approaches. It can also infuse capital, decrease overhead expenses, enable you to share the activities involved in running a business, and provide you with another person with whom you can brainstorm. It could also be a nightmare. A written partnership agreement is crucial.

Corporations

The major categories of business corporations are C Corporations, S Corporations, and Professional Corporations. The type of business you operate and your tax requirements determine which structure is the best for you. Many people incorporate because they think it gives them an air of legitimacy—without considering all the legal implications.

A corporation provides a business entity that's separate from the owner as an individual. That distinction assists in creating clear boundaries between your work and the rest of your life—an important consideration—since wellness practitioners have a tendency to become so enmeshed in their work that it becomes difficult to "switch off." Owners who work in an incorporated business are considered employees and are paid as such.

My relationship to my work dramatically shifted when I incorporated my business: I became more detached (which is good); the ups and downs of business are a bit easier to take; and I pay myself regularly. Now there is Cherie, the person, and Sohnen-Moe Associates, Inc., a company which I happen to own. Of course, I always knew there was a difference between my company and me, but I hadn't really experienced the separation on an emotional level.

A corporation tends to be the most costly legal structure to form and dissolve in terms of finances and time. There are required filings with the IRS, as well as with the state in which the corporation is formed. Though there are no federal fees involved, the state may require an initial filing fee and annual report filing fees. Contact your state Corporation Commission or Secretary of State to ascertain the specific requirements and fees for incorporation. The minimal components of the incorporation process are:

- Adopting and filing Articles of Incorporation
- Developing corporate Bylaws
- Holding the first board of directors and shareholders meeting and preparing meeting minutes
- Issuing stock certificates
- Filing for an IRS Employer Identification Number (EIN, Form SS-4)
- Filing Subchapter S status if so adopted within 75 days of incorporation or start of business (IRS Form 2553 which requires your new EIN)
- Setting up your corporate book that contains all corporate documents

Myriad details are involved in each step. The incorporation process varies from state to state according to each state's regulations, and so do the requirements for the content of your bylaws. Be sure your bylaws include the approval of telephone or cyber meetings for shareholders and directors. This saves time and helps to minimize travel expenses.

The general minimal requirements for maintaining a corporation are conducting annual meetings and filing the minutes in your corporate book, as well as filing required documentation with the state on an annual basis. In the event your corporate status is questioned by the IRS or the state, the first thing they do is inspect your corporate book to make sure you've followed all the requirements. If you haven't, your status as a corporation can be nullified, which could result in severe tax consequences. Keeping your corporate book up to date is essential. Even though there are do-it-yourself incorporation kits, it's strongly recommended that you consult with an accountant and an attorney.

IRS Publication 542

www.irs.gov/publications/p542/index.html

Incorporation Services

www.incorporate.com
www.mynewcompany.com
www.legalzoom.com

One of the primary motivations for incorporating is to limit liability. If your business is a sole proprietorship, you could lose your personal assets, such as your home or car, if your business is sued. Wellness practitioners in partnerships often incorporate to shield individual owners from possible losses and lawsuits stemming from actions (e.g., a malpractice suit) of the other partners. In most cases, incorporation protects your personal assets from being taken by creditors; but it doesn't shelter you from lawsuits.

Other popular reasons for incorporating include the ease in which the business can be transferred, the ability to raise capital by selling shares of stock, potential tax advantages, and fringe benefits, such as health and life insurance premiums, tuition reimbursement, and tax-sheltered retirement plans, which can be deducted partially (and often fully!) as business expenses.

C Corporations

C Corporations are subject to a corporate income tax on the net business profits. Although there is the potential for double taxation (the corporation as well as an individual), most small business owners use all the profits as tax-deductible salaries and fringe benefits, or they retain money to expand the business. Income can be divided between paying money to shareholders (salaries and dividends) and keeping the rest of the profits in the business. This process is called income-splitting. The retained earnings are taxed at a rate that is usually lower than the individual income tax rates of the owners. C Corporations must file annual returns (Form 1120) by the 15th day of the third month after the close of their fiscal year and make quarterly estimated tax payments.

S Corporations

S Corporations are taxed like partnerships but retain the liability protection of C Corporations. They have the same basic structure as C Corporations and file corporate tax returns, but the corporation doesn't pay federal income tax, as the profits are passed on to the owners who pay the taxes at their individual rates. Losses are treated in the same manner. A primary tax advantage of an S Corporation is reducing the potential for double taxation. Another financial consideration is that start-up businesses often show a loss in the first year or so. Given those circumstances, an S Corporation might be the most appropriate choice, because it allows the owners/shareholders to directly declare business losses on their individual tax returns.

One of the prime eligibility requirements for S Corporations is that the number of stockholders be 75 or less. To form an S Corporation, fill out IRS Form 2553 (Election by a Small Business Corporation) within 75 days after incorporating. S Corporations must file annual returns (Form 1120-S).

Personal Service Corporations (PSC)

Wellness providers, as well as other service professionals (e.g., accountants, attorneys, engineers, business consultants, performance artists), often opt for this status. In some states, these types of service providers are required to choose this incorporation designation. The benefits include the separation of the owners from the business entity (which also makes it easier to carry on the business should one shareholder withdraw), fringe benefits similar to those under C Corporations, and limited liability protection. If you're a sole business owner, a PSC might not be advantageous. This designation is more common with group practices, particularly given that most states require all owners of a PSC to be licensed to render the same type of service.

Professional corporations lost their popularity in the late 1980s when tax laws changed. Now they're taxed at a higher rate than other corporations, and income-splitting isn't allowed. Limited Liability Companies are usually preferred where available.

Figure 15.5 **Legal Entity Status Comparison**

	Sole Proprietor	Partnership	C Corp	S Corp	LLC
Ownership	One Owner, cannot be transferred	Multiple Owners/ Partners, transfers may be restricted	Separate Entity from Individual Owner(s), easily transferred	Separate Entity from Individual Owner(s), easily transferred but may be restricted	Separate Entity from Individual Owner(s)/ Member(s), transfers may be restricted
Liability	Unlimited	Unlimited for General Partners	Limited	Limited	Usually Limited, varies state to state
Formation & Admin, Regulation	Easiest, Minimal Regulation	Moderately Simple, but Regulated	Difficult & Expensive, Highly Regulated	Difficult & Expensive, Highly Regulated	Moderately Simple, but Regulated
Taxation	Owner pays personal income tax on profits. Subject to SE tax.	Partners pay personal income tax on profits. Subject to SE tax.	Corp income tax on net profits (possibility of double taxation for owner-employee dividends). Dividends not subject to SE tax.	Shareholders pay personal income tax on net profits (no double taxation). Not subject to SE tax.	Depends on the type of designation chosen.
IRS Forms & Publications	Schedule C, Form 1040, Pub 334	Form 1065, Pub 541	Form 1120, Pub 542	Form 1120S, Pub 542	Form 1065, Pub 3402
Advantages	Minimum legal restrictions, easy to discontinue.	A good way to combine skills/ finances of different people.	Limited liability, perpetual life, ability to raise capital through issuing stock, ease of transfer of ownership.	Limited liability, no double taxation, profits not subject to SE tax.	Easier to form, choice of designation, less paperwork.
Disadvantages	Unlimited liability, can't bring in new owners or outside capital, can't defer tax by retaining profits.	Hard to get out of, general partners are liable for actions of others.	Double taxation, corp charter restrictions, subject to state and federal controls.	Shareholders pay tax on undistributed earnings, retirement plan contributions are limited to shareholder-employee wages.	Inconsistent treatment state to state, relatively new entity with little regulatory case law to follow.

§5

Limited Liability Companies (LLCs)

A Limited Liability Company (LLC) is a hybrid of a partnership and a corporation. The main benefits of an LLC is that it provides you with a choice regarding taxation, has fewer state requirements, and provides you with a limited personal liability shield. Most states require a minimum of 2 owners (they can be spouses) and these owners are generally called members (membership title and status changes depending on the type of LLC chosen). In setting up an LLC, you have the choice of the following designations: Disregarded Entity (single member LLC wherein you use your Social Security Number); C Corp; S Corp; or Partnership (more than 1 member). All entities, other than Disregarded Entities require a separate IRS Employee Identification Number (EIN).

The paperwork isn't as complicated as with corporations. You must file Articles of a Limited Liability Company and develop an Organizational Agreement. Make sure that the Organizational Agreement specifies the designation for taxation. (Consult with an accountant before choosing the LLC designation for taxes and work with an attorney to draw up the Articles and Organizational Agreement.)

Professional Limited Liability Companies (PLLC)

Some states require service and wellness professionals who hold a license to form a Professional Limited Liability Company (PLLC), rather than the more general LLC. These options and requirements vary state to state, so check with your Corporation Commission or Secretary of State. The formation of a PLLC is similar to a LLC, except that you may be required to have your articles of organization (or similar company documents) approved by your profession's licensing board. As with a LLC, a PLLC gives the individual owner a separate entity from the actual business and provides a limited personal liability shield. However, forming a PLLC doesn't protect you from malpractice claims.

Business Name

Choosing an appropriate name for your business takes some contemplation. Most wellness practitioners are their business and thus need not go further. If you choose this route, I recommend that you also include a title, such as Tracy Jones, D.C.; Steve Smith, L.M.T.; or Terry Richards, Licensed Esthetician.

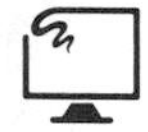

Check available business names

www.corpnet.com/corporate-name-search

You may want a separate business identity, particularly if you have a group practice. If so, choose your name carefully and avoid anything gimmicky. Select a name that conveys the essence of your business in a manner that inspires people to find out more about your services. Names such as Riverside Wellness Clinic are okay, but they lack oomph. One of the best names for a massage center is The Right Touch (located in Tucson). The Relaxation Center, Just Feet, Transformations Day Spa, and The Athletic Edge are examples of names that convey a company's mission or identify target markets.

When you've selected a potential company name, say it out loud several times to be sure it's easy to pronounce and understand. Test the name out on your friends and potential clients. Verify that your business name doesn't mean something unfortunate in another language.

Naming a business can be an arduous process. In over 3 decades, I still haven't found a name that encompasses the many facets of my business. If I were to decide to change my company's name, the transition would be bumpy because Sohnen-Moe Associates is well known (even though it's extremely difficult to understand over the phone).

Trademark: Legal Care for Your Business & Product Name by S. Elias and R. Stim

If you choose a business name other than your own, request a name search with the Corporation Commission or Secretary of State. Most have a search option on their website. They may also do this by phone and let you know if the name is available for use. Regulations and fees vary, as do forms. In some states, there is a difference between a "trade name" and a "trademark." Each has its own form and fees. With the trade name, you're registering the actual name of your company (e.g., Hands That Heal). A trademark is the registration of your logo and its description, which can be a design or set of words. If you plan to use a company name, specific word(s), or a logo in interstate commerce, consider obtaining a federal trademark. This is a somewhat complex process. The fees vary per mark and per classification (depending on whether or not you file online). The fee is nonrefundable regardless of the results.

Whenever your business name is different from your personal name, most states require that you publish a DBA ("Doing Business As"), also referred to as a Fictitious Name Certificate, in the classified section of at least 1 newspaper in the county where you operate. Contact your county clerk for forms and procedures.

As a sole proprietor, you don't need an employer identification number (EIN) unless you have employees or a retirement plan. (See IRS Publication 583 for specifics.) Otherwise, you can use your Social Security number. To get an EIN, file form SS-4 with your local IRS. You can complete the application online at www.irs.gov, mail it, or fax it. Contact the IRS directly to get the fax number for your region.

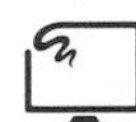

Internet Trademark Search

tmsearch.uspto.gov
trademarks.thomsonreuters.com
www.corsearch.com

U.S. Trademark Office

www.uspto.gov/trademark

Figure 15.6 Tips for Choosing a Business Name

Marketing expert Healy Jones[3] says your business name should be:

1. Simple to remember.
2. Easy to pronounce.
3. Easy to spell.
4. Illustrative of your service.
5. Have the same Internet domain name.

§5

Domain Name

In today's digital world, a website functions as an extension of your business card. We discuss the importance of a website and the details about it in chapter 27, but while you're choosing a business name, you should also be choosing a domain name (an address for your website). Your domain name should match your business name. It makes it easier for people to find you, and your clients can easily direct their friends and family your way. If at all possible, choose ".com" for your domain extension. Many additional extensions exist, still .com is the most commonly used and remembered. Although my website, Sohnen-Moe.com, has a dash in it, I don't recommend using dashes. They are confusing and make it harder to share your website over the phone. Keep your domain name short, and like your business name, make it easy to spell and pronounce.

Verify that your potential business name is available on your desired social media platforms.

Laws and Regulations

Business owners need to comply with the laws and regulations that apply to them. These fall into two main categories: professional regulations that relate to you being a wellness practitioner; and the local, state, county, and federal requirements that apply to starting or relocating a business.

Professional Licenses and Requirements

Many wellness practitioners are required to be licensed or certified to provide their services, some aren't. Laws vary by state or province, so you must find out the regulations defining your scope of practice. Regulatory methods for professional credentials are described in Chapter 5.

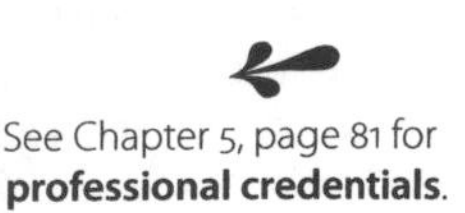

See Chapter 5, page 81 for **professional credentials**.

Healthcare providers must abide by many laws above and beyond just doing business. Many states enforce Federal Anti-kickback laws that prohibit practitioners from taking referral fees from other practitioners, and from receiving money from third-party group buying companies (who split the fees they collect with the practitioner). A useful online resource to simplify your research is the FindLaw for Small Business website, which provides extensive information about licenses and permits specific to each profession and the associated board regulations.

Business Licenses and Permits

State Guides for **Licenses and Permits**

smallbusiness.findlaw.com
business.usa.gov

www.sba.gov/content/what-state-licenses-and-permits-does-your-business-need

Business laws and regulations aren't the same as your professional laws and regulations, and the fees are usually separate. For example, if you're a massage therapist, then your professional license to practice (which is often granted by the state) is separate from a business license to operate your practice in a specific city. Depending on where you practice, you might not be required to get a business license.

The U.S. Small Business Administration (SBA) has a great website for finding licensing requirements. Its Business Licenses and Permits Search Tool allows you to search by location (city, state, or zip code), combined with your type of business. Massage is one of the 15 types of business listed! Once you put in the information and click "Search" you get a results page that lists the federal, state, and local requirements (permits, licenses, and registrations) needed to run that business. It also provides links to web pages, contact information, application forms, and instructions. Your local City Hall, Secretary of State, or the Consumer Affairs office can also provide you with information and resources.

See Chapter 16, pages 218-220 for details on **zoning**.

Whether you do your research online, in person, or by phone, be sure to contact your city or county Business Licensing Division for their requirements. Government rules and regulations can change at any time. Figure 15.7 provides an overview of the basic required licenses and permits, and who to contact for specific information and forms. This list doesn't cover every possible situation, as your business may have special site requirements or industry regulations.

Figure 15.7 **Licenses & Permits — Quick Reference**

Business License: Allows you the privilege of doing business. Contact your Business Licensing Bureau.

Occupational License: Allows you to work in a specific industry as long as you comply with that profession's regulations. Contact the State Agency of Consumer Affairs or the local Business Licensing Bureau.

Transaction Privilege Tax License: Allows you to collect (and remit) sales tax. Contact your State Department of Revenue.

Planning and Zoning Permits: These permits are issued after your location has been assessed and shows that the business operation conforms with area plans, has proper zoning, and has adequate parking. A Certificate of Occupancy is an example of this type of permit. Contact your City or County Hall Planning Department.

Building Safety Permit: This permit is issued after your location is inspected and has met the minimum safety requirements, and complies with fire and building codes. Contact the Fire Department.

Insurance Coverage

Obtaining proper insurance coverage is imperative for any small business. Discuss your specific needs with an insurance agent (or three) to determine the appropriate types and amount of insurance needed. You may need more than 1 insurance carrier, since very few companies offer all of the types of coverage. Check your office lease thoroughly. Your leaseholder may not be responsible for providing complete (if any) coverage. Also, if you work out of your home, be certain to review your homeowner's or renter's policy. While the standard homeowner's policy protects you from personal liability if a guest is injured at your home, it doesn't cover you if the visit is related to business.

Determine which types of insurance are required by law and purchase those policies first.

Figure 15.8 Types of Insurance Coverage

Liability Insurance: Covers costs of injuries that occur to business-related visitors on your property. It doesn't cover you or your employees.

General Liability Insurance: Covers negligence resulting in injury to clients, employees, or the general public while you're on their premises. This is particularly important if you do office calls or teach classes.

Malpractice Liability Insurance: Protects you from claims due to a loss incurred by your clients as a result of negligence or failure on your part to perform at a professional skill level.

Small Business Insurance: Offers umbrella coverage for business losses in terms of general liability, business interruption, errors and omissions, and product liability.

Product Liability: Protects you from claims by clients who use products designed, manufactured, or sold by you. Wellness providers rarely need this coverage, as the product manufacturers should carry this insurance.

Automobile Insurance: Make sure you have the correct policy if you use your car in your business. Be sure to carry full coverage including disability, business interruption, and loss or damage to business-related items.

Fire and Theft Insurance: Covers business equipment, furniture, supplies, and documents. If you work out of your home, you may need to purchase a rider to get adequate protection for a home office.

Business Interruption Insurance: Pays you approximately what you would have earned if your business closes due to fire or other insurable causes.

Permitted Incidental Occupancies-Residence Premises: Deletes the liability exclusions for business activities conducted on the main residence premises and modifies the business personal property special limit. Doesn't cover Professional Liability.

Personal Disability Insurance: Safeguards you from loss of income if you cannot work due to illness or injury. You receive a certain monthly amount if you're permanently disabled or a portion if you're partially disabled.

Medical Health Insurance: Helps cover medical bills, particularly for complicated illnesses, injuries, and hospitalization.

Workers' Compensation Insurance: Required by law if you have employees. It covers all of the costs that you as an employer would be required to pay for any injury to an employee. It also provides the employee with disability and death benefits if injured or killed on the job.

Partnership Insurance: Protects you against lawsuits arising from actions or omissions by any of your business partners.

Setting Your Fees

Fee structures vary greatly depending on the type of work you do and where you're located. Setting an appropriate fee structure and fee increase strategy is necessary in any business. No matter which method you choose for determining your rates, be certain your fee structure promotes credibility.

Carefully consider all of the costs involved in running your business before you finalize your fee structure. This includes your fixed costs (e.g., rent, utilities, phone, equipment, loan payments, maintenance, insurance, licenses, promotion, staffing), as well as the amenities that vary depending on the number and type of clients (e.g., providing free samples and educational materials, sales tax collection, supplies). Then there's your time: keeping client records, networking, planning, extended business hours, traveling, practice management, continuing your education, and client follow-up.

Figure 15.9 Four Major Fee-Setting Strategies

1. **High-end rate**: Set rate significantly higher than industry standard rate to target a small percentage of the population. This usually only works if your service is innovative, in demand, and has no competition.
2. **Industry standard rate**: Determine the industry standard rate and align with it.
3. **Low-end rate**: Set rate significantly lower than the industry standard rate to attract a larger market share.
4. **Time-limited introductory rate**: Offer introductory rates for a limited time or package deals reflecting reduced rates. Beware of the tendency to overextend introductory rates.

Figure 15.10 illustrates how to determine your fees. It's based on a 40-hour workweek, which leaves a maximum of 25 billable hours per week. Since overhead varies greatly from one business to another, it isn't included in this breakdown. Note that this chart can have an unsettling effect.

Let's say that you want to earn $40,000 this year before taxes. If you plan on working 50% (billing 12.5 hours per week), then you need to charge $61.50 per hour. If you want to work 90% (bill 22.5 hours per week), then you only need to charge $34 per hour. But, you also must include the costs in running your business. Imagine that your fixed costs are $15,000 per year plus $6 per session. So, at a 50% workload, you need to cover $40,000 income, $15,000 fixed expenses, and $3,900 per session cost (650 sessions), which equals $58,900. Looking at the chart, you find that to bring in gross revenues of $60,000, you need to charge approximately $92 per hour. Yet, if you plan on working 90%, then you need to cover $40,000 income, $15,000 fixed expenses, and $7,020 per session cost (1,170 sessions), which equals $62,020. In this instance, you only need to charge about $53 per hour.

> "The difference between the top money winners on the PGA golf tour and the bottom money winners can be as little as one stroke a day.
>
> —Steve Miller
> former PGA tour player

You may be wondering how you can possibly earn the income you desire while charging a fair and equitable price. Several possibilities exist for increasing your income potential. First of all, you can increase the number of billable weekly hours by working more than 40 hours per week (which isn't uncommon with small business owners). Another alternative is to reduce your overhead costs—but be certain this doesn't cause clients to experience a decrease in benefits. You can also diversify your practice by selling products, subcontracting work (or hiring other practitioners to work for you), and leading workshops. Finally, one of the most viable options is to delegate some of your business activities, which frees you to increase the number of hours of direct client contact (billable hours).

Determining your appropriate fee structure involves more than simply deciding what you want to charge per hour. Balance your desired income and requisite expenses with what's realistic. Set fees that you feel comfortable with and confident about that are also fair and instill trust. Even if you're considered to be the best practitioner in your field, it's futile to charge more than what the market will bear. Just because you desire a specific income level and feel you deserve to charge a certain rate doesn't necessarily mean people will pay it. Choose your market(s) carefully and strategize your fee structure.

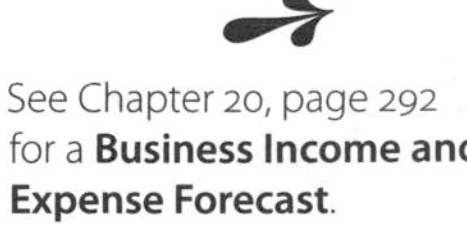

See Chapter 20, page 292 for a **Business Income and Expense Forecast**.

When someone inquires about your fees, state them with confidence. If the client indicates in some way that he cannot manage that fee, you get to choose in that moment if you want to offer a lower fee to accommodate the client. You may want to offer a person-to-person sliding scale as you see fit and as your budget allows. Many practitioners know how many clients they need to see at full price and then how much room that leaves for other clients to pay less. I base my decision to lower a fee on necessity and desire to make positive change.

Figure 15.10 **Time/Income Factor Analysis**

One Year	=	365 days
	–	*104 days (weekends)*
	–	*8 days (holidays)*
	–	*10 days (health)*
	–	*10 days (vacation)*
	=	233 days
233 days x 8 hours/day	=	1,864 hours/year
	–	30% (promotion, operations, professional development)
	=	approximately 1,300 hours
1,300 hours	=	approximately 25 billable hours/week

Desired Annual Income*	50% 650 hrs *(12.5 hr/wk)*	70% 910 hrs *(17.5 hr/wk)*	90% 1170 hrs *(22.5 hr/wk)*	100% 1300 hrs *(25 hr/wk)*
$25,000	$38.50	$27.50	$21.50	$19.25
$30,000	$46.00	$33.00	$25.75	$23.00
$35,000	$54.00	$38.50	$30.00	$27.00
$40,000	$61.50	$44.00	$34.00	$31.00
$50,000	$77.00	$55.00	$42.75	$38.50
$60,000	$92.00	$66.00	$51.25	$46.00
$75,000	$115.50	$82.50	$64.00	$58.00
$100,000	$154.00	$110.00	$85.50	$77.00

**Does not include allowance for overhead and income taxes*

§5

Sliding Fee Scales

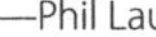

Money will not add to your self-esteem, it works the other way around.

—Phil Laut

A sliding fee scale allows people who cannot afford your full fee to pay a lower one. Sliding fee scales can be awkward and tough to set up in advance of the first session unless a client has said something to you while booking the appointment. I don't advocate advertising a sliding fee scale unless you know that your target market is going to need it (e.g., people on meager fixed incomes). Usually what works best is to give parameters. A frequently used model that seems least offensive and fair is determining fees based on income level. This depends on trust, although I suppose you could require to see a copy of a client's tax return. Here is an example of a sliding scale statement:

> *My standard rate is $60 per session. If this presents a hardship for you, I accept a sliding scale fee based on your combined family annual income level. If the total annual income earned is less than $15,000 annually, the fee per session is $30; $15,000-20,000 = $35; $20,000-25,000 = $40; $25,000-30,000 = $50; and over $30,000 = $60.*

Prepaid Package Plans

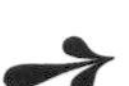

See Chapter 30, pages 472-479 for additional ideas on **client incentives**.

Prepaid package plans encourage people to book sessions more frequently and infuse extra income into your bank account. Some ideas are: purchase 3 acupuncture treatments and get a $5 savings per treatment; 7 counseling sessions qualify for a 20% discount; and purchase 5 massages and receive the sixth one free. Keep it simple—don't overwhelm yourself and your clients with too many options. Also, consider putting the majority of that money in a savings account and transfer it into your main checking account when the client actually has a session.

Raising Your Rates

If you're a self-employed practitioner, you have ultimate control over when and how much to raise your fees. When you've determined a fee increase is required, be certain the amount is appropriate. You will probably lose credibility (and clients) if you raise your rates more than once per year. Do a 1-year financial forecast. Ascertain the amount of money you need to charge per session should you experience no growth in your business. Raise your fees accordingly, with a caveat against an increase of greater than 15%.

Inform your clients of your rate changes at least 2 weeks in advance via a personalized letter or pre-printed postcard. Springing a higher charge on them at the last moment, particularly right after a session, is disrespectful. If you offer package discounts, promote goodwill by allowing your clients the opportunity to sign up for a package at the "old" rates. Of course, they need to make this commitment before the new fee structure goes into effect. In fact, you may want to let them purchase as many future treatments as they want at the old rate, as long as they pay for them up front.

In her article, "How to Raise Your Session Fees",[4] Jenny Hogan says that raising your prices is necessary for the advancement of your professional career. She offers these tips:

1. Place signs in your treatment room.
2. Send an email or mail an announcement to your client list.
3. Use professional and positive language in your announcement, taking the time to appropriately thank your clients for their business.
4. State the exact date of the rate increase.
5. Consider offering a value-added service, discount, or special gift.
6. Describe any changes in services.
7. Provide client education about the benefits of your services.
8. Be ready with references to a few trusted colleagues, for those clients who decide not to return after your increase.

Value-Added Service

Keep in mind that raising your rates isn't the only way to increase your income. Most wellness providers have a rather extensive repertoire of techniques and services they use on a regular basis. Even though these modalities may usually be incorporated into treatments without additional charge to clients, you may want to consider expanding some of those services and charging a fee. For instance, instead of doing a 3-minute energy balancing technique at the end of a treatment, you could do a full 20-minute energy balancing session.

Using massage therapy as an example, other techniques that can be full sessions in and of themselves are: modalities such as reflexology, acupuncture, and craniosacral therapy; crystal or stone therapy; sound treatments; chakra clearing and balancing; breath work; stretching and exercise; biofeedback; and vibrational treatments. Many complementary services such as facials, pedicures, and hypnotherapy can be performed after the massage or even at the same time by another practitioner.

> "It is common sense to take a method and try it. If it fails, admit it frankly and try another. But above all, try something.
> —Franklin D. Roosevelt

Another arena to consider is the use of products or equipment that take very little of your time yet are of immense benefit to your clients. This includes hydrocollator packs, hot pads, ice packs, ginger fomentations, herbal compresses, paraffin treatments, aromatherapy, heated gloves and booties, as well as special equipment such as steam units, passive movement tables, anti-gravity machines, flotation tanks, and "brain-gym" equipment. Some of these treatments can be part of your primary treatment or done before or after the session. Utilizing these products and equipment allows you to do other things such as paperwork, phone calls, or exercising while your client is receiving the treatment. They provide you with an innovative means to serve your clients' wellbeing and earn money without much of your hands-on time. Also, most of these items are a pure profit-generator after the original cost of the equipment. For instance, you can purchase a paraffin unit for $150. It would only take between 15-20 sessions to recoup your initial outlay for the cost of the unit plus the extra wax. A great side benefit is that you can utilize the equipment to take care of your own hands and feet. A steam canopy is another example of a tool which provides a profitable adjunct service to your practice. For less than $1,000, you can own a piece of equipment that virtually costs nothing to use and takes very little of your time. This is my idea of working smarter—not harder.

§5

Gauge what is a billable modality and what isn't. For instance, some massage therapists charge extra for using aromatherapy oils or hot packs while others don't—they consider it a way of differentiating themselves from other therapists. The questions to ask yourself to determine whether to charge an additional fee for a service are: Does this cost me much in time or money? Are others charging for this service? Will my clients easily perceive the benefits? Does this make my job easier (e.g., a hot pack loosens muscles so I don't have to put in as much effort or pressure to achieve the same results)? Will offering this service at no extra charge increase the number of referrals and enhance client retention? Is incorporating this service the most effective use of my time?

See Chapter 21 for **retailing**.

Figure 15.11 illustrates how the discounts increase with the number of services included in the package. The beauty of this customer service-based marketing approach is that the client receives a wide variety of services without costing the therapist much in time or product (the steam treatment is done without the therapist needing to be present, and the paraffin treatment can be done during the massage). Using the Total Health Session as an example, the time required for Francine to directly work with a client is approximately 2 hours. She is earning more than her standard hourly massage rate, and the client receives an incredible treatment. This is what win-win is all about. Offering adjunct services and treatments to your primary service is beneficial to both you and your clients. It increases your clients' awareness of the scope of available modalities and gives them the power to take more responsibility for their wellness by designing their ideal treatment sessions. Most people appreciate options as long as the list of choices isn't too overwhelming. It also helps you avoid burnout from doing one session after another, gives you a competitive edge, and increases your income potential.

Figure 15.11 Package Example

Francine Feelgoode is a massage therapist who is trained in several energy balancing techniques and aromatherapy. In addition to her massage equipment, Francine has a steam canopy, a paraffin unit, and a set of heated gloves and booties. She offers several different packages to her clients:

- 1-hour Massage, $60
- 90-minute Massage, $80
- 20-minute Steam Treatment, $15
- 20-minute Aromatherapy Steam Treatment, $20
- 30-minute Energy Balancing, $25
- Hand and Foot Paraffin Treatment, $20 (included in the session time)
- Deluxe Session (1-hour Massage and Aroma-Steam), $70
- Mini-Spa Session (90-minute Massage, Aroma-Steam, and Paraffin), $100
- Total Health Session (90-minute Massage, Aroma-Steam, Energy Balancing, and Paraffin), $125

Buying a Practice

The idea of buying an existing practice may seem very appealing. After all, you avoid much of the process entailed in building a strong business foundation. Although it may be easier and faster to buy an established practice, you also inherit the previous owner's problems, and there is no guarantee the clients will stay on with you.

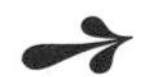

See Chapter 23, pages 341-343 for tips on how to **price a business**.

Practice Sale Scenario

A seller is asking for $15,000 for her practice. She has been in business for 5 years, and, during that time, her clientele has steadily increased. She sees an average of 15 clients per week and charges $50 per session. Her office is in a small professional building. Her monthly operating expenses run approximately $1,000. She is making a major life change and has decided to move to a tropical island. She is including her equipment and supplies as part of the package.

If the assets are items you want and you could retain the majority of her clients, this would be a reasonable price. You can minimize your risks by requiring that, in addition to the hard assets, the remainder of the selling price be based on the actual number of clients who stay with the business. Two examples are: making payments only if the business meets certain client retention requirements (e.g., at least 50% of the clients stay); or you only have to pay the seller a set percentage of the fees received from the current clientele (e.g., 40% of fees collected until the original loan is repaid).

Points to Ponder

How comfortable would you be with the risk of poor client retention in a sale such as this? What other benefits of an established practice would offset poor client retention?

Figure 15.12 Steps to Buying a Practice

1. Evaluate your reasons for buying.
2. Determine the "fit."
3. Conduct a preliminary evaluation.
4. Analyze documentation.
5. Evaluate the business premises.
6. Clarify legal agreements.
7. Have an attorney review all documents.
8. Open negotiations.
9. Offer a letter of intent.
10. Have an attorney finalize the purchase agreement.
11. Purchase the business.
12. Begin the transition stage.

Evaluate Your Reasons For Buying

There are many advantages and disadvantages to buying an existing practice. Before you jump into a purchase, do the following exercise to assess your reasons for taking this route.

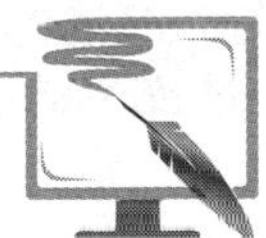

Should I Buy an Existing Business?

Ask yourself the following questions:

- Why do I want to buy an existing business?
- What are the potential risks versus the perceived benefits?
- What liabilities will I incur (e.g., lease, unclaimed gift certificates, payroll)?
- What conditions need to be present to make it worthwhile?
- Does the business generate enough money to meet my financial goals and loan repayment?
- Are the practice's image and philosophy compatible with mine?
- Why might buying this practice be inappropriate?
- Would it be more cost-effective to set up my own practice?
- What are my other options?

All businesses aren't created equally. Clarify exactly what you're buying. Determine if you're purchasing one or more of the following: rights to use a well-known business name; a client list; established contracts; goodwill and reputation; an office location; and equipment.

The most common instance of a wellness provider buying another practice is when that practitioner is just starting out, or moving to a new location. An established practitioner might purchase a practice if she is interested in expanding her current target markets or wants to branch into another area.

Determine the Fit

When meeting with a potential seller, attempt to discover the true reason for the sale. This could dramatically influence your decision. For instance, if the seller is moving to another state or retiring, that's one thing; but if the move is within 30 miles, you may not be buying anything, because the majority of the clients may still continue to see the practitioner at the new location.

The seller may not be versed in the protocol for selling a business. Usually, sellers view their practices in terms of the work they've invested in making it successful. It may not be set up for someone to easily take over. It's rare to just step in and retain all the clients. They may not like you and vice versa. More than anything else, assess the "fit" you would have with the business.

Your chances for success are much greater if your knowledge, training, personality, modalities, and style are similar to that of the seller. One way to determine this is by receiving a session from the seller. Ask to be treated as though you were a typical new client. Although the seller will most likely be on her best behavior, this experience gives you insight into her style, as well as what the current clients are accustomed to receiving. If the company's policies and procedures don't suit you, or the types of treatments offered are outside your desired scope of practice, it most likely isn't in your best interest to buy the practice.

Conduct a Preliminary Evaluation

Many factors come into play in judging the viability of a business. The seller should have a fact sheet that encompasses the company's history, mission statement, business description (including the number of clients, the services offered, the equipment and products used, location description, fee structure, client profile, position statement, competition analysis, and differential advantage), assets, financial history, reason for sale, and pricing terms.

Obtain this fact sheet and samples of promotional materials before making an offer. Ask to view the current appointment book. Check to see how many appointments are scheduled each week and how far in advance the practitioner is booked. After reviewing these materials and receiving a session, you're in a better position to decide whether to make an offer.

Analyze Documentation

When you make a written offer, be sure to state that it's contingent upon verification of the detailed documentation. This documentation should include the following: a detailed business description; a copy of the lease; names of all owners, associates, and staff members; profit and loss statements for the past three years; tax returns for the past 3 years; copies of current contracts; a listing of accounts payable and receivable; a list of fixtures, equipment, and inventory with their replacement value noted; a list of outstanding liens; and a portfolio of promotional materials about the company and owner. Another positive consideration is whether the business has outside contracts to provide ongoing wellness services to a business or seasonal work for conferences. Review contracts to make sure there are no clauses regarding cancellation of the contract if the business is sold or transferred.

Assess the Business Premises

One of the most beneficial aspects of buying a practice can be obtaining a lease in a "prime" location. Sometimes, this is more important than the actual number of clients. Let's say a massage therapist has a concession in a very busy, upscale gym, but this therapist hasn't been marketing his practice very well. If you're willing to invest the time in marketing, you could probably do quite well, and it would be worth a reasonable selling price. Do the proper research before you allow a location to inflate the selling price of a business.

First, verify the building is zoned for your particular profession; don't assume that because someone is currently running the same type of business in that location, it's therefore legal. Zoning may have changed or the current business might have somehow slipped through without anyone noticing (yet).

Next, find out if the current lease can be subleased or assigned, or if a new lease needs to be negotiated. Be sure to verify the particulars about the lease. Determining the worth of a lease during the negotiations of a selling price is a rather subjective process. After researching the property, weigh your findings with the perceived importance of the space to the current clients.

Open Negotiations

Deciding on a fair price for a practice is difficult at best. The seller sets what he feels is a realistic price. You must do the math. Calculate how much time, energy, and money it would cost you to build your practice to the same point as the seller's, remembering that there's no guarantee the current clients will stay with you.

Most buyers take out loans (from friends, a bank, or the seller) to finance the purchase of a business. When a service business is sold, the seller often becomes the loan holder.

Brokers

Many brokers work on either an hourly consultation rate or a flat transaction fee. A qualified broker knows what questions to ask and can identify potential problems. In your initial interview, ask if the broker has ever negotiated a sale for the type of practice you desire (or a similar type of sale). The most crucial factor is that you communicate well with each other. Also, have your accountant interview a potential broker. Your accountant already knows your business, has your best interests at heart, and can determine if the broker is qualified. After the sales contract has been negotiated, have an attorney review it before you sign.

International Business Brokers Association
www.ibba.org

Final Stages

The final two stages are the completion of the purchase and the transition time after the sale. The ideal situation would be to work as an associate for several months before actually purchasing the business. This way the current clients would get to know you, and you could assess whether you like working in that environment, particularly if an office space or working with other practitioners is part of the sales agreement. In addition, this gives you an opportunity to discover little nuances of the business and become familiar with the logistics of running the business. It also makes the actual transition much smoother.

As a buyer, it's wise to understand the process a seller goes through, so please refer to the section on selling a practice. Buying an existing practice is very risky, yet the potential benefits can be rewarding. Keep in mind that even if the practice is a strong one, you need to continue nurturing it through marketing and incorporating an active client retention program.

See Chapter 23, pages 338-345 for information on how to **sell a practice**.

§5

Purchasing a Franchise

With the rise in popularity of wellness related franchise businesses, buying a franchise may be an option for practitioners who wish to own their own business. Among the 2015 Entrepreneur Magazine Franchise 500 list, 42 are healthcare-related businesses.[5] Franchises are businesses that have a blueprint for operation and training programs that help you get started. Most healthcare franchise business plans include a multi-practitioner operation. This option requires you to be a business owner first, and a practitioner second, because the start-up and operation of a fully-functioning business can be a full-time job. There is usually a higher start-up investment in purchasing a franchise than starting your own practice, or even buying an existing practice, because the franchise brand reputation and marketing power come with a much larger value.

16

Location, Location, Location

"There are three things that matter in property: location, location, location."
—Lord Harold Samuel

Zoning Regulations
- Home Office Requirements
- Variances

Leasing Agreements
- Negotiate a Fair Lease

Office Design
- Ambiance
- Professionalism
- Sensations
- Layout
- My Ideal Session Room

Relocating Your Practice
- Moving Within the Same City
- Moving to a New City

Key Terms

Ambiance
Chamber of Commerce
Commercial Zoning
Feng Shui
Industrial Zoning
Lease
Networking
Professionalism
Residential Zoning
Sensations
Special Exemption Permit
Variance
Zoning Ordinance
Zoning Variance

You spend a lot of time in your office, so it's critical to choose a location that you like and that also attracts clients, fits your business image, accommodates your business needs in terms of size and layout (and potential expansion), is properly zoned, and is priced within your budget.

Many practitioners have home offices as their main business site. Some practitioners who operate out of a commercial space may still see clients at home. You may be comfortable in your home, but your clients might not feel the same. You need to take extra steps to ensure the space lends a professional atmosphere for your clients. This includes keeping any space the client comes in contact with (e.g., parking area, entrance, restroom, hallway, treatment space), clean and free of clutter. Also, limit the amount of personal items displayed.

Choose an office location that's convenient to the majority of your clients. While it may be handy to have an office near or even in your home, that might not be the best option for your target market(s). For instance, let's say one of your target markets tends to use public transportation, and the space you're contemplating using as your office is located blocks away from the nearest stop. This choice will hamper your marketing efforts, particularly if you live in an area with inclement weather. Many potential clients will simply look for another practitioner whose office is more conveniently located.

Most practitioners don't generally have a large walk-in clientele—although locating a business in a high-traffic area can provide exposure. They tend to choose office buildings where the tenants are wellness practitioners or other service providers. The exception to this is a business that has multiple practitioners and offers services that can easily be done "last-minute" (e.g., chair massages, chiropractic adjustments, quick-fix pain relief treatments). This type of business needs to be in a high-traffic area.

Office prices vary greatly depending on the actual location and the local economics. Check out the going rates on comparable office space. "Comparable" is the key word. Read the fine print. The quoted price might not include such things as utilities, parking, leasehold improvements (lighting, decorations, and structural changes to the floors and walls), maintenance, and signage.

Zoning Regulations

Once you find a site that seems excellent, you must determine if you can actually practice there. Zoning ordinances can be a potential source of frustration and financial cost. You must know the local zoning requirements before opening up a business, buying an existing practice, or even remodeling your current office space. Wellness providers are often required to obtain several types of licenses and permits. It can be difficult to discover the requirements, because each locale has different zoning laws, and it isn't always clear which departments issue the various permits.

Warning! Get your information in writing. It isn't unusual for 2 different people in the same office to give conflicting information.

The two main purposes for licenses and permits are raising revenue and protecting the health and safety of the public. Zoning ordinances essentially divide an area into sections in which various activities and businesses are allowed or prohibited. The 4 major types of zoning are residential, commercial, industrial, and agricultural. Within these categories are subsections which define the types of allowable activities. For example, a commercial area might be zoned for professional businesses only, retail, a combination of professional and retail, light industry, or major manufacturing. Some residential areas allow certain types of businesses (mainly professionals) but not others. The level of enforcement varies widely. Some areas have negligible standards of operation and others are strict. Often it becomes important only if someone complains.

In some cities you're required to meet certain codes before you open your business (e.g., building, health, safety). Health practice items commonly regulated in zoning ordinances are off-street parking, signage, wheelchair accessible, shower facilities, and types of business activities. For example, hydrotherapy is an area in which many practitioners encounter restrictions. A touch therapist in the Southwest was told that unless his office had a shower he could not do light steam treatments—even though he was using professional equipment. Before investing money in adjunct equipment, make certain that the zoning regulations allow its use. If the zoning doesn't, do your best to get a variance.

Keep in mind that ordinances are amended frequently, and just because a similar business is in operation, doesn't mean that yours will be allowed. The other business could have been in place before a zoning change was made, and, as such, is allowed to stay in operation. But any new business, or one that changes hands, would have to meet the new requirements. Any time you apply for a business permit, license, or building permit, it can tag your business for scrutiny.

Consider this case in point.

Zoning Scenario

Susan Smith, L.Ac., decides to open an office in a well-established professional building. The tenants are a mixture of accountants, attorneys, counselors, and a reflexologist. The office she wants formerly belonged to a massage therapist. She assumes that she won't encounter any problems since the businesses are similar and a wellness practitioner previously rented the office. She proceeds to sign a lease and decorate the office. Within a month Susan opens the doors, only to be served with a cease-and-desist order. She wonders how this could possibly happen.

If she had researched the zoning ordinances, she would have discovered that 2 years ago, the regulations had changed. Since the previous therapist had already been there before the new regulations, he didn't have to comply with the changes. But the moment Susan applied for an occupation license, it set off a chain of events that resulted in the zoning board discovering that she didn't make the necessary changes to legally operate an acupuncture practice in that building.

Points to Ponder

Besides researching zoning ordinances, what other issues should you investigate if you find yourself in this situation? What types of professionals could you consult? How can you be sure you're getting the answers you need to proceed?

§5

Talk with your state licensing board to ascertain if there are any additional regulations you must meet, particularly in terms of size, entrances, bathrooms, and shower facilities. Ask for a list of the profession-specific requirements and the permits you need. If they are unable to supply you with all of the information, they should at least have the appropriate contacts.

If you still don't have all the information you need, talk with people at city or county hall. Then meet with the planning department and the health department. If you experience any difficulties in obtaining the necessary information, go to the library, the office of economic development, or the state office of industrial development.

Home Office Requirements

Home office requirements are often more stringent than those for commercial office space. Check your deed covenants and homeowner association's documents (i.e., articles of incorporation, bylaws, CCRs) for any specific limitations. Residential offices are often restricted to the amount of vehicular traffic generated, parking, the numbers of clients allowed in the home at any one time, signage, hours of operation, the percentage of floor space devoted to business, and storage facilities. Many permits require a separate office entrance with an

See Chapter 11, pages 157-158 for details on **home offices**.

attached bathroom. In some locations, home businesses aren't allowed to have employees or sell products.

Now that many households have members who work at least part time in their homes, city officials are beginning to ease up on home office restrictions. Still, it's risky to open a practice in a location where zoning is questionable. If possible, get the zoning changed before it's a necessity. If you operate a home business, you may opt to take a "let's wait and see attitude" and not worry about the zoning ordinances. This can put you in a precarious position, particularly if you're investing a lot of money in remodeling your home office.

Variances

If you're found in violation of a zoning ordinance, you're sent a notice ordering you to cease your business. You must file an appeal immediately or cease operations, because every day you continue to operate can be considered a separate violation. Remember, a decision from a zoning official isn't necessarily written in stone. You can often appeal that decision, get a conditional use permit, or even obtain a zoning variance.

When meeting with any official, it's best to have garnered support from adjacent business owners, your neighbors (for home offices), and other members of the community. (This is an example of why it pays to be involved in your chamber of commerce, business networking organizations, and local trade associations.)

If you need to alter the current zoning requirements to legally run your business, begin by meeting with city officials to ask for a zoning variance or "special exemption" permit. This requires the cooperation of neighbors or nearby businesses. Get letters or have them sign a petition that says they support your business use. If your business is already established, bring photographs that illustrate the scope of your business.

If this doesn't work, take your request to the zoning board. It's very helpful if you can get your neighbors or adjoining business owners to go with you and speak on your behalf. The next step would be appealing to the city council. If all else fails, you can take your case to court.

Wellness providers are often required to meet very stringent conditions founded upon antiquated regulations. I recommend that practitioners in each city get together and decide what requirements they feel are reasonable and submit them to the zoning board. Start a lobbying campaign now. Create a structure that you want—not one that's dictated by officials who may not understand your profession.

Leasing Agreements

Before signing a lease, make sure the office space is right for you. Research the office's historical information: find out why the space is vacant; ascertain the number of tenants who have held the space in the past 10 years; and get a listing of other current tenants, including their types of businesses, office hours, and schedule of lease expiration dates. Visit the area at different times of the day and night to get a sense of the traffic flow. Ask the landlord or leasing agent for a copy of the operating rules and regulations to ensure compatibility with your practice. Determine if the building is properly zoned for your type of work.

Inspect the physical structure: make sure the roof is sound, the heating and cooling system is in good condition, and the building is secure (e.g., appropriate exterior lighting, stable stairs, lockable lobby door). Check with building and fire inspectors to see if the space has been cited.

Before signing a lease, find out the restrictions and actual costs of any necessary adaptations (e.g., custom build-outs) and miscellaneous requirements (e.g., signage, hours of operation) and restrictions. For instance, I have heard many tales of woe from practitioners who signed leases without realizing that the cost to install the required signage was thousands of dollars. Refer to the Office Leasing Checklist (Figure 16.1) for common lease agreement categories.

Negotiate a Fair Lease

The last step before finalizing a lease agreement is to review all legal documents with an attorney or leasing consultant. The relatively few dollars spent with counsel can save you thousands later, should disputes arise.

Dale Willerton, founder of "The Lease Coach" and author of *Negotiate Your Commercial Lease*, gives these tips to wellness practitioners:[1]

1. **Negotiate to win.** Don't accept every position the landlord's agent presents, because you can be sure they are negotiating to win.
2. **Be prepared to walk away.** Set aside your emotions and be objective.
3. **Ask the right questions.** Do your homework on the deals that the other tenants are getting and position yourself for the same or better deal.
4. **Remember that the broker is working for the landlord, not you.** When researching multiple properties, try to deal with the listing agent for each property directly, he is most likely to be able to give you the best deal.
5. **Never accept the first offer.** In real estate, most things are negotiable and the landlord expects you to counteroffer.
6. **Ask for more than you want.** Counteroffers are all part of the game. If you want 3 months free, ask for 5 months.
7. **Negotiate the deposit.** Deposits are negotiable too, and large deposits are usually not legally required.
8. **Measure your space.** Most tenants pay per square foot, but often don't receive as much space as the lease agreement says.
9. **Negotiate, negotiate, negotiate.** Leasing is a process, so take your time.
10. **Educate yourself and get help.**

Remember, you don't get what you deserve, you get what you negotiate!

The Lease Coach
theleasecoach.com

See Chapter 24, pages 360-367 for information on **targeting markets**.

Office Design

§5

The major elements involved in office design are ambiance, professionalism, sensations (scent, sight, touch, and sound), and layout. Make this a space that is mutually healing to yourself and others. The basic tenet is: Appeal to the majority of your clients while being inoffensive to all. The main sources of offense are forcing your personal or professional beliefs on others and invading people's sense of smell, sight, sound, and touch. Oftentimes people are affronted by things we don't even consider as potential problems.

For instance, you may hold strong spiritual or religious beliefs that aren't shared by everyone. Most people would be fine with seeing one or two symbols in your office, but would probably feel ill at ease if they walked into a room filled with icons and artifacts. Your clients are much more comfortable if your office space is client-centered. In other words, create a space that's comfortable for them. This might not be your personal favorite decor; be sure to find some way to balance both your clients' needs and yours—after all, you're there day in and day out.

The first thing to do is review your client base and identify your major target markets. Next, consider what would be an ideal space for them. You can also survey your clients and representatives of future target markets for direct feedback. After you've completed your research, the next stage is the actual creation of the session room.

Your office design may need to be developed in stages. Begin by identifying the "must have" items and elements and include them as soon as possible. You don't have to own top-of-the-line equipment, just be sure it's high quality and in good condition.

If you're sensitive to energies, consider hiring a feng shui consultant to enhance the energy flow and to create an overall sense of wellbeing throughout the office. Feng shui is the ancient Chinese art of creating harmonious environments. Although methods and schools of teaching

Feng Shui Your Life by Jayme Barrett and John Cooledge

Feng Shui and Health: Using Feng Shui to Disarm Illness, Accelerate Recovery, and Create Optimal Health by Nancy SantoPietro

Interior Design with Feng Shui: New and Expanded by Sarah Rossbach

Figure 16.1 Office Leasing Checklist

Logistics

- ❑ Is the building in an area that is easily accessible to your target markets?
- ❑ Is there adequate parking, storage, and space for signs?
- ❑ Do other allied professionals work nearby?
- ❑ Will your clients feel comfortable transitioning from your office to the outside—or will it be culture shock?

Ambiance

- ❑ Does the location and the building itself fit your image?
- ❑ Are the other businesses in the building compatible with your practice?
- ❑ Is the noise level suitable? (It's difficult to mask the sounds and vibrations if an aerobics class is in the adjacent room or if a band rehearses next door.)

Comfort & Safety

- ❑ Is the building in a safe neighborhood?
- ❑ Is the building accessible to the physically challenged?
- ❑ Does the space provide privacy and security?
- ❑ Are the utilities sufficient (e.g., do the air conditioning and heating units have adequate capacity)?
- ❑ Do you have direct access to the temperature controls?

Safety Note: If you work at night, make sure other tenants also keep evening office hours.

Remodeling & Improvements

- ❑ Can you alter the layout?
- ❑ Do the premises need major improvements or remodeling in order to be appropriate for your practice?
- ❑ Once you've furnished and organized the space, will it blend in with the style and decor of the rest of the building?
- ❑ Does the premises provide space to expand your business?

Business Terms

- ❑ What are the terms of the lease?
- ❑ Who is responsible for the repairs and maintenance of the premises?
- ❑ Who is responsible for upkeep or possible replacement of major items, such as the roof or air conditioning unit?
- ❑ What type of insurance coverage is provided?
- ❑ Who pays the utilities, taxes, and insurance?
- ❑ What are the sales options or renewal provisions?
- ❑ By what formula are lease increases determined?
- ❑ Can you sublease, and, if so, are the terms the same as the original lease?
- ❑ What are the signage requirements?

vary, all are based on improving the flow of "chi" or life-force energy and aligning harmoniously with nature. Simply put, feng shui is all about a good flow of energy that supports wellbeing, vibrant health, and prosperity.

Feng Shui Resources
www.fengshuidirectory.com

When interviewing a potential feng shui consultant, ask to see an educational résumé. Be careful of those who share only a biography of themselves. Pretty words can't compare to an in-depth education, no matter what feng shui method is practiced. Be aware that the current trendiness of feng shui has attracted some fly-by-night practitioners. Would you hire a doctor, lawyer, or other professional who refused to answer your questions about their professional qualifications? Continue your search for the right consultant if your request for information is met with a less than an enthusiastic response or a lack of solid credentials.

Keep in mind that the foremost reason your clients come to you is for wellness services. Until you can establish your "ideal" office, make sure your space offers a warming energy with a tranquil ambiance—whatever shape that may take for you. Avoid letting clutter or other encumbrances creep into your space and detract from your desired image.

Ambiance

Ambiance is a rather amorphous concept. It is a special atmosphere created by your environment. It arises from all of the previously covered factors and impacts your image and the mood you set. Establishing the appropriate ambiance isn't always an easy feat; although, an unlimited budget would certainly help.

Beware of "theme" rooms. They often have limited appeal and in time can become boring to both you and your clients.

You always create a mood—intentional or not. Consider the image you wish to portray and the characteristics associated with it. Do you want your office to project a clinical feeling (which would be appropriate if many of your clients are insurance referrals)? Do you want a calm, quiet, soothing atmosphere to appeal to those wanting stress reduction? Do you want a cheery room with toys and lots of color for infants? Do you want a high-tech look for executives?

Professionalism

§5

A professional office establishes credibility and demonstrates concern for the client. You validate your credibility by conspicuously posting your business license, policies, educational certificates, awards, interview clippings, business cards, brochures, and letters of appreciation and recommendation. These items represent the time you've invested in your career and the goodwill you've generated in your community.

You express concern for your clients by the ways in which you design your office to assist them in feeling comfortable, appreciated, and that they are the center of attention. Creating a sense of privacy is essential. You may need to be inventive to accomplish this. For instance, some massage therapists and estheticians work in salons in which the walls don't even reach the ceiling or are paper thin. If remodeling isn't an option, it helps to pad the walls or enclose the room with a false ceiling or canopy.

Make your clients feel important by providing a special area for their belongings (e.g., a small closet, a shelf, a chair behind a screen, a hook with hangers); keeping supplies handy (e.g., linens, tissues, blankets, bolsters); and maintaining a comfortable temperature. If you don't have easy access to the temperature controls, place a portable heater and fan in the room. Keep notes about clients' preferences in their files, and refer to the file before the session so you can properly prepare the room.

Nothing detracts more from a pleasant atmosphere than a dirty office space, especially the bathroom. Keep your room clean and free of clutter. Make sure there are no product spills, trash cans overflowing with garbage, sinks filled with dirty dishes, soiled linens piled in a corner, and dust-bunnies hiding under the furniture, on fan blades, in vents, or around moldings.

Sensations

We're all sensual beings. Incorporate as many of the senses as possible—particularly touch, sight, smell, and sound—into your design plans. Engaging multiple senses subconsciously links your client's experience to you and your services.

Touch

Physical sensation plays a pivotal role—especially in touch therapy practices. In addition to the actual hands-on treatment, consider the tactile sensations from your equipment and linens. A treatment table is one of the most important pieces of office equipment. Does it inspire feelings of safety and comfort? Can you make necessary adjustments? Is it wide enough? Is it well padded? Does it squeak? Do your clients need to pole vault to get onto it? Use a secure, well-padded table or futon; make sure your sheets, towels, and gowns are soft; and cover bolsters with a towel or sheet.

Most people like to touch things, so have items available for your clients to play with, such as a skeleton, a replica of the foot with reflexology points, a model of a muscle, samples of products you sell, and professional publications they can peruse.

Sight

Designing the physical appearance of your treatment room can be fun. Most people are visually oriented and are affected by the colors, textures, and artistry of your room.

Creativity specialists contend that the key to creativity is to get out of your normal frame of reference. One technique is to lie on your treatment table or sit on your chair and notice what you see. Include all positions: face up, face down, and side to side. This is how your clients view your room. You might be surprised at what they can see at those angles. For example, if you have a bookshelf, note which shelves are at eye level and be sure to place appropriate books in that line of vision.

> "Design is not just what it looks like, it's how it feels.
> —Steve Jobs

Simple changes to alter the visual impact of your ideal session room include painting the walls, texturizing the ceiling, suspending a mobile, hanging artwork and charts, furnishing the room stylishly, installing unique window coverings, and including potted plants or fresh cut flowers (exercise caution with aromatic flora).

Make sure the floor covering is constructed of high-quality materials. Avoid light colors as they get dirty quickly. If the flooring is less than ideal, you can use throw rugs or an area carpet—just be certain they're skid-proof.

Lighting is another important element in the design of a session room. Ideally you would have a source of natural light from a window or a skylight. If not, place lamps in different areas of the room to give balanced, indirect illumination.

Smell

In terms of scent, a clean, crisp, barely discernible fragrance is usually preferred. If your office is in a salon, you must eliminate or conceal the harsh chemical odors from nail polish and hair treatment applications. Some solutions to odor problems are to insulate your room, use an unscented air freshener, run an air purifier, or diffuse essential oils. But be careful with fragrances, because your clients may suffer from allergies, or your next client may want the opposite results of the aromatherapy essence used by the current client.

Sound

Recorded sound, or the absence thereof, is the most commonly used means of creating a mood. Invest in a good system that's programmable. Purchase a wide variety of music and make sure you can easily adjust volume or change selection. Some offices might have piped-in music, but still you can often access the controls. I used to go to a dentist who played a style of music which I abhorred. I was always apprehensive about check-ups, not because I feared he might discover cavities, but because I dreaded listening to the music.

Regardless of the atmosphere you desire, it can be undermined if you don't block out external noise, so be sure you silence your phone and soundproof thin walls. You can also create other auditory experiences with chimes, an aquarium, or even an indoor water feature.

Layout

The most comfortable and inviting offices are organized, clean, and free of clutter. Decorate the room with appropriate furniture and equipment. Don't put your favorite recliner in the corner if it takes up so much room that clients have to walk sideways to get to the table. Consider the ways in which you interact with your clients and design your office accordingly. For instance, if you like to teach clients how to stretch, make sure there's adequate, obstruction-free floor space. Also, keep supplies such as tissues, blankets, and water at hand.

My Ideal Session Room

My vision of the ideal session room is one in which I feel comfortable and pampered. The room is located in a small professional building that is nicely landscaped. I enter through the front door and find myself in the waiting room that's painted with pastel colors and the floors are tiled. There are several stuffed chairs, a couch, a magazine table, end tables with lamps on them, and vases of fresh flowers.

Directly to my left is a desk where the receptionist works. Next to the desk is a beautiful ficus tree. Against one wall is a bookshelf with brochures about the various practitioners and literature on wellbeing. Along an adjacent wall is a display case filled with unique health-related items such as books, essential oils, diffusers, hot and cold therapy packs, relaxation tools, ergonomic support devices, and CDs. In the corner is a water dispenser and a stand with cups and a pot of herbal tea.

The actual session room inspires a sense of deep relaxation the moment I enter. The lighting is diffused, the temperature moderate, the walls are painted a soothing color, the ceiling is vaulted, and I can feel a soft breeze from an overhead fan. I experience a sense of total privacy no outside noises whatsoever.

The practitioner guides me to a little alcove where I can get ready for my session. This dressing area has hangers for clothes, a shelf for belongings, a mirror, and a chair. The natural sunlight gently streams through a skylight.

I proceed to get on the extremely comfortable table that is thickly padded and hydraulic with adjustable angles. I notice how good the soft linens feel, and appreciate that they're also fragrance-free. The table has a shelf that I can easily reach and on it I find tissues and a bottle of water. I look around the room and see certificates on one wall, artwork on another, and anatomical charts on the third wall. The window is covered with wooden shutters, and several large potted plants are positioned in the corners. The room is uncluttered, clean, and exudes professionalism. Then I hear faint sounds emanating from the stereo, lulling me into a state of deep relaxation....

Visualize Your Ideal Session Room

Close your eyes and imagine yourself as a new client about to step foot in the perfect session space. Use all your senses to visualize the setting. Now, take out a piece of paper and describe the following:

- What does the ideal session room feel like? Describe the texture of the decor, the temperature, the equipment, and products with which you come in contact.
- What does the ideal session room look like? Describe the furniture, equipment, artwork, and supplies. Be sure to include colors.
- What does the ideal session room smell like? Describe the bold and subtle scents.
- What does the ideal session room sound like? Describe the sounds and the music in the room, as well as any sounds emanating from outside the space.
- How does being in that room make you feel emotionally?

Relocating Your Practice

At some point over the course of your business you will most likely need to relocate. Regardless of whether it's down the street, to the other side of town, or across the country, moving can be a stressful event. Before you actually relocate, set a foundation for success and ease your stress level by establishing a network of professional resources in the new community, thoroughly researching regulations, and becoming well informed about any unique aspects of the new locale. Any move provides you with an opportunity to re-evaluate your life and business, implement changes, meet new people, and revitalize your practice.

Moving Within the Same City

One of the most critical factors to consider in choosing a new location is the potential impact on your clients. You risk losing clients whenever you move more than several blocks from your current location. This chance is heightened if a large portion of your clientele is based on geography. Let's say your office is in a downtown skyscraper and the majority of your clients are attorneys who work in that building. Attorneys tend to keep chaotic schedules, and, most likely, one of the reasons they utilize your services is that you're convenient. If they can't simply take the elevator to your office (or at the most, walk across the street), they may not see you as frequently—if at all. Regardless of how good a practitioner you are, many people won't travel far to see you, especially on a regular basis. Who wants to drive 45 minutes through traffic after getting relaxed? Other people may only have a limited amount of time they can take from work and thus need to schedule after hours or find another practitioner.

> "There is nothing permanent except change.
> —Heraclitus

Retain Clients By Communicating Benefits

Help retain clients and foster goodwill by taking the time to communicate the benefits of your office relocation to your clients. Do this by sending a promotional mailing or welcome letter offering special pricing. An office move may result in the following: more space; improved ambiance; a location adjacent to other wellness providers; and proximity to public transportation. In some cases, a move may provide: a more intimate, relaxed, private space (good way to describe downsizing); a safer location; a greater variety of practitioners in the same office; space for classes; more convenient parking; and lower overhead to keep prices down. Whatever the case may be, when clients feel valued and the location is convenient, clients usually welcome a move to a better locale.

Figure 16.2 Moving Checklist

- ❑ Personally talk with regular clients (after the decision is set).
- ❑ Send moving notification (3 weeks prior to moving date).
- ❑ Review files.
- ❑ Organize paperwork into active and archival boxes.
- ❑ Make an inventory list.
- ❑ Clean the new office before moving.
- ❑ Hire movers.
- ❑ Schedule an open house.
- ❑ Send a second announcement (1 week prior to move).
- ❑ Call current clients.
- ❑ Introduce yourself to your new neighbors.
- ❑ Forge alliances with businesses.
- ❑ Gain visibility in the local community.
- ❑ Post new address at previous location.
- ❑ Send a final announcement (once you're settled in the new location).

Revitalize Your Practice

Moving provides you with an excellent opportunity to reconnect with your clients, particularly those you haven't seen lately. Many wellness practitioners avoid contacting inactive clients due to the time involved in reviewing their files and writing individualized letters. A form letter without something specific to each client is usually ineffective in generating interest. But moving announcements don't require personalization! You can even offer an incentive for them to come back.

See Chapter 18, page 258 for details on the **paperless office**.

Take the time to go through your files as you box them (unless you have a totally paperless filing system). Note who hasn't been in for a while and send them a special letter (if they don't attend your open house). Think about what you could do to provide further service to each client. For instance, a client has been diagnosed with fibromyalgia. You haven't worked with her in more than a year. Several months ago you read an excellent book on the subject and could share some information with her. Place a reminder in your tickler to send her a note about the book and invite her to your new facilities.

§5

Notification

Notify all of your clients, colleagues, and associates as soon as possible. Send out email announcements, postcards, or flyers at least 3 weeks before the move. Include the date of the move, your new address and phone numbers, any changes in hours, and a map detailing directions to your new facilities. Consider sending your active contacts another notice closer to the moving date. If your office accepts last-minute appointments or walk-in clients, call your current client list one week before the actual move to inform them of your new address.

After you've relocated, go through your client files and send out one personalized letter or postcard each day.

Once you relocate, post a note on the door of your previous office with the address, phone number, and directions to your new location. If that option isn't available, perhaps you can leave a stack of flyers with the new tenants. Be sure to confirm all appointments and remind clients of the address change. Keep track of who has been reminded about the new location by coding your clients' files with colored dots (or if you're computerized, create a special field). Finally, you may want to send one more announcement to your client list now that you are in the new location.

If you use a cell phone for your business, you can easily keep your same phone number (recommended). But, if you have a landline, you should note that most phone companies wait

3-12 months before reassigning business numbers. Right after that time comes, call your old number and tell the new holder your new phone number and address. Send a thank-you card and a gift (flowers, plant, or gift certificate) to thank them in advance for forwarding your calls. Deliver additional thank-you notes as long as they continue to forward your information.

Figure 16.3 Sample "We're Moving!" Flyer

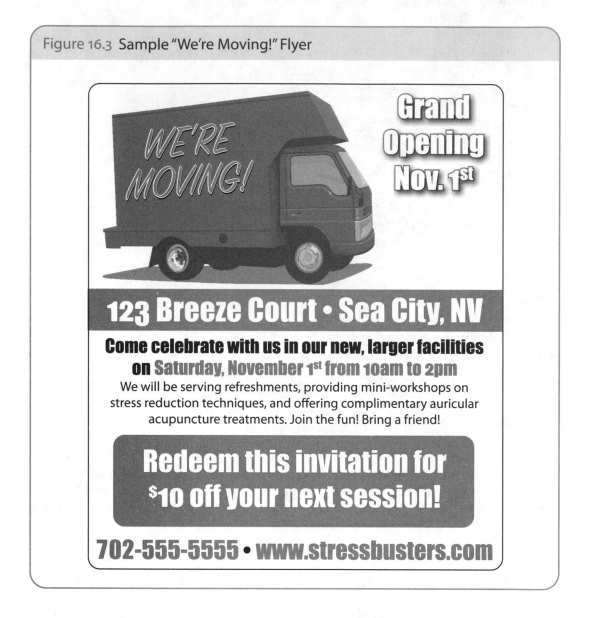

Generating New Clientele

Relocation furnishes you with a splendid opportunity to generate new clientele. Survey the surrounding area for other businesses that could be a source of referrals (mutual referrals are even better). Get to know your neighbors. Hand-deliver flyers or brochures to adjacent businesses, hold a special open house just for the people nearby, and make yourself visible in the community. Get involved in local business association meetings (e.g., the Downtown Business Owners Alliance). If there's a local publication, advertise in it or offer to write an article or a wellness column.

Most large buildings have a newsstand or coffee booth in the lobby. Ask to place your cards and flyers near the counter. Perhaps you can leave a container in which tenants place their business cards to win a free session. In addition to generating visibility, this provides a means to obtaining the tenants' names, phone numbers, and email addresses for future marketing ventures. If you're a somatic practitioner, you can offer the stand owner a free weekly 15-minute session (preferably right in the stand area) in exchange for displaying your materials.

Forge alliances with other business owners for the purpose of cooperative marketing. Let's go back to the attorney example. You're a massage therapist who wants to increase the number of attorneys in your client pool. To heighten your differential advantage, you decide to relocate to a building that is populated mainly with attorneys. A restaurant down the block offers free delivery service to tenants in your building. Together, you could plan several marketing activities that would increase the range of people you reach and reduce the cost of reaching them:

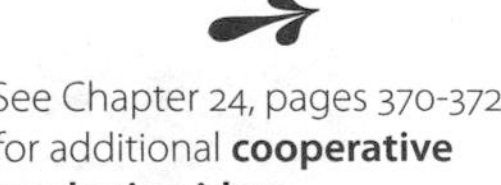

See Chapter 24, pages 370-372 for additional **cooperative marketing ideas**.

1. Share the cost of hiring someone to hand-deliver your brochures and the restaurant's menus to each office.
2. Offer a joint special, such as "Receive a certificate for a free 15-minute chair massage with your 10th delivery" and "Receive a 10% food purchase coupon with every massage."
3. Keep a stack of menus by your office door. At the restaurant, place your cards and brochures (in a professional display holder) near the cash register.
4. Get the restaurant to cater your open houses (at cost or for free). Offer free massages for special events hosted by the restaurant.
5. Have monthly drawings at the restaurant for a free massage, and at your office for a free dinner for two.

Moving to a New City

For most people, moving to a new city means starting a business from scratch. You can create a smoother transition and actually develop a strong referral base and network by doing legwork before the actual move.

Research

Research your new location to determine what it has to offer economically, socially, politically, culturally, and climatically. Start by asking the Chamber of Commerce to send you a relocation packet with information on the city, population, demographics, and major industries. Request that they send you the following: any directory listings on your specific service, health services, stress reduction, and holistic wellness providers; listings of business and professional associations; and anything else that piques your interest. Not all chambers are so accommodating—you may need to do some of this research at the library and over the Internet.

Another method for gathering information about the community and your specific profession is talking with people in that city. If you're a member of a professional association, contact members in the area. If you aren't a member, or if no other members live there, contact the officers or directors of allied professional associations. Also, contact several people in your same profession. Request information from any local wellness schools.

Some questions to ask are: What position does your type of service hold in this community? What are the attitudes toward the profession and the practitioners? How much publicity does this profession garner? What is the range of fees charged and what is the scope of practice? What is the average annual yearly income for a practitioner in your specific profession?

Call the relevant business, zoning, and health licensing agencies to ascertain their requirements and obtain the number of licensed or registered wellness practitioners in the area. You may need to contact state agencies to learn the specific regulations for wellness providers. Get in touch with a commercial real estate agent to obtain information on the types of available office space and the going rates. Order copies of the local newspapers(s), holistic magazines, and special interest publications—all of which provide valuable information about your new city.

Network

Begin to network even before you move. Ask your friends, relatives, and colleagues if they know anyone in that city. Send a letter of introduction to allied professionals such as physicians, counselors, chiropractors, massage therapists, and other wellness providers. Let them know who you are and what you do, including your abilities and qualifications. Address the potential mutual benefits of your association. Close the letter by telling them how to contact you and inform them that you will be calling them within the next few weeks. When you do, ask for any advice, suggestions, or contacts they might recommend. Be sure to thank them for their time and consideration with a follow-up note.

Scouting Expedition

If you're considering a place for relocation and it isn't definite that you will actually move there, visit the city during the worst (hottest, coldest, wettest, driest, and most crowded) part of the year to see whether you can tolerate it. This is also a good time to meet with colleagues and explore potential associations.

17
Create a Dynamic Business Plan

"Efforts and courage are not enough without purpose and direction."
—John F. Kennedy

Business Plan Fundamentals
- Getting Started

Business Plan Outline
- The Basic Business Plan
- Business Plan Supplement

Key Terms

Advertising
Breakeven Analysis
Business Plan
Community Relations
Executive Summary
Financial Analysis
Marketing Plan
Mission Statement
Owner's Statement
Promotions
Publicity
Return on Investment (ROI)
Risk Assessment
SCORE

If the thought of writing a business plan conjures up images of endless hours of drudgery, you aren't alone. Many business owners don't relish this time-consuming, yet vital, task. Several things can help ease the way. Keep in mind that building a business without a business plan is a lot like building a house without a blueprint. The house may get built, but the budget may go through the roof and the project may take a lot longer than expected. What's worse, "on the fly" construction doesn't lend itself to longevity. The house may look good for a while but may not last as time and stress work their magic.

Business Plan Fundamentals

Creating a business plan makes good sense. Most importantly, it dramatically increases your chance of success. According to business expert David M. Anderson, "There is no single omission that bodes worse for a start-up's future than the lack of a comprehensive business plan."[1] In short, develop a business plan if you want to tilt the odds in favor of your success.

Although you may lack the financial resources to hire a highly paid business consultant to prepare a business plan—an ideal solution that many of us dream about—recognize that you don't have to approach this task alone. Those who have traveled the path before you have created numerous resources. Browse an online or local bookstore and purchase a few books on business plan writing that catch your interest. Search the Internet for sample business plans and useful articles. Some tech-savvy business owners prefer to work with a business plan writing software that includes sample business plans, along with forecast and cash flow models.

You can find help through business organizations such as local business schools, centers for entrepreneurs, and SCORE. SCORE is a nonprofit association dedicated to helping small businesses through education and mentorship. They also offer a free online workshop "Developing a Business Plan" and free business plan templates. Advisors in local chapter offices meet with you to review your plan and can provide valuable feedback to fine-tune your rough draft. In addition, many local Chamber of Commerce organizations offer free consultations for new business owners as well as low-cost small business seminars.

A business plan serves many functions. It's a powerful declaration of your goals and intentions, a written summary of what you aim to accomplish, and an overview of how you intend to organize your resources to attain those goals. Developing an effective business plan generally requires a considerable amount of time. You have to do a lot of honest thinking in addition to some technical research. However, if you've completed the exercises throughout *Business Mastery*, you already have the groundwork for a business plan!

If you're opening a private practice or clinic, a business plan assists you to clarify your vision and values, evaluate the marketplace, identify your goals, calculate your costs, forecast your growth, and identify your risks. For those of you who have been in business for a while, a new or updated plan can rejuvenate your practice.

A business plan addresses these issues: What are you offering? Who will your clients be? What needs do your services satisfy? How will your potential clients find you? How much money do you plan on making? What actions do you intend on taking to ensure success?

As you navigate through your career, a business plan reminds you to celebrate milestones.

Although business plans vary in scope and content, the major components of a business plan are an owner's statement, executive summary, mission statement, business description, long-term and short-term goals, a financial forecast, operations overview, risk assessment, success strategies, and a marketing plan. Each of these components need not be a novel, in fact, if you're succinct in your thinking and writing, you can cover each subject in a paragraph or two.

Use your business plan to keep you inspired and on track. Many business owners get overwhelmed by the minutiae of running a business and miss valuable opportunities to plan strategies for future success. Clearly describing where you want to go and how you intend to get there encourages you to be more realistic. It also assists you to anticipate and avoid problems, or at least be prepared so that you can overcome them, thus minimizing your risks. Written goals give you solid criteria to evaluate progress. A financial forecast illustrates exactly what finances are required to launch and maintain a thriving business.

Schedule periodic "reality checks" with your business plan on a monthly, quarterly, and annual basis to help you to adjust course when needed and identify new ways to grow your business. A business plan can help you discover vital steps to your success and happiness that you may have otherwise overlooked.

When your business plan is complete, print it and put it in a 3-ring binder. This type of binder allows you to easily update your plan and add information (e.g., copies of reports and sample promotional materials) and keeps all major business documents in one place. If you're submitting the business plan for a loan, consider taking your documents to a printing facility and having them professionally copied and bound.

Business Plan Resources

www.sba.gov/category/navigation-structure/starting-managing-business
www.bplans.com
www.score.org/resources/business-planning-financial-statements-template-gallery
www.planware.org

Getting Started

Avoid getting stuck on attempting to create a perfect first draft of your business plan. Most business owners create a rough first draft and spend a good bit of time fine-tuning subsequent drafts. Once you know the key ingredients of a business plan, you can start with a mission statement and let the rest flow from there. Think of your first few hours of work on a business plan as a brainstorming session. If you're having trouble getting started, plan an initial 2-hour work session with a business advisor, colleague, or business coach.

One of the toughest challenges in writing a business plan involves financial projections. Make informed estimates for sales, expenses, and profits. Know that no one does it perfectly. Lean toward the conservative: include "wiggle room" for unexpected expenses.

Figure 17.1 Business Plan Tips & Insights

- Business plans must be based on facts, so do your research.
- Business plans for internal use average about 10 to 15 pages; business plans to raise funds typically span about 40 pages or more.
- Talk to other business owners about their business plans. Ask what they would do differently or what they found most valuable about the process.
- Be realistic and use a conservative approach for your financial projections. Being overly optimistic can set you up with unreasonable expectations.
- Consult with an accountant to look at your financials, and help you put them in a standard business format.
- Find an experienced business person and share your plan. Ask for feedback. Listen, but don't follow advice that doesn't ring true for you.
- Take your time and don't rush through the business plan process. The time you invest is well spent.
- Do your homework when it comes to competitive analysis and pricing. Gather as much supporting data as possible. Back up any statements you make with statistics from a reputable source.
- If you're looking for investors, make sure you proofread and spell check everything (business plans with errors won't be taken seriously), avoid gimmicks and superlatives (e.g., amazing, outstanding, unbelievable), and stick to the facts.
- Revisit your business plan quarterly to make sure you're on track.
- Celebrate when you've completed writing your business plan. It's the first key milestone of many to come.

Business Plan Outline

Before you go to your journal or computer, scan through this section. It highlights the key components and scope of a business plan. Use this outline to refine what you've already written in the activities from the other chapters, and to clarify any other details that are requisites for your success.

The Basic Business Plan

The basic business plan isn't lengthy or complicated. You simply need a description of your business and plans for marketing, management, and financials. The categories in Figure 17.2 help you keep this information organized.

The One Page Business Plan by Jim Horan

Business Plans for Dummies by Paul Tiffany and Steven Peterson

Figure 17.2 **Basic Business Plan Components**

- Cover Page
- Table of Contents
- Owner's Statement
- Executive Summary
- Mission Statement
- Purpose, Priorities, and Goals
- Business Description
- Marketing Plan
- Risk Assessment
- Financial Analysis
- Operations
- Success Strategies
- Appendix

Cover Page

The cover page is simply the first page of the business plan. Include a title (e.g., "Business Plan for The Healthy Alternative"), and below it put your name, address, telephone numbers, website address, and email address.

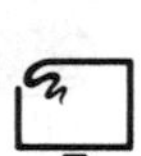

Create Your Business Plan

www.sba.gov/writing-business-plan

Online **Business Plan** tool

www.liveplan.com

Build Your Business Plan

.https://sohnen-moe.com/products/tools/#product-business-plan

Table Of Contents

The table of contents lists all of the business plan sections with corresponding page numbers. It also lists the titles of each document that you include in the appendix.

Owner's Statement

This is a one-page description of the business and the owner, which includes: the business name, address, phone numbers, email address, and website address; your name, home address, home phone number; a summary of your business experience and philosophy; and a brief business status description (the year the business was established and current financial status).

Executive Summary

The executive summary consists of business plan highlights. This section is critical if you apply for financial backing, as it must convince lenders and investors that your business will succeed. Although the summary appears at the beginning of the business plan, it's best to write it last (and keep it to 3 pages or less).

Mission Statement

A mission statement conveys the essence of your business—why your business exists and what values underpin everything you do. Values are beliefs that guide you and your organization. The best mission statements focus on the benefits your customers receive. For instance, an acupuncture clinic's mission may be: "We help clients achieve their wellness goals and enjoy vibrant health. We're committed as a team to values of integrity, compassion, and excellent customer service." Approaches to writing mission statements vary. Some experts suggest keeping your mission statement short and memorable—a sentence or two at most. However, many owners and organizations like to say more, elaborating on who they are, why they do what they do, and what values and vision guide the company.

See Chapter 1, page 7 for more information on **values**.

"How to Write a Mission Statement"

successnet.org/files/B-Mission.htm

Purpose, Priorities, and Goals

This section is a detailed description of your business activities and career plan in terms of short-term and long-term goals. State your overall career purpose and at least 6 priorities. List at least 6 long-term (3-5 year time frame) priorities and at least 2 goals per priority. List at least 6 short-term (1-2 year time frame) priorities and at least 3 goals per priority. Many of these declarations assist you in being clear and motivated, and they can be quite personal. You may want to censor some of these statements if you're submitting this plan for a loan.

See Chapters 2 and 3 for **goal setting** and **strategic planning strategies**.

Business Description

This section provides background about your practice. Begin by writing a brief history of your company and which business activities your company pursues to accomplish its mission. Describe the services you offer and products you sell; special products used; equipment; the physical location; and the features that distinguish your practice from others (e.g., experience, range of services, pricing, location, product sales, equipment, management abilities). If you sell products, include a product register with the suppliers' names and specify the types of clients who purchase these products.

§5

Marketing Plan

Marketing is the pivotal component of a business plan. Begin by depicting the image you wish to convey. Next, describe your target markets and clarify your differential advantage. Follow with a competition analysis, including steps you'll take to meet any challenges. The major section is the strategic action plan. Outline your marketing goals for all 4 areas: promotion, advertising, publicity, and community relations. Delineate a timeline, budget, and rationale for each strategy. If you sell products, include a description and cost for the following: inside displays; additional sales staff (include training); equipment; and special promotions, discounts, and sales. Set a marketing budget per year. Tabulate the cost to market your services and the cost to market your products. Determine the total marketing costs and calculate the actual cost per potential client. Close this section with a summary of how your marketing strategies will enable you to succeed.

See Section 7 for details about **marketing**.

Figure 17.3 **Marketing Plan Components**

- Company Image
- Target Markets
- Differential Advantage
- Competition Analysis
- Strategic Action Plan
- Marketing Budget

Risk Assessment

Risk assessment is a demonstration of your ability to anticipate and manage risks. Detail the effects your competition has on all phases of your business. List possible external events that might occur to hamper your success, such as a recession, new competition, shifts in client demand, unfavorable industry trends, problems with suppliers, and changes in legislation. Identify potential internal problems such as income projections not realized, long-term illness, or serious injury. Then generate contingency plans to counteract the most significant risks.

Financial Analysis

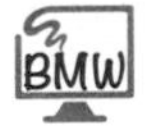

Business Plan Checklist
https://sohnen-moe.com/resources/free-resources/

This section consists of statements about your income potential, fees, current financial status, and financial forecast. The financial analysis section differs if the plan is for a new or established business. For instance, financial data for a new business includes a projection of working capital for start-up expenses (e.g., equipment, office supplies, inventory), as well as an estimate of capital reserves required to keep the business afloat until it makes a profit.

For an established business, the financial analysis includes extensive historical data related to financial reports (e.g., balance sheets, profit and loss statements, cash flow projections, tax returns) and sales data. For more details about a financial analysis for an established business, see the *Business Mastery* workbook for the extensive business plan checklist. The following guidelines focus on financial data for a new business:

- **Determining income potential** for a new business can be tricky. Contact your professional association or several major teaching institutions (for your specific field). You may have to do some informal research because this data has not been compiled for every profession. Describe the existing business conditions. Where do you stand in the current state of the art? Describe the projections and trends for your specific profession both nationally and locally. List the average income for practitioners in your field, both nationally and locally, for the first 6 months of practice, the first year, the second year, and the third year. If possible, include the average number of clients for those same times.

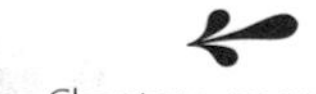

See Chapter 3, pages 47-49 for **the art of risk-taking**.

- **List your service fees**, including introductory offers, prepaid package discounts, professional courtesy discounts, and sliding fee scales. Enumerate the amenities to be absorbed in pricing (e.g., credit offered, outcalls, parking, consultations, educational materials, samples, supplies). Describe your competition's effect on pricing.
- **Determine the equipment**, supplies, and inventory needed for the next 12 months. Clarify your acquisition plan (buy, consign, or lease), and prioritize the purchases.
- **Calculate how much money is needed** to open your business and the annual operations budget for each of the next 3-5 years. Generate this information from a computerized accounting program or written worksheets. Include the actual worksheets in this section or in the business plan appendix.
- **List your potential funding sources**, describe exactly how you anticipate spending the money received, and note how loans (if any) are to be secured. Calculate a breakeven analysis. Determine at what client (or sales) volume your business moves into the "black." This is the point at which total costs equal total income. You may need to update this every few months to accurately reflect your business growth.

Figure 17.4 Financial Plan Components

- Income Projections (3-5 years)
- Start-Up Costs
- Annual Budget (3-5 years)
- Funding Sources and Spending Plans
- Breakeven Analysis

Operations

This section is an overview of your business organization, procedures, and policies. Identify the management qualifications needed to run the "business" part of your practice, and assess your strengths and challenges. Specify the legal form of ownership you've chosen and the reasons why. Cite the requisite licenses, permits, and insurance coverage.

For businesses that have a staff, list the various functions and estimate the number of people needed for each function. Describe the training required, and state your compensation plan. If you have a group practice, describe the various functions and the person(s) responsible. Indicate the level of authority for each person (e.g., hiring, firing, scheduling, purchasing).

> "Genius begins great works, labor alone finishes them.
> —Joseph Joubert

Write a brief overview of your company policies and procedures. Include details on safety precautions. Determine your security needs (consider client screening, location safety, ample lighting for the parking lot, and night travel), and develop a plan to reduce these types of risks.

Close this section with an accounting and control summary. Clarify who does the bookkeeping. Set a production schedule (e.g., daily, weekly, monthly, quarterly, annually) for the following types of management reports: checking account balance; service reports such as the total number of return clients or the number of clients in relation to the time spent per client; product sales reports; balance sheets; profit and loss statements; condition of client accounts; expense reports; insurance reimbursement aging; forecasting; and inventory reports.

Figure 17.5 Operations Components

- Management Description
- Legal Status, Licenses, Permits, Insurance Coverage
- Staff Functions and Responsibilities
- Company Policies and Procedures
- Accounting and Reports

§5

Success Strategies

List your goals for developing your success strategies. Specify your methods for implementing your business plan and having a prosperous practice. Include activities, such as developing strategic plans, creating monthly flow charts, identifying decision points, reviewing and revising your plans, creating a business support system, networking, and choosing appropriate advisors.

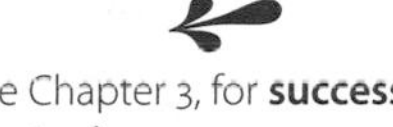

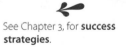

See Chapter 3, for **success strategies**.

Appendix

The types of additional information or documents (if any at all) to be included in this section depend upon the nature of your business plan. If your business plan is mainly for your personal use, you may not need to add anything else. If you intend on using your business plan to obtain financial backing, consider including the following data. (Note: This list is only a guide. Check with the specific lending institutions or investors for their requirements.)

- Personal net worth statement
- Copies of income statements and balance sheets from the last 2 years
- List of client commitments
- Copies of business legal agreements
- Credit status reports
- News articles about you or your business
- Photographs of your location
- Copies of promotional material
- Letters of recommendation from your clients
- Key employee résumés
- Personal references

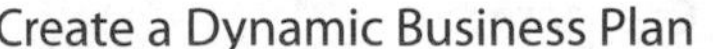

Business Plan Supplement

If your business plan is for securing a loan, it's recommended to incorporate the following additional information into the previous sections of the business plan.

The Executive Summary

In addition to your executive summary in the previous section:

- State the type of business loan(s) you're seeking (e.g., line of credit, mortgage).
- Summarize the proposed use of the funds.
- Calculate the projected return on investment (ROI).
- Write a persuasive statement of why the venture is a good risk.

> "It's never too late, in fiction or in life, to revise.
> —Nancy Thayer

The Financial Analysis

In addition to your financial analysis in the previous section:

- Describe the loan requirements: the amount, the terms, and the desired date.
- State the purpose of the loan, detailing the facets of the business to be financed.
- Provide a statement of the owner's equity.
- List any outstanding debts. Include the balance due, repayment terms, purpose of the loan, and status.
- Document your current operating line of credit: the amount and security held.

References

Add this information to your Success Strategies section, or create a new References section with the following:

- A list of all pertinent information regarding your current lending institution: branch, address, types of accounts, and contact person(s).
- A list of the names, addresses, and phone numbers of your attorney, accountant, and business consultant.

§6
Business Operations

Section 6 of *Business Mastery* focuses on the nuts and bolts of business operations, including tips and information to help you run your business smoothly and efficiently, and how to transition it. While much of the information in this section is geared toward practitioners who are self-employed, some of the topics are key to all practitioners.

Even if you plan to be an employee, this information helps you understand what's involved in establishing a business and the costs of running it, thus giving you a better appreciation of what an employer offers. This knowledge is also crucial if you plan on moving into management.

Chapter 18 focuses on office management. We start with policies. Although not many people thrill at the thought of developing policies and procedures, this chapter shows how they're like the frame of a house—a necessary part of building a house that lasts, and a business that thrives. You'll find tips on how to write policies and procedures, organize your office, and make smart technology choices.

Chapter 19 examines the aspects of actually managing a practice, including complying with HIPAA regulations and handling insurance reimbursement. Also included are useful insights into contract basics, effective negotiation, and conflict resolution.

Chapter 20 presents the essentials of financial management. It provides concrete information to help you keep the books, prepare financial reports, and understand tax laws. You'll also learn how to use barter to exchange goods and services with others. Finally, the chapter covers the basics of retirement planning and offers a number of helpful resources to assist you in planning for your future financial stability.

Product sales is a great diversification method and the profits boost your bottom line while serving your clients. Additionally, many employees are required to sell products. **Chapter 21** explores how to ethically sell products. It covers how to choose appropriate products, provides ideas on selling and marketing products, and closes with tips on effective displays.

For growing practices, **Chapter 22** provides insights into when and how to hire support or professional staff. It also explores the characteristics of a good employer, examines the regulations regarding employees and independent contractors, and guides you on ways to successfully manage your staff.

Chapter 23 provides guidance as you consider transitioning your practice. It starts by highlighting major decision-making pinnacles, and discusses exploration and evaluation techniques. The first option covers the variety of ways you can transfer or sell your practice, and provides a step-by-step process for achieving the best outcome possible. The chapter concludes with a checklist for closing your practice, including steps to take prior to closing and after the officially closing.

18

Office Management

"We are what we repeatedly do. Excellence, then, is not an act, but a habit."
—Aristotle

Policies and Procedures
- Policy Manual
- Procedure Manual

Smart Technology Choices
- Telephones
- Computers and Tablets
- Business Software
- Internet Service
- Copiers, Printers, and Fax Machines

Office Organization
- The Paperless Office
- Get Organized Now!
- Protecting Your Records

Key Terms

App
Ambiance
Barter
Benefits
Bounced Checks
Boundaries
Client Interaction Policies
Cloud Technology
Compensation
Confidentiality
Conflict of Interest
Continuing Education
Co-workers
Credit Terms
Desktop Publishing
Documentation
Dual Relationships
Etiquette
Exit Interview
Fee Structure
Gift Certificates
Goals
Gratuities
Grievance Protocol
HIPAA
Insurance Reimbursement
"I Owe You" (IOU)
Mission Statement
Occupational Safety and Health Administration (OSHA)
Online Scheduling
Package Plans
Paperless Office
Performance Review
Personnel
Policy Manual
Procedure Manual
Risk Management
Safety Protocol
Scope of Practice
Sliding Fee Scales
Standards of Behavior
Termination
Tickler File
Values

The foundation of a well-managed office is built upon having clearly defined policies, comprehensive written procedures, appropriate technology and equipment, and efficient organizational systems. This doesn't have to be difficult if you allot the required time to set up this structure. Keep in mind that you can always update and revise these items as your business grows.

Policies and Procedures

If you look behind the scenes of any smoothly running and successful business, you're likely to find clearly defined policies and procedures. A Policy and Procedure Manual provides a framework for your business by defining expectations, values, and standard business practices. Policies direct your decisions and actions; they're built on the philosophy and values that guide your practice. Procedures are specific steps that detail how you want to run your business day to day.

Formulate your policies and create a written manual, even if you're the only person in your business. By going through this process, you may discover conflicts or potentially risky situations, and thus address and resolve these issues before they actually arise. Also, if you decide to expand your practice and hire staff (or bring in an associate), the transition is easier if the operational guidelines are already established. If you work for someone else, discuss the current policies and procedures with your employer. You may find that you can add to or alter them.

> "Lots of folks confuse bad management with destiny.
> —Kin Hubbard

Establishing policies and procedures is critical for group practices. Ideally, this is done collaboratively. Some details may appear trivial, such as rules about parking lots and bathrooms, but they reflect the daily realities of shared space and time. A successful practice identifies potential problems before they arise and creates values-based and orderly methods for their resolution. Rules and regulations ought not be arbitrary, but based on the desire to create a working atmosphere where respect for one another, and for the business, can flourish. When a group creates working policies on such a basis, they're in fact creating ethical guidelines for conducting the business. Of course, even though a Policy and Procedure Manual may not mention applicable laws and regulations, these still govern the conduct of the business owners, practitioners, and staff.

Policy Manual

Policies are generally divided into two branches—internal company policies and client interaction policies. In designing a policy manual, begin with a statement of your company's purpose, priorities, and goals. Figure 18.1 highlights the main policy categories. The depth of detail required depends on whether you have employees, how many different practitioners or partners are present, and how many different types of services you provide.

Internal Company Policies

Internal company policies are those that define the rules of operation, the conduct of personnel, and the procedures for getting things done effectively and efficiently. These are the policies that you and your employees or partners know about and follow, but that you don't necessarily share with clients. For example, you may have a policy that defines the practitioner hierarchy for new client scheduling, or describes who is responsible for the care and maintenance of the facility, or lists the procedures for the organization of client records. But your clients don't need access to those policies. On the other hand, some of your internal policies may overlap with your client policies if the policy pertains to both you and your clients, such as a fragrance-free office policy.

Figure 18.1 **Policies Checklist**

Company Mission Statement
- ❑ Values
- ❑ Purpose, Priorities, and Goals
- ❑ Customer Service Statement

Scope of Practice
- ❑ Laws and Regulations
- ❑ Training and Background
- ❑ Scope for Each Separate Type of Practitioner at the Company
- ❑ Continuing Education and Training Requirements

Documentation
- ❑ All Forms Used

Finances
- ❑ Fee Structures, Gratuities, and Gift Certificates
- ❑ Product Sales
- ❑ Credit Terms
- ❑ Bounced Checks
- ❑ Insurance Reimbursement
- ❑ Guarantees and Returns
- ❑ Barter

Communication
- ❑ Boundaries
- ❑ Confidentiality
- ❑ Hours and Availability
- ❑ Discharge and Referrals

Ambiance and Etiquette
- ❑ Noise, Children, Food, and Drink
- ❑ Clothing, Fragrance, and Hygiene
- ❑ Cancellation and Lateness
- ❑ Inappropriate Client Behavior (e.g., cell phones, smoking, altered states)

Personal Relationships
- ❑ Dual Relationships
- ❑ Social Activities

Personnel
- ❑ Qualifications (e.g., training, license, insurance)
- ❑ Compensation and Benefits
- ❑ Performance
- ❑ Scheduling and Time Off
- ❑ Conduct, Behavior, and Conflict of Interest
- ❑ Relationships
- ❑ Separation (e.g., termination, notice requirements, exit interviews)

Specific statements for office policies are beyond the scope of this chapter, but the following elements should be considered, and guidelines created, as appropriate. The elements that mostly relate to internal company policies are listed here, with the client interaction elements discussed in the next section.

Company Mission Statement

As suggested earlier, start with your purpose, priorities, and goals. Asserting your mission and values at the beginning of your policy manual keeps all subsequent policies in line with your mission. Include a specific statement regarding the level of customer service your company prioritizes, and any interest you have in community involvement or giving back.

Scope of Practice

Your policies should define your scope of practice, including applicable laws, regulations, and industry standards. Include background and training, and any required licensing and continuing education. If yours is a multi-discipline practice, define the scope for each of the different types of service offered. Also, describe the various expectations for practitioners and employees regarding correct billing practices, and the handling of taxes and other financial regulations.

Documentation

Describe your policies on the use and maintenance of business records, as well as client records. If you track certain business operations (e.g., number of clients per day, gift certificate redemptions), describe your policy on maintaining those records in an accurate and confidential manner. Include a blank master copy of each form in your policy manual (e.g., sign-in, intake, health history, informed consent, HIPAA).

Finances

Describe your policies on fees for products and services, receiving gifts and gratuities, and the various payment terms you will accept. Your internal company policies on finances may include the handling of credit terms and bounced checks, the hierarchy of client collection actions, and sample collection letters.

Personnel

See Chapter 22, pages 332-334 for more on **employee relations**.

If you have partners or employees, or you share your space with other practitioners, you should have detailed personnel policies for the use of the space, as well as expected conduct and behavior. Figure 18.2 highlights a few elements and questions to consider when creating your personnel guidelines.

Client Interaction Policies

Client policies are about setting boundaries that encourage trust, safety, and comfort. Policies explicitly define the parameters of expectations for both clients and practitioners. They make running a business easier, circumvent potentially awkward situations, provide means for conflict resolution, and demonstrate professionalism. These are the policies you share with your clients in the form of a client policy statement.

Client policy statements can take various forms, such as a letter, a page with bulleted items, or a combination of the two. The major areas to cover in your policies are scope of practice, finances, communication, ambiance and etiquette, and personal relationships.

Because change is a given, periodically review your client policies to delete any outdated ones and clarify new requirements. It may be helpful to discuss potential changes with colleagues before updating your policy statement and sharing it with clients.

The main caveat with policies is: Don't create a policy you won't enforce. If you alter a policy for a client, either on a one-time basis or if you change that specific policy permanently,

Figure 18.2 Creating Personnel Guidelines

Relationship between the Organization and the Practitioner

- How does the business ensure practitioners have proper licensure, credentialing, insurance coverage, and continuing education?
- What procedures are in place for regular peer or employee review?
- What is the expected use of parking facilities by practitioners and clients?
- What constitutes overlap of services or retail competition among practitioners?
- What pricing policies exist to prevent undercutting of other practitioners?
- What recordkeeping responsibilities do practitioners have?
- What situations constitute a conflict of interest?
- What responsibilities do team members share for the care of common areas such as lobbies, waiting rooms, bathrooms, kitchen, or break room?
- What procedures are established to create a healthy, safe, and secure working environment?
- How does the organization encourage community involvement?
- What guidelines are provided regarding personal relationships between practitioners and clients?
- What policies govern client/practitioner relationships when the practitioner leaves the practice?

Standards of Behavior for Practitioners

- What Is the dress code?
- What is the policy regarding use of fragrances?
- What are the expectations regarding timeliness?
- How are absences handled?
- What are the expectations concerning noise in the office?
- What are the expectations regarding sobriety in the office?
- What are the expectations regarding language in the office (e.g., profanity, offensive language, innuendo)?
- In what off-site situations are practitioners considered representatives of the office? What kind of image should practitioners exhibit in these situations?
- Are there limitations to practitioners advertising in a common waiting room to all clients, or to an individual client who is waiting for a different practitioner?

Relationships with Co-workers

- What hierarchy exists among group members? In what circumstances is this hierarchy invoked?
- What referral patterns are acceptable among practitioners? What behaviors are considered poaching clients?
- What lines of communication exist for resolving internal conflicts between practitioners?
- What are appropriate reporting avenues when practitioners suspect or know of unethical behavior on the part of a co-worker?
- What policies exist regarding trading services with co-workers? How are discrepancies in value handled?
- What guidelines are provided regarding personal relationships between co-workers?

make it clear to the client your intention is to address the specific situation and that you would appreciate her continued adherence to all other policies.

Written policy statements set a professional tone and help build positive relationships with clients, even if you don't have specific policies for every situation.

Scope of Practice

These statements define the type of work you do and assist your clients in knowing what to expect. Consider prefacing your policies with a short paragraph describing your work, the types of clients you work with (or don't work with), your training and background, any conditions that are your specialty, and your procedures. Often, these don't lend themselves to precise policies, yet are vital in setting the tone for a safe, enjoyable experience for both practitioner and client. Some specific scope of practice policies cover draping, diagnosing, and charting.

Finances

When creating your financial policies, include the following: your fee structure; sliding scale schedules; package plans; credit terms; gratuities; insurance reimbursement; product guarantees and returns; bounced checks; gift certificates; and barter.

Fee Structures vary greatly depending on the type of work you do and where you're located. Once you've determined your fees, communicate the following to your clients: your basic session rate and duration of the session; alternatives such as longer sessions; options for other services (e.g., hydrotherapy, paraffin treatments, acupuncture, aromatherapy); and types of payments accepted (e.g., cash, check, credit cards).

See Chapter 15, page 210 for details on **sliding fees** and **package plans**.

Sliding Fee Scales can be awkward. It's tough to set one up in advance of the first session unless a client has said something to you while booking the appointment. It may be enough to state that you offer sliding fees for special circumstances, and then negotiate those fees should the opportunity arise.

Package Plans encourage people to receive treatments more often and infuse advanced income into your bank account.

Insurance Reimbursement is a time-consuming, detailed process. Many wellness providers prefer not to deal with it at all, some help clients by filling out the forms (but require payment at time of service), while others do direct billing. If you offer third-party billing, require the client to sign a statement saying that the client is responsible for payment if a claim isn't paid within a specified time (e.g., 60 days), or if the claim is denied. Whichever method you choose, clearly state it in your policies.

See Chapter 19, pages 267-273 for details on **insurance reimbursement**.

Product Guarantees and Returns instill consumer confidence. Check with your suppliers to determine their return policies. Your customers may need to return defective or unwanted goods to the manufacturer. I recommend offering a money-back guarantee on all services and products. Of course, to take a stand such as this, you need to carry quality products. You may want to include a time limit on returns, such as within 10 days of purchase. Service guarantee can be a bit more complicated. Some practitioners offer dissatisfied clients a partial or a full refund. In order to make this type of guarantee, the practitioner must do a thorough intake interview and set realistic goals with the client, otherwise a client might say something like "I'm still in some pain, so the treatment didn't work."

> "Common sense is not so common.
>
> —Voltaire

Credit Terms are rare in service professions. The three most common reasons for extending credit are: the fees are billed to a third party, such as an insurance agency, attorney, or a client's employer; a client forgets his checkbook; or a client has cash flow difficulties. For those with a cash flow difficulty, create a formal IOU with a payment schedule. Let's say a regular client recently got laid off from work. She has another job lined up, but won't be starting for 2 months. She wants to continue receiving her biweekly treatments but is unable to afford them and doesn't have anything to barter. Ideally, she would pay a nominal fee with each session, but that might not be a viable option. Figure 18.3 is an example of a written payment agreement that both parties sign.

Figure 18.3 Sample IOU

I, Darlene Dunning, agree to pay the sum of $70 per session for each treatment I receive between May 1, 2020 and July 11, 2020 in the following manner: Beginning July 14, 2020, I, Darlene Dunning, pay the sum of at least $30 every two weeks until the entire amount is repaid. This amount is in addition to any charges for treatments received after July 11, 2020 (which are payable in full at time of service).

In the event of nonpayment, I, Darlene Dunning, agree to pay reasonable attorney's fees and costs for making such collection.

Bounced Checks happen to the best of us. Unfortunately, as the recipient, you must deal with the repercussions. In most states you can go to the bank where the check is drawn and obtain preferential status in getting the check cashed as soon as funds are deposited into the account. Many businesses charge a fee (ranging from $25 to triple the check's amount) for bounced checks to cover their bank's charges and time involved in settling the account. Note that this fee can be contested if it isn't stated in your policies.

See Chapter 26, pages 423-426 for more on **gift certificates** and **expiration dates**.

Gift Certificates can be handled in various ways. Some people advocate assigning a 3-month expiration date. Others recommend 6 months or a year, and some suggest no expiration date at all. All these options have pros and cons. You can also create an automated workflow that sends an email or reminds you to call a client at specific intervals (e.g., 6 months), to use the certificate or apply it to other services or products. Whichever you choose, make the conditions clear. Keep in mind that in many states you cannot put an expiration on a gift certificate that was purchased. I also suggest that the certificate be transferable. Clients often appreciate the added convenience and flexibility.

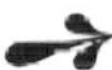

See Chapter 20, pages 300-302 for details on **barter**.

Barter is one of the most commonly misused and abused areas of financial management. Although it isn't necessary to include barter in your written policy statement, it's advisable to set guidelines ahead of time for the types of bartering and the amount of bartering you allow. Keep accurate records, particularly if you aren't doing a direct trade.

Communication

Policies relating to communication apply to the environment you intend to create, the language and terminology you use with clients, your attitudes toward clients, the types of questions you ask, the degree of honesty and self-disclosure you require of your clients, and your physical space boundaries.

Confidentiality must be maintained in a therapeutic relationship to promote an atmosphere of safety. Describe your procedures for maintaining confidentiality and the circumstances that require breaking confidentiality.

Availability to your clients includes your business hours, location, and the time allotted before and after sessions to answer questions or offer support. Follow-up tends to be a weak area in most practices. While it's a good idea to place appointment reminder calls, emails, or text messages, it's also important to find out if your clients want you to contact them, when they prefer to be contacted, and how they want to be contacted. Some practitioners call new clients within 48 hours of their first session just to check in with them. Others also like to call clients who've experienced a major shift during the session. Regardless of the type and frequency of follow-up, always discuss it first with your clients.

Ambiance and Etiquette

This topic concerns behaviors that generally fall under the heading of good manners. Policies need to address the following: late clients; clients who cancel appointments with less than 24 hours notice or don't show at all; hygiene (e.g., bathing, fragrances); and personal habits, such as smoking on the premises, eating prior to a session, or arriving in an altered state. It's also common to include a policy on cell phone and text use in the office and in the treatment room.

Personal Relationships

See Chapter 5, page 74 for more information on **dual relationships**.

Dual Relationships continue to be one of the most talked about subjects. As mentioned in Chapter 5, the term dual relationships describes the overlapping of professional and social roles and interactions between two people. The classic depiction of a dual relationship is when two persons who interact professionally develop other roles of social interaction.

Some people claim that dual relationships should be avoided at all costs. But let's be real: they happen, especially in small towns or rural communities (because of the limited numbers of people and choices for professional services). It usually isn't a question of whether you'll have them, but how you'll handle them. And this is where policies come in.

Think about who your first clients were—most likely friends and family. Many people find that at some point, it becomes awkward juggling the roles of being a relative or friend, as well as a wellness care provider. When I was in practice, one of my clients was my best friend. We had absolutely no problems for several years. Then the roles started blurring. We began chatting too much during sessions and discussing what occurred during a treatment when we were in a social setting. I created a simple ritual to transition our roles that proved to be extremely effective. Right before going into the treatment room, I would take a big step to the right and say, "Now I'm your therapist and not your friend. And you're my client." After the session was over, I would take a big step to the left and say, "Now we're no longer therapist and client, but friends." That simple statement with the physical movement did the trick.

The Ethics of Touch by Ben E. Benjamin, Ph.D., and Cherie Sohnen-Moe

Some people have very stringent policies about not working with friends or family members. There is no right or wrong here, although it's much easier if you don't have to accommodate dual relationships. You're the only one who can gauge your ability to keep clear boundaries. Even if you can work effectively in a dual relationship, you need to ask yourself if the other person can manage multiple roles. Another aspect of working with family and friends is that they're more likely to test your policies and limits—although not always on purpose or consciously. Having clear policies makes enforcement less awkward.

Sexual Activity in a therapeutic context is never appropriate (unless you're a licensed sex therapist). Sexual inappropriateness on behalf of the client or practitioner isn't always easily defined. In addition to being clear with your own boundaries, it helps to set guidelines for your clients that include interactions and scope of practice.

Create Client Policies

- List your client interaction policies for scope of practice, finances, communication, ambiance and etiquette, and personal relationships (see Figure 18.4 for a Sample Client Policy Statement).
- Specify what your clients can expect of you.
- Clarify how you will handle the "bending" of policies (e.g., a client forgets her checkbook or a client thought you were going to bill the insurance company).
- Determine how you will present your policies (e.g., handout, verbal).

Procedure Manual

A procedure manual defines operational best practices and methods to accomplish daily, weekly, and monthly business tasks. It clarifies what needs to be done and how to do it. Written procedures aid in the training of new personnel, and ensure a comfortable and consistent experience for your clients. You may choose to have a separate procedure manual, or simply add these types of items to your policy manual under procedures.

Figure 18.5 Procedures Checklist

General Procedures
- ❑ Opening and Closing
- ❑ Cleaning and Maintenance
- ❑ Equipment Use and Repair
- ❑ Safety Protocol
- ❑ Purchasing Supplies and Retail Inventory

Front Desk Operations
- ❑ Phone Etiquette
- ❑ Scheduling
- ❑ New Client Protocol
- ❑ Maintenance of Client Records (HIPAA Compliance)
- ❑ Payment Collection and Processing
- ❑ Bookkeeping
- ❑ Client Interaction Instructions

Personnel
- ❑ Documentation Requirements (e.g., license, insurance, CE)
- ❑ Work Hours and Scheduling
- ❑ Dress Code, Hygiene, and Scents
- ❑ Parking
- ❑ Charting
- ❑ Performance Reviews
- ❑ Disciplinary Actions
- ❑ Grievance Protocol

General Procedures

Describe your ideal process for general office tasks. In addition to the procedures detailed below, include procedures for cleaning, maintenance, and determining what supplies and products need to be purchased (and when).

Opening and Closing

Describe how you want to start each day: what needs to be done the moment the first person arrives to open the facility. For example, turn on the hydrotherapy equipment, check phone messages, check email, adjust the thermostat, and anything else that needs to be done before the first client arrives.

In this way, identify any other important daily activities that should be done at a specific time, including how to close the office at the end of the day. Many of the closing tasks may be the opposite of the opening tasks (turning off the hydrotherapy equipment), but should be listed independently as well.

Equipment and Facilities

Office furniture and equipment lasts longer if it's well maintained. If you don't put these things on your list of procedures, there will always be something else to prioritize until you wake up one day to worn and broken equipment. Proper use and care of equipment used in treatments is especially crucial when you share your equipment with other practitioners. Create procedures for the proper operation of all equipment. Include a maintenance and cleaning schedule, and a protocol for repair when necessary.

Figure 18.4 **Sample Client Policy Statement**

My requirements of clients

1. Sessions begin and end at scheduled times. Sessions that begin late because the client arrived late end at the appointed time and are full price.
2. Clients are present (not under the influence of alcohol or drugs).
3. Clients provide a health history and update when necessary.
4. If cancellation is necessary, client gives 24-hour notice or is charged for the appointment (unless it can be filled). Emergency cancellations are determined at the practitioner's discretion (e.g., client is running a fever, has a contagious condition, was in an accident).
5. Payment is due at the time of service unless other arrangements have been made prior to treatment.
6. On outcall appointments, if a client does not arrive within 15 minutes of the appointed time, he is charged for the appointment.
7. Sexual harassment is not tolerated. If the practitioner feels her safety is compromised, the session is ended immediately.
8. This office is a nonsmoking environment.

For touch therapists, also include

9. Clients are clean, having showered the same day as the treatment.
10. Clients do not eat a heavy meal less than 2 hours prior to the treatment.

What clients can expect from me

1. I provide my clients with a competent and professional session each time they come for an appointment, addressing the client's specific needs for that session.
2. I am available to my clients between the hours of 8 a.m. and 6 p.m., and clients may reach me through my answering service on a 24-hour basis.
3. I return calls within 24 hours, unless I am out of town.
4. Clients are treated with respect and dignity.
5. I charge a fair price for my services and offer a sliding fee scale when appropriate.
6. I accept cash, checks, and credit cards.
7. I do not provide direct billing for insurance. I will gladly assist clients in filling out the appropriate forms for reimbursement.
8. Appointments are confirmed the day before the session.
9. I perform services for which I am qualified (physically and emotionally) and able to do, and refer my clients to appropriate specialists when work is not within my scope of practice or not in the client's best interest.
10. I keep accurate records and review charts before each session.
11. I customize my treatment to meet the client's needs.
12. I stay current with information and techniques by reading, receiving regular sessions (of the same service I provide), and taking at least 1 workshop per year.
13. I respect all clients regardless of their age, gender, race, national origin, sexual orientation, religion, socioeconomic status, body type, political affiliation, state of health, or personal habits.
14. Privacy and confidentiality are maintained at all times.

15. If I need to cancel an appointment, I do so within 24 hours whenever possible. If an emergency arises and I cannot keep an appointment, I provide a 50% discount on that client's next session. For non-emergency cancellations of less than 24 hours, the next session is at no charge.
16. My equipment and supplies are clean and safe.
17. Personal and professional boundaries are respected at all times.
18. If a client is dissatisfied with a treatment, and no other arrangement can be agreed upon, a 50% refund of the treatment is honored.
19. Clients may return for refund any unused products (in saleable condition) within 10 days of purchase.

For touch therapists, also include

20. Clients are draped with a sheet or towel at all times during the session. Only the parts of the body being worked on are uncovered at any time.

Safety

Safety procedures minimize the risk a company may encounter for physical, emotional, and mental liability involving its employees, clients, visitors, and products. These activities also pertain to insurance liabilities for loss due to theft, fire, chemical hazards, neglect, and misuse. Many large companies have Risk Management Departments, whose sole purpose is to analyze the physical layout of buildings, prepare ergonomically designed work space, assist employees in being comfortable (therefore more productive) in their working conditions, look for potential hazards, make sure comprehensive and liability insurance coverages are adequate, and assess and develop plans for any other problems that may put the company "at risk."

Occupational Safety and Health Administration
www.osha.gov

Within the realm of a small business, careful attention is required to manage and minimize risks (see Figure 18.6). Implementing effective risk management practices and policies saves time and money, and may help to avoid costly lawsuits. It's also crucial to have a clear procedure for what to do in case of an emergency.

After analyzing your working and client conditions at all levels, take care of any problems which can be eliminated, and make plans to minimize any that you cannot completely resolve. In a nutshell, manage your risks before they become crises.

§6

Figure 18.6 Risk Management Factors

- Building condition
- Escape routes in case of fire
- How you position yourself as you work
- Ergonomic safeguards to avoid or minimize repetitive use syndrome
- Adequate malpractice, liability, and medical coverage
- Ample lighting (particularly if people work at night)
- Potential hazards for clients as they use your facilities
- Clearing parking area and walkways during inclement weather
- Employee stress levels
- Proper use of equipment

Front Desk Operations

Even if you handle your own front desk duties, writing down your desired protocol helps clarify your intentions and provides consistency. Start with your procedures for answering the phone and returning messages. If there is more than one practitioner in the practice, define how to handle scheduling. Also, establish a new client protocol: include questions to ask (screening), scheduling, policy disclosures, and recordkeeping.

Describe the proper use of all your business documents, as well as the proper maintenance and storage of client records. Create a list that helps you and any other personnel understand what is considered HIPAA-compliant (discussed in the next chapter).

Define all other front desk activities such as: marketing, handling sales, processing payments, tracking gift certificates, as well as routine business activities and everyday bookkeeping.

Client Interactions

This is different than client interaction policies. Client policies are the "what" and sometimes the "why." The procedures are the "how" to interact with clients. Part of this involves phone etiquette, as well as every other interaction with clients, from the way you want clients greeted, to the presentation of client forms, to the rescheduling of appointments. This section should also include information on how to dispense educational materials, how to discuss financial arrangements, and how to refer out.

Personnel

Your personnel policies state expectations and responsibilities, while procedures describe how to accomplish the required tasks. For partners or employees who provide treatments to clients, define the specific documentation that is required to verify licensing and continuing education (if applicable) and describe exactly when and where to provide that documentation.

Work hour expectations can be different for everyone, so be specific about things, such as: when they need to show up for an appointment (e.g., 30 minutes prior); what to wear (if there is a dress code); how to present themselves (e.g., clean and scent-free); and where to park. Describe how to request time off or make schedule alterations. For employees, describe the frequency and the process of performance reviews, and how you deal with inappropriate behavior and poor performance. Also clarify your grievance protocol.

Policy and Procedure Manual Draft

- Describe your philosophy toward your profession in general.
- Describe your philosophy and attitude toward your business in particular.
- Describe how you want to run your business.
- Outline your internal policies (also create client policies if you didn't complete the previous activity).
- Sketch your procedure manual.

Smart Technology Choices

Smart technology choices help simplify business logistics, reduce overhead, and cost-effectively market your wellness services. From computers to copiers to cellular phones and answering systems, the tools you rely on each day to communicate with clients and operate your business can provide a competitive edge and boost productivity. Web-based capabilities such as online scheduling and marketing promotions are strong competitive differentiators, especially for group practices. They can increase revenues and repeat business. In fact, studies show that customers who can serve themselves on a website are 30-40% more loyal.[1]

As with everything you purchase, check the warranties and keep all documentation.

Figure 18.7 Assessing Technology Needs

- Will it reduce my expenses?
- Will it increase my income?
- Will it save me time?
- How much do maintenance and supplies cost?
- How long will it take me, or how much will it cost to install?
- Am I willing to make the effort to learn how to properly use and maintain the equipment and software I need?

Online Product Reviews
www.consumersearch.com

Telephones

What could possibly be said about a telephone besides the obvious: every business needs one. They have come a long way from the rotary dial, single line phone. Yesterday's optional phone services—such as caller ID, call waiting, call forwarding, and voice messaging—are today's standard features. If you lean toward high-tech solutions, smartphones offer combined access to phone, text, social media, web browsing, email functionality, and even credit card processing.

See Chapter 6, pages 107-109 for ideas on **telephone etiquette**.

Headsets and speakerphone options are handy when making lengthy calls or several calls in a row. This is far more comfortable than holding a phone to your ear, especially if you need to write while talking. These options are ergonomic as they help you avoid muscle strain and headaches. Your phone system is your primary link with clients, associates, and vendors—in effect, all aspects of your business. Choosing the services and appropriate phone system is paramount. Research the different models and consult with a phone representative to assist you in making the best choices for your circumstances.

Messaging Systems

For those times in session or away from the office, there must be a system in place to receive your business calls. Some people simply use their voicemail, while some use answering machines or a combination of both. Many practitioners utilize answering services so their business contacts can speak with a person. Keep in mind, when people are trying to schedule a same-day appointment, they will often call different places until they get a live person to answer a phone. Ideally, have a live person who is knowledgeable and can schedule appointments.

Answering Services

Answering services provide a human touch, which is often lacking in the business world, but also leave things open to human error. Find a service that has a track record for accuracy, dependability, and timeliness. Provide all pertinent information regarding your practice so questions can be answered correctly. Give your service up-to-date scheduling information and stay in communication with the service on a regular basis throughout your day.

Voicemail Services

Voicemail comes standard with most phone services today and is usually more dependable and more easily accessible than an answering machine. One of the prime benefits is that many people can call at the same time and not receive a busy signal. Most services can receive at least 15 simultaneous calls. If there is a monthly service fee, it's well worth the uninterrupted service and ease of retrieving messages. Be sure to create a brief, welcoming informational greeting (be aware of background noise), providing necessary information. Consider announcing the available appointment slots for that day—just remember to update it throughout the day.

Computers and Tablets

There is more to owning a computer than simply buying it and plugging it in the wall. You need to learn the special terminology (e.g., gigabyte, RAM, hard disk), perform regular maintenance (e.g., file organization, cleaning, backups), install a good anti-malware program, and buy accessories. Fortunately, today's plug-and-play software makes it easier than ever for a computer novice to get up and running fairly easily.

> "Once technology is out of the jar, you can't put it back in.
> —Ervin L. Glaspy

While the Apple MacIntosh software and operating system rules when it comes to graphics and is extremely user-friendly, it isn't as popular as the Microsoft Windows operating system for personal computers. Windows dominates the business market, and the programs for PCs are generally less expensive than for MacIntosh. The system speed and storage requirements depend on how you plan to use your computer.

First, determine what you want the computer to do; this will help you decide which software you need to accomplish those goals. Software choices often determine computer choice due to factors such as the amount of disk and memory space the programs use, and the CPU speed you want. Some programs are only available for one platform (either PC or Mac).

Online computer stores can be a good source for saving on computer hardware and software costs. However, you need to be fairly computer literate to choose what you need, install additional hardware, load programs, and learn how to use the software. If you aren't confident about your computer expertise, establish a relationship with a local supplier who can furnish you with recommendations and continued support after purchases are made.

Computer consultants can design systems based on your needs, help you get the best prices, provide tutoring, and troubleshoot problems. Of course, you pay for their services in addition to the costs of hardware and software.

Once you know what you want, get supplier referrals from associates and friends. Call each one and explain your needs. Ask for price quotes, clarify what software comes bundled with the system (some include office software and games), determine warranty information, and ascertain service time frames. Obtain pricing on each component of your system; ask for a package deal to include the entire system, training, maintenance agreement, and support. Be sure to shop around to get the best price.

Laptop Computers

Today's laptops offer many of the same features as a desktop computer with added mobility. Most people adjust easily to the smaller keyboard and don't mind using a trackpad instead of a mouse. A notebook may be a good choice if you travel outside of your office often or work in multiple locations. Consider the following features:

Battery Life: Your battery will usually last 2-6 hours with constant access to the hard drive. However, most portables come with software that helps manage power use to maximize battery life, generally doubling the minimum time.

Pointing Device: Your choices include trackballs, trackpads, or keyboard buttons called trackpoints. The trackpad is the most popular (utilizing your finger as the means to get around the screen). Next are trackpoints and then the trackball. The standard mouse is awkward on the lap.

Touch Screen Technology: Many laptop computers are equipped with touch screens. This blends the ease of use of a tablet with the functionality of a full computer.

Power Supply: While most portables come with an AC adapter and power cord, consider buying a second one so you can have one at home and one at the office.

Weight: You're looking at carrying around between 2-7 pounds, plus the weight of an adapter, a cord, the carrying case, and whatever else fits in the case. If weight is an issue for you, you may want to look into a tablet.

Tablets

For many business people, even notebook computers are unwieldy. Tablets are compact (handheld), travel easily, and provide nearly as much computing and electronic communication capability as a laptop. You can connect them to your computer and transfer information, or share information wirelessly if you're connected to a cloud-based network. These lightweight assistants can help you schedule meetings while on the run, take notes during meetings, track expenses, write letters, make airline reservations, check your email, read books, and do market research on the Internet.

Business Software

Save time and energy in running the business side of your practice by using the right business software. Some programs are custom-designed for wellness practices, others are created for multipurpose business use. Listed below are some core business functions that you may want to automate using business software.

Figure 18.8 Software Capabilities

- Client scheduling
- Client forms
- Client database
- Client charting notes
- Accounting and taxes
- Human resources recordkeeping
- Insurance billing
- Project tracking
- Website setup and maintenance
- Automatic hard-drive backup
- Marketing materials design
- Automated marketing campaigns

§6

First, decide what functions you want to computerize. Then expect to spend a few hours exploring options. One of the best ways to find user-friendly software is to ask other wellness practitioners what has worked well for them. Articles in trade magazines that focus on making smart technology choices are another good source of practical tips and insights. You can also check out customer reviews on Internet sites such as Google and Amazon.

As you shop for software, make sure it's compatible with your computer's hardware, especially if you own an older model computer or handheld device. Check the minimum software specifications against your hardware capabilities. Ideally, you would plan to attend hands-on training to learn new software. However, don't despair if this isn't possible or practical. Many software programs include online tutorials or help menus that you can use to master basic skills. Although your learning curve may seem steep in the beginning, the key to mastery is hands-on practice and a little coaching from tech-savvy friends or colleagues.

Before you purchase software or hardware, call the manufacturer's toll-free help line. How they handle your call (e.g., if you can't get through, are put on hold for what seems like an eternity, or they don't promptly return messages) helps you determine whether you want to deal with them.

If you aren't computer savvy, consider hiring a technical expert to install the software on your computer and give you a basic tour of how it works. In most cases when you purchase software, install it, and register it, updates are automatically downloaded to your computer.

Business Software

squareup.com
www.getinform.com
www.myreceptionist.com
specialtyansweringservice.net
www.noterro.com
www.handshealehr.com
www.microsoftstore.com
quickbooks.intuit.com
www.paypal.com
www.spaboom.com
www.frontdeskhq.com
zenplanner.com

Finally, explore options for automatic backup of your computer data to an external hard drive that doubles as a fully compatible replacement drive with a complete system image. In the event that your hard drive fails, this replacement drive can be installed in its place, avoiding many headaches and ensuring business continuity.

Cloud Technologies and Apps

Many businesses today are choosing to use cloud-based software, rather than purchasing programs to install directly on their computer or mobile device. Cloud-based means that you access software through a web browser or mobile application, and thus you must be connected to the Internet to use it. This also means you can access your software and associated data from anywhere with an Internet connection. With the pervasiveness of WiFi connections, that's pretty easy to accomplish these days. Some simple services are free to store information, like the Google Calendar and Google Drive apps. But more sophisticated cloud-based software usually comes with an annual or monthly fee. There are online programs that handle accounting, scheduling, marketing, and human resources. There are also online programs that backup your computer hard drive, adding another option for ensuring your data does not disappear if something happens to your computer, or to your office where your backup hard drive exists.

Mobile application software (APPS) can be used to communicate with your clients as well. For example, certain APPS allow you to send texts using your landline number, become a point of sale (POS) cash register or credit card machine, and post informational content to your various social media accounts.

Accessing Information

Utilize a database program to provide accurate analysis of any part of your business by setting up fields for the information, compiling them into reports, and printing them out—all in a matter of minutes. For example, you can choose a single client or group of clients to contact with information (all based on certain criteria you select, such as locale or profession), analyze how often certain modalities are being requested, and evaluate marketing effectiveness (by setting fields to tell you which resources referred clients).

Recordkeeping and Financial Analysis

Simplify your bookkeeping efforts and reduce the amount of time spent in recordkeeping. This type of software allows you to print checks (or send online payments) from your computer and it automatically puts the information in all the appropriate places. You can examine expenses by category and do financial projections. Preparing taxes becomes a matter of a simple command stroke and Voilà!, everything you or your accountant needs is in a printed report.

Calendars, Tasks, Reminders

Computer calendars and address books help you manage your time and can automatically remind you about appointments, birthdays, and follow-up calls.

Client Management

These programs range in features from keeping client charts, preparing insurance billing forms, analyzing information, invoicing, and sending follow-up correspondence.

Marketing Strategies

See Chapter 27 for more on **online marketing strategies**.

Once you establish your marketing strategies, the computer can become your best ally in implementing your plan. With the ability to set criteria, select appropriate clients, and handle functions such as mail merge and labeling, you can quickly get communications out to your target market(s). Online applications for email marketing, such as MailChimp® and Constant Contact,® can manage your client list and marketing newsletters for you.

Desktop Publishing

Many programs can design business cards, brochures, flyers, and newsletters. Some word processing software programs even include basic desktop publishing. Most of these programs come with templates, so all you need to do is type in the text. Several paper companies design products to work with these templates. Many online printing companies, like VistaPrint,® have templates you can choose and customize online during the ordering process.

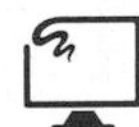

Email Marketing

mailchimp.com
www.constantcontact.com

Custom Printing and Preprinted Paper

www.paperdirect.com
www.vistaprint.com

Online Scheduling

Online scheduling is a great tool to enhance customer satisfaction and help you work smarter. It can minimize frustrating rounds of telephone tag, and save both you and your clients valuable time. Practitioners often find that online scheduling increases bookings from clients who appreciate the added convenience. It's an easy and affordable way to increase productivity and enhance customer service. Plus, you can check and update your calendar from anywhere.

Using this software capability, clients can schedule appointments 24 hours a day at their convenience. Likewise, you can easily set single or standing appointments for clients when you see them in your office. If clients need to cancel or change an appointment, it's easy for them to do so online. In a spa or group practice environment, a receptionist can use the ease and flexibility of online scheduling to book and track appointments. You can also use online scheduling software to manage client contact information.

Another time-saving feature applies to tracking a client's package use. For instance, if your business sells packages, such as a package of 10 sessions, the software lets both staff and clients know the number of remaining sessions. Usually the type of packages that can be set up are number of sessions, dollar amount, or flat monthly fee.

Setting up service is simple. You don't need to install any scheduling software on your computer to use the system. All you need is an Internet connection and some time to locate and evaluate companies with a track record of success and outstanding customer service. Because your critical scheduling and operational data is stored on the company's remote server, be sure to evaluate what data security measures are in place to protect your data from harm—whether from natural disasters or data center events such as fire. Plus, the data needs to be secure to meet HIPAA regulations. Ask questions about these aspects of a company's operations before you sign on the dotted line.

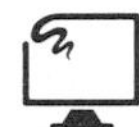

Online Schedulers

www.fullslate.com
www.appointment-plus.com
www.flashappointments.com
www.acuityscheduling.com
www.genbook.com
www.bookeo.com
bookedin.com
www.findjoo.com
www.schedulicity.com
www.mindbodyonline.com
www.bodyworkbuddy.com
clienttracker.weebly.com

Internet Service

The Internet offers a wealth of resources for your business. First, you need to set up a high-speed service account with a local cable or telephone company. Monthly service fees and access vary, so it's a good idea to shop around. Once you get your high-speed connection in place, you can connect to the Internet via web browser software such as Google® Chrome, Apple® Safari, Opera,® Mozilla® Firefox,® or Microsoft Internet Explorer.® Keep in mind, connections can get lost and service can be interrupted for extended periods of time.

You can easily and quickly communicate with clients and co-workers through email software installed on your computer or through an Internet email service such as Yahoo or Google. Whether your email contact is in your hometown or halfway around the world in India on vacation, you can seamlessly coordinate business logistics or share insights into challenging case studies. You can also use the Internet to order supplies, manage online banking and bill paying tasks, access trade journal articles, locate the latest research, register for continuing education seminars, and post job openings.

Copiers, Printers, and Fax Machines

Photocopiers range from very simple, relatively inexpensive desktop units to machines that do everything except go to the post office for you. You can spend a couple hundred dollars or many thousands depending on what you need. Having quick access to a copier can save time (not having to run out to make a few copies) and provide clients with important information without having them wait. Choosing a copier can be an adventure since there are so many that do different tasks at varying speeds. Again, deciding on your needs will narrow the field. Copier companies are willing to bring machines to you for a trial period. Pick out several brands and see how they work. Compare features, cost per copy, maintenance agreement coverages and costs, trade-in allowances for the future, speed, and service availability. In many cases, having a full maintenance agreement covering all parts and labor is a good investment that saves you time and money.

EFax

www.myfax.com
www.efax.com
www.rapidfax.com
www.nextiva.com

The two most widely used **printers** are laser and inkjet printers. Inkjet printers spray tiny droplets of ink into patterns on a page. Inkjet printers are primarily used for color and very economical. If you mainly use your printer for black-and-white printing (e.g., correspondence), consider the basic laser printer. Laser printers use a laser to electrostatically imprint information on a page (this eliminates the smudging problems often encountered with inkjet printers). They're faster, quieter, and provide the clearest print. Color laser printers are becoming more popular, although the cost is usually quite a bit more.

FAX machines come in two major styles; a stand-alone model or a hardware/software combination you install on your computer. Even with the advent of eFAX, a stand-alone FAX machine still comes in pretty handy. It's usually easier to put a document through the FAX machine to send it, than to scan it into the computer, attach it to your email, and send it.

All-in-One

For small offices, you can't beat the all-in-one units that combine printing, copying, scanning, and FAXing all together in one machine. They're a bit more expensive than the basic printers, but affordable if you don't have to also buy a copier and a FAX machine. This option offers the biggest benefit to those with limited office space.

Office Organization

While it might take some time to organize your office for maximum productivity, once you get the systems in place, you're free to concentrate on working with clients. The major areas involve planning, managing paper, and operations. Two keys to avoiding clutter are to designate a proper place for keeping your records and establish a routine for when and how you attend to specific tasks.

The Paperless Office

The paperless office is still a dream for most of us. Even with the advent of PCs, scanners, email, e-faxing, and cloud-based tools, a lot of paper passes through our hands on a daily basis. Many practitioners rely on paper for their client records and financial management. Use a tablet or computer as much as possible. Time is the most crucial commodity practitioners possess. The increased productivity, time savings, and enhanced service that technology provides, more than compensate for your learning-curve efforts and expenditures.

Notes and Receipts Organizers

www.shoeboxed.com
www.evernote.com

First, review your files and purge outdated or irrelevant materials. Discard instruction manuals on equipment you no longer use. A common contributor to clutter is keeping numerous copies of the same item. Usually one copy is enough, although you might keep a duplicate if the item has an artistic value (e.g., a beautifully designed, multicolored brochure).

Use a paper shredder if the information to be disposed of is related to clients or finances. Put inactive files and past records in storage boxes. Label the boxes and put them in a secure place. Archived files should be kept in a separate filing cabinet or storage box. Store your critical financial records in a fireproof case, or take them to a place that specializes in archiving documents (this also holds true for computer files). See Figure 18.9 for tips on going paperless.[2]

Figure 18.9 Tips for Going Paperless

1. Commit to a paperless scheduling experience.
2. Track client progress electronically.
3. Go cashless with smartphone credit card processing.
4. Trade your shoebox of receipts for Shoeboxed.com.
5. Manage your todo list in the cloud.
6. Thumb your nose at the 80's with eFax.
7. Sign documents electronically.
8. Invoice via email.
9. Invest in a good shredder.
10. Keep important documents in Evernote.

Get Organized Now!

The first step to getting organized is to establish a space that's dedicated exclusively to your business. This area would include a writing surface (preferably a desk), an ergonomic chair, a desk lamp, a filing drawer or cabinet, and a collection of office supplies.

See Chapter 20, page 283 for a list of **how long records should be kept**.

Having difficulty finding needed information is the most common form of office inefficiency. This applies to paper systems as well as computers. Consider the various business activities you engage in and design a structure to deal with them.

Minimize handling paper. Begin by dividing all paperwork into 4 initial categories: take action; file; get rid of it; and read or review later. The primary purpose of a filing system is easy retrieval, not storage. Ideally, you would have at least 3 separate filing drawers: client records; current projects, upcoming events, and financial management; and resources.

Mail

We spend an incredible amount of time dealing with mail. Set a specific time of day to open mail. Avoid going through your mail if you don't have the time to appropriately process it. The goal is to handle mail once. First, choose a place for opening mail that's next to a filing center, trash can, and paper-recycling bin. Use a letter opener—it saves time, keeps things neat, and alleviates paper cuts. Whenever possible, take immediate action such as write a return letter, file the information in resources, or trash it.

Phone Calls and Messages

The key to managing the telephone is to be prepared logistically and mentally. You don't want to keep callers waiting while you search for supplies or information. Store needed provisions (e.g., paper, pen, appointment book, new client checklist) within reach. Keep a message pad next to the phone and return calls within 24 hours.

Projects

Create a separate file for each of your projects. Whenever you come across information pertaining to a particular project, immediately put it in the proper folder. Once the project is complete, sort through the file and put into your resource folders any information that could be useful in the future. Then archive or throw away (if possible, recycle) the rest of the file's contents.

Upcoming Events

Develop a tickler file for upcoming events. A tickler file reminds you of your commitments and assists in follow-through. Essentially, a tickler system contains 12 separate sections (one for each month) and a set of dividers numbered 1-31, for each day of the month. You can put these in a 3-ring binder, an accordion file, or hanging files. Place the 31 dividers in the "Current Month" section. Then, if someone asks you to contact them in 2 weeks, you go to your tickler file, turn to the corresponding date, and make a note to call that person. Check your tickler file daily. Look at the current day and possibly the next 2 days. If you own a computer, you can purchase planning software programs that include tickler systems, or use your calendar software to track events for you.

The true beauty of a tickler file is for keeping track of future events. For example, a client is going out of town for the summer and asks you to call back on September 12th. You put a note in the September section of your file. When it's the end of August and you transfer your 31 dividers to September, you would put the note under 12. Using this system helps ensure that you won't forget your commitments. Various computer programs do this automatically. Even if you use a computerized tickler system, a physical tickler folder is handy for keeping paperwork associated with the activities on the various dates.

Contacts

Keep track of contacts and potential business resources. Use your computer contact manager or place pre-designed contact forms in a binder with alphabetical dividers. Give each contact a separate sheet. Some of the information to include is the person's name, company, title, work address and phone number, home address and phone number, email addresses, referral source, where you met, any personal or professional information that you want, and action to be taken. Transfer the items from the action to be taken section to your tickler file or appointment book. You might also want to list the dates and times of any actions directly onto the contact form. This is particularly helpful as a document to record business interactions. For example, you get a bid for supplies over the phone and you place an order. Then you get your bill, and it's for a different price. You're more likely to resolve the difference in your favor if you can say, "I talked with Ann Alleby on Tuesday, August 17th, at 3:20 p.m. and was told...."

Review your contacts at least every 2 months.

Storing business cards can be frustrating. They can be filed by name, company, or type of business. Choose a method and stick to it. Otherwise, you'll spend a lot of time attempting to remember which way you filed that specific card. If you have extra cards, then you can file by each category (the downside to this option is that your business card holder gets filled extremely quickly). Options for storing business cards include using a Rolodex® type of system, inserting cards in binder sleeves, or stapling the cards to contact sheets. Remember, you could always manually enter this information in your computer contact manager or use a business card scanner for the paperless route.

Client Files

Keep client files in alphabetical order. Determine what client information and forms you want included in each client folder. Design a one-page checklist and staple it to the left side of the folder (unless your files are computerized). On the top of the form put the client contact information. Then include other details that you deem important, such as who referred the client; insurance data; and physician contact information.

Designate a section that lists completed forms to be put in the folder (e.g., client intake, insurance verification, treatment plan, HIPAA forms). Be sure to leave space next to each item to put the date when the form was placed in the file. If you don't have a computerized tickler file, consider putting a follow-up section on the bottom of the page so you can easily see when you last made contact.

Review all client files at least twice a year. See if you can re-establish connections and if not, consider these inactive files and archive them. There is no federal guideline for how long client records must be kept, although some states do have specific laws. In general, keep all records at least 10 years (indefinitely is ideal).

If you do a lot of work on the road, purchase a portable file carrier. Stock it with your promotional materials, client materials, a receipt envelope, and supplies (e.g., a calculator, receipts, pens, paper clips). Each morning, go to your master filing system, pull the client files on the specific clients you'll be seeing that day, and add those files to the portable carrier. Return them to your master filing system at the end of the day. Keeping electronic files simplifies this process.

Financial Management

The rule of thumb for financial recordkeeping is: Keep all receipts. A corollary is: Jot down expenses when receipts are unavailable. Keep all receipts in one place, and post them in your ledger on either a daily, weekly, or monthly basis to ease the paperwork burden at income tax time.

The two major ways for keeping financial receipts are: by the category (place receipts in separate folders according to type, such as "Marketing Expenses"or "Supplies"); or by the date (one file folder for each month of the year). Keep in mind that even though you do your bookkeeping on a computer, you still need to keep hard-copy receipts for tax purposes (hopefully those rules will change given the vast amount of purchase receipts being sent through email).

Resources

This group of files can easily get unwieldy. What may work well is to store magazines and journals on a shelf, and put newsletters into a binder. Sort loose papers by subject. Oftentimes an article or piece of information could go in several places. A solution is to make copies and put them in the various places. A paper-conserving idea is to put the information in one folder, and then make a note on the inside of the other folders referencing the folder where the information is stored. Significantly reduce the amount of paper you accumulate (such as magazine articles), by scanning them into your computer using a good cross-indexing program. If you need materials from your master files to go into a project folder, either make a copy or note in the master folder as to where the resource material has been moved.

Figure 18.10 Filing Tips

Managing Paper

- File materials immediately with the most current materials in the front.
- Files should be in use or put away.
- Label and color code file folders.
- Separate active files from archive files.
- Don't overstuff folders—create subfiles.
- Ease filing by reducing oversized documents to letter size.
- When a project is finished or a client is inactive, remove extraneous material from the file and archive the rest.

Organizing Computer Information

- Use the same names for computer directories, folders, and files that you label your paper documentation storage.
- Eliminate or archive inactive files on a monthly basis.

Data Protection

www.epa.gov/records

www.techrepublic.com/article/10-things-you-can-do-to-protect-your-data

humanresources.about.com/od/healthsafetyandwellness/a/protect_data.htm

oag.ca.gov/privacy/facts/online-privacy/protect-your-computer

Protecting Your Records

Any number of mishaps and catastrophes can occur in a place of business. One of the most common is damaged or lost computer data due to viruses, hard drive failures, spilling liquids or food onto the computer, or energy spikes. Other culprits are theft or property damage due to vandalism, critter infestation, broken water pipes, fire, smoke, and acts of nature. The good news is that you can take proactive measures to limit damages caused by an unforeseen catastrophe and speed recovery. For instance, an uninterruptible power supply (UPS) comes in handy to keep your equipment running long enough to save data during a power outage.

Figure 18.11 How to Protect Your Records

Emergency Contact List: Keep a list of who should be notified in the event of a disaster: insurance agent; lawyer; clients; colleagues; suppliers; employees; property manager; or owner.

Key Documents: Maintain a copy of key documents (e.g., bank account, loan papers, tax records, backup files) off-site in a bank safety deposit box.

Computer Back-Up: Regularly back up your computer information onto a flash drive or external hard drive, and archive off-site or in a fire-proof box (a bank safety deposit box is good for this). Also, consider cloud-based back-ups. Regularly perform a minor restore operation to stay familiar with how it works; rather like a fire drill.

Insurance Recordkeeping: Store insurance related information such as photographs, major receipts, and identifying information of your insured assets (e.g., model number, year purchased) in a fire-proof box or off-site.

19
Practice Management

"The worst days of those who enjoy what they do, are better than the best days of those who don't."
—E. James Rohn

Health Insurance Portability and Accountability Act
- The Four Facets of HIPAA
- Who Must Comply with HIPAA Regulations?
- Myths
- Steps to Implement Now

Insurance Reimbursement
- Insurance Claim Processing Overview
- To Bill or Not to Bill
- Types of Insurance Providers
- Licensing Regulations
- Procedure and Modality Codes
- Basic Steps for Submitting Claims
- Electronic Billing
- The Affordable Care Act

Anatomy of a Contract
- What to Include

Negotiations

Conflict Management
- Mediation and Arbitration

Key Terms

Affordable Care Act
Arbitration
Breach of Contract
Business Associate
Comorbidity
Confidentiality
Conflict
Conflict Management
Confrontation
Contract
Current Procedural Terminology (CPT) Codes
Diagnosis
Health Insurance Portability and Accountability Act (HIPAA)
Health Maintenance Organization (HMO)
Insurance Claim
Insurance Reimbursement
International Classification of Diseases-Tenth Revision-Clinical Modification Code Book (ICD-10-CM)
Lawsuit
Litigation
Managed Care Organization
Mediation
Medicaid
Medicare
Modality
National Provider Identifier (NPI)
Negligence
Negotiations
No-Fault Insurance
Occupational License
Personal Injury Insurance
Personal Injury/Med-Pay Insurance
Preferred Provider Organization (PPO)
Prescription
Procedure
Protected Health Information (PHI)
Uninsured Motorist Insurance
Workers' Compensation Insurance

The previous chapter focused on creating the necessary documentation and tools to run your office. This chapter covers the special circumstances that can occur in the day-to-day managing of your practice: complying with regulations; handling insurance reimbursement; negotiating contracts; and resolving conflicts. We begin by exploring HIPAA.

Health Insurance Portability and Accountability Act

Health Information Privacy

www.hhs.gov/hipaa

The Health Insurance Portability and Accountability Act of 1996 (HIPAA) is intended to protect the privacy of healthcare consumers and establishes compliance rules for healthcare providers. Further revisions have added security protection guidelines for the use of health information technologies.[1] HIPAA has three major purposes:

1. Protect and enhance the rights of consumers by providing them access to their health information and controlling the inappropriate use of that information;
2. Improve the quality of health care in the United States by restoring trust in the healthcare system among consumers, healthcare professionals, and the multitude of organizations and individuals committed to the delivery of care;
3. Improve the efficiency and effectiveness of healthcare delivery by creating a national framework for health privacy protection that builds on efforts by states, health systems, individual organizations, and individuals.

The Four Facets of HIPAA

Get your **Assigned National Provider Identifier**

https://www.cms.gov/Regulations-and-Guidance/Administrative-Simplification/NationalProvIdentStand

1. **Electronic Health Transactions Standards**: When billing insurance, practitioners are required to use the Standard Code Sets of the International Classification of Disease (ICD-10) codes and the Current Procedural Terminology (CPT) codes.
2. **Unique Identifiers for Providers, Employers, Health Plans, and Clients**: Each practitioner who transmits information electronically is assigned a National Provider Identifier (NPI).
3. **Security of Health Information and Electronic Signature Standards**: All practitioners must provide uniform levels of protection of all health information that is stored or transmitted electronically. This includes your computer, along with any faxes and email messages sent. An electronic signature is required for all HIPAA transactions.
4. **Privacy and Confidentiality**: Limits the nonconsensual use and release of private health information; gives clients new rights to access their medical records and to know who else has accessed them; restricts most disclosure of health information to the minimum needed for the intended purpose; institutes criminal and civil sanctions for improper use or disclosure; and establishes new requirements for access to records by researchers and others.

Who Must Comply with HIPAA Regulations?

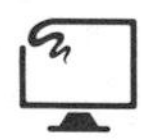

HIPAA Covered Entity Charts

https://www.cms.gov/Regulations-and-Guidance/Administrative-Simplification/HIPAA-ACA/AreYouaCoveredEntity

Unfortunately, the answer isn't straightforward. Journalist Julie Bryant stated, "What was to be a simple federal rule, designed to lift the healthcare industry out of antiquated paper-based systems and into the bright, organized world of high-speed technology, has instead spawned hysteria, predatory opportunists, and outright befuddlement."[2] Many companies charge thousands of dollars to provide businesses with training, guidelines, and forms to ensure HIPAA compliance. Caution is advised before investing in these programs.

The current emphasis of HIPAA compliance centers on electronic transmission of a client's Protected Health Information (PHI). When you go to the HIPAA site, review the readiness checklist to determine if you're a Covered Entity. Many wellness practitioners (unless they bill insurance) will find that, indeed, they aren't required to be HIPAA compliant.

Following the HIPAA guidelines actually makes good business sense, and the requirements are fairly easy to implement. Consumers are used to receiving privacy policy statements from other healthcare providers as well as from a myriad of other businesses, such as insurance carriers and credit card companies. Your clients might find it disconcerting if you don't follow suit. Also, failure to heed the HIPAA regulations can result in civil and criminal penalties.

HIPAA Resources

www.sohnen-moe.com/resources/resource-directory/

Sample Business Associate Contract

www.hhs.gov/hipaa/for-professionals/covered-entities/sample-business-associate-agreement-provisions/

Note that even if you don't need to be HIPAA compliant for your own practice, you still need to be compliant if you work with other covered entities. The term for this is a "chain of trust." If you're a Business Associate, you must meet the same requirements for privacy and security as a covered entity.

According to the HIPAA regulations, a Business Associate is defined as "a person or entity that performs certain functions or activities that involve the use or disclosure of protected health information on behalf of, or provides services to, a covered entity."[3] Thus, if a primary care provider refers a client to you or you send a client's progress report to her doctor, then you're considered a Business Associate. There is a form that Business Associates must sign. Also, be aware that your state regulations might be more stringent than the federal requirements.

Greg Neely, a medical massage therapist who is certified in Insurance Massage Billing and HIPAA Certified Security Training, says to ask yourself questions like these to help you determine if you should voluntarily become HIPAA compliant:[4]

- Do you complete an intake form for clients?
- Do you write session notes on clients?
- Do you work in a wellness establishment with more than 10 employees?
- Do you have general liability insurance or malpractice insurance?
- Do you want to be covered if your session notes are subpoenaed for legal reasons?
- Do you want protection if your client decides to sue you for any reason?
- If you answer yes to either of these questions, you **must** become HIPAA compliant:
  Do you work for someone who files insurance claims, or do you file insurance claims?
  Do you file claims with any clearinghouses, such as Availity or Office Ally?

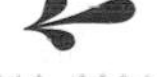

See Chapter 6, pages 97-100 for information on **charting**.

Myths

Some of the confusion about client privacy has led to unnecessary changes. Myths abound regarding using a client's name and client paperwork such as sign-in sheets and files. It's fine to greet your client by name even if others are in the waiting room. You can still have client sign-in sheets as long as they don't disclose any PHI. You can put clients' charts on the treatment room doors as long as the clients' names don't show and unauthorized people can't access the charts. For instance, if people must walk past a treatment room to get to the bathroom, then it might not be wise to put a chart on that treatment room door.

Steps to Implement Now

If you work with insurance reimbursement, it's wise to immediately follow the HIPAA compliance guidelines. If you're a covered entity, compliance is mandatory. Regardless of insurance issues or HIPAA regulations, it's vital that you take appropriate measures to ensure the privacy, confidentiality, and security of clients' PHI.

Figure 19.1 HIPAA Tips

- Designate someone in your office (or hire an outside party) as a Privacy Officer. This person is responsible for creating a process to handle PHI. If you work alone, you're the privacy officer.
- Train office staff on how to handle PHI, including what circumstances PHI may be disclosed.
- Use consent or authorization documents that clients sign.
- Don't discuss any medical information with any third parties unless written consent or authorization has been obtained.
- Be careful when discussing a client's PHI with office staff. Be aware of who may overhear conversations.
- Assign User IDs and passwords to anyone with access to electronic information.
- Verify that your software has effective security features allowing you to comply with HIPAA regulations.
- Use passwords and security programs to protect and maintain electronic files.
- For email, obtain written consent from the client and use secure transfer methods (encryption). Use electronic signatures to authenticate who sent the email.
- Use auditing software to monitor who sent what and when.
- Develop a policy and procedure manual that delineates how you handle all aspects of HIPAA compliance. Also, designate your policy for the destruction or retention of client records that includes email communications.
- Design a client information sheet that explains the following: how you use clients' information; the storage method for client files; the circumstances under which you may disclose client information; and the procedure for clients to see or obtain copies of their files.
- Store all client files in a locked room or in a locked cabinet. Only allow authorized employees access to these files.
- Don't leave files in an area that is accessible by clients or unauthorized staff.
- Keep appointment books from view of anyone except those directly dealing with client care.
- Get authorization from clients about marketing (including greeting cards, flyers, and newsletters) and communications, such as appointment confirmation notices.
- Present each client with a "Notice of Privacy Policies" form.
- Have new clients sign a separate form indicating that they've received the Notice of Privacy Policies.
- Have each client sign a form giving consent for treatment, payment, and healthcare operations.
- When applicable, have clients sign an authorization for any and all releases of PHI.
- Put confidentiality notices on all faxes and emails.

Insurance Reimbursement

Accepting insurance can be an incredible boon to your business. However, if not properly managed, it can bring extra stress and negatively impact your profitability. Many practitioners who accept insurance hire outside help to handle this part of the business so they can stay focused on clients, and not get bogged down by the mounds of paperwork that inevitably accompany insurance processing.

> Words have the power to both destroy and heal. When words are both true and kind, they can change our world.
> —Buddha

Oftentimes your policy on accepting insurance can be the determining factor in whether a potential client chooses you as her wellness provider. In addition, during economic downturns, clients with insurance can help keep your income stream steady.

The best way to decide if you would like to become involved with insurance companies is to do the math and figure out if it will help your bottom line and help your business be more profitable. Figure out your cost per client for doing business by adding up all your income and expenses and dividing by the number of clients you have. Then find out what insurance companies are paying in your area and run the numbers again to see if taking insurance would help your business. Additional factors to consider include:

- Do you need more clients?
- Do you have the time to spend learning the ropes and keeping up with the details of billing insurance?
- Does it fit in with your business vision?
- Does it fit in with your healthcare philosophy?

Massage Insurance Billing 101 by Julie Onofrio

Insurance Billing and Practice Building by Vivian Mahoney

Points for Profit, Fifth Edition by Honora Wolfe, Marilyn Allen

Hands Heal, Fourth Edition by Diana L. Thompson

Many practitioners pin a lot of hopes on the insurance industry. Look what it has done to enhance the medical profession in terms of recognition and financial compensation. The most recent example of this benefit is evidenced in the chiropractic field. People claim that wellness providers' credibility increases as more and more insurance companies cover their services. Perhaps so, but at what cost? Keep in mind that many consumers see the value of alternative methods in their healing process and want CAM providers to be covered by their insurance.

Your cost of doing business may increase with the additional management required to bill and track clients. When working with health insurance companies, the small practice doesn't have the negotiation power that hospitals or large medical clinics have, so basically you must abide by the rules and accept the fees that the insurance companies set.

The business cost for a non-insurance case is less than that for a medically related case. A medical case involves far more time spent on documentation, processing paperwork, coordinating payment conditions, tracking payment, and appealing rejected claims. When determining fees for medically related sessions, it's best to consult a business advisor, legal advisor, or reference manual.

§6

When it comes to determining best treatment options for clients, you will find that insurance companies are increasingly dictating to the healthcare community the types of treatments they can perform. Since the insurance companies are paying for these procedures, they're imposing stricter guidelines about what they consider acceptable care and under what conditions.

As we progress in this arena, we must strive to keep the integrity and diversity of our work intact. I think it's possible to have the whole spectrum of allied wellness covered by insurance and to provide varied techniques. To accomplish this, we must make a concerted effort to educate the primary care providers and the members of the insurance industry, as well as employer groups, about the different therapies, techniques, and their specific benefits. This is why we also need more evidence-based research.

See Chapter 4, pages 62-63 for information on **research**.

This section provides an overview of insurance processing, insights into the pros and cons of accepting insurance as payment, descriptions of the types of insurance, key definitions, and the basic steps for submitting a claim. Because this vast topic could span thousands of pages, if you decide to accept insurance, it's best to seek specialized training—either by attending a course, working with a consultant, or studying a reference manual.

Insurance Claim Processing Overview

Let's look at the insurance industry itself. From a consumer's point of view, most of us think about health insurance as a way to ensure that our healthcare costs are covered in case of a serious illness or accident and as a means to assist in the payment for our wellbeing to prevent major illness. What we tend to forget is that insurance companies are just that—companies. And as such, one of their major priorities is to make a profit. Very few insurance companies hold altruistic beliefs as their main purpose for being in business; we must always remember that motivation when contemplating the role of the insurance industry.

The three main types of insurance claims are:

1. Motor Vehicle Collisions (MVC) also known as Motor Vehicle Accidents (MVA). Accidents are also now being called incidents or being referred to as a motor vehicle collision so that fault isn't implied.
2. Workers' Compensation (sometimes known as Labor & Industries or L&I) which involves injuries that happen while a person is at work.
3. Private health insurance companies such as a Health Maintenance Organization (HMO) or a Preferred Provider Organization (PPO).

Workers' Compensation

List of **Workers' Compensation Boards**

www.dol.gov/owcp/dfec/regs/compliance/wc.htm

Workers' Compensation is a form of insurance that provides wage replacement, medical benefits, and compensation for permanent physical impairments to employees injured in the course of employment. Workers' Compensation insurance is mandated by law in the United States, and claims account for a significant amount of money that goes toward health care. If you decide to accept clients with Workers' Compensation insurance, find your state's contact information on the online list of workers' compensation boards.

Personal Injury Claims

Personal Injury Claims are claims made when an injury occurs in an automobile, at home, in a business space, or in a space that is covered by some sort of liability insurance. In most states there is Personal Injury Protection Insurance (PIP) or Medical Payments (Med-Pay) coverage on your own insurance plan that covers the cost of care up front (within policy limits) without having to wait until the claim settles. The person who is injured starts a claim with their own insurance company and their insurance company may later collect from the other party who caused or is responsible for the injury.

Typically, you submit the bill directly to the claims adjustor or the attorney. In most instances, everything is covered unless the injured party's insurance requires a co-pay or deductible. If you aren't the primary care provider, you need a prescription from one. Care must be medically necessary and reasonable to be covered. The claim process is fairly straightforward for minor injuries (and that can be lucrative for a small clinic).

Third-Party Insurance Claims

Currently, insurance reimbursement is a bit erratic, particularly with third-party claims. A lot seems to depend upon the unique perspective of the claims adjustor as well as the policies of the specific insurance company. A company might honor a claim one time and refuse payment on the next. Each company has different general rules that apply to coverage and payment. Each insurance company offers a variety of insurance coverage policies, and each of those policies has its own rules and benefits. As a result, you may have conflicting experiences from the same carrier due to a difference in the terms of the policies. This is why you must verify coverage and ascertain what is needed to get paid for each client.

Most people use this insurance for their overall care, but it's sometimes used for injury claims. For instance, when PIP/MedPay claims are complex because of the severity of the injury, the claimant may use up the initial benefits and then the claim moves into a Third

Party Claim, where the insurance company of the person at fault pays for care when the case is settled. This can involve waiting a few years for the claim to settle.

Financial Responsibility

In short, you can't always predict if an insurance company will authorize payments, the total amount it will cover, or the number of sessions it will allow. Worse, verifying the coverage of a specific policy doesn't always guarantee payment. The best way to ensure payments are made is to have the client sign a contract that she will pay no matter what. You can also ask the attorney to sign the contract, but he may refuse in case he wants to ask you for a reduced fee in the future. Reneging on a contract would be an ethics violation for attorneys. A contract increases the likelihood of getting paid and getting paid the billed amount.

In view of the uncertainties surrounding insurance reimbursement, it's wise to create a statement of financial responsibility for all new clients. When working with motor vehicle, liability, and homeowners insurance, signing a contract is usually the best way to go. This clearly communicates that even with insurance, a client is ultimately responsible for any unpaid balance for sessions. This approach may not apply in certain cases, such as Workers' Compensation.

Determine how much credit you're willing to extend to a client, and over what period of time, before requiring the client to provide payment for a specified amount of the outstanding balance. Some practitioners require the client to pay up front and provide the appropriate documentation for the client to submit to his insurance company for reimbursement.

To Bill or Not to Bill

Choosing whether to accept insurance reimbursement clients (or even developing associations with primary care providers to gain referrals) is a major decision. Sometimes it becomes a spontaneous decision if a potential client comes to you with a prescription in hand; you must decide right then if you will help this client and possibly earn extra income from this source, or refuse to work with the client's insurance.

The potential advantages are higher fees and an increased number of client sessions. The disadvantages include paperwork, possible regimentation, the potential of not receiving compensation for your work, and the time lag between provided service and remittance (payment). This can be alleviated by knowing what you're doing and by obtaining proper training in working with insurance.

Keep in mind that you or your staff could spend a lot of time verifying policies and filling out paperwork. There is also the added HIPAA requirements that must be implemented and maintained. That is why many practitioners don't accept insurance claims. They require clients to pay them directly for the services, and then the clients must submit a voucher to their own insurance company (or attorney) for reimbursement. This can pose a problem in those cases in which you would in fact be reimbursed but the client cannot afford to pay up front for the number of treatment sessions a week that the referring physician prescribed.

In the best of all possible worlds, all wellness practitioners would be fairly and promptly reimbursed for delivering a competent service of proven effectiveness. Until (and even after) we reach that stage, you must weigh the tradeoffs inherent with the insurance bureaucracy, realizing that as your business grows, you may change your mind. You can also get clients involved in this process and let them do most of the work of dealing with the insurance companies.

Figure 19.2 Types of Insurance

Fee for Service: General health insurance coverage offered by an employer or other entity to an individual or a group. With this type of coverage, an insurance provider reimburses directly to the healthcare provider as long as they accept an assignment of benefits to the provider (you) from the insured person. The amount of reimbursement to a healthcare provider is based on what is termed "usual, customary, and reasonable" charges.

Workers' Compensation: This insurance coverage is required in almost every state. Most employers must carry this coverage to protect employees in case of injuries on the job.

Personal Injury: Covers a multitude of situations. For the most part, it means that someone was injured in an automobile accident or during a slip-and-fall accident.

No-Fault: This is referred to as personal injury protection. What this means is that in No-Fault states, if one is injured, the injured party can obtain medical treatment and have the bills submitted to her own insurance company for remittance regardless of who is at fault.

Personal Injury Protection/Med-Pay: Refers to medical payment for motor vehicle collisions. This is additional coverage a person can purchase when first purchasing or renewing an auto insurance policy. This is coverage above and beyond the usual $10,000 coverage that is on a no-fault policy.

Uninsured Motorist: If an uninsured driver injured the party, the injured party must have previously purchased "uninsured motorist protection" (UM) on her policy to be covered for the injury the uninsured person caused.

Medicare: A federal program that provides health benefits for those 65 years of age or over, and for those under 65 who are permanently disabled.

Medicaid: Medical coverage for those unable to pay for medical services because of financial hardships. Medicaid is run by both the state and federal government, with the federal government covering 55% and the state paying the remainder. Some states, such as Tennessee, don't utilize the Medicaid System. These states offer other methods of providing medical coverage.

Types of Insurance Providers

To help you get acquainted with some common terminology, listed below are descriptions of the major types of insurance providers. Arrangements made between insurance companies and employers must comply with state regulations. In addition, some states now require individuals with Workers' Compensation claims to be processed through Managed Care Organizations.

Managed Care Organization (MCO)

These entities manage costs by contracting with providers who agree to charge predetermined fees. They're administered by a gatekeeper; a physician who oversees the services supplied by the organization. All providers must be contracted by the MCO and approved by the gatekeeper prior to providing services to the patients. Some MCOs include complementary wellness providers.

Health Maintenance Organization (HMO)

A type of MCO, HMOs provide healthcare services for a fixed fee to subscribers in a specific geographic location. Plans usually cover preventive services with little or no out of pocket expenses. In most cases, members must use the physicians and facilities authorized by the HMO. They typically don't reimburse complementary wellness providers unless it's written in the state law.

Preferred Provider Organization (PPO)

A type of MCO, PPO contracts with a group of preferred providers to deliver health care to members. Unlike HMO members, PPO members are free to choose any physician or hospital for services, but they receive more benefits (or pay less of the cost themselves) if they choose a preferred provider. A PPO plan usually requires filing claims and paying deductibles and copayments.

Licensing Regulations

An occupational license is a license required by a city or county to sell a product or perform a service for money at a certain location. A licensed provider of healthcare services is a professional who obtains a state license by passing a state examination and has received a license to operate from his state professional board. Most wellness providers are allowed to see a client without a physician referral or prescription. However, for the service to be reimbursed by an insurance company, it must be considered medically necessary and prescribed. Additionally, you must have a physician's diagnosis written on the prescription as well as the frequency and duration of treatment.

Unlicensed states often have restrictions and requirements to operate within their cities or counties. It's strictly up to the person providing treatment for compensation to know the specific state licensing laws, rules, and regulations. In these unlicensed states, practitioners can sometimes provide services if they hold a certification in their profession. When it comes to licensing requirements, it's best to ask the insurance company for specific requirements, and to check the state statutes for both automobile and Workers' Compensation cases.

See Chapter 15, pages 205-206 for more information on **laws and regulations**.

Procedure and Modality Codes

Procedure and modality codes are critical pieces of the insurance puzzle. All insurance carriers require these codes to process insurance claims. Procedure codes are also known as Current Procedural Terminology (CPT) Codes. They indicate the type of services performed during the session to improve function. These codes are defined and maintained by the American Medical Association. A *procedure* is the main service you provide, such as massage therapy. A *modality* is an adjunct to that procedure, based on the the device used (e.g., ultrasound), and can only be used one time per session, regardless if used for more than 15 minutes. For example, CPT Code 97124 refers to massage therapy, each 15 minutes; CPT Code 97140 is for manual therapy techniques (e.g., manual lymphatic drainage), each 15 minutes; CPT Code 97810 is for a basic acupuncture treatment of 15-minutes duration. Thus, if you' re a massage therapist and your session is 60 minutes, then you list the main procedure code 4 times (e.g., 97124, 97124, 97124, 97124).

CPT codes will be changing soon and moving away from timed codes like 97124 and 97140. The codes will be based on the level of complexity of the client's condition and the clinical decision-making process, comorbidities, and complexity of how you approach a client's care. Comorbidity is the presences of other diseases and conditions, like having diabetes and a hamstring pull. Physician codes already do that. When the new codes do come out there will be much to do in working with the insurance companies to set the allowable fees.

Diagnostic Codes

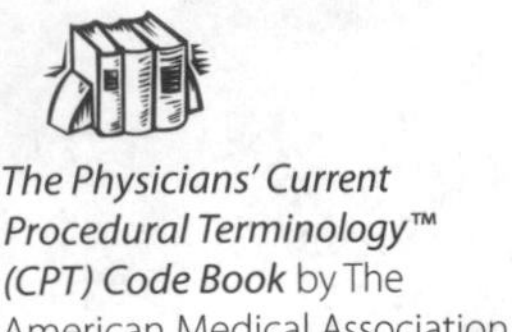

The Physicians' Current Procedural Terminology™ (CPT) Code Book by The American Medical Association

The diagnostic codes for licensed healthcare providers are listed in an ICD-10-CM (International Classification of Diseases-Tenth Revision-Clinical Modification) Code Book. The diagnostic codes are used by physicians to indicate a medical condition for diagnosing and prescribing treatment and therapies for their patients. A nonphysician provider cannot diagnose a medical condition. Be sure to check with your state professional board for detailed requirements for your profession.

Basic Steps for Submitting Claims

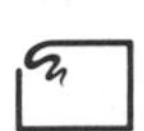

Coding Resources
www.cdc.gov/nchs/icd.htm

1. **If you aren't considered a primary care provider**, you must have a written prescription from a referring physician. The prescription must indicate the following: the procedures or modalities to be performed; the number of visits per prescription (e.g., how many times per week for how many weeks, or the total number of visits allowed); and the diagnosis (e.g., 847.2: lumbar strain and sprain).
2. **Verify coverage**. During the call to the adjuster, confirm the following: the client does indeed have insurance; what, if any, are the deductibles; has the deductible been met, and if not, when is it due; does the patient have copayments that need to be collected, and if so, how much.
3. **Prepare the claim form**. The latest version is the CMS 1500 form 02/12.
4. **Submit the completed claim form**. There are also now many companies offering online submission of claim forms which makes the process much faster. You must be HIPAA compliant when using this type of company.
5. **Record the treatment session**, amount billed, and total amount due.
6. **Copy all checks when received**, record payment and balances due. In instances of a personal injury case, bill the client for any amounts due if you haven't agreed to send balances to the attorney for payment at time of settlement.

Ensure Efficient Claim Processing

When processing an insurance claim, it's advisable to check with the insurance carrier or adjuster for each client. When a client arrives to complete his initial evaluation and intake form, he should provide this contact information for you. If not, it can be obtained from the treating physician.

Medical Forms Processors
www.availity.com
cms.officeally.com

Obtaining verification for services can be very helpful in receiving payment. Always note the name of the insurance company representative you talk with and (if possible) get a code for verified service. Obtaining written insurance verification provides you with the most protection. When it comes to Workers' Compensation claims, you must obtain authorization from the insurance adjuster prior to treating the client.

Figure 19.3 Reasons for Denials, Delays, or Reductions

1. Prescription is outdated or not included in the claim.
2. Documentation isn't accurate.
3. Claim isn't submitted in a timely manner.
4. CPT Codes aren't in scope of practice.
5. Fees are more than usual, reasonable, and customary.
6. Accepting a type of case that wouldn't be covered by the policy.
7. Pertinent information isn't included on the claim form.

Electronic Billing

The best reason to utilize electronic billing is that this type of insurance claim gets processed and paid much more quickly. It can simplify recordkeeping and decrease the time spent processing claims. Those who submit electronic claims have fewer denials, reductions, and disputes. In short, electronic billing can save you time, money, and enhance your cash flow.

If you aren't HIPAA compliant, don't submit claims electronically.

Nearly all insurance companies have implemented electronic claims submission to streamline operations and lower costs. Some commercial carriers don't yet accept electronic billing, even though they do accept electronic claims reports for notice of injuries. Electronic billing usually involves submitting a claim to an insurance provider through a clearinghouse (this often speeds up claim processing and minimizes errors). An electronic claim is typically submitted to the insurance provider in a digital format via a secure website or as a digital FAX.

Figure 19.4 **Top 10 Billing Tips**

1. Submit your claims "personal & confidential" to the adjuster in charge.
2. Check your prescriptions often to make sure they haven't expired.
3. Be sure the client has provided a completed history form with all required contacts.
4. The best time to contact insurance companies for verification or authorization is during the middle of the week and not around lunch or closing time.
5. Have a pre-printed prescription sheet so the physician knows which services you provide.
6. Ask the client to advise you whenever a new physician or attorney is involved in his case.
7. Use black or blue ink for all documentation or claim forms if not printed.
8. Know that medical cases are legal cases, so document them accordingly.
9. "If it isn't documented, it wasn't done."
10. Document and submit claims for only that which is written on the prescription.

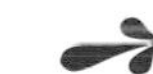

See Chapter 25, page 392 for a **sample prescription pad**.

The Affordable Care Act

The Affordable Care Act includes a section that could change the future for CAM providers. 2706 states:[5]

SEC. 2706. NON-DISCRIMINATION IN HEALTH CARE.

(a) Providers- A group health plan and a health insurance issuer offering group or individual health insurance coverage shall not discriminate with respect to participation under the plan or coverage against any health care provider who is acting within the scope of that provider's license or certification under applicable State law. This section shall not require that a group health plan or health insurance issuer contract with any health care provider willing to abide by the terms and conditions for participation established by the plan or issuer. Nothing in this section shall be construed as preventing a group health plan, a health insurance issuer, or the Secretary from establishing varying reimbursement rates based on quality or performance measures.

(b) Individuals- The provisions of section 1558 of the Patient Protection and Affordable Care Act (relating to non-discrimination) shall apply with respect to a group health plan or health insurance issuer offering group or individual health insurance coverage.

It's very similar in nature to the Every Category Provider Law in Washington State that mandates that all CAM providers are allowed to become contracted providers with health insurance companies. The Integrative Healthcare Policy Consortium created a website for consumers and practitioners to gather information on implementing 2706. Their main project, Cover My Care, offers a toolkit for letter writing and help with implementation.

Integrative Health Policy Consortium

www.ihpc.org

Cover My Care Project

www.covermycare.org/cmc

It will be a long, difficult road as each state has such different licensing requirements for all of the different CAM providers. Some aren't yet licensed as healthcare providers. The first step is making sure your profession is licensed as a healthcare provider. The next step is to get your Office of the Insurance Commissioner involved and find out what is required to make sure that your profession is allowed to become contracted providers or to bill insurance in your state. The insurance companies will also have to implement the steps to becoming contracted as well as set up fees and contracts.

The Anatomy of a Contract

Legal forms and agreements are an integral part of any business relationship, yet all too often people avoid written contracts. Whether you're interested in a one-time only interaction or a long-term affiliation, it's wise to delineate in writing your roles and expectations. Clear written agreements serve several purposes: they keep you focused on your goals, help avoid problems, and provide a predetermined method for resolving conflicts.

Figure 19.5 is a contract checklist to help you make informed choices and protect yourself legally. It defines the major elements of any contract. Sometimes this information may appear in separate documents, although it's best to combine it in one contract signed by all parties. Too many horror stories abound about people terminating business relationships and filing lawsuits because of misunderstandings that could have been averted with a solid contract. Your contracts should reflect the specific nature of your business and clearly define the expectations of all parties involved. Keep in mind that contracts are negotiable.

> "A verbal contract isn't worth the paper it's written on.
> —Samuel Goldwyn

Ideally, you would come to the negotiating process with a sample of your own contract and the checklist, review the other party's contract, and create a contract mutually agreeable to both of you. If the other party insists on only using their contract, make sure you have responses (preferably in writing) to all the items in the checklist.

Sample Contracts

https://corporate.findlaw.com/contracts.html

Most issues can be addressed in a 1-2 page contract document. Sometimes an informal letter of agreement serves the same purpose, sans legalese. You may be tempted not to use a contract for presumably simple transactions, particularly if it's just a "one-time" deal. Yet it's usually those seemingly negligible events that you live to regret! Invest the time in clarifying what is truly important to you in a business relationship. Even if you're currently involved in a business relationship and don't have a contract, you can always design one now. Each situation is unique, and one contract doesn't suit all situations. Once you've crafted a basic contract, you will find it much simpler to alter any subsequent contract.

What to Include

Start with the basics: legal names and contact information, timeframes and locations, a description of the parties or companies involved, and a summary of the desired roles and responsibilities. Contracts may be for a single specific event (e.g., hiring a company to paint your office), a series of events (e.g., providing wellness care at all the bike races for a particular team for the next 6 months), or ongoing until either party decides to terminate the contract. If it's an employment contract, it may include a description of additional benefits such as health insurance coverage, facilities privileges, sick time, paid vacation, and discounts on products and services.

Figure 19.5 Contract Checklist

- ❑ Names and addresses of all parties involved
- ❑ A short description and mission statement of the companies involved
- ❑ A statement summarizing the desired role of the contracted party
- ❑ A classification of the business relationship
- ❑ A detailed description of what each party agrees to provide
- ❑ A timetable for the work to be performed
- ❑ Location of where work is to be performed
- ❑ The duration of the contract
- ❑ Payment method and schedule
- ❑ Additional benefits
- ❑ Opportunities for increases in financial remuneration
- ❑ Insurance coverage provided
- ❑ Insurance coverage required
- ❑ Guarantees
- ❑ Financial obligations of the contracted party
- ❑ Conditions for termination of the agreement
- ❑ Guidelines for transfer of the contract
- ❑ Arbitration
- ❑ Designate who is responsible for legal fees if a breach of contract occurs
- ❑ The location and contact to send communications regarding the contract
- ❑ Signature lines and date the contract is signed

If the contract is for providing wellness services, find out if the hiring company provides workers' compensation, premise liability insurance, fire and theft insurance, and medical health insurance. If you provide services as an independent contractor, it's wise to obtain general liability insurance that covers negligence toward clients, employees, and the general public while you're on their premises. General liability insurance is good to have anyway—particularly if you do any on-site work or even public demonstrations. Unfortunately, none of these policies cover you personally, so be sure your health insurance and personal disability insurance provides adequate protection. Most companies also require practitioners to provide their own malpractice/professional liability insurance. Malpractice liability insurance is usually limited to protecting you against claims due to loss incurred by your clients as a result of negligence or failure on your part to perform at a professional skill level.

See Chapter 22, pages 328-331 for more on **employment** and **independent contractor agreements**.

§6

When the contract involves subcontracting, a financial obligations description is usually included. This is mainly to protect the hiring party in case you don't adequately perform your services. For example, let's say a convention coordinator contracts a local company to provide 10 massage therapists for their convention. The local company hires you as a subcontractor, but for some reason you don't show up. The convention coordinator could require compensation from the local hiring party, and then the local hiring party would pass that charge to you.

Conditions for termination and guidelines for transfer are common sections. Some termination conditions to consider are: violation of the hiring company's policies and procedures, poor or non-work performance, mismanagement of funds, and untimely payment of fees due.

The ability to transfer your contract to another person or company is desirable, although it won't work in all cases. Since wellness is such personal work, the hiring party may be reluctant to have a different practitioner provide the service. You can most likely include a transfer clause if you're truly an independent contractor. For example, let's say you were hired by a company to provide their staff with on-site yoga classes for 8 hours per week. After a while you decide that it isn't in your best interest to do this anymore (perhaps you've moved or the other aspects of your practice are requiring all of your time). Since you were the one responsible for getting the contract (marketing, negotiating the original contract, and providing the services for a time), you could easily charge a fee to another practitioner for the privilege of taking over the contract.

Arbitration, mediation, and breach of contract are additional legal terms that should be defined within the contract. Most contracts state who is responsible for legal fees if a breach of contract occurs (usually the party who breaches the contract).

Negotiations

Throughout your career, you will experience situations in which negotiation skills serve you well—such as negotiating an employment contract, vendor agreement, or working arrangements with team members. On the client side, you may encounter problematic situations such as repeated cancellations, bounced checks, or an unhappy customer for whom you must set boundaries and negotiate a solution agreeable to all parties.

Fearless Negotiating: The Wish, Want, Walk Method to Reaching Solutions That Work by Michael C. Donaldson

Beyond Reason: Using Emotions as You Negotiate by Roger Fisher and Daniel Shapiro

When it comes to unhappy clients, do your best to appreciate their feedback—even if it lacks tact or diplomacy. Many times you garner a kernel of useful information that may help you retain that client, or perhaps another in a similar situation. At other times, clients may be unreasonable or inconsolable due to causes beyond your control, and you must set clear and firm boundaries for what you will or won't do in response to their discontent. In all cases, thank clients for their feedback, listen carefully, and explore solutions that may work best.

The goal of all negotiations is to find a rewarding and mutually satisfying outcome for all parties. For this to occur, each person must feel truly heard and valued as an individual. Start with a set agenda. Make introductions, summarize the purpose of the negotiation, and allow ample time for each party to present their position. Then discuss the details. If possible, come to agreement, or schedule a follow-up meeting and set an agenda for the follow-up meeting.

"Honest disagreement is often a good sign of progress
—Mahatma Ghandi

Sooner or later you may run into thorny situations and unpleasant characters—such as the bully, screamer, or a less than honest person—that require special skills. Fine-tune your skills by reading books about the art of negotiation. You may also find trade magazine articles that offer useful and practical insights. Like any skill, the more you practice, the more your expertise grows.

Logistics Count. Give careful thought to choosing the right time and the right place. Negotiate in person, if possible.

Prepare. Start by diagnosing the situation. Be crystal clear on what you want, get a sense of what the other party wants and how he or she will push for results. Define your bottom line and determine where you will draw the line that you won't cross. Set an agenda and practice stating your key points concisely. Be careful what you eat and drink before and during the meeting. In general, it's best to avoid alcohol.

Negotiate Styles and Personality Dynamics. Learn about personality types so you can adjust your communication style and better understand the person with whom you're negotiating. Control the back and forth tempo by taking as much time as you need. Know when to talk and when to listen. Be cautious with your questions, as they could reveal concerns you may have that you would prefer to keep to yourself. Ultimately, seek to develop an appreciation for the healthy differences we all have.

Use Active Listening Skills. Listen carefully to the other person and restate what he or she has said, using your own words. This helps the other party to feel heard and prevents misunderstandings. Encourage both parties to consider non-monetary, valuable additions.

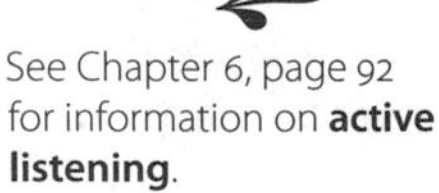

See Chapter 6, page 92 for information on **active listening**.

Walk Away for Awhile. If you come to an impasse, don't hesitate to take a break. You can say something like, "It looks like we're both bogged down here, so let's take a break to do more homework and talk again in a day or two." Negotiations can be emotional, but refrain from responding emotionally. Avoid appearing overly eager to come to an agreement.

Set Time Limits for Complex Negotiations. Allot a specific amount of time for hearing each other's view (e.g., 20 minutes), brainstorming solutions (e.g., 20 minutes), and finalizing a solution (e.g., 20 minutes). Otherwise, the process could go on for a long time.

Pause and Reflect. Before you sign on the dotted line, take a couple of hours or a few days to think things over, especially when signing contracts or agreements that involve large dollar amounts or time commitments.

Conflict Management

Most people hate conflict, some seem to thrive on it. Conflict can be a good thing. It can bring sensitive and controversial issues—and subtle counterproductive behaviors—to the surface so they can be resolved. The ability to skillfully navigate frustrating situations and people offers many benefits, such as more self-confidence, less anger, and greater enjoyment of life. Learning conflict resolution skills is like turning on the light in a dark room. You can see your way more clearly and get to where you're going much faster.

The Coward's Guide to Conflict: Empowering Solutions for Those Who Would Rather Run Than Fight by Tim Ursiny

Crucial Conversations: Tools for Talking When Stakes are High, by K. Patterson, J. Grenny, R. McMillan, A. Switzler

Conflict occurs when individuals or groups aren't getting what they need or want. Sometimes an individual isn't aware of an unmet need and unconsciously starts to act out by exhibiting annoying or counterproductive behaviors. The highly effective individual is aware of what she wants and then acts to achieve a goal—using clear communication and mutual give-and-take to find a solution that satisfies all parties.

Figure 19.6 Common Sources of Conflict

- Poor communication
- Not involving people in decision-making that directly affects them
- Clashes in chemistry—rooted in either conflicting values or personality styles
- Inconsistent leadership
- Broken promises
- Lack of fairness (e.g., favoritism toward certain employees or family members)
- Lack of openness
- Violated expectations
- Poor behavior (e.g., boundary violations, not honoring commitments, disrespect)

§6

Although uncomfortable at times, confrontation is necessary to hold people accountable for actions or inactions. Whether it's a difficult employee or co-worker, or a family member slacking off on chores, learning how to generate a positive outcome from confrontation helps strengthen relationships while solving problems. Here are some tips and techniques to help build your knowledge, skills, and confidence:

- Agree to a mutual give-and-take in which both parties create a mind-set focused on finding a solution that meets the needs of both parties.
- Take time to gain some perspective on the conflict before entering into a conversation about the conflict.
- Identify one thing you can do about the conflict.

- Identify the issue, including what you want that you aren't getting or what you're getting that you don't want.
- Explore the conflict by talking to a friend or putting your thoughts in writing. Does the issue bother you because you're tired or angry about something else? Determine your role in the conflict.
- After you take a good look at the conflict and potential solutions, wait at least a day before you do something to address the conflict.
- Use "I statements." Avoid the use of "you statements" that place blame.
- Give your full attention to the other person when they're speaking. Don't interrupt or judge what is said. Also, listen for the emotion behind the words.
- Practice "active listening." Acknowledge and reflect back the person's concern and feelings. For example, "It sounds like you're really frustrated right now. If I understand correctly…." Ask the other person to rephrase what he heard you say.
- Talk in terms of the present as much as possible.
- Identify the things on which you agree and disagree.
- Refrain from venting at the person with anger or frustration. Stay centered.
- Don't pacify or over-apologize. Upset people respond much better to a genuine apology that comes from strength, not weakness.
- Focus on the issues and solutions, not the person. Don't get sidetracked by unimportant details.
- Ask: "What can we do to fix the problem?"
- If possible, identify at least one action that each of you can take to move closer to a solution.
- Ask for a "cooling off period" if you come to an impasse.
- In business situations, consider seeking a third party to mediate if there's difficulty resolving a conflict.

Mediation and Arbitration

National Arbitration and Mediation

www.namadr.com

Resolute Systems

resolutesystems.com

Mediation Resources

www.mediate.com
www.nolo.com

Arbitration Resources

www.adr.org
www.adrforum.com

Mediation is a popular method small businesses choose to resolve business disputes; it's cheaper and faster than litigation, and, oftentimes, leads to a settlement that all parties find agreeable. Although some disputes wind up in arbitration, mediation is popular among those who prefer to find quick and cost-effective solutions to their problems. By relying on expert mediators trained to negotiate many types of disputes, business owners can avoid costly, time-consuming lawsuits and achieve more win-win results. Because of the growing popularity of mediation, you can easily find local, national, and online resources. In fact, you may even resolve the conflict itself through online mediation services.

Arbitration usually takes place when a business dispute or contract negotiation comes to an impasse or when mediation fails. Traditionally, each side takes a turn to present their case to an arbitrator, who makes a final decision. There are two kinds of arbitration—binding and nonbinding. In binding arbitration, both parties agree to accept the arbitrator's final judgment. In nonbinding arbitration, both parties are free to go to court if one or the other disagrees with the result. Typically, an arbitrator is a neutral third party.

20 Financial Management

"The universe operates through dynamic exchange… giving and receiving are different aspects of the flow of energy in the universe. In our willingness to give that which we seek, we keep the abundance of the universe circulating in our lives."

—Deepak Chopra

Key Terms

Accountant
Accounts Payable
Accounts Receivable
Assets
Balance Sheet
Barter
Budget
Capital
Canadian Taxes
Cash Flow Projection
Corporations
Credit Score
Deduction
Depreciation
Disbursement
Drawing Account
Equity
Expense
401(k)
Form 1040
Gift Certificates
Gratuity
Gross Income
Income Tax
Ledger
Liabilities
Net Profit
Overhead
Partnership
Petty Cash Fund
Pro Bono Work
Profit
Profit and Loss Statement
Recession
Retirement Plan
Roth IRA
Schedule C Profit or Loss from Business
Schedule SE
Self-Employment Tax
Shareholders' Equity
SIMPLE IRA
SEP-IRA
Small Business Administration (SBA)
Sole Proprietor
Tax Credits
Traditional IRA
Transaction Privilege Tax License
U.S. Taxes

Some people naturally handle money well while others find it difficult to balance their checkbooks. For many of us, money matters get tangled in a web of emotions because we don't know how to relate to money in a healthy way, or because we didn't have the opportunity to learn money smarts when we were growing up.

In fact, many passionate and talented wellness practitioners struggle financially. Whether they own their own business or work as an employee, they find it a challenge to get ahead. According to many money management experts, the first step to enhancing your financial prosperity is to transform your attitude toward money. As Suze Orman, author of *The 9 Steps to Financial Freedom*, so aptly states:

Money Attitudes Quizzes

www.moneyharmony.com/moneyharmony-quiz

https://www.nerdwallet.com/article/finance/money-personality

> *Before we can get control of our finances, we must get control of our attitudes about money, feelings that were shaped by our earliest experiences with it. Opening ourselves to abundance—not only of the pocketbook but also of the heart—is what's necessary for true balance and freedom.*[1]

An odd phenomenon sometimes happens in the helping professions. This takes the shape of practitioners who proudly wear the "poor but pure" badge because they're uncomfortable with money or fear that financial prosperity will somehow corrupt them. Besides contributing to financial insecurity, this attitude can lead to questionable business practices. These same practitioners can experience difficulty in charging appropriate fees for their services and many are uncomfortable charging anything at all.

Financial Literacy

https://www.annuity.org/financial-literacy/

On the flip side, employees can become resentful over the disparity in their wages versus the charged fee. This misconception can occur because they haven't factored in the true costs the business owner incurs in setting up and running the business. They only look at the $100 the company charges per session versus the $35 they receive. They forget about the thousands or even millions of dollars the facility costs to build and maintain.

Although we may wish money didn't play such a central role in our lives, money skills are crucial to creating personal and professional success. By working with this book you can easily master the basics of money management—and pave the way to your future success.

Personal Budgeting

The first step to financial freedom is to know where you stand. With the fast pace of life and the many demands on our time, it's easy to be in denial about finances. A simple and time-tested antidote to this common experience is to develop and work with a budget. A personal monthly budget can prevent a lot of financial stress and build a solid financial future. A budget gives you a realistic picture of what you need to earn to cover your expenses.

The following checklist gives you an idea of the personal expenses to track. Your individual situation may include only some of these items, or it may include all of these and more. Be as thorough as possible in estimating the monthly costs for each. If it's an expense you only have once per year, divide that amount by 12 to get your estimated monthly expenses.

Figure 20.1 Personal Budget Expense Checklist

- ❑ Rent/Mortgage
- ❑ Home Insurance
- ❑ Utilities
- ❑ Telephone
- ❑ Household (supplies, repair, maintenance)
- ❑ Food
- ❑ Health Care
- ❑ Auto Expenses (payments, fuel, repairs, maintenance, insurance)
- ❑ Clothing (purchases, laundry, dry cleaning)
- ❑ Debt Payments (loans, credit cards)
- ❑ Education and Self-Development
- ❑ Entertainment and Travel
- ❑ Miscellaneous

Where Do You Actually Spend Your Money?

Keep track of everything you spend your money on for 1 month, whether it's a fixed monthly expense such as rent or variable expenses like dining out. If you buy a pack of gum, record that, too. Be as honest and thorough as possible to get the best overall picture of your spending patterns. Once you gather this information, compare your actual spending with your personal budget and what your current income allows. Are you exceeding your planned monthly expenditures? Do you need to make adjustments to your current spending patterns? What changes can you implement to include savings and long-term investments?

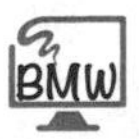

Monthly Personal Budget Worksheet

https://sohnen-moe.com/bm5-workbook-request/

Your personal financial needs play a pivotal role in determining your business finances. If you intend to be self-employed, you need to do similar estimating and forecasting for your business expenses. Knowing both your personal expenses and your business expenses helps you define the minimum amount of income you need to generate from your business.

Use your budget as a tool to forecast your daily, monthly, and annual expenses, for both personal and business, and plan accordingly. Forecasting is a great tool to help keep expenses on track and avoid the tendency to let "extra cash" slip away. For instance, it's natural for many people to spend "extra cash" when they experience an unexpected windfall such as having a higher than usual number of clients for the week. Avoid this pitfall by checking your cash flow forecast before spending that extra income, as you might have a large one-time expense coming up soon. Another useful strategy is to put at least half of the extra money into a savings account.

Rich Dad, Poor Dad by Robert Kiyosaki

The 9 Steps to Financial Freedom by Suze Orman

Your Money or Your Life: 9 Steps to Transforming Your Relationship with Money and Achieving Financial Independence by Vicki Robin, Joe Dominguez, Monique Tilford

Saving Money

In *Your Money or Your Life: 9 Steps to Transforming Your Relationship with Money and Achieving Financial Independence*, the authors talk about creating a new road map for generating fulfillment, satisfaction, and value in your life. They suggest making peace with your past relationships with time and money, give you instructions for tracking your energy and expenditures in the present, and help you save money by minimizing spending and maximizing income. A large part of budgeting, both for personal and business, is to understand your spending habits to save the money you do earn. Figure 20.2 gives the above mentioned authors' money saving suggestions.[2]

§6

Figure 20.2 Money Saving Tips

- Don't Go Shopping
- Live Within Your Means
- Take Care of What You Have
- Wear It Out
- Do It Yourself
- Anticipate Your Needs
- Research Value, Quality, Durability, Multiple Use, and Price
- Buy It for Less
- Meet Your Needs Differently

Credit Scores

Credit Reporting Agencies

www.equifax.com
www.experian.com
www.transunion.com

Business Credit Score

www.dnb.com

Opt out of Pre-Approved Offers

www.optoutprescreen.com

Personal credit scores impact your business, especially if you operate as a sole proprietor or partnership. Making smart choices with your money and your use of credit can make that effect a positive one. Making bad credit choices, however, can be disastrous to your business plans. The first step in managing your credit score is to be aware of your various credit reports. There are three major credit reporting agencies, and they're required to provide you with one free report per year.

If your credit rating is poor before you start your practice, you can do certain things to improve that score. First, make sure you pay your bills on time. Also, keep your credit card balances low, pay more than the minimum balance, and avoid transferring balances and closing accounts. Financial institutions usually look at your total debt compared to your overall credit limits, and closing accounts reduces your credit limits. Opening new accounts may also lower your scores, so use caution when trying to repair your credit.

If you operate as a corporation, your business can have its own credit report. Register with Dun & Bradstreet to get a DUNS number (which is the recognized standard for tracking business credit activities). This can help you establish as a reputable business with vendors.

You should always try to keep your personal and your business finances separate. If you need financing for your business start-up or for business activities, avoid using personal credit cards as business loans. There are much less expensive loans available, and you should only be using credit cards for purchases you can afford to pay for in full when you get the bill.

Financial Recordkeeping

Financial recordkeeping, particularly bookkeeping, is often viewed as an evil chore or an arcane art designed to deaden the psyche. Since most people will do almost anything to avoid chores, many practitioners keep minimal records, if they keep any records at all. Thus, they miss numerous legitimate tax deductions. Keeping records is a habit that must be developed. Ideally, consult with an accountant or bookkeeper prior to setting up your books. Definitely confer with an advisor when it's time to file tax returns. The manner in which you keep your records can be simple and straightforward despite complex tax laws that seem to change every other week.

Disclaimer!

This is **not an accounting book**. The material in this chapter is provided to assist you in developing your bookkeeping system and inform you about basic Internal Revenue Service (IRS) tax regulations. It has been streamlined to highlight key points. For more detailed information please visit the IRS website, read accounting books, or speak to an accountant.

Maintaining accurate records is vital for any small business. Bookkeeping entails more than keeping a ledger for tax purposes. The information you glean from your records assists in running your business smoothly and achieving optimal profits. It's difficult to make prudent decisions without all of the facts. The checkbook alone doesn't always give an accurate account of the business' financial standing. Many business owners make the mistake of believing they're generating a profit because they have plenty of funds in their checking account, while unpaid bills accumulate and upcoming expenses are forgotten.

In addition, many people find themselves in a precarious financial position come tax time because they haven't set aside money for taxes. I advocate opening an interest-bearing business savings or money market account and regularly depositing money into that account. Accountant Robert Decker, says, "The two most common mistakes that people make are doing their own taxes, and not setting aside money to pay for taxes." He suggests putting away 20 to 30% of the amount you pay yourself. For instance, every time you write yourself a check for $1,000, immediately write another check for at least $200, and deposit it into a savings account that you designate specifically for paying taxes. If you practice online banking, it can be as easy as a few clicks to transfer that money into your savings account.

What Types of Records Should I Keep?

Your bookkeeping can be quite simple if you operate a small sole proprietorship with no employees. All you really need is a bank account, a ledger system with income and expenditure sheets, and a file to store receipts. It isn't necessary to spend a fortune on a bookkeeping system. Sometimes a simple columnar record book from an office supply store will suffice, or use a basic spreadsheet application on your computer or tablet. The records required and the complexity involved escalate with added business dimensions such as employees, product sales, partnerships, and corporations.

IRS Guidelines

www.irs.gov/Businesses/Small-Businesses-&-Self-Employed/Small-Business-and-Self-Employed-Tax-Center-1

www.irs.gov/publications/p583/

Some people use hand-posted ledgers for all their bookkeeping activities. I highly recommend using a computer as much as possible. Several inexpensive, user-friendly accounting programs are available for personal computers. These software programs can print your checks and post the information in the appropriate places. The software usually includes a tutorial that walks you through setting up your accounts—it poses questions, and your responses enable the program to determine how to organize your files. If you're familiar with cloud-based software, you can choose to do your bookkeeping from any of your devices (desktop, laptop, tablet, or smartphone), without having to install the software on each individual device.

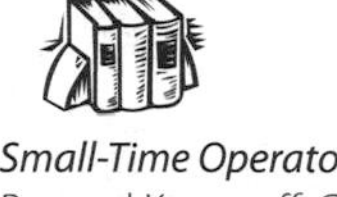

Small-Time Operator by Bernard Kamoroff, CPA

Minding Her Own Business by Jan Zobel, EA

It's so much easier to know where you stand and to plan the future because the information is right there. In most applications, you simply go to the "Reports" section where it lists all the major standard reports. All you do is select the dates (e.g., "Last Month" or "Current Fiscal Year to Date"), and, in a matter of seconds, a report is prepared—one that could easily take hours by hand. You can also examine expenses by category, such as creating a report of all your automobile expenses for the year. The reports can combine information from all of your accounts (e.g., checking, credit cards, petty cash). Let's say that XYZ Supplies sends you a notice for an outstanding invoice. You're fairly sure you paid for it, but you don't remember the payment method. If you only kept manual files, it could take you 20 minutes (or more) to sort through all the various ledger sheets and receipts. It takes moments with a computerized accounting package.

IRS regulations require taxpayers to keep records and receipts for as long as they may be applicable to the enforcement of tax law.[3] Bank statements and other documents, such as inventory records, canceled checks, expense records, and payroll records, should be kept at least 7 years (see Figure 20.3). Tax returns and records related to the basis (cost) of property should be kept indefinitely (e.g., papers related to the purchase of real estate and equipment). Also, archive a copy of your accounting software record at the end of each year.

§6

Figure 20.3 How Long Do I Need to Keep My Business Records?

Document	Retention
General correspondence	5 years
Bank statements	7 years
Receipts	7 years
Canceled checks	7 years for most
Year-end financial statements	Indefinitely
Contracts	Indefinitely
Licenses and permits	Indefinitely
Insurance claims	Indefinitely
Tax returns	Indefinitely

Figure 20.4 Recordkeeping Tips

- Keep all business-related receipts.
- Pay bills when they're due—unless you receive a discount for early payment.
- Have a separate business checking account.
- Keep thorough financial records as discussed in this chapter.
- Keep lists of inventory, equipment, and furniture.
- Maintain thorough and professional client files.
- Make cash flow projections.
- Keep automobile mileage logs.
- Maintain daily records (e.g., appointment book, activity tracking sheets).
- Prepare monthly bank reconciliations.

Create a Separate Identity

Standard Industrial Classification (SIC) Directory
siccode.com

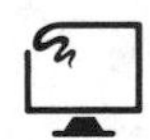

Financial Planning Association
www.onefpa.org

A separate business identity is important for personal and financial reasons. Corporations have regulations that require financial divisions between the business and the business owners, yet many sole proprietors are lax about setting business boundaries. One of the best ways to set boundaries is to keep business and personal finances separate. Open a business bank account. This can be a "personal" account with your name (e.g., Mary Jones, D.C.), although it's best to establish yourself with a "business" account. Deposit all income (checks and cash) into the business checking account. If you accept credit cards, the monies collected should be directly transferred to the business checking account.

Pay your business bills by check or credit card. This provides better documentation than cash. If you use credit cards for purchases, note the charges on a ledger sheet and pay the monthly statement with a business check. Avoid paying for business expenses with cash or personal checks. If you find yourself in a store with only a personal check, don't worry. Just make sure that when you return to the office, you post the expense under Petty Cash and note which checking account was used and the check number. Then write a check to "petty cash" for the same amount.

Business Income

Business income includes all monies received: cash, checks, credit cards, and barter. Record income at least twice a week; daily is preferred. Also, make sure your bank and credit card processor properly code your business. For instance, most non-primary care wellness providers should use the SIC/MCC code 8099 (Health and Allied Services, Not Elsewhere Classified) and the NAICS code 621399 (Offices of All Other Miscellaneous Health Practitioners).

Credit Cards

Merchant Credit Card Services
www.paypal.com
www.merchantone.com
www.clover.com
www.squareup.com
www.cellcharge.com
www.merchantseek.com

We live in a society that relies heavily on credit, and many clients appreciate the convenience of this payment option. From a business standpoint, the advantages of accepting payment cards usually outweigh the disadvantages. In fact, marketing research shows that people are often willing to spend more if they can pay with a credit card—plus there's the impulse buy factor. Advantages that come with accepting this form of payment are: added convenience for your regular clients; increased appeal for your gift certificate program; more high-dollar product purchases; and an increased likelihood of clients purchasing a package deal for a series of sessions. In most instances, you don't even need special equipment—you can process the payment with your smartphone or tablet.

Managing Gift Certificate Finances

I recommend that you put at least half of all gift certificate revenue into a savings account and transfer the funds into your checking account when the certificate is redeemed. Otherwise, if you sell a lot of gift certificates, you could find yourself in the position of working for an extended period of time without receiving "new" income.

Keeping track of gift certificates is easy when you design a system and stick with it. This can be done on a computer in a spreadsheet program, accounting software, or client management software. You can also use a manual register system.

Gratuities

The topic of accepting tips is complex. Due to the power differential, it's unwise and often unethical to take extra money. This includes extravagant gifts such as the use of a vacation home. The gray area concerns gifts that are more symbolic, such as garden produce or homemade cookies. Graciousness is a delightful skill. It recognizes and affirms positive intentions. However, if a client always brings something extra for you or offers you an expensive gift, it would be prudent to state that you're well compensated for your time and nothing else is needed.

Most people feel awkward about tipping. They aren't certain when it's appropriate or how much to give. Are you supposed to tip mail carriers, hair stylists, pet groomers, auto mechanics, estheticians, gardeners, and physicians? Do you tip them if they work for someone else, but not if they're the owners of the business?

Another downside to accepting tips is that it creates expectations: you don't want clients worrying about whether to give you a tip. Even worse is the anxiety clients might experience if they give you a tip one time and not the next. Will you think they didn't like the session as much? Will they receive the same level of service next time? This tension defeats the therapeutic value of the work.

If you decide that in your setting a professional doesn't accept tips, you can make a clear choice. If someone asks you about tipping, you can say something like, "I appreciate the acknowledgment, but a tip isn't expected in a therapeutic relationship." You can also give the client options such as donating the tip to your favorite charity or starting a scholarship fund for people who normally cannot afford your services. Another idea is to thank the client and ask her instead to tell her friends about your services. Remind the client that gift certificates are a wonderful way to introduce individuals to your services.

Gratuities can make you feel appreciated, yet money isn't the only way to express appreciation. Given that many people have money issues, it isn't necessarily the best form of gratitude. Encourage people to simply say, "Thank you!" and have that mean something.[4]

If you decide to accept gratuities in your practice, remember that tips and most gifts are considered taxable income.

Business Deductions

Business deductions reduce your net profit which in turn reduces your tax liability. Business owners are entitled to numerous deductions. Most of these expenses (except for those such as draw) are recognized as full deductions—although some of these allowances have strict guidelines and ceilings.

Each year, many small businesses overpay their income taxes. According to Bernard Kamoroff, author of *Small Time Operator* and 475 *Tax Deductions For Businesses & Self-Employed Individuals*, "The overpayments are made because businesses fail to take tax deductions they're legally entitled to take. Many of these businesses are still unaware of their errors. They overpaid their taxes and don't even know it."[5]

According to the IRS, a legitimate expense must meet the following guidelines: it must be incurred in connection with your business; be ordinary (similar expense to others in your profession); and be necessary.

Consider the following example for a sole practitioner's business that generates $40,000 in income from client sessions and product sales and has $20,000 in expenses from items such as rent, supplies, marketing, and inventory.

Gross Income	$40,000	*Deductions*	$20,000
Taxable Income	$20,000	*Taxes Due*	$6,000
Total Cash in Pocket	$14,000		

Depending on your tax bracket, the combined tax rate of your Federal, State, and Self-Employment Tax rates can vary from 20% to well over 50%. Thus, in this example, the taxes due would be between $4,000 and $10,000! Now you can see why every penny counts. Even just an additional $1,000 in expenses saves you between $200-$500 in taxes. However, to reap these benefits you must develop a system to accurately track your expenses.

Educational expenses can only be deducted if they relate to improving your current line of work. In general, you cannot deduct educational expenses for starting a new career. For instance, if you're a physical therapist or a chiropractor and you want to expand your practice by offering massage, it would most likely be deductible. But if you're an artist and want to sculpt muscles instead of clay—enrolling in a massage program wouldn't be deductible.

Expenses most often questioned during an audit are claimed expenses that aren't usually associated with your profession, as well as extravagant travel, entertainment, and transportation expenses. The latter are also areas that rarely receive full expense deductions.

Business Use of Home

You can deduct expenses related to using a part of your home regularly and exclusively as either a principal place of business or as a place to meet clients. The percentage of business use of a home is determined by dividing the square feet of the business space by the total square feet of the home. If the space was used for less than a full year, you must prorate expenses for the number of months used for the business. If you file a Schedule C tax return, you must also file Form 8829 (Expenses for Business Use of Your Home).

All of the costs of decorating, furnishing, repairs, and maintenance of the business-use space is deductible or depreciable. The business percentage of permanent improvements that benefit the entire home (e.g., new roof or temperature control unit) is depreciable. Deductions for the business use of a home may not be used to create a business loss or increase a net loss from a business. Deductions in excess of that limit may be carried forward to later years (subject to the income limits in those years). Also, if you deduct office space in your home, you may be subject to a capital gains tax upon the sale of your house.

Travel, Entertainment, and Gifts

Keep accurate records to substantiate travel and entertainment expenses. In addition to receipts, keep a journal that denotes the following for each expense: a description of the expense; the amount spent; date, time, and place; business purpose; names and business relationship of person(s) entertained or gifted; and any other pertinent information. In regard to gifts for clients, you're limited to a certain amount per client per year. The deduction for business-related meals and entertainment is limited to a maximum of 50% (the IRS frowns upon lavish meals that include magnums of Dom Pérignon). If you must travel any distance for business, the transportation and lodging costs are usually wholly deductible (although an unusual number of trips to exotic locales might spark an audit).

Transportation

The customary and necessary expenses incurred on operating and maintaining a vehicle for business purposes are deductible according to the actual percentage of business use. The two methods for computing allowable expenses are the actual expenses (at the business-use percentage) or the total business mileage (using the IRS determined allowance). You must use actual costs if you use more than one vehicle in your business. The best evidence to support a transportation deduction is a spreadsheet or journal that shows the date, business purpose, destination, and mileage of all business travel.

Depreciation

Depreciation is a tax term that describes the loss in value of an asset over time. An asset is a tangible commodity that will last for more than one year (e.g., a computer, a building). When you purchase more than a certain dollar amount of assets in any given year, the IRS requires the cost to be deducted over years (since the asset's life is greater than one year). The amount of depreciation allowed depends on the category of the asset and its value. Depreciation rules frequently change and can be quite complicated to calculate. This is a prime example of why you need an accountant.

Assets Owned Prior to Business Establishment

A common question asked by new business owners is, "Can I deduct the expenses of the equipment and books I bought while I was a student?" As a sole proprietor, anything that was your personal property and is now being used solely for your business can be declared as owner's equity (e.g., inventory, merchandise, supplies) or as a fixed asset (e.g., massage table, office furniture, stereo equipment), which then gets depreciated as of the date you place it in service in your business. The basis used for depreciation is the lower of the actual cost or the fair market value of the item when placed into service, not the original cost.

Pro Bono Work

Many people wonder if they can legally take a deduction for their *pro bono* work. Alas, no. Such work doesn't "cost" you money. What it does cost is your time. Even though we know time is money, the IRS doesn't view it in those terms. So choose wisely to whom you give your *pro bono* work, be it for an individual, organization, or event. Most people do *pro bono* work to help a needy individual, support a specific cause or group, or to further establish themselves in the community. The services you give to charity should be considered an act of goodwill, motivated by compassion. Any expenses associated with the *pro bono* work, such as supplies should already be taken as a general business expense.

Figure 20.5 Common Fully Deductible Business Expenses

- Bank Service Charges
- Maintenance and Repairs
- Business Books and Trade Publications
- Marketing
- Business Insurance
- Office Supplies
- Credit Card Fees
- Online Fees
- Dues
- Postage
- Continuing Education
- Printing and Copying
- Furnishings, Decorations, and Equipment
- Professional Fees
- Interest on Business Debt
- Rent
- License/Certification Fees
- Sales and Excise Tax
- Inventory Cost of Goods
- Samples
- Linen Service
- Telephone and Utilities
- Software Subscription Fees

§6

Figure 20.6 Common Estimated Business Expenses

Initial Expenses	Estimated Cost
Opening Business Checking Account	$100
Telephone Installation/Activation	$200
Equipment	$1,500
First & Last Month's Rent & Security Deposit	$1,500
Business Cards	$100
Stationery & Envelopes	$200
Brochure	$250
Logo	$250
Website	$250
Opening Promotion Package (ads, direct mailers)	$750
Decorations	$250
Office Supplies	$500
Furniture, Music System, Clothes	$1,000

Annual Expenses	Estimated Cost
Property Insurance	$175
Business License & Permits	$125
Liability Insurance	$250
Professional Association Membership	$300
Legal & Accounting Fees	$400
Networking Club Dues	$100

Average Monthly Expenses	Estimated Cost
Rent	$500
Utilities	$50
Telephone	$75
Internet Services	$45
Bank fees	$12
Supplies	$75
Education (seminars, books, journals)	$50
Marketing	$150
Postage	$25
Repair & Maintenance (also cleaning service)	$70
Travel Expenses	$30
Inventory	$30
Business Loan Payments	$??
Staff Salaries	$??
Personal Draw/Salary	$??

Calculate Your Business Budget

Fill out the Start-Up Cost Worksheet and the Monthly Business Expense Worksheet. Combine the totals to determine how much money your practice needs to open the door and operate for the first year. Next, add the total from your personal budget. The sum total is how much money you need to generate for the first year in practice. Next, identify how much money you plan to earn from the different aspects of your practice (e.g., sessions, product sales, classes). After completing these worksheets, note how you feel. What are some steps you can take to help ensure your success?

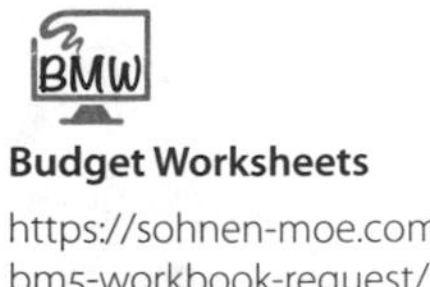

Budget Worksheets

https://sohnen-moe.com/bm5-workbook-request/

Figure 20.7 Accounting Definitions

Assets: The total resources (current, fixed, or other) of the sole practitioner or business—tangible and intangible. Assets may include cash in the bank, inventory, goodwill, accounts receivable, and equipment.

Capital: Essentially it's the net worth of a business—the difference between the assets and the liabilities.

Accounts Receivable: The amounts owed to you by another person or business.

Accounts Payable: The amounts you owe another person or business.

Capital Account: The total money invested by the owner.

Depreciation: The loss in value of an asset over time.

Disbursement: The act of paying out funds.

Drawing Account: Sole proprietors may withdraw cash for personal use. It's similar to a salary except you don't take out withholding taxes (instead you pay self-employment taxes). Withdrawals can reduce the owner's equity.

Equity: the monetary value of a property or business beyond any amounts owed on it in debt (e.g., mortgages, claims, liens).

Journal: A book for recording complete information on all transactions as they're incurred (e.g., Monthly Expense Disbursements Journal).

Ledger: An account book of financial transactions.

Liabilities: Current and long-term debts of the practitioner or business. Liabilities may include accounts payable, long-term debts (e.g., a car loan), payroll taxes, and credit card balances.

Petty Cash Fund: Cash on hand to pay for incidental expenses. Put a voucher in the petty cash drawer and record each transaction. Don't put cash received from a client into the petty cash fund. When the fund is low, make a "petty cash" deposit by cashing a check to bring the fund back to the desired level (most likely between $20 and $100). Be sure to transfer the transactions to your Petty Cash or Disbursements Journals.

Shareholders' Equity: The amount owners invested in the company's stock plus or minus the company's earnings or losses since inception.

§6

Financial Statements

Financial statements are formal records of the financial activities of a business. They provide an overview of a practice's profitability. They show where a company's money came from, where it went, and where it's now (e.g., assets, profits).

Income and Disbursement Ledger Sheets: They provide detailed, categorized information on income and expenses. These ledger sheets can be recorded manually or by using accounting software. Ideally, update them daily. (See Figures 20.8 and 20.9.)

Profit and Loss Statements: Also called Income Statements, they tell you how much a company earned or lost over a specific period of time (usually for a month, quarter, or year). They show how much money a company generated over a specific time period, as well as the costs and expenses associated with earning that money. (See Figure 20.10.)

> "The reaction of weak management to weak operations is often weak accounting.
> —Warren Buffett

Business Income and Expense Forecasts: These forecasts project the income derived from an estimated number of clients you expect to utilize your services, how often they will schedule appointments, as well as how many will also purchase products and the dollar amount of product they will purchase. (See Figure 20.11.)

Cash Flow Statements: Cash flow statements document the timing of how income and expenses occur throughout a year. They're best used as forecasting tools so you can gauge how to manage your finances. For instance, you discover that every April your income decreases by 30%. You can either save money to cover your expenses for that month or increase your marketing efforts in February and March to boost April's revenues. Using another example, let's say you've completed your forecasting for the next year and discover a one-time $2,000 expense in June. You then go back to the forecast and add another category titled "Savings for June Expenses" and split up the $2,000 over the previous 5 months (and, of course, actually put that money into a savings account). (See Figure 20.12.)

Balance Sheets: They provide summary information about a company's assets, liabilities, and net equity as of a given point in time. A company's assets must equal, or "balance," the sum of its liabilities and shareholders' equity. The following formula summarizes what a balance sheet shows: **Assets = Liabilities + Equity**. (See Figure 20.13.)

Figure 20.8 Sample Weekly Income Ledger Sheet

Month/Year: April 2020 **Week:** 1

Date	Client Name	Amt Paid	Ck #	Services	Products	Type	Location	Company	Notes
4/2	Perry Winkle	$20.00	911	$20.00	$0.00	O	Outcall Office	ABC Corp	
4/2	Astria Ames	$20.00	123	$20.00	$0.00	O	Outcall Office	ABC Corp	
4/2	Sandy Lott	$35.00	709	$25.00	$10.00	O	Outcall Office	ABC Corp	
4/2	Maureen Dock	$25.00	312	$25.00	$0.00	O	Outcall Office	ABC Corp	
4/2	Brad Jones	$35.00	1947	$25.00	$10.00	O	Outcall Office	ABC Corp	
4/2	Amy Allen	$50.00	417	$50.00	$0.00	N	Office	Humane Society	
4/2	Bill Peters	$0.00	Prepay	$0.00	$0.00	O	Outcall Home	Attorney	Prepaid Services
4/3	Warren Piece	$55.00	Cash	$55.00	$0.00	N	Office	Evans & Assoc	
4/3	Shirley Ujest	$0.00	Prepay	$0.00	$0.00	O	Office	T&J Accounting	Gift Certificate
4/3	Weldon Rod	$75.00	Cash	$40.00	$35.00	O	Office	Artist	
4/3	Les Moore	$0.00	Promo	$0.00	$0.00	N	Office	Stars R Us	Knows many people
4/3	Helena Montana	$55.00	653	$55.00	$0.00	N	Office	Thornton Co	
4/4	Gail Windser	$47.00	712	$7.00	$40.00	O	Outcall Home	Mattson Corp	Prepaid Services
4/4	Hope Esperanza	$0.00	Prepay	$0.00	$0.00	O	Outcall Home	N/A	
4/4	Holly Fields	$100.00	211	$60.00	$40.00	N	Office	N/A	
4/5	Morris Katz	$55.00	506	$55.00	$0.00	O	Office	School District	
4/5	Grover Funk	$45.00	614	$35.00	$10.00	O	Office	TMJ Corp	

Total Income:	$617.00
Services:	*$472.00*
Products:	*$145.00*

# Sessions:	17
New Clients:	5
Ongoing:	12

Figure 20.9 Sample Monthly Disbursement Ledger Sheet

Month/Year: **April 2020**

Date	Description	Amt Paid	Ck #	Rent Utilities	Repair Mainten	Equip Supplies	Phone	Ads Promo	License Ins/Fees	Educ Dues	Travel	Misc Draw
4/2	ABA	$250.00	140						$250.00			
4/2	Joes Cleaning	$27.00	141		$27.00							
4/2	Paul 'd Auto	$17.30	142								$17.30	
4/2	Sunset Bld	$350.00	143	$350.00								
4/3	Gas To Go	$9.00	Cash								$9.00	
4/4	RJ Office	$6.21	144			$6.21						
4/4	Pace Printer	$29.50	145					$29.50				
4/4	Last Café	$12.70	Cash									$12.70
4/10	The Garden	$18.40	146									$18.40
4/12	Phone Co.	$65.90	147				$65.90					
4/12	Success 1st	$20.00	148							$20.00		
4/17	Career Sem	$50.00	149							$50.00		
4/17	Draw	$800.00	150									$800.00
4/18	Discount Sup	$8.14	Cash			$8.14						
4/19	Western Bank	$8.20	--						$8.20			
4/20	Ace Ins.	$200.00	151						$200.00			
4/21	USPS	$25.00	152			$25.00						
4/25	Earth Time	$60.00	153					$60.00				
4/25	AAA Util	$50.00	154	$50.00								
4/26	Discount Sup	$20.00	155			$20.00						
Totals:		**$2,027.35**		**$400.00**	**$27.00**	**$59.35**	**$65.90**	**$89.50**	**$458.20**	**$70.00**	**$26.30**	**$831.10**

Figure 20.10 Sample Abbreviated Profit and Loss Statement

This report covers June 1, 2020 to June 30, 2020			
Income			
	Sessions	$	4,000.00
	Product Sales	$	300.00
	Workshops	$	400.00
	Room Rental to Associate	$	300.00
	Total Income:	**$**	**5,000.00**
Expenses			
	Rent	$	800.00
	Inventory	$	200.00
	Utilities	$	50.00
	Supplies	$	120.00
	Phone	$	80.00
	Marketing	$	200.00
	Misc.	$	350.00
	Total Expenses:	**$**	**1,800.00**
Net Profit*			**$ 3,200.00**
	*Note this is earnings before taxes.		

§6

Figure 20.11 **Sample Business Income and Expense Forecast**

One Year Estimate Ending 31-Dec-2020

Projected Number of Clients	Estimate
For Your Services Only	30
For Your Products Only	15
For Your Services and Products	55
Total Number of Clients	100

Session Frequency	Estimate
Weekly: 5 clients	260 = 5 X 52
Twice per Month: 20 clients	480 = 20 X 24
Monthly: 30 clients	360 = 30 X 12
Quarterly: 30 clients	120 = 30 X 4
Other: 15 clients	15
Total Number of Sessions	1235

Projected Income	Estimate
Sessions (at $55 per session)	$67,925
Product Sales	$4,000
Other (workshops)	$1,000
A: Total Income	$72,925

Projected Expenses	Estimate
Start-up Costs (include if this is your first year)	$10,000
Monthly Expenses (x 12)	$18,000
Annual Expenses	$3,000
B: Total Expenses	$31,000

Projected Income Needed to Generate	Estimate
C: Total Operating Profit (or Loss) (A – B)	$41,925
D. Personal Expenses	$??
E: Actual Money Left Over (C - D)	$??

Figure 20.12 Sample Cash Flow Projections

	A	B	C	D	E	F	G
1			**May**	**June**	**July**	**Totals**	
2							
3	**Beginning Cash**		$1,000	$2,690	$1,890	$1,000	
4							
5	**Plus Monthly Income From:**						
6		Fees	$3,000	$2,400	$3,200	$8,600	
7		Sales	$300	$200	$300	$800	
8		Loans	$0	$0	$0	$0	
9		Other	$0	$0	$0	$0	
10	**Total Cash and Income**		**$4,300**	**$5,290**	**$5,390**	**$10,400**	
11							
12	**Expenses:**						
13		Rent	$400	$400	$400	$1,200	
14		Utilities	$50	$55	$50	$155	
15		Telephone	$75	$75	$75	$225	
16		Bank Fees	$10	$10	$10	$30	
17		Supplies	$75	$10	$65	$150	
18		Marketing Materials	$100	$300	$250	$650	
19		Insurance	$0	$650	$0	$650	
20		Dues	$75	$0	$325	$400	
21		Education	$25	$200	$0	$225	
22		Postage	$25	$0	$40	$65	
23		Entertainment	$40	$30	$60	$130	
24		Repair & Maintenance	$80	$50	$80	$210	
25		Travel	$0	$70	$0	$70	
26		Business Loan Payments	$0	$0	$0	$0	
27		Licenses & Permits	$0	$0	$75	$75	
28		Salary/Draw	$500	$1,000	$500	$2,000	
29		Staff Salaries	$0	$0	$0	$0	
30		Taxes	$0	$0	$600	$600	
31		Professional Fees	$35	$50	$25	$110	
32		Furniture, Fixtures, Décor	$70	$0	$0	$70	
33		Equipment	$0	$0	$425	$425	
34		Inventory	$50	$500	$0	$550	
35		Other	$0	$0	$0	$0	
36	**Total Expenses**		**$1,610**	**$3,400**	**$2,980**	**$7,990**	
37							
38	Ending Cash (+ or -)		$2,690	$1,890	$2,410	$2,410	
39							

§6

Figure 20.13 Sample Abbreviated Balance Sheet

	A	B	C	D	E	F	G	H	I
1	**Balance Sheet as of December 31, 2020**								
2		**Assets**							
3			Current Assets						
4				Cash/Bank Balance				$ 5,000.00	
5				Accounts Receivable				$ 500.00	
6				Inventory				$ 1,000.00	
7				Supplies				$ 1,000.00	
8			Fixed Assets						
9				Property				$ -	
10				Equipment				$ 3,500.00	
11							**Total Assets:**	**$ 11,000.00**	
12		**Liabilities**							
13			Current Liabilities						
14				Accounts Payable				$ 500.00	
15				Credit Card Charges				$ 500.00	
16			Long-Term Liabilities						
17				Bank Loans				$ 3,000.00	
18							**Total Liabilities:**	**$ 4,000.00**	
19									
20		**Net Worth (Owner's Equity)**						**$ 7,000.00**	
21									

Taxes

> "This [preparing my tax return] is too difficult for a mathematician. It takes a philosopher.
>
> —Albert Einstein

The information provided here is a general overview. Tax laws change regularly, so keep apprised of current regulations. IRS Publication 334 (Tax Guide for Small Business) is published annually and contains comprehensive tax information for small business owners. I highly recommend you consult with an accountant or tax professional regarding tax matters. Unless your financial affairs are extremely simple, chances are that you'll overlook deductions and credits to which you're entitled. A professional tax preparer knows what to look for and what's available to reduce your tax bill. While it's important for you to be familiar with the general workings of tax planning and the tax law—leave the technical details to your accountant.

Think of this in terms of your own practice. The general public might adequately handle their wellbeing on their own, but they come to you because you offer a higher degree of knowledge, experience, objectivity, and techniques than they possess. Similarly, it makes sense to rely upon the expertise of a tax professional and other business experts.

Preparing Income Tax Returns

The three primary methods for preparing tax returns are to do them manually, use a tax software program, or engage the services of a tax professional. The two major drawbacks to preparing taxes yourself (either manually or with a software program) are: tax preparation isn't always as straightforward as it seems; and there are thousands of codes related to deductions that frequently change, although the tax forms list only a few standard deduction categories.

You need to know what expenses are deductible, and they aren't always obvious. For instance, there are options for declaring deductions for business-related meals and incidentals. Currently, the standard per diem rate in the United States is $46-71 per day (depending on the specific city) for meals and incidental expenses. As an employee of your own corporation or another business, you may also claim the per diem rate for lodging. If you have receipts that are higher than the per diem, you can use those receipts (remember that you can only claim 50% of the total meal bill, including tip). The exciting part is that you can take the per diem rate even if it's more than your actual expenses. Loopholes aren't just for the wealthy! Working with a knowledgeable tax professional can ensure that you take advantage of all eligible deductions. Keep in mind that a tax deduction is what you can deduct, not necessarily what you spent. Sometimes this works in your benefit, as in the above per diem example. The flip side of this is that there are legitimate business expenses for which you cannot deduct the full cost (e.g., 50% of business entertainment and meals) and others for which there are limits (e.g., $25 per person ceiling on gifts).

The main problem with using tax software programs is that they aren't necessarily designed to handle the complexities of a business. They're great for wage earners who receive a W-2. So if you work solely as an employee, then a software program might work well. Not every practitioner must utilize an accountant, but it's wise to meet with an accountant at least once to determine what deductions you may be overlooking, and to plan for ways to legitimately write off future expenditures.

Current U.S. Tax Information
www.irs.gov

How to Find the Right Accountant

A good accountant looks into ways to save clients money through tax savings, shifting how and where money is spent, increasing revenues, and reducing overhead. The problem areas in tax returns are depreciation and "underuse" of eligible deductions. There are hundreds of legitimate tax deductions, and even the best accountant cannot spend the time going through each one with you to make sure you're aware of them all.

Find an accountant who takes the time to work with you, not just someone to whom you hand your paperwork and get a tax return to send to the IRS. You also need to feel comfortable with this person. Some accountants take an aggressive approach to tax return preparation while others are conservative. It's also crucial that you can communicate clearly and easily. Your accountant can profoundly affect your business success, so choose wisely. Ask for recommendations from people you trust: other business owners; your insurance agent, and your bank associate. Still, check their references and credentials yourself. Look for someone whose primary practice serves small businesses like yours, with expertise in your specific type of accounting needs.

If you document your work and keep accurate accounts, tax preparation becomes a natural extension of your bookkeeping activities.

U.S. Federal Tax Reporting

§6

The following information provides an overview of federal tax reporting requirements. Check the IRS guidelines to determine filing dates for tax returns. Generally, state tax returns are due at the same time as federal returns. Some states follow the same tax law as the IRS and others don't. Check with your state tax agency to verify requirements.

Employees

Employees receive a Form W-2 (Wage and Tax Statement) from their employers. They're issued in January for the previous calendar year. Form W-2 combines all wages and reported tips. It lists the amount of taxes withheld and paid throughout the year.

Form 1040	U.S. Individual Income Tax Return
Form 1040ES	Estimated Tax For Individuals (quarterly—if you will owe taxes)
Form 2106	Employee Business Expenses
Form 4070	Employee's Report of Tips to Employer (given monthly to your employer)
Form 4137	Social Security and Medicare Tax on Unreported Tip Income

"Taxes, after all, are dues that we pay for the privileges of membership in an organized society.
—Franklin D. Roosevelt

Employee Business Expenses

According to the IRS regulations, employee expenses are generally listed on Form 2106 and the total amount is carried forward to line 20 of Schedule A on Form 1040, or line 9 of Schedule A of Form 1040NR. This is only applicable if you itemize. Also, don't file Form 2106 if none of your expenses are deductible because of the 2% limit on miscellaneous itemized deductions.

Note: Check if the standard deduction amount is greater than your itemized deductions. If so, use the standard deduction.

Gratuities

All tips you receive are income and are subject to federal income tax. The IRS Publication 531 discusses reporting tip income. You must include in the gross income all tips you receive directly, charged tips paid to you by your employer, and your share of any tips you receive under a tip-splitting or tip-pooling arrangement.

Reporting your tip income correctly isn't difficult. You must do 3 things.

1. Keep a daily tip record.
2. Report tips to your employer.
3. Report all your tips on your income tax return.

You must report tips to your employer so that:

- Your employer can withhold federal income tax and Social Security and Medicare taxes.
- Your employer can report the correct amount of your earnings to the Social Security Administration (which affects your benefits when you retire or if you become disabled, or your family's benefits if you die).
- You can avoid the penalty for not reporting tips to your employer.

If your total tips for any 1 month from any 1 job are less than $20, you don't need to report the tips for that month to that employer. Also, you don't need to report the value of any non-cash tips (such as tickets or passes) to your employer. You don't pay Social Security and Medicare taxes on these tips, although you need to list their value as miscellaneous income on your tax return, and those monies are subject to income tax.

If your employer doesn't give you any other way to report your tips, you can use Form 4070 (Employee's Report of Tips to Employer). Fill in the information requested on the form, sign and date the form, and give it to your employer.

If you don't use Form 4070, give your employer a statement with the following information.

- Your name, address, and Social Security number.
- Your employer's name, address, and business name (if it's different from the employer's name).
- The month (or the dates of any shorter period) in which you received tips.
- The total tips required to be reported for that period.

You must sign and date the statement. You should keep a copy with your personal records.

If you received tips of $20 or more for any month while working for 1 employer but didn't report them to your employer, you must figure and pay Social Security and Medicare taxes on the unreported tips when you file your tax return. If you have unreported tips, you must use Form 1040 and Form 4137 to report them. You may not use Form 1040A or 1040EZ to file your tax return. If you don't report tips to your employer as required, you may be charged a penalty of 50% of the Social Security and Medicare taxes due on the unreported tips unless there was reasonable cause for not reporting them.

IRS Publication 531 discusses **Reporting Tip Income.** It is updated each year.

Sole Proprietors

A sole proprietorship isn't an independent entity from its owner, so the business does not file a separate tax return. Income or loss is reported on the owner's personal tax return. Sole proprietors must file:

Schedule SE	Self-Employment Tax
Schedule C	Profit or Loss From Business (Sole Proprietorship)
Form 1040	U.S. Individual Income Tax Return
Form 1040ES	Estimated Tax For Individuals (quarterly—if you will owe taxes)

Practitioners who operate as an LLC can be a sole proprietor, a partnership, or a corporation for IRS purposes, and should file taxes based on the rules for that entity.

Generally, you must pay estimated tax if you expect to owe (after subtracting your withholding and credits) at least $1000 in tax for the current year, and you expect your withholding and credits to be less than:

1. 90% of the tax to be shown on current year tax return; or
2. 100% of the tax shown on the previous year tax return (given the return covered all 12 months).

Plan ahead: If your income level requires you to pay taxes (even if you can avoid making prepayments to the IRS this year), set up a "savings" account for that money.

Partnerships

Partnerships are taxed similarly to sole proprietors. A partnership doesn't pay taxes. Income or loss is reported on the individual partner's tax returns. The partnership must file the following:

Form 1065	U.S. Partnership Return of Income
Form 1065 K-1	Partner's Share of Income, Credits, Deductions, etc.(given to each partner)

Corporations

Corporate annual returns are due by the 15th day of the third month after the close of the corporation's fiscal tax year. Corporations must file the following:

Form 1120	U.S. Corporation Income Tax Return (or short form version, 1120A)
Form 8109	Federal Tax Deposit Coupon (corporation estimated tax payment)

Employer's Forms

As an employer, you're required to file the following:

Form 941	Employer's Quarterly Federal Tax Return
Form W-2	Wage and Tax Statement
Form W-3	Transmittal of Wage and Tax Statements
Form 940	Employer's Annual Federal Unemployment (FUTA) Tax Return
Form 1096	Annual Summary and Transmittal of U.S. Information Returns
Form 1099	Miscellaneous Income (a business that pays more than $600 to a self-employed person must report that payment to the IRS and the sub-contractor)

Tax Credits

The IRS advises that taxpayers consider claiming eligible tax credits when completing their federal income tax returns. A tax credit is a dollar-for-dollar reduction of taxes owed.

Business Tax Credits

Tax credits differ from business deductions in that most tax deductions are the actual costs incurred in running a business and the categories tend to stay the same year after year. Tax credits are government incentives to encourage business owners to take socially responsible actions or to stimulate the economy. The regulations regarding tax credits can frequently change. Historically, business tax credits have included hiring people with disabilities, using

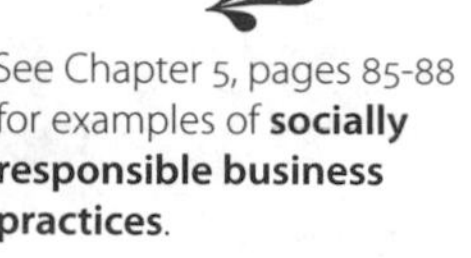

See Chapter 5, pages 85-88 for examples of **socially responsible business practices**.

renewable energy sources, renovating buildings, purchasing alternative fuel vehicles, operating a business in an empowerment zone or renewal community, and investing in certain types of equipment.

Tax Credit for Disabled Access

ADA Materials Specifically for Business and Non-Profits

www.ada.gov/ta-pubs-pg2.htm#titleiii

Possible tax credits are available for the purchase of equipment such as hydraulic tables. Practitioners may benefit by Section 44 Disabled Access Credit (Forms 8826 and 3800), which applies to costs incurred by small businesses to comply with the applicable requirements under the Americans with Disabilities Act of 1990 (ADA). In addition to access expenditures such as ramps, the definition includes, "To acquire or modify equipment or devices for individuals with disabilities." These expenses must meet the standards issued by the Secretary of the Treasury.

To qualify as a small business, the practice must meet the following requirements: the annual gross receipts for the preceding year did not exceed $1 million or had no more than 30 full-time employees during the preceding tax year.

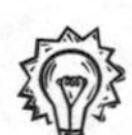

A **tax credit** is subtracted from your tax liability after you calculate your taxes, while a tax deduction is subtracted from your total income before taxes, to establish your taxable income.

If you work with clients who fit into this category (such as physically challenged or elderly), then you could be eligible for a rebate. This credit can only be applied to reduce an existing tax liability down to zero, but not to the point at which the business would show a loss.

Personal Tax Credits

Many types of tax credits are available, ranging from the Earned Income Tax Credit (EITC) for people who work and have an earned income under certain thresholds, to Child and Dependent Care Credit, to Education Credits. Since many of you reading this book are in school or plan to further your education, we've included an overview on education tax credits to help save you some money.

Education Tax Credits and Education Deductions

The American Opportunity Credit (AOC) and Lifetime Learning Credit (LLC) for "qualified tuition and related expenses" provide potential tax savings on higher education costs incurred by you, your dependents, or your spouse. The AOC is for the payment of the first 2 years of tuition and related expenses for an eligible student. The LLC is available for all post-secondary education for an unlimited number of years. A taxpayer cannot claim both credits for the same student in 1 year.

U.S. State Tax Reporting

In the United States, most states and the District of Columbia require you to file a state return if your income is above some minimum requirement. State tax returns are usually due at the same time as federal returns. Contact your State Department of Revenue or a tax professional to ascertain your state's specific requirements and the way they determine your tax liability.

Sales Tax

A taxation area that practitioners sometimes ignore is state sales tax. Unless you live in a state that doesn't levy sales tax, you're required to collect (and remit) sales tax on product sales—regardless of the volume. Some states also tax services. Sometimes, a sales tax license is bundled with a Business License. Keep in mind, in most states a Business License isn't the same as an Occupational or Professional License. Many states don't even require service businesses to have a Business License; you only need to apply for a Transaction Privilege Tax License.

Contact your State Department of Revenue to apply for a Transaction Privilege Tax License. Most states charge a one-time fee of less than $20. Some cities require a separate Transaction Privilege Tax License or Resale Permit.

Discuss tax collection requirements with the state, as well as the company from which you buy products for resale (e.g., certain food-based products are not taxed). Also, if you purchase products to resell, you don't need to pay sales tax to the company that sells you the product. The companies from which you purchase products often ask for your Resale Number (which is on the Transaction Privilege Tax License).

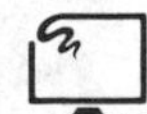

State Tax Forms

www.taxadmin.org/fta-directory-of-state-tax-administrators

Sales tax is calculated by multiplying the purchase price by the applicable tax rate, and is collected by the seller at the time of sale. Technically, you don't have to "collect" it, but that is the amount you must remit to the government. If you don't charge your clients the sales tax, that money comes out of your pocket.

If you experience any difficulty getting the information you need from the above sources, go to your State Department of Revenue (DOR) website. I searched a couple of different states and found that the DOR websites had the most complete, clear information–and include local requirements, too. Compile the information in Figure 20.14 before filling out the Transaction Privilege Tax License form.

Figure 20.14 Information Needed to Get a Transaction Privilege Tax License

- Business name
- Business entity (e.g., sole proprietor, LLC, PSC) and date it was established
- Employer Identification Number (EIN) or Social Security Number (SSN) if you're a sole proprietor without employees
- The starting date for collecting sales tax in your state
- The type of products or services to be sold
- The amount of sales tax you estimate you will collect
- If you have more than 1 location, whether you will be filing consolidated returns

Reports

The frequency of how often you must submit reports and the collected sales tax varies. Usually you're required to fill out a form on a monthly basis for the first year. If the volume is low, the state might reduce it to quarterly or even annually. Note, while it's called State Sales Tax, the percentages usually vary by the type of taxable activity and the city.

Once you know the sales tax rate you need to charge, you're on your way! If you use an accounting or office-management software program, it should calculate the amount of sales tax to charge for each sale and prepare your sales tax reports.

§6

Canadian Tax Resources

As in most countries around the world, tax regulations in Canada are complex and change frequently. Regulations and requirements vary among the provinces and territories. To ensure compliance with the most current Canada Revenue Agency (CRA) tax laws, readers are advised to consult with their accountant or financial planner for specific advice prior to making any business decisions.

Canadian Taxes

www.cra-arc.gc.ca/menu-e.html

sbinfocanada.about.com/cs/taxinfo/l/bltaxindex.htm

www.canadabusiness.ca

When it comes to business expenses, some are fully deductible and some are only partially deductible. Any reasonable expense that you incur to earn business income should be treated as a potential deduction. Many expenses can be fully claimed in the year of purchase.

The CRA is responsible for collecting federal, provincial (except Québec), and territorial income taxes. The Canadian tax system is also based on self-assessment. Under the self-assessment system, nonresidents with Canadian income and Canadian residents are responsible for making sure they've paid their taxes according to the Income Tax Act. Income tax rates are set annually. Income and deductions are listed on the income tax and benefit return so both the tax filer and the CRA can calculate the taxes the tax filer has to pay. Similarly, Canadian corporations and nonresident corporations with Canadian income pay corporate income tax according to the Income Tax Act and provincial and territorial legislation. Corporations file a corporate income tax return.

For those who want to get familiar with the general workings of the CRA tax requirements and tax planning, refer to the Internet websites listed in the margin. They're a good starting point and can help answer many frequently asked questions. The following information is an overview of various tax requirements.

Provincial and Territorial Tax Rates

Provincial and territorial tax rates vary. Under the current tax on income method, tax for all provinces (except Québec) and territories is calculated the same way as federal tax.

Goods and Services Tax (GST)

The Goods and Services Tax (GST) was implemented by the Federal Government in January 1992. Some services which had been tax-free became taxable, including wellness services such as massage therapy, chiropractic, and acupuncture services. However, not every wellness practitioner has to charge the GST. Refer to the CRA for current requirements and rates.

Provincial Sales Tax (PST)

When you must charge GST and PST, calculate GST on the price excluding PST. Readers are advised to contact their provincial sales tax offices for more information. Keep in mind, in the participating provinces, PST includes both the federal and provincial parts.

Harmonized Sales Tax (HST)

The participating provinces of Nova Scotia, New Brunswick, Newfoundland, Labrador, Ontario, and Prince Edward Island harmonized their provincial sales tax with GST to create the Harmonized Sales Tax (HST). HST has the same basic operating rules as GST and is applied at a single rate on the same base of goods and services that are taxable under GST.

Work Smarter with Barter

Barter is a cashless exchange of goods and services. This method isn't confined to primitive societies. It's the preferred method of managing finances for some, while others use barter only occasionally to enhance their cash flow. Bartering isn't a casual activity. According to the International Reciprocal Trade Association (the oldest and largest trade organization representing the reciprocal trade industry), over 400,000 of their worldwide member-companies used the "modern trade and barter" process last year to earn an estimated $12 billion dollars in revenues.[6]

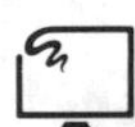

International Reciprocal Trade Association

www.irta.com

Technological advances in electronics (e.g., computers, email, websites, cloud-based software) have expanded barter from a face-to-face interaction to a global transaction. This enables a small business owner the opportunity to participate in an arena previously dominated by large corporations.

Barter affords you a simple, legal method to conserve cash outlays. If you can trade for something you need, then you can use your cash for other purposes. Common business bartering includes office supplies, printing, advertising, cleaning, repairs, and accounting services. Bartering is also an excellent method for expanding your client base. Many people who've never received the services of a complementary wellness provider might be more open to scheduling an appointment if they didn't need to pay in cash. I've made several training contracts with companies that probably would not have hired me or anyone else if it meant dipping into their cash reserves. Even though I didn't receive cash, the trade was useful and those clients referred cash-paying clients to me.

Keep in mind that barter is considered the equivalent of cash. If you barter your services for a business related purchase, then the "income" is offset by the business "expense." Ideally, you would record the amount of your service in your income ledger and the equal amount for the business item or service in your expense ledger, although most people don't record it at all if it's an even trade. However, if you barter for a personal purchase, then you're required to list the value of the service you bartered as "income."

Direct Barter

Many wellness providers already barter on a direct basis. They identify services and products they need and approach appropriate business owners with a trade proposal. Quite often, too, a client is the one to initiate a barter transaction. These direct trades work best if the items or services are of equal value. You can use gift certificates for trades and get gift certificates or vouchers from the person with whom you're trading. For instance, if you barter chiropractic services with a printer, have the printer give you a voucher for the amount you normally charge for an office visit. Then, when you're ready to do a printing job, you can redeem your vouchers. In this example, your barter is essentially a wash, as the "income" you generated from your services was used to pay for business expenses. Still, you need to record the vouchers as income and post the printing costs (paid with vouchers instead of cash) as an expense.

Barter is considered **taxable income** like cash, credit cards, and checks.

Here's another example: Let's say a restaurant owner wants to trade you meals for acupuncture treatments. You charge $65 per visit. One method is to have the restaurateur provide you with a $65 voucher for each treatment. Another idea is to transact a trade for a set amount, such as 10 acupuncture certificates for $650 worth of restaurant vouchers (in varying denominations). The beauty of the latter idea is that the certificates and vouchers can be redeemed by anyone. If you don't want to eat $650 worth of food at that restaurant, you can give the vouchers as gifts or use them for trading with someone else. Your client can do the same with the acupuncture certificates you give, which can ultimately bring you additional cash-paying clients.

Two major problems with direct barter arise from inequitable trades and trading for things you don't really need. The following scenario demonstrates the first concern: You want to have someone clean your office. You don't really have the cash to pay for that service so you consider approaching someone to barter. Although you may find an office cleaner, it probably won't work for long. The person is likely to become resentful when 5 hours of labor (at $10 per hour) equal 1 hour of your services.

The second problem relates to setting good boundaries. It can be so tempting to accept a barter offer from a potential client, particularly if you feel that the only way the person will utilize your services is if you agree to trade. If this occurs, remind yourself that your time is valuable. If the trade isn't for something you want or that you can give to another, then you essentially give away your session if you agree to trade. Both of these problems can be eliminated by membership in a barter network.

Developing your own direct barter network takes some thought and a bit of research. Start by listing all the goods and services you need in your business. Then make a second list of the items you would like for personal use. Make a third list of friends, colleagues, and clients and the services and goods they offer. Then compare all 3 lists. You may match a lot of your needs with people you already know. Build your network by telling people that you're interested in bartering—let them know your needs and what you can offer in return.

Barter Exchanges

Join a barter exchange if you plan to incorporate more than the occasional barter into your practice. Contact the National Association of Trade Exchanges or the International Reciprocal Trade Association for listings of barter organizations in your city. Approximately 500 barter exchanges operate in North America.[7] The International Trade Exchange (ITEX) and International Monetary Systems (IMS) are two of the largest exchanges.

Barter Exchanges
www.itex.com
www.imsbarter.com
www.natebarter.com

Essentially barter organizations work by members selling their goods and services to other members in exchange for trade dollars, which are valued at the equivalent of cash dollars. With each transaction, trade dollars are debited from the buyer's account and credited to the seller's account. The seller can then spend these trade dollars with other exchange members.

Barter exchanges function like a bank. They handle transactions, debit and credit accounts, charge fees, and send monthly statements. They may even offer a payment plan or extend a line of credit. You get either a credit card or checkbook with which to make your transactions. A client getting a treatment from you either charges it and you call it in to the exchange office (a similar procedure to processing bank credit cards), or writes you a barter check which you deposit (just like a bank check). Barter organizations often charge 10-15% commission (in cash) on the value of the actual trade. Usually the commission is applied against the buyer's account, but some exchanges split the charge between buyer and seller.

Before you join an exchange, check how many other people in your specific profession and geographic location are members. If the total local membership of a prospective exchange is under 200, and if 5 of the same type of practitioners are members, you may want to consider a different group because there might not be a large enough potential client pool.

Retirement Planning

When you have bills to pay and other priorities demanding your time and money, saving for retirement may seem like a distant goal. No matter the size of your business or your age, it's important to take the first steps toward saving for your retirement and developing an investment plan.

> "Prosperity is the fruit of labor. It begins with saving money.
> —Abraham Lincoln

It all starts with the realization that you're not going to work forever—and that you need to save now to pay for future living costs. These concerns require that you act today so you can enjoy a comfortable and worry-free retirement. Whether self-employed or an employee, the steps to a successful retirement are simple:

- Develop an effective savings plan: save the right amount; save regularly; save in the right accounts.
- Create an investment strategy: choose the best mix of investments based on your retirement goals and comfort with potential risk.

The first step is to understand what retirement investment options are available. You can either work with a financial planning advisor or spend some time with a good resource book to get the information you need. The next steps are to set retirement goals, estimate what your living expenses will be when you retire, and develop a strategic savings and investment plan to meet your financial goals. Financial experts agree that it's best to treat Social Security retirement income as a supplemental source of retirement income—not the primary source.

Retirement Plan Options

Tax-deferred retirement plans are valuable because, while saving for your retirement, you delay paying taxes on money you earn and contribute to these plans. Additionally, the interest and dividends earned on the money in the retirement plan are tax deferred. Tax-deferred means that you pay no taxes on the money until it's taken out of your retirement account.

Theoretically, when you take the money out of the account, you're retired or working part time, which puts you in a lower tax bracket than you were in when you invested the money. As a result, the money you contributed and the earned interest or dividends are taxed at a lower rate than they would have been if you hadn't put the money in a tax-deferred account and instead had paid tax on it when it was earned.

Due to compounding interest, the earlier in life you begin contributing to a retirement plan, the less total amount you'll need to deposit to accumulate a substantial amount of retirement money. The money you contribute to a retirement plan, however, should be money that you don't expect to need until you're at least 59½ years old. When you take a distribution from your retirement account, you're taxed on that money in the same way as you're taxed on other income. With few exceptions, the IRS also assesses a 10% penalty if money is taken out before you're 59½. Your state may have a similar penalty, which means that if you take the money out prior to reaching the minimum age, you may lose nearly 50% to federal and state taxes and penalties. No matter how little you contribute, get into the habit of making an annual contribution to your retirement account. Following is a brief overview of retirement plans.

Small Business Retirement Plans

Employer-Sponsored Plans

- 401(k) Plan
- 403(b) Tax-Sheltered Annuity
- Tax-deferred Annuity Retirement Plan

Contributing to these types of plans gives you an immediate tax deduction and tax-deferred growth on your savings. Deductions are taken from your paycheck and put into your designated retirement account. Many employers offer matching contributions. Distributions in retirement are fully taxable.

SIMPLE IRA Accounts

SIMPLE IRA accounts (Savings Incentive Match Plan for Employees) are available to some employees. Their employers are required to match employee contributions up to a certain percentage. These plans also can be beneficial to self-employed small business owners as they may make SIMPLE contributions as both an employer and an employee.

Self-Employed 401(k) Plans

These are retirement plan for business owners with no employees. They allow you to put the most away annually but must be opened by December of the year in which you want to contribute.

§6

Traditional IRA

AN IRA (Individual Retirement Account) can be set up at a bank, brokerage house, mutual fund company, or other financial institution. You get a deduction in the year in which you contribute and pay taxes on the amount you withdraw in retirement. Tax regulations may prevent high-income earners from contributing to a traditional IRA, particularly if they also have another retirement plan.

Roth IRA

These plans, which can also be set up at a bank, brokerage house, mutual fund company, or other financial institution, offer tax-free (not tax-deferred) growth, and distributions in retirement aren't at all taxable. Contributions are post-tax and not taxable.

SEP-IRAs

SEP-IRA Accounts (Simplified Employee Pensions) are available to sole proprietors and partnerships. Contributions are based on a percentage of net (after business expenses have been deducted) self-employment income. Employers are required to make a contribution on behalf of anyone over age 20 to comply with SEP-IRA account guidelines.

Recession-Proof Your Practice

A substantial number of talented and dedicated wellness practitioners find it difficult to earn enough money to adequately support their families. One of the biggest drawbacks is the finite number of hours you can work directly with clients. Depending on the type of work you do, you may only have the physical and emotional stamina to work directly with clients for 25-30 hours per week. Imagine that you see 25 clients per week, 50 weeks per year. At $50 per session, that's $62,500 per year. Not bad, except that figure is before expenses. Depending on your setup, you may clear less than $25,000 per year after deducting business expenses.

> "Good fortune is what happens when opportunity meets with preparation.
> —Thomas Edison

It's unwise to rely on your hands-on work as your only source of income. You can increase your income potential in several ways: reduce your overhead, increase your number of billable hours, increase product sales, hire support staff to free up your time, or raise your rates.

More than anything else, diversification is the key to long-term financial success. The saying goes, "Don't keep all your eggs in the same basket," and it's true. When you develop multiple streams of revenue, you don't have to rely solely on your hands-on work to generate income. The most common methods of diversification are to vary the scope of your practice by incorporating additional billable modalities, hiring other practitioners, or teaching.

You could also consider investing in your future business success with specialized equipment and advanced training certifications. These become assets to your practice that help you to solve health issues with your current clients, set you apart from other therapists who don't have the same assets you do, and help you to generate new clients. Advanced training can help with the additional billable modalities, as well as with potential teaching opportunities, if you learn how to teach those advanced techniques.

The following chapters address diversification by hiring others or selling products.

21

Retail Management

"Nobody likes to be sold, but everybody likes to buy."

—Earl Taylor

Boost Your Bottom Line While Serving Clients
- Extend Session Benefits
- The Importance of Retailing
- Retail Reality

Ethical Concerns
- The Power Differential
- Product Knowledge
- Nutritional Supplements

Choose Appropriate Products
- Product Research
- Distributors
- Pricing Products
- Inventory Control

The Art of Selling Products
- The Three C's of Effective Sales
- Sales Methods
- Creative Ideas for Selling Products
- Closing the Sale
- Fostering Ongoing Sales

Merchandising
- Visibility
- Design

Drive Your BUS to Success

Key Terms

Analgesics
Baking
Bottom Line
Bundling
BUS
Distributor
Ergonomic
Ethics
Inventory
Keystoning
Manufacturer
Merchandising
Nutritional Supplements
Point-of-Sale (POS) Displays
Power Differential
Product Knowledge
Retailing
Shelf Talkers

Product sales is a great diversification method and profits from them can defray overhead expenses. It's hazardous—physically, emotionally, and financially—to rely on your hands-on work as the sole source of your livelihood, particularly if your work requires intensity. Product sales adds value to your sessions, extends the session benefits to home, and increases your bottom line. Product sales is a natural extension of the standard of care and healing already associated with wellness practitioners. You have a relationship with your clients and retailing is simply another avenue of supporting your clients in their wellness.

Clients like to get products from you, and appreciate the convenience of purchasing from you. You save them time when they don't have to make a special trip to buy an item or wait for it to be delivered. They expect you to have more knowledge than they do about these products and will trust your recommendations, especially those products that are used in the session itself. By selling clients the right products, you help them reduce their stress and improve their health.

Boost Your Bottom Line While Serving Clients

Product sales offers clients a valuable service, because you have access to many products that aren't easily available to the general public. For instance, there are wonderful self-care products your average clients can't find at their local health emporium. Many of these products aren't even directly available to retail consumers, they must be purchased by a practitioner and then sold to the client.

I believe that you do your clients a disservice if you don't have products they can purchase. Many people are overworked and time management is a problem. If you can save them the time of having to stop to buy a product, then you've simplified their lives—and that's priceless. Also, clients with tight schedules may not have the time to fit in a treatment and purchase wellness products, and you don't want them to have to choose one over the other (they might not choose the treatment!). I've received sessions where the practitioner used a really nice product or had great music playing, but didn't offer those items for sale. This was a missed sales opportunity for the practitioner—and disappointing to me.

Massage therapist Robert Flammia of Berkeley, California, sells a variety of gels, balms, books, and massage tools. He also sees product sales as a way to introduce people to massage and increase his massage practice:

> *Selling touch is perhaps one of the hardest things to sell because of being so invasive on the psyche and body of the unknowing recipient. Selling items, whether physically or psychologically related to touch, is a much easier icebreaker.*

As a wellness practitioner, you already have a unique position with your clients, and retailing is simply another avenue of supporting your clients in their wellness. Some of the contributing elements to this unique position are your knowledge, experience, the built-in trust you have with your clients, the time you spend with clients, and the power you have to help and recommend. Also, you can keep your retailing efforts simple and you don't need a large storefront.

Extend Session Benefits

Extend the session benefits at home by providing clients with products that they can use between appointments. This can be from a direct therapeutic point of view, such as a self-massage tool or a book on stretching, to recreating a relaxation response. Ideally, you use some of these items in your sessions so your clients associate those items with their experience of your work.

Sounds and scents are strong triggers for memories. This is particularly applicable to somatic practitioners and skin care specialists. Let's say that in your session you played a certain CD, placed an eye pillow on your client's eyes, infused your massage lubricant with an essential oil, or used a special foot balm while massaging the client's feet. Those are all items clients can purchase for home use; every time they feel, smell, or hear those items, they most likely are transported back to the last time they experienced them—which would be while in a state of relaxation on your table. Although it isn't the same as receiving a treatment from you, it certainly helps extend the benefits of your work in-between sessions. Depending on the type of work that you do and your clients' goals, some of the products for clients to use at home can also be for a direct therapeutic result, such as keeping muscles loose, addressing trigger points, increasing flexibility, or reducing pain.

Clients see wellness practitioners for many reasons, ranging from stress reduction to injury rehabilitation to getting fit to pure pampering. Regardless of the reasons clients work with you, it's nice when they leave with that "AAAAHHH" feeling. You can extend that feeling of bliss by sending your clients home with products. Spas understand this, and garner a large percentage of income from product sales. Because you're educating clients on self-care rather than doing hard sales, you can sell retail products as part of your practice, just like spas in your area do.

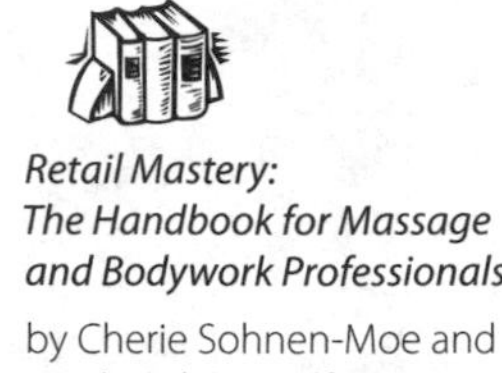

Retail Mastery: The Handbook for Massage and Bodywork Professionals

by Cherie Sohnen-Moe and Lynda Solien-Wolfe

As a bonus, retailing can actually increase the frequency of clients booking sessions. When clients use a product at home, it reminds them of the treatment they received, and that usually inspires them to book another session. Plus, if they share those products with friends, those friends are more likely to become clients.

Figure 21.1 The Four Requirements to Effectively Extending Session Benefits

1. Properly assess clients' needs.
2. Take the time to match up potential products to meet those needs.
3. Educate clients on the proper use of those products.
4. Inspire clients to use the products at home.

The Importance of Retailing

The three major ways to increase revenue in your practice are to increase the number of clients you see by working more (or hiring other practitioners to work for you), increase the amount you sell (in services and products) to the same number of clients, and raise your prices.

Yet, you can easily increase your income with add-on services, gift certificates, and product sales. One of my favorite sayings is "Do the Math!" Let's say your client base consists of 100 people. If you averaged selling $50 in products to each client per year, that would increase your income by $5,000. After you factor in the cost of the goods, shipping, promotion, and time, you should still see a net profit of at least $2,000. That's pretty good for just stocking a few items that your clients would like and would probably buy something similar from another company anyway. Now imagine bringing in a few higher-end items or increasing the average amount that you sell each year.

Retail Reality

If you're in private practice or work in a group setting, you control what you sell and how you sell. This is usually not the case if you work in a spa or wellness center. Many of these companies require their practitioners to sell products. They know that retailing is a critical element in client satisfaction and rely on the income generated by product sales. The sales volume increases when the practitioners have input on products carried and the products are within their scope of practice. According to the International Spa Association (ISPA), retail sales account for almost 20% of a spa's total revenue. Plus, the profit margin on products is typically higher than services. Thus, even a small increase in the revenue from retail sales can make a tremendous difference in a spa's bottom line.

Employers commonly expect wellness practitioners (such as massage therapists) to generate between 10 to 20% of their total sales in home-care products or supplies. As a side note, most estheticians are required to generate upwards of 50%. Salaries, bonuses, and seniority are often based on the amount of products sold. Before taking a job at one of these establishments, clarify their product sales requirements, and make sure that you feel comfortable and confident in their product lines. If you currently work in such a setting and don't like the products, then talk with management. Offer input on the product lines so that the company can carry items that you feel comfortable selling. This makes it a win/win/win situation for you, the clients, and the company. Perhaps you can develop a different client check-out system so that you don't feel like you're hawking products or rushed for time.

See Chapter 7, page 116 for **practice setting statistics**.

Some practitioners are reluctant to sell products. One concern relates to having to "push" products. If you view products as an extension of the treatment and a value-added service, then sales become a natural part of the client/practitioner relationship (without pressure), particularly when you use the product within the session.

The lack of product knowledge is another aspect that contributes to sales reluctance. Make sure you know the major details about and how to apply any product you sell. Also, make sure you learn about all of the products that you're expected to sell. If training isn't provided, then at least read the materials that accompany the products and research the items online.

Another common concern is the lack of time between sessions to sell products. Whenever possible, schedule at least 15 minutes between sessions. This allows you time to discuss questions with clients, review their treatment plans, sell appropriate products, and book the next session. When you consider the revenue that generates, how can you afford not to allot that extra time?

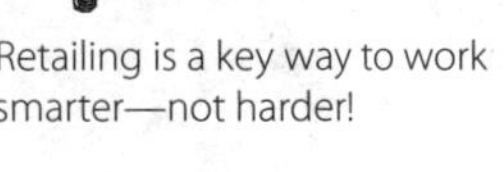

Retailing is a key way to work smarter—not harder!

Retailing does have its challenges, particularly determining what products to sell, how much inventory to carry, the potential to get stuck with stuff that nobody wants, products going bad, and having to schlep around products if you operate a mobile practice. Also, retailing takes a time investment on your part to thoroughly learn about the products, deal with increased paperwork, collect and remit sales tax, create attractive displays, and market the products.

Figure 21.2 Advantages and Disadvantages of Retailing

Advantages:	Disadvantages:
• Adding value to your sessions	• Doing extra paperwork
• Extending the benefits at home	• Collecting and remitting sales tax
• Providing convenience to your clients	• Handling inventory management
• Increasing your bottom line	• Investing time and energy

Ethical Concerns

The focus of ethical products sales is providing your clients with easy access to high-quality products that help enrich their wellbeing. At times, unethical practices such as aggressive sales techniques or misinformation can characterize product sales. Fortunately, in most wellness professions, this is the exception rather than the rule. Nevertheless, you must be cautious when selling products. If product sales are not handled well, they can negatively impact your practice. The major issue here is: are you influenced more by the money that product sales generate, or are you selling products to clients because they need or want them? Exercise caution and check your motives to make certain that you aren't "pushing" a little harder because your income is down or because you're required to meet a targeted sales volume.

A conflict doesn't need to exist, as long as a few guidelines are followed. If you currently run a professional, ethical practice, then retailing can naturally follow suit. If you keep good boundaries, treat people with respect and fairness, and remain client-centered, then you will manage product sales in the same manner that you manage the rest of your practice.

The Power Differential

The power differential is the key factor in ethical product sales. As a wellness practitioner, a power differential exists between you and your clients. You're the authority figure whose actions, by virtue of your role, directly affects your clients' wellbeing. Clients may feel uncomfortable about raising concerns or making requests. They may find it difficult to say "no" or refrain from communicating anything that could possibly be construed as negative for fear of reprisal or loss. Clients may feel influenced to purchase products out of a need to please you or in deference to you being an authority figure. Even if you take great care not to exploit this power differential, it still exists.

> "Most people think 'selling' is the same as 'talking.' But the most effective salespeople know that listening is the most important part of their job.
> —Roy Bartell

Don't manipulate or coerce your clients. It's one thing to display a product, mention it in your marketing materials, and even use that product in the session. It's crucial that you invite clients to see if they're interested in learning more about a product. Don't assume that they're interested.

Reduce the possible abuse of the power differential by restricting your conversation about products to before or after sessions. It's fine to mention the product during a session, such as, "Now I'm going to use XYZ product on you. If you're interested in learning more information about it, we can discuss it after the session."

Actually, when your selection of products closely relates to your session, product recommendation becomes easier. Give your clients the power to learn more about maintaining their health and making better decisions. Remember, you provide a solution for your clients.

The post-session interview is a good time to reference products. It's natural to recommend products that are appropriate to the client's goals when you review the treatment plan and any "homework" you might have for a client. This is also the time to ask for feedback on any of the products you used during the session.

Product Knowledge

Ethical sales are based upon educating your clients on the benefits of certain products and then allowing them the opportunity to purchase them from you. Only sell products you know are reliable, professional grade, suitable for use by your clients, within your scope of practice, a natural extension of your business, and congruent with your image. Remember, you have access to products that most consumers can't easily find!

Clients depend on you to provide them with accurate information and guidance. You must know every one of your products well and convey the proper use, benefits, limitations, and possible side-effects or contraindications to your clients. For instance, if your client really enjoyed the cervical hot pack you used during the session and wants to purchase one, you would educate the client how to use the pack and under what circumstances not to use it. Your clients will lose faith in you (and then no longer be your clients, not to mention the loss of goodwill) if you fail to adequately inform them about the products you sell. Also, don't make product claims that the manufacturer doesn't make or would not support.

Nutritional Supplements

In the quest to diversify their practices, many practitioners sell nutritional supplements. The major concern is that practitioners may be working beyond their scope of practice, unless they're a nutritionist or herbalist (or extremely well versed in this subject).

The industry term of "nutraceuticals" has been coined due to the prevalence of the use of herbs and vitamins. And given that it sounds like medical-ese, you can be sure that the government has its eye on regulating it. The Food and Drug Administration (FDA) has attempted to reclassify certain herbs as narcotics, and, on more than one occasion, has said that certain supplements aren't safe.

Rumors cycle through about pending legislation to require these types of nutritional supplements to be prescribed by a physician. These bills haven't come to fruition, but the idea is frightening. Most consumers don't want anyone to take away their freedom to choose and purchase supplements from wherever or whomever they desire. Unfortunately, the more that people haphazardly sell products without proper education, the more likely the government will intercede.

I've been in some wellness practitioners' offices where the waiting room looks like a small health food store. It is highly unlikely that those practitioners know much about all the various products they carry. You might be thinking that store clerks don't know that information either, so what's the problem? Essentially, the problem is that you have a client/practitioner relationship, which differs from a consumer/retailer relationship.

But what happens when you've taken a product that changes your life or someone you know has experienced profound change? How can you not sell it? After all, your role is to support your clients in their overall wellness. If there's a product that you really believe in and want to make available to your clients, educate yourself on the product: the contents, suggested usage, possible adverse reactions, and contraindications. Keep in mind that just because something works for you doesn't mean it's beneficial to the next person. Also, "works" is a tricky word. Beware of anecdotal evidence. Results aren't always proven or reliable. The possibility exists that the product could even be harmful to someone else. When discussing nutritional supplements with clients, you need to discuss the potential side effects (such as a healing crisis) in addition to explaining the benefits.

The more informed you are about the products you carry, the less risk there is for you and your clients. If you're interested in herbs and vitamins, consider taking courses on the subject—or even pursue a degree in nutrition or herbology. Another option to help ensure that you provide your clients with information and products that are in their best interest is to team up with a nutritionist or herbologist.

The U.S. market is flooded with nutritional supplements, and the general public is looking for direction. As wellness providers, your clients naturally rely upon you to provide them with information, products, and services to enhance their wellbeing. Proceed cautiously when it comes to incorporating nutritional supplements into your practice.

Ensuring Ethical Sales

Reflect on the types of questionable sales approaches that you've experienced and list the key aspects of those experiences. Note if they share anything in common. Next, identify how those experiences could have been handled better. Finally, create a list of behaviors, policies, and procedures that you'll take to set a strong ethical foundation for your product sales.

Figure 21.3 Ethical Product Sales Do's and Don'ts

Ethical Product Sales: Do's

- Make sure the products you carry are appropriate and wanted.
- Find products that meet clients' goals and needs.
- Know the products well.
- Educate your clients on the proper use, benefits, and possible side-effects.
- Restrict discussion of products to before or after the session.
- Ask for client feedback.
- Clearly label the cost of products.

Ethical Product Sales: Don'ts

- Don't overuse products.
- Don't make product claims that the manufacturer doesn't make.
- Don't manipulate or coerce your clients.

Choose Appropriate Products

There are so many products that you can sell. You just need to make sure there aren't any local statutes or specific industry guidelines forbidding the sale of certain items. In addition to healthcare products designed to assist in the relief of pain and promote wellbeing, it's fine to sell ancillary items that are fun or make for unique gifts. It's also appropriate to sell products that help clients feel pampered (and we can all use that from time to time). Just imagine how lovely it would be for your clients to create a mini-oasis of tranquility in their homes. I've interviewed many people on the types of products they sell and what seems to work best. The most successful items are those that help clients with their pain issues, home self-care products, and gift items. (See Figure 21.4 for a list of general product ideas.)

> "Ninety percent of selling is conviction and 10 percent is persuasion.
>
> —Shiv Khera

In addition to the general products that wellness practitioners could sell, there might be some industry-specific items to sell. For instance, a yoga practitioner might also sell mats, blocks, and bands. A reflexologist might also sell pumice stones, tea tree oil, wallet-sized reflexology cards, foot sprays, loofah pads, foot bath equipment or products, and arch supports. A counselor might also sell hypnosis CDs and batakas. A personal trainer might sell fitness equipment, bands, and monitoring gear. An acupuncturist might also sell herbs, nutritional supplements, decoctions, and linaments.

§6

Carefully consider the products you sell. When choosing the right product, ideally choose one that is NOT commonly sold, is unique, and, if possible, is an extension of your work. Ideally, you would use some of these items in your sessions so your clients associate those items with their experience of your work.

See Chapter 5, pages 85-88 for details on **socially responsible businesses**.

Select products that have a healthy profit margin, are beneficial, you believe in, and your clients need or want. Occasionally, you might carry an item that is easy to find, but you make it available for convenience—so that you client doesn't need to make a stop on the way home. A prime example of this is Epsom salts. Many practitioners recommend clients go home and take an Epsom Salt bath after the session—particularly after a vigorous session or if the client had a lot of holding patterns or trigger points.

Figure 21.4 Items to Sell

- Bath salts
- Body butters
- Books
- Candles
- DVDs
- Ergonomic devices
- Essential oils
- Eye pillows
- Foot balms
- Gifts
- Hot and cold packs
- Music
- Oils, lotions, creams, gels
- Pain erasure balls
- Relaxation tools
- Scrubs
- Self-care items
- Self-massage tools
- Slippers
- Support pillows
- Topical analgesics

Product Research

Research is the first step in determining which products to carry. Start with identifying the types of retail products that correspond to the specific services you provide. Keep track (for about a month) of all the products that you recommend your clients buy somewhere else. Note which of those items you could potentially sell. The next step is to get feedback from clients on the types of products they would like you to carry. Combine the 3 lists and find specific products (do online research, attend expos, and ask other practitioners for their input). Then find out details of the potential products (e.g., where do you buy them, how much do they cost, what's the suggested retail cost). Be sure to read the product information sheets.

The final step is to purchase products and test them yourself. Make sure you know how to use any product you sell. Something might sound good on paper, but could be cumbersome to use, smells weird, has negative side-effects, or isn't very effective. After testing the product on yourself, ask a few key clients to test the product. Give the testers a form to fill out that asks questions about their experience with the product. In addition to helping you ascertain if you should carry a specific product, their feedback can help you determine how to market it and the depth of client education needed. Anita Shannon of ACE Massage Cupping states,[1]

> *This is also a wonderful way to collect testimonials and before-and-after photos in advance and include them in your presentation materials. In client retention, a photo really is worth a thousand words.*

Distributors

Distributors
www.massagewarehouse.com
www.universalcompanies.com
www.optp.com
www.yogadirect.com
www.360fitnesssuperstore.com
www.acu-market.com

Financial success in retailing requires that you purchase products at wholesale prices and mark up those prices appropriately. Many practitioners purchase items from a distributor that carries a wide selection from a variety of manufacturers (e.g., Massage Warehouse, Orthopedic Physical Therapy Products). Sometimes practitioners buy bulk products directly from a manufacturer or publisher. Sometimes you can get a better price if you go directly to the manufacturer. Also, the manufacturer might offer you free items. Yet, many manufacturers only sell through distributors. The main benefits of buying from a distributor are that you only have to place one order for multiple product lines, and the minimum quantity orders might be more flexible than the manufacturer's requirements.

The bottom line is you need to find companies with which you feel comfortable and ideally are socially responsible. Also, consider working with local companies for specialty products.

Whenever possible, work with companies that provide marketing materials (e.g., brochures, eye-attracting posters, point-of-sale displays) and samples. Some provide these types of items for free while others charge a fee or require a minimum order.

Ideally, work with companies that understand the nuances of your specific industry and actively support your industry. Also, look for companies (and products) that have worked to brand themselves and are consumer driven. Some other considerations to factor into your choice of what companies to work with are the following: their level of customer service; how quickly products ship; how shipping charges are assessed; their return policies; if they offer the best price; and if they provide price guarantees.

A Twist on Traditional Sales

Traditional sales involve a practitioner buying products at wholesale and reselling to clients. This involves an investment of time and money. Here are two creative ways to work with manufacturers or distributors (particularly for high-end items).

1. The item is displayed and clients place orders with the practitioner. The item is either delivered directly to the client or the practitioner. This involves some time and paperwork, but lessens your financial risk.
2. The item is displayed, clients are provided with order information, clients order directly from the manufacturer, and the manufacturer sends you a commission check. This option takes almost no time and incurs no risk.

Most wholesalers require a minimum order. If you're just starting out and can't afford the minimum, consider joining forces with others to make cooperative purchases.

Pricing Products

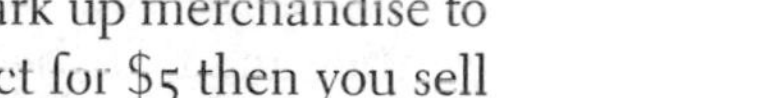

See Chapter 20, pages 298-299 for details on **sales tax**.

When it comes to pricing, charge a fair but profitable price. Your distributor, or the product's manufacturer, should guide you with suggestions of the proper selling prices. They will usually provide you with the MSRP (Manufacturer's Suggested Retail Price). This is the price the company suggests you charge for its products. In general, you can charge whatever you want, although some companies may not allow you to price an item below the MSRP.

Most retail sales use the keystoning method, which means that you mark up merchandise to an amount that is double the wholesale price. Thus, if you buy a product for $5 then you sell it for $10. You will find that some products offer an even better mark-up than that and others less. In most instances, you also have to pay shipping and that can add up if the item is heavy.

The cost of selling products isn't limited to purchase price and shipping. You must consider the time involved in research, placing orders, displaying products, and marketing. Also factor in the time to manage the paperwork involved in collecting sales tax and submitting tax reports. And then what do you do with inventory that doesn't sell?

Inventory Control

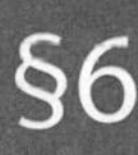

Practitioners who sell products need to keep track of what has been ordered, how long it takes to receive merchandise, how long it takes to sell merchandise, and what's in stock. You don't want to run out of your best-selling item—particularly if it takes weeks to obtain more. Also, it isn't wise to carry too much stock that has a relatively short shelf life—oils that can go rancid or magazines that are published monthly.

If you carry a limited selection of products, daily inventory can be checked visually and a written tally (often referred to as a physical inventory) taken at least twice per year. A more formal approach to inventory is recommended if you stock a wide variety of goods. Most accounting software packages include inventory recordkeeping. These programs keep track of inventory on hand and alert you when stock gets low (even so, doing a physical inventory at least once a year is recommended). The programs can output a variety of reports to track sales trends. This also assists you in determining what products to sell and how to sell them. For instance, if you only sell 1 unit of a certain product in 6 months, then perhaps it should be eliminated from your product line. Also, if you have an item with a quickly approaching expiration date, you might consider reducing the price or giving it away as an added-value promotion.

Forgetting to place an order can easily happen when you're busy with all the other aspects of running a practice. Charting inventory activities (either manually or computerized) reduces the chances for errors and provides you with a quick overview.

Create Your Product List

Make a list of products that you want to sell in your practice. Identify where to purchase those items. Note the retail price, and the wholesale discount structure for varying quantities (including any applicable shipping). Identify the quantity of each product that you want to purchase initially and determine the cost for your initial stock. Do a breakdown analysis (determine how many units you must sell to recoup your initial investment). If you're in practice already, make a list of which clients are likely to purchase each product.

The Art of Selling Products

Selling products isn't about hype or "hard-sell" tactics. The income you receive from the items your clients purchase isn't going to make you rich, but it can be a decent source of supplemental income. Just carrying a product doesn't guarantee it will sell. Because people are more inclined to buy something they've experienced, incorporate your products into your practice and take the time to educate your clients. Always keep in mind that the major focus of product sales is to provide your clients with easy access to high-quality products that enrich their wellbeing.

> "For every sale you miss because you're too enthusiastic, you will miss a hundred because you're not enthusiastic enough.
> —Zig Ziglar

Ultimately, selling products is like "selling" your services—simply share your enthusiasm about them. If you make your products visible, accessible, attractive, and affordable, your clients will buy them when it's appropriate.

For those of you who haven't been selling products, I encourage you to give it a try. Start out small and gradually increase the types and quantity of products you carry. For those of you who already are comfortable with product sales, I hope that you will revamp what you do and look for ways to increase those sales, and perhaps even work with some higher-ticket items.

If you're reluctant to incorporate product sales, start out simply. Perhaps sell just a few products until you're more comfortable with the process and are more attuned to what your clients want to purchase. Ideally, you would have products on hand, but if you have major concerns about carrying inventory, you can have a sign-up sheet where clients place orders. You would then purchase those items when you've reached the minimum amount needed for a wholesale order. Some wholesalers will even drop-ship products directly to your clients.

There are many ways to incorporate product sales in your practice to support your clients' wellbeing and the wellbeing of your bottom line. This section highlights the concepts behind effective retailing, overviews three sales methods, and provides specific suggestions for creative ways to sell products.

The Three C's of Effective Sales

Building relationships is the foundation of effective sales in the wellness field. Consider the Three C's of Effective Sales (Consultation, Convenience, and Compliance) in fostering those relationships.

Consultation

Product recommendation becomes easier when your selection of retail products closely relates to what you do in your sessions. Give your clients the power to learn more about maintaining their health and making better decisions. Remember, you're ultimately providing a solution to your clients. When you provide the right products to clients, their satisfaction and the value of your advice grows. This is one reason a thorough intake interview and a post-session interview are crucial.

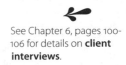

See Chapter 6, pages 100-106 for details on **client interviews**.

The intake interview is when you identify clients' concerns and goals. The post-session interview is when you summarize the session, establish the long-term wellness care plan, and recommend any reference materials, relaxation tools, support devices, books, and other items that are appropriate to the client's goals.

Remember to educate your clients about the benefits and features of your products. This can be done with verbal descriptions, demonstrations, signs, literature, brochures, articles, DVDs, and product testers. Most people like to smell and feel products before purchasing them.

Convenience

Clients have the immediate satisfaction of knowing they can obtain and use products recommended by a wellness practitioner. They would rather not have to decide between multiple, unknown products on a retail shelf.

By sending clients home with samples, they're more likely to make future purchases when they return for treatment. Keeping your business at the top of clients' minds creates passive revenue that builds your practice. This is all about time management. Most people are extremely busy. This is where even selling an item that they could easily buy elsewhere is helpful.

Compliance

You know what treatments work for clients and what they can do to maintain better health. Many of the services you offer aren't completely effective unless you can extend and enhance the benefits post treatment. Self-care is most successful when clients do what a practitioner instructs. When you recommend a product for home use and explain how to apply it, chances are greater the product will be used properly. Remember, you're the expert! Selling clients the right products helps them achieve their wellness goals.

Sales Methods

This sections explores three methods of selling products: making recommendations, baking, and direct sales. Most practitioners incorporate a mixture of these methods in their retailing ventures.

Recommending

Recommending is the most common form of communicating about product sales. If you refer back to what we covered earlier about assessing your client's needs and having the appropriate products, then recommending is easy and natural. Utilize the products you sell in your sessions: play a CD; apply a hot or cold pack; use specialized gels, creams, or liniments; incorporate strength and agility items; or include aromatherapy applications. Then you can easily sell those items to your clients because they've already enjoyed them.

You can also provide clients with product recommendation sheets. These are handy, particularly if you don't have a lot of time between clients, and are often experienced as less invasive than if you talked directly with the client about the products (see Figure 21.5).

Figure 21.5 Sample Product Recommendation Sheet

WELLNESS ASSOCIATES

123 BREEZE • ANYWHERE • 555-5555 WWW.WELLNESSASSOCIATES.COM

Jane Doe	3/7
CLIENT NAME	DATE

HOME CARE SUGGESTIONS*	DAILY AM	DAILY PM	WEEKLY TIMES/WEEK
Product 1 Topical	√	√	daily
Product 2 Self-Massage Tool	as needed		
Product 3			
Product 4			
Activity 1 Shoulder Stretches		√	daily
Activity 2 Relaxation Exercises			3x/week
Activity 3			
Activity 4			

*Only add products and activities when appropriate and within your scope of practice.

FOLLOW-UP CARE	WHEN
Next Session	Tues 3/14
Talk to PCP regarding skin condition	ASAP

Mary Massage, LMT

PRACTITIONER

PRODUCT RECOMMENDATION SHEET (EXAMPLE)

Baking

Baking is done by creating a special treatment that includes using a products in the session and sending the client home with the products. For instance, a massage therapist could create the "Weekend Warrior Pain Relief Treatment" that includes a massage with the use of a topical analgesic and a hot pack. After the treatment, the client goes home with the remainder of the topical analgesic and the hot pack. Let's say that this practitioner's normal session rate is $70, the retail price of the topical is $15 and the retail price of the heat pack is $20. The practitioner sets the price for this special treatment at $90. The practitioner's cost of the products is $17.50. The client saves $15 and the practitioner earns an extra $2.50. It's a win/win experience for everyone, particularly when the package includes a product that needs to be replenished. If the client really likes it, you now have set it up for ongoing sales.

Direct Selling

Direct selling requires taking a proactive role in marketing your products. In addition to the methods involved in recommending and baking, directly inform your clients about your products. Post signs in your office. I've even seen practitioners post product special flyers in their bathrooms. Print flyers that describe all the products you carry. Give these to your clients and mail (or email) them for special promotions. Mention product sales in your newsletter. Send email blasts about any new product you carry or if you run a special. Promote your products on your website and Social Media sites. Create educational videos and post them on YouTube. (While you don't have to take online orders, it's still wise to let people know about the items they can purchase from you.) You can also place ads in specialty publications that your target markets read, and through online services.

> "To sell a product or a service, a company must establish a relationship with the consumer. It must build trust and rapport. It must understand the customer's needs, and it must provide a product that delivers the promised benefits.
>
> —Jay Levinson

Creative Ideas for Selling Products

Have fun with retailing. As with any type of marketing, the more interesting you make it, the more likely you are to do it, and the more likely it will be effective. Several creative ideas for selling products include spotlighting products, bundling products, and public speaking.

Spotlight Products

Choose a limited number of products to highlight on a monthly basis. Put those items on a focus area in your waiting room or a tray in your office, make a sign about the special product(s), and mention your top products in your promotional materials.

Also, use products throughout your office building. For example, if you carry a line of soaps or lotions, place them in the bathroom for your clients to use. Always display a retail sized product in your treatment room. For instance, you might have an extra large bottle of lotion that you use for your treatments, but it's wise to nicely display the size bottle that a client would be likely to purchase.

Bundle Products

Bundling products together with other products or certificates is an effective sales technique. These bundles can be designed for clients to purchase for themselves or to give as gifts. People are always looking for unique gifts year round! Bundling products with a gift certificate provides instant gratification (the products) and something for later (the session).

Some examples of theme bundles are self-care, relaxation, pain management, new mom, traveler, and stress-buster. For instance, if one of your target markets is executives who travel frequently, you could assemble a travel kit consisting of an eye pillow, essential oil, and a small self-massage tool.

You can also create seasonal bundles. This could be for holidays, the actual seasons (winter, spring, summer, or fall), or health-related seasons (e.g., flu season). Consider pairing items that you sell in your practice along with other festive items. For instance, in February (Valentine's Day) you could bundle a self-care tool, an essential oil, a mug, and chocolate.

When assembling bundles, offer a variety of packages that range in price, so your clients can feel good about the purchase while staying in their financial comfort zone. Consider putting together a basic kit that costs approximately $25, a pampering kit in the $50 range, and a deluxe kit that costs $100 or more. If a gift certificate for your services isn't included in the kit, make a sign that encourages people to add a certificate. For instance, your $50 kit could say something like, "$50 for the kit. Add a gift certificate for a 1-hour session for only $50 more!" Package the products attractively. You can use baskets or pretty bags. Sometimes, simply attaching a ribbon makes a purchase seem special.

See Chapter 25, pages 394-397 for more on **public speaking**.

Public Speaking

Include products whenever you host open houses or give public presentations or demonstrations. These can be part of the presentation itself, where you explain how the products align with your work. Educate the audience about the products. Ideally, you would have the participants experience the products. After the presentation, the participants can purchase those items. Even if the products aren't an integral part of your presentation, you could simply have a nice product display for people to look at (and hopefully purchase) before and after the presentation.

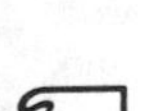

Present Yourslf Powerfully

sohnen-moe.com/prodinfo/pyp.php

Closing the Sale

For some practitioners, selling products is as natural as booking the next session. Others struggle with both. If you've done a thorough intake interview and truly listened to your clients, you have a fairly accurate knowledge of their needs and wants. After the one-on-one segment of the session is finished (and if you do massage, the client is dressed), give a very brief overview of what took place in the session, highlight some of the client's major goals, assign homework, give the client an opportunity to ask questions, make any necessary referrals, discuss which products might be helpful to purchase (and sell those products or provide samples), and schedule the next appointment.

See Chapter 6, page 102 for details on asking **open-ended questions**.

Fostering Ongoing Sales

The key to working smarter—not harder is to develop long-term product sales relationships with your clients. Follow up on product sales, especially after the initial sale. Contact clients several days after their session. Ask them how they're enjoying the product, what results they notice, and what questions they might have. If you gave them samples, ask if they would like you to reserve/order a larger size. Also, consider sending thank-you notes after the first sale or a large sale. Some practitioners offer a modified type of frequent buyer plan that rewards clients for their purchases. It could be a free product, a free service, or a special discount.

Make notes in your client files about their purchases and product preferences. Also, review those files for important dates that could lead to future purchases (e.g., birthdays, anniversaries, seasonal changes, vacations). If clients purchase consumables (items that get used up, such as scrubs and topicals), make a note in their files as to the estimated date those products will need to be replenished, and send a follow-up reminder. Also, when making appointment confirmations, check to see if they're running low on any products and offer to put those items aside for them. Take the time to design a plan of action that fosters ongoing sales and then be sure to notify current and potential clients through your website, newsletters, print materials, and office signage.

Merchandising

The *Merriam-Webster Dictionary* defines merchandising as "the activity of trying to sell goods or services by advertising them or displaying them attractively."[2] This section explores how to display products in a manner that draws clients to check them out and inspires them to buy. Humans are sensitive. Appeal to all the senses: sight, smell, hearing, touch, taste. The more you can do this, the easier it is for the products to essentially sell themselves.

Visibility

Make sure people can easily see what you offer for sale. Don't place product behind a receptionist's desk where it might be unnoticed or inaccessible to clients. Display retail products throughout your office space in addition to a specific area that is dedicated to displaying your merchandise. Also, consider displaying retail sizes of certain products (e.g., the lotion you use in the session) in your treatment room.

Shelf Talkers

www.shelftalkers.com

Regardless of the size of your office, you want your retail area to be attractive. Keep the space organized, clean (regularly wipe down all testers and make sure there are no dust bunnies or rancid product), well-lit (so people can read labels, prices, and instructions), and appeal to all of the senses. If you don't have a waiting room, display products on a mirror or small glass shelf inside the session room, or on top of a rolling case if you do on-site work.

Identify all products with price tags or signs. People might assume that the product is too expensive and not even ask. Also, utilize shelf talkers (signs or clips that draw attention to a product) to spark interest and boost sales.

Design

Display your products in an eye-catching manner. In general, it's best to avoid just putting items on a shelf as they can easily get disorganized. Point-of-sale (POS) displays (also known as point-of-purchase, or POP) are effective ways to attractively display products. Get POS displays that fit easily onto a countertop, on a shelf, in a front room, or even on a table in the classroom (for when you do public speaking). If you're unable to purchase POS units that are specifically designed for the product lines you carry, you can purchase them from companies that make attractive, generic units. Some of those companies can even customize your display unit.

POS Display Units

www.cardboarddisplays.com
www.displays2go.com
www.displaywarehouse.com

You can also put products in baskets or other containers. In one of my retailing workshops, participants had to design a marketing and merchandising plan for a specific product. The winning group displayed an arrangement of foot balms, foot rollers, and other foot care products in a shoe.

Arrange seating areas around product testing stations (e.g., essential oils, skin care products, self-care tools), and create a feature area to highlight new products and seasonal items. This feature area can be a separate section of the waiting area or an area created by using decorative items, rolled towels, baskets, or plants.

Eye Appeal = Buy Appeal
Eye Level = Buy Level

Consider putting a pitcher of water (perhaps with lemon slices, cucumber slices, or mint leaves) and glasses in the same area as your retail products. This way, when clients walk over to get a drink, they see your products. Also, if you encourage clients to arrive a few minutes before your session to update any paperwork and transition from the rest of their day to getting a session, it's likely that they will check out your products while waiting. The same is true for encouraging them to spend some time in the waiting room after a session before transitioning back into the world.

Display smaller impulse items, sale products, or new items on the front desk area. Change the general retail displays at least 3 times per year, placing new or seasonal items in featured areas. Change the items in the feature areas every 4-8 weeks.

Some other specific ways to be creative with your merchandising is to have themes for holidays and special events. You might put up signs or decorations or even carry special "seasonal" types of items (e.g., products that evoke the smell of pumpkin pie). Jenny Hogan, media director for Marketing Solutions Inc., suggests, "Use holiday decorations as a backdrop for retail sales. You can put gift certificates or holiday coupons in transparent ornaments and hang them on wreaths, garlands, or a Christmas tree."[3]

Product Sales Tips

www.retailmastery.com

www.facebook.com/RetailMastery

Drive Your BUS to Success

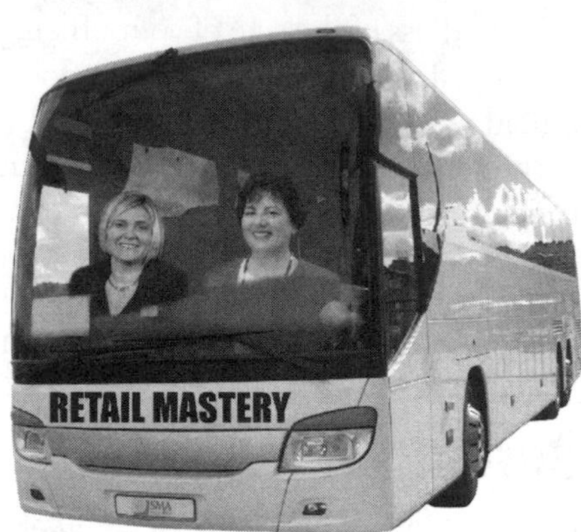

I've been collaborating with Lynda Solien-Wolfe, Vice President of Massage & Spa at Performance Health, for several years on the topic of retailing. We've facilitated workshops, written articles and blogs, and have a website and a Facebook page on this topic. She coined a phrase that has inspired us throughout this adventure:

When it comes to retailing, you need to drive your BUS to selling success!

B Believe in the products you use.
U Use the products in your sessions.
S Supply samples to your clients.

I wish you good fortune and safe travels on your retailing journey!

Figure 21.6 Retail Mastery Tips

- Conduct product research before you offer products for resale.
- Try a product before offering it in any session or for retail in your practice.
- Sell only products that fit into the type of work you do or gift items that align with your image.
- Choose products you believe in and trust.
- Find products that aren't easily accessible to your clients.
- Educate yourself and your staff on the products you use and sell.
- Focus on a few product lines.
- Purchase products from a distributor/manufacturer that offers marketing support.
- Charge a fair but profitable price.
- Encourage questions about the products used during sessions.
- Ask clients for their reaction to, and opinions on, the products being used.
- Make recommendations for homework and products during the post-interview.
- Display your products and promotional literature in your waiting area.
- Make the products visible and attractive.
- Put the products on display so clients can see, feel, and smell the product.
- Bundle items.
- Put price stickers on your products.
- Utilize Shelf Talkers.
- Put testers on display.
- Keep the display area clean, organized, and well lit.
- If you carry self-care DVDs, play them before and after sessions in the waiting area.
- Utilize products during the session.
- Print flyers that describe all the products you carry.
- Promote specials in your waiting area, newsletters, social media, and website.
- Make price sheets and recommendation sheets available for clients.
- Keep track of your sales and inventory.
- Know your local, state, and federal tax laws.
- Offer samples to your clients. If a client tries and likes a product, the product will sell itself!

22
People Management

"Always treat your employees exactly as you want them to treat your best customers."
—Stephen R. Covey

What Makes a Good Employer?

Hiring Help
- Administrative Support Staff
- Sources for Finding Help
- Employment Regulations
- Independent Contractor Status
- Interviewing Practitioners

Managing Your Staff
- Employment Policies
- Performance Reviews
- Cultivate Camaraderie

Key Terms

Administrative Support Staff
Camaraderie
Common Law Rules
Employee
Employee Policies
Employer
Employer Identification Number (EIN)
Employment Forms
Employment Regulations
Federal Insurance Contributions Act (FICA)
Federal Unemployment Tax Act (FUTA)
Independent Contractor
Job Description
Performance Reviews
Workers' Compensation

It might not be completely obvious when it's time to consider hiring help. You may be ready to take that next step if you find yourself working a lot of hours just to keep up with your clients' scheduling needs, working late hours to get administrative tasks done, or you simply want to take an extended vacation or regular time off.

As your business builds, you may find that it's more cost-effective for someone else to handle the administrative, accounting, and housekeeping tasks, or to take on some of the client load. This is the time to hire outside help; either as employees or independent contractors.

Once you make the decision to add employment relationships to your practice, you must step out of the role of practitioner and into the role of employer. The attitudes and skills that make someone a good employer aren't necessarily the same as that of a practitioner.

What Makes a Good Employer?

Becoming an employer requires dualistic thinking. You must simultaneously hold the best interests of your company and the best interests of your employees in equal measure. *The Ethics of Touch* states, "The reality of the power differential means that, ethically, a business should take a protective role towards its employees."[1] That means, you're now responsible for the success of your business and for your employees.

> "A good manager is a man who isn't worried about his own career but rather the careers of those who work for him.
> —H.S.M. Burns

A good employer is one who understands the mutual benefits of the employment relationship. Just as you, the employer, provide an opportunity for others to do their work, the employees are providing you with growth and success opportunities by doing good work. When you successfully demonstrate your understanding of this mutually beneficial relationship, your employees are satisfied and everybody wins.

To demonstrate your "good employer" skills, you don't have to veer far from your practitioner skills. Good employer skills include the ability to:

- Be a direct communicator.
- Keep accurate and thorough records.
- Investigate issues and make fair decisions.
- See the strength in diverse beliefs, skills, and thought-processes.
- Provide a safe and secure work environment.
- Maintain honesty and integrity.
- Expect commitment and loyalty.
- Encourage cooperation.
- Provide clear policies and procedures.
- Deal with difficult situations swiftly and confidently.

These may sound simple and obvious, but it takes considerable time and excellent communication skills to be a good boss. Train your staff to understand the type of work you do so they can explain it to potential clients. You need to organize your business to make certain there's enough work to be done, hold staff meetings, give employees regular feedback, and be willing to delegate. You earn respect as a good employer if you let your employees know you care about them and their success.

Hiring Help

If you find yourself working a lot of hours just to keep up with your clients' scheduling needs, or you work late hours to get the administrative tasks done, you may be ready to hire someone to help you.

Expanding your practice by bringing in other practitioners or support staff can free you to focus on what you do best. This relates to honoring yourself and valuing your time. Often we do everything ourselves instead of delegating tasks, and this usually isn't the wisest use of our time. For example, let's say you charge $60 an hour for your services and it takes you 3 hours per week to clean your office. Most cleaning services charge about $20 per hour. If you were to hire a service rather than do the cleaning yourself, you could spend those 3 hours working with clients. It would cost you approximately 1 hour's worth of service ($60). This leaves you with 2 extra hours in which to make a profit of $120.

I realize this isn't as simple as it sounds. Often it means taking a risk, because you might not get those extra appointments. Consider, though, that the more you focus on income-producing activities, the more profitable your practice becomes.

> "Give me a stock clerk with a goal and I'll give you a man who will make history. Give me a man with no goals and I'll give you a stock clerk.
> —J.C. Penney

Hiring office support staff can free you up to spend more time with clients or focus on marketing tasks to help grow your business. Administrative tasks (e.g., scheduling and confirming appointments, organizing client records, purchasing supplies), can usually be handled efficiently and cost-effectively by someone other than yourself. Financial matters (e.g., bookkeeping, tax preparation, payroll, filing insurance claims), can easily be assigned to another person or firm. Many of the maintenance duties in your practice can be handled by janitorial and laundry services.

Some wellness providers hire a marketing consultant to coordinate their promotions and advertising, organize special events, oversee the graphic design and printing of promotional materials, and schedule speaking engagements. The most common manner in which practitioners enlist additional help is by including other wellness providers in their business. This usually occurs when a practice has grown to the point at which there is a client overflow or the owner wants to expand the scope of modalities and services offered to current clients.

Figure 22.1 The Hiring Process Steps

1. Identify your needs.
2. Write a clear job description.
3. Recruit and advertise in appropriate media.
4. Choose 3-5 applicants to interview.
5. Involve other team members in the interview process (if applicable).
6. Select the best candidate or continue the search until you find the right one.

Administrative Support Staff

§6

Administrative support staff are key team members in any small business. They're often the first point of contact that a potential client has with your business. In those first few minutes (as well as in the continuing relationship with established clients), your support staff establishes the persona of your business: its image and philosophy. Therefore, hiring the right type of person with the proper skills for your particular job requirements and client service is critical.

The first step is to identify what type of support you need. What are the job duties? Are you looking for a receptionist, secretary, bookkeeper, administrative assistant, or operations manager? Each type of position has differing job duties and responsibilities. Some common office tasks are filing, answering the phones, taking messages, producing monthly reports, submitting insurance claims, analyzing data, marketing, maintaining databases, managing inventory, and proofreading. Determine whether the position is part or full time, the hours you require, and the wage rate according to the demands of the position and skill level required.

Schedule ample time to screen candidates, interview effectively, and hire intelligently. The better you can clearly and concisely communicate job requirements to an applicant, the better prepared the applicant will be to realistically assess if the job is a right fit. A well-written job description helps define your needs and provides a better chance to avoid hiring the wrong person.

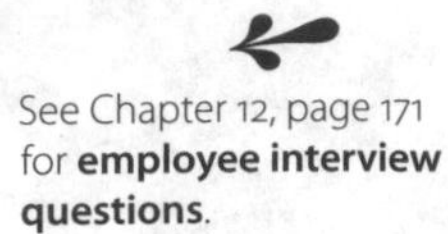
See Chapter 12, page 171 for **employee interview questions**.

Once you've established the position's duties, responsibilities, and the personality you need to project the persona of your business, design your interview questions to elicit the most information about your candidates and ascertain whether they fit into the mold. Consider the following scenario:

A manager had gone through 5 secretaries in 1 year. She finally admitted that obviously something was amiss, otherwise, why would 5 different secretaries quit within a one-year period? The manager established that she needed to know what would make an individual person quit. Hence, in the interview, 1 of the questions she asked was simply, "What would make you quit a job?" She also got feedback from her previous employees and established a certain "personality" that she knew was needed to work together effectively and harmoniously.

Points to Ponder

What other questions would you ask during an interview with a potential employee? From whom else could you gather information about your own management style and personality?

By identifying your position well and designing your interview effectively, you enable yourself to choose the best possible support staff—not just for yourself and your business persona, but for those you serve.

Sources for Finding Help

There are many options to explore when looking for quality people to assist you with your business. You can hire independent contractors, consultants, or employees. You may even find someone to work as an intern or apprentice. You can contract with a company that provides specific business services (e.g., secretarial, answering service, laundry, bookkeeping, janitorial). Or you may hire a "temporary employee" through an employment agency or even an employee leasing company—then you won't have to worry about all the paperwork, because those agencies are responsible for withholding taxes, paying appropriate fees such as workers' compensation, and filing all the governmental forms. Another option is to form associations with other business owners to share tasks and expenses.

As for where to find good people, many cities have online employment resources such as Craigslist or Careerbuilder. You may also want to check your local Chamber of Commerce for resource listings and tap into local business networking groups. Often, local or regional industry trade association websites or trade publications include job listings (these are particularly useful if you're looking for a wellness practitioner or independent contractor). Community newspapers can be a good source for finding cleaning and laundry services. If you're looking for part-time help, check with career centers or job boards at local colleges and universities. Lastly, you may want to search the Internet using keywords, as each city offers different types of resources.

Employment Regulations

Deciding whether to hire an employee or subcontract for the services you need can be a difficult decision. You may want to incorporate a variety of people and service providers in your business support team. Most small businesses prefer to hire independent contractors, consultants, or service firms rather than employees.

The IRS guidelines for determining employment status are fairly clear when it comes to administrative staff: in most instances, an office support person is an employee. A gray area exists in hiring other wellness providers.

IRS publication 15, (Circular E) **Employer's Tax Guide**
www.irs.gov/pub/irs-pdf/p15.pdf

Generally, it's much easier and less risky to terminate a contract than to fire an employee. Also, your liability is reduced in terms of malpractice if you hire independent contractors, because you can require they carry their own insurance. The potential pitfalls of working with non-employees include paying a higher price for their services and not having control over their work in terms of timeliness and quality.

I may seem to be making a strong case for not hiring employees. Au contraire! Many practitioners and clinic owners claim they couldn't have achieved their level of success without employees. It can be extremely helpful and comforting to know that someone is going to be at your office every day taking care of business. A strong bond tends to develop between employees and the business owner, particularly in a small business. The peace of mind and sense of stability this creates is invaluable. You also receive the other benefits as previously mentioned when you can focus on your high priority activities.

I've interviewed and consulted with many business owners, and the majority prefer to have practitioners work as employees rather than independent contractors. The benefits far outweigh the drawbacks. Practitioners who are employees tend to be more committed, and there's a heightened sense of camaraderie. Employees are there to help build your business, while independent contractors are attempting to build their own businesses. If you decide to hire an employee but are concerned about the regulations and paperwork, you can pay an accountant or payroll service to do it for you.

U.S. state and federal law require all employers to report each newly hired employee to the **State Directory of New Hires**.

In addition to the responsibility of having enough money for employee paychecks, you need to comply with various payroll requirements. In the U.S., you must match their FICA (Social Security and Medicare) deductions; pay FUTA (Federal Unemployment Tax Act); pay state unemployment taxes; provide workers' compensation; withhold state and federal taxes; deposit withheld taxes; file regular returns; and send W-2 forms to employees annually. In many instances, to stay competitive with other employers, you need to offer benefits such as health insurance, paid time off, sick leave, and retirement plans. Consider these costs when calculating how much it really costs to hire an employee, as the total costs could be more than 40% above pay cost.[2]

Two of the employment forms you need are SS-4, Application for Employer Identification Number, and Form W-4, Employee's Withholding Allowance Certificate. Check with your state employment department for requirements, fees, and forms. In addition to a Federal Employer's Identification Number (EIN), you need a state EIN. All employees must also fill out Form I-9, Employment Eligibility Verification (from the U.S. Department of Justice, Immigration, and Naturalization Service).

§6

You don't have to withhold income tax or Social Security tax from independent contractors. But if you pay an independent contractor $600 or more during the year in the course of your trade or business, you must file a form 1099-MISC at the end of the year. That form is optional if you've contracted with a service company.

The sample Employment Agreement in Figure 22.3 is for illustrative purposes only and not intended for use as a legal document.

Independent Contractor Status

IRS: ***"Independent Contractor (Self-Employed) or Employee?"***
www.irs.gov/Businesses/Small-Businesses-&-Self-Employed/Independent-Contractor-Self-Employed-or-Employee

As an employer, you take a considerable risk by deeming a worker an independent contractor. If the IRS determines that your independent contractors are (or were) indeed employees, you may be required to pay fines of up to 100% of the tax, in addition to the back income taxes and Social Security taxes. This easily adds up to a sizable amount. In the eyes of the IRS, it makes no difference if you signed an agreement that states you're contracting with an independent contractor—although a written agreement is advisable. Many spas, clinics, and group practices

SBA: *"Hire a Contractor or an Employee"*

www.sba.gov/content/hire-contractor-or-employee

IRS Form SS-8

www.irs.gov/pub/irs-pdf/fss8.pdf

walk a very thin legal line. A significant number of the so-called independent contractors they have working for them would most likely be classified as employees under the IRS guidelines.

You can minimize the risks of your independent contractors being reclassified as employees by taking the following steps: make certain independent contractors have multiple sources of income; sign "independent contractor" agreements which clearly state the requirements of all parties while making it clear the contractors are free to pursue other clients; require contractors to provide their own tables, linens, products, music, and other supplies; allow contractors to set their own schedules (ideally, no more than 10 hours per week or on an as-needed basis for special events); have clients pay contractors directly; request copies of the contractors' tax returns; and require contractors to provide their own insurance and Workers' Compensation coverage.

Complying to these suggestions still doesn't guarantee independent contractor status. If in doubt, you can have the IRS determine whether a worker is an employee by filing Form SS-8. Get legal counsel to develop an independent contractor agreement. Include a work description for each subcontracting assignment along with a policy and procedure statement.

Figure 22.2 Employee vs. Independent Contractor in the Wellness Industry

The key elements that differentiate between employee status and independent contractor status in the wellness industry are:

- Who regulates the type of work done and how it's performed
- Where and when the sessions occur
- Who determines the fee structure
- Who receives the money from the clients
- Who provides the equipment and supplies
- Who pays for client-related expenses
- Who generates the clientele

Common Law Rules

Under common-law rules, anyone who performs services subject to the will and control of an employer, as to both what must be done and how it must be done, is an employee. It doesn't matter that you allow the employee discretion and freedom of action, so long as you have the legal right to control both the method and result of the services.

The IRS looks for evidence of control in three categories: behavioral, financial, and the type of relationship. Do you have the right to control how they do their job? Do you have the right to determine how they're paid? Do you offer employee-type benefits? Is the work they perform a primary aspect of your business?

In general, it's wise to consider an individual as an employee unless you can prove otherwise.

Just because the employee provides his own specific tools and supplies, doesn't necessarily mean they're independent. "Tools" is a broad term that can include the equipment required in running a practice, such as telephones and copiers.

From an IRS viewpoint, if an employer-employee relationship can be established through evidence of control, it's irrelevant how it's described. It doesn't matter if the employee is called an employee, associate, partner, or independent contractor, you must have evidence to support the classification you choose. It also doesn't matter how the payments are measured, made, or what they're called. Nor does it matter if the individual is employed full time or part time.

The key is to evaluate control and independence in each of the three categories, determine a classification, and most importantly, document the factors that you used to determine that classification.

Other Government Agency Guidelines

State workers' compensation, unemployment compensation, and tax agencies use various tests to determine worker status. Many use the common-law right of control test, but emphasize different factors than the IRS. Each agency is concerned with worker classification for different reasons, and has different biases and practices. Thus, it's possible for one agency to view an individual as an employee, while another agency may view the same individual as an independent contractor.

The sample Independent Contractor Agreement in Figure 22.4 is for illustrative purposes only and not intended for use as legal document. Please confer with an attorney before finalizing any legal agreements to ensure the document meets IRS guidelines.

Interviewing Practitioners

Screening applicants and interviewing potential employees can be tricky. You usually get a good (or bad) first impression rather quickly, but finding out how someone will perform on the job can be a difficult task. If you run a touch therapy practice, professional and effective treatments are essential to your success, and how your employees interact with clients is a critical factor. A well structured interview helps you avoid employee issues down the road.

During the hiring process, many employers require applicants to give a practical session in addition to the interview. This may or may not be an entire treatment session, but enough to evaluate hands-on skills and quality of touch. What many employers forget to evaluate is the interactions before and after a treatment.

I recommend having the potential employee complete an entire client interaction routine with you. Have her greet you in the lobby, discuss the intake process with you (e.g., client forms, expectations), describe the treatment plan, and then provide the treatment. After the treatment, continue in "client" mode and have her discuss the treatment and rebooking (if appropriate), and any other things she would normally discuss with clients as they complete their time at your office. This helps you get a much better idea of her professionalism and communication skills.

Then return to the hiring process interview to ask any follow-up questions. Ideally, complete the interview process in a separate physical space from the treatment room, as this helps the applicant transition from practitioner persona to interview persona.

Figure 22.3 Sample Massage Therapy Employment Agreement

This agreement, dated July 4, 2020, is by and between Holistic Health Clinic ("Employer"), with principal offices located at 1776 Independence Way, Washington, D.C., and Frank Benjamin ("Employee").

Services to Be Provided by Employee

Employee agrees to provide massage therapy services within the scope of licensure. Employee is responsible for maintaining appropriate certification and licensure (including all costs thereof). Employee agrees to dress in a style consistent with the Employer's image and as stated in the Employee Manual. Employee shall maintain client records in the manner prescribed by employer.

When Employee isn't engaged in treatments, Employee shall assist with other office duties as directed, including but not limited to:

a. Assisting other practitioners with clients.
b. Performing clerical duties.
c. Cleaning and organizing the clinic.

This form is for illustrative purposes only. It is not intended for use as a legal document.

Services to Be Provided by Employer

Employer shall provide the following: a safe, clean environment; a room furnished with a chair or settee, stool, hydraulic table, hydrotherapy equipment, and storage area; receptionist services; appointment scheduling; insurance billing; marketing; and all necessary supplies and materials used in the performance of services (e.g., oils, lotions, linens, music).

Other Provisions

a. Employee has the right to perform services for others during the term of this Agreement, however such services are not to be performed on Employer's premises.
b. Employee shall not solicit or provide services to Employer's clients for private practice while employed or for 6 months after termination of employment, except as noted in "c."
c. Upon termination of employment, Employer and Employee shall discuss which clients, under what conditions, and with what compensation, Employee may maintain continuity of service.
d. All client records shall remain the property of the Employer.
e. All Employee's non-clinic marketing materials that include any information about Employer, must be approved in advance by the Employer.

Fees, Terms of Payment, and Fringe Benefits

Employee shall be compensated at the base rate of $10 per hour, with an additional $7 per half-hour massage and $17 per hour massage, not to exceed 30 hours per week. Employee shall be paid biweekly. Employee shall receive payment on all services performed regardless of the collection time. Employee is eligible to participate in any of the following fringe benefits: health insurance, vacation time, and employee pension plan (see Employee Manual for eligibility requirements).

Local, State, and Federal Taxes

Employer is responsible for withholding all required income, Social Security, and Medicare taxes.

Workers' Compensation and Unemployment Insurance

Employer will provide Workers' Compensation and Unemployment Insurance.

Insurance

During the term of this agreement, Employee shall maintain a malpractice insurance policy of at least $2,000,000 aggregate annual and $1,000,000 per incident. Employer shall maintain insurance coverage for liability, fire, and theft.

Terms of Agreement

Either party may terminate this agreement, given reasonable cause, as provided below, or by giving 30 days written notice to the other party of the intention to terminate this Agreement:

a. Material violation of the provisions of this Agreement.
b. Action by either party exposing the other to liability for property damage or personal injury.
c. Violation of ethical standards as defined by local, state, and/or national associations and governing bodies.
d. Loss of licensure for services provided.
e. Employee fails to maintain the standard of service deemed appropriate by Employer.
f. Employee engages in any pattern or course of conduct on a continuing basis which adversely affects Employee's ability to perform services.
g. Employee engages in any pattern or course of conduct on a continuing basis which adversely affects Employer's or other Employees' ability to perform services.
h. It is agreed that any unresolved disputes will be settled by arbitration, including costs thereof.

This constitutes the entire agreement between Employee and Employer and supersedes any and all prior written or verbal agreements. Should any part of this agreement be deemed unenforceable, the remainder of the agreement continues in effect. This agreement is governed by the laws of the District of Columbia.

Signatures, Dates

Figure 22.4 **Sample Massage Therapy Independent Contractor Agreement**

This agreement, dated July 4, 2020, is by and between Mobile Holistic Health Services ("Company"), with principal office located at 1776 Independence Way, Washington, D.C., and Frank Benjamin ("Contractor"), with principal office located at 1912 Thomas Jefferson Blvd., Washington, D.C.

Status as Independent Contractor

Contractor is an independent contractor and not an employee of the Company. As an independent contractor, Company and Contractor agree to the following:

a. Contractor has control of the means, manner, and method by which services are provided.
b. Contractor furnishes all necessary supplies and materials used in the performance of services (e.g., oils, lotions, linens, music).
c. Contractor has the right to perform services for others during the term of this Agreement. Contractor shall not solicit services to Company's clients for private practice during the term of this Agreement or for 1 year after termination. Upon termination of Agreement, Contractor and Company shall discuss which clients, under what conditions, and with what compensation Contractor may maintain continuity of service. All client records shall remain the property of the Company unless otherwise agreed.
d. Contractor shall indemnify and hold Company harmless from any loss or liability arising from services provided under this agreement.
e. Contractor is responsible for maintaining appropriate certification and licensure, including all costs thereof.

This form is for illustrative purposes only. It is not intended for use as a legal document.

Services to Be Provided by Contractor

Contractor agrees to provide massage therapy services within the scope of Contractor's license. Contractor agrees to dress in a style consistent with the Company's image. Contractor shall maintain client records in a mutually agreed manner.

Services to Be Provided by Company

Company shall provide the following: a safe, clean environment; appointment scheduling according to Contractor's stipulated hours; and marketing.

Other Provisions

All Contractor's marketing materials, which include any information about Company, must be approved in advance.

Fees and Terms of Payment

Company shall pay the Contractor $35 per massage. Contractor acknowledges that Contractor is not eligible to receive employee benefits.

Local, State, and Federal Taxes

Contractor is responsible for paying and filing all applicable income, Social Security, and Medicare taxes.

Workers' Compensation and Unemployment Insurance

Company is not responsible for payment of Workers' Compensation and Unemployment Insurance. If Company is a corporation, Contractor must provide Company with a certificate of Workers' Compensation Insurance prior to performing services.

Unemployment Compensation

Company shall make no state or federal unemployment compensation payments on behalf of Contractor. Contractor is not entitled to these benefits in connection with work performed under this Agreement.

Insurance

During the term of this agreement, Contractor shall maintain a malpractice insurance policy of at least $2,000,000 aggregate annual and $1,000,000 per incident.

Terms of Agreement

Either party may terminate this agreement, given reasonable cause, as provided below, or by giving 30 days written notice to the other party of the intention to terminate this Agreement:

a. Material violation of the provisions of this Agreement.
b. Action by either party exposing the other to liability for property damage or personal injury.
c. Violation of ethical standards as defined by local, state, and/or national associations and governing bodies.
d. Loss of licensure for services provided.
e. Contractor engages in any pattern or course of conduct on a continuing basis which adversely affects Contractor's ability to perform services.
f. Contractor engages in any pattern or course of conduct on a continuing basis which adversely affects Company's or Company's associates' ability to perform services.
g. It is agreed that any unresolved disputes are to be settled by mediation. Any costs and fees, other than attorney fees associated with the mediation, shall be shared equally by the parties. If the dispute is not resolved within 30 days after it is referred to the mediator, any party may pursue further action.

This constitutes the entire agreement between Contractor and Company, and supersedes any and all prior written or verbal agreements. Should any part of this agreement be deemed unenforceable, the remainder of the agreement continues in effect. This agreement is governed by the laws of the District of Columbia.

Signatures, Dates

Managing Your Staff

As a manager or owner, you're responsible for "supporting" all the members of your team, including your support staff. Simply establishing positions and hiring the appropriate people isn't the end, it's the beginning of a working relationship. A crucial concept to grasp is that you're working "with" your staff, not managing your staff from an ivory tower. This establishes a sense of teamwork and camaraderie. Quality intercommunication is essential, since you work with your staff many hours during the work week. If issues arise regarding job performance, they need to be handled diplomatically and quickly.

> "Motivate employees, train them, care about them, and make winners of them. At Marriott we know that if we treat our employees correctly, they'll treat the customers right. And if the customers are treated right, they'll come back.
> —Bill Marriott Jr.

Carefully listen to all team members' input, as they're the ones who deal with daily tasks and generally have some very creative, imaginative, and efficient methods of conducting their work. Never underestimate your staff. Your staff is one of the greatest assets to your business. While they may not all have college degrees or be versed in the intricacies of your profession, they may provide valuable insights and practical solutions to everyday problems.

When managing your business, allow plenty of individual autonomy; avoid micromanagement (i.e., an over-controlling approach to things). Give your staff the authority to make decisions. Make certain your team understands company policies and procedures, and knows when to take initiative and when to confer with you before taking action. It's important to oversee your staff and review their actions, yet refrain from monitoring their every move. You can enhance teamwork by identifying and eliminating barriers that limit employees' responsibilities and decision-making abilities.

Employment Policies

See Chapter 18, page 252 for more on **personnel guidelines** to include in a **policies and procedures manual**.

Employment policies cover the requirements and expectations of your staff. These are often included in your general policy manual, or you may decide to have a separate staff handbook. This is your opportunity to set clear expectations for conduct, behavior, procedures, and communication, as well as the defined roles for you and your employee(s).

Figure 22.5 Employment Policies Checklist

- ❑ Expectations of work quality and customer service standards
- ❑ Chain of command
- ❑ Work hours and schedule
- ❑ Salary, raises, overtime, pay dates, leaves of absence, tardiness, sick leave, and bonuses
- ❑ Benefits package and eligibility requirements
- ❑ Personnel records, grievance procedures, and performance reviews
- ❑ Dress code, hygiene, smoking, and phone use
- ❑ Parking
- ❑ Employee discounts (of services and products) and purchasing procedures
- ❑ Actions requiring discipline and specific consequences
- ❑ Disciplinary procedures and grounds for termination

Performance Reviews

Institute annual performance reviews that evaluate job performance and establish goals and objectives for the coming year. Review the position duties and responsibilities and make adjustments according to the changing needs of your office operations. Make this performance review a two-way communication. Ask your staff members to clarify:

1. What are their perceptions of their duties and responsibilities?
2. What contributions have they made to the position other than the mechanics of the job?
3. What are their goals and objectives for the coming year?
4. What additional seminars, lectures, or outside activities would they like to attend?

Answer these questions from your own perspective and then sit down together to review them. This allows each of you to jointly assess the previous year, while lessening the opportunity for misunderstanding and poor communication about each of your expectations and needs. Included in this performance evaluation should be an objective review of performance (e.g., quality of work, quantity of work, communication, timeliness).

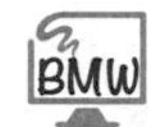

Sample **Employer Checklist for Performance Evaluation**

https://sohnen-moe.com/bm5-workbook-request/

A well-designed performance evaluation is an excellent management tool that promotes effective, clear communication and establishes a sense of teamwork. This helps form a satisfying working relationship. Avoid waiting until the end of the coming year to informally discuss progress and concerns. Conduct informal reviews quarterly, if not monthly. This provides an occasion for you to affirm exceptional performance, correct minor difficulties before they become major problems, and initiate changes in operational needs in a timely manner. It also allows your staff the opportunity to discuss matters of concern they may have in their working relationship with you or your clients.

Cultivate Camaraderie

In addition to reviews, hold regular staff meetings. These should be at least once per month and preferably once per week. These meetings serve to build camaraderie, as well as provide a forum to discuss problems, learn new skills, brainstorm ideas, and set goals. It also keeps everyone informed and fosters better understanding and teamwork when people are aware of each other's projects and deadlines. Ideally, limit these meetings to less than one hour.

Every business has the "Jobs That Nobody Wants To Do." These tasks are either boring, unpleasant, or difficult to accomplish. Resentments can easily arise around these noxious tasks. As a manager, you need to find a way to balance these duties among your staff. This can be difficult when you only have one employee or if you're the only person in your business. If you're lucky, you will find someone who loves to do those tasks that everyone else hates. Alas, such people are rare. So, the next best option is to hold a staff meeting and brainstorm ideas for dealing with these tasks. Conducting brainstorming sessions and including your staff in some of the decision-making processes enhances teamwork. When people feel that they're working as a team, they're less apt to feel resentful over having to do those "awful" assignments.

One of the outcomes of a brainstorming session might be a change in the company's operations and procedures. Sometimes a slight alteration in the execution of a task can alleviate the dread associated with it. Frequently, tasks can be simplified or even eliminated. Changes don't occur very often because people rarely take the time to evaluate policies, procedures, and goals. Another outcome of the brainstorming session may be that the staff decides to rotate these unpleasant tasks. Whatever the results of this session are, it's imperative that you follow through by monitoring progress.

> "One of the reasons people stop learning is that they become less and less willing to risk failure.
> —John W. Gardner

People are motivated most by recognition, appreciation, and participation. Each person on your team requires a different type of encouragement. Get input from your staff and develop incentive programs. By skillfully managing your staff, you create a happy and harmonious team, an efficient workplace, and an environment that fosters good relationships with both employees and clients—all of which adds up to a healthy bottom line.

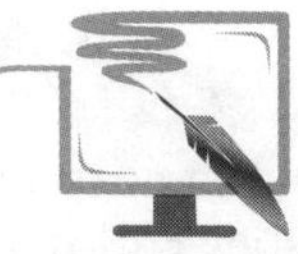

People Management Skills

1. Review the "Good Employer" skills at the beginning of this chapter. Which do you excel at and which are challenging for you? Ask a mentor for feedback regarding your potential challenges on this list of skills. Make a plan for enhancing any weak skills.
2. Get together with one or more colleagues and practice an employee interview. Develop a list of 10 questions to ask the potential employee during the interview. Take turns being the employer, focusing on asking questions and waiting for the answer without interruption.
3. Create a scenario in which your employee needs to be reviewed on a performance issue. With a colleague, practice 2 discussions: the initial discussion with the employee regarding the performance issue; and a follow-up discussion (that would happen a week or two later) to review how or if the employee's performance has changed. Reflect on the practice discussions and update your procedure manual with suggestions, key phrases, and perhaps even a specific protocol (so that you will feel more confident doing actual performance reviews).
4. Create an agenda for regular staff meetings. What subjects need to be discussed on a regular basis? How do you allow for discussion of special circumstances or brainstorming of new ideas? Think of ways to limit the amount of side-conversations and personal discussions, to maintain the specific meeting timeframe.

23
Transitioning Your Business

"Trust your instincts, and make judgments on what your heart tells you. The heart will not betray you."

—David Gemmell

Choose Your Direction
- Decision-Making Pinnacles
- Exploration and Evaluation
- Options

Selling a Practice
- Four Ways to Leave Your Business
- The Eight Selling Stages

Closing a Practice

Key Terms

Acceptance
Adjusted Cash Flow
Affordability
Analyze
Assets
Attention
Capitalized Earnings
Carry Back
Cash Flow
Contingency Clause
Due Diligence
Duplication Cost
Liquidation
Net Present Value
Price
Transition
Value

Businesses take on a life of their own. Throughout the life of your business, you may encounter pivotal moments when it's necessary to reassess your direction. For instance, one day you may look around and ask yourself, "Just how did I get here? This wasn't exactly what I had in mind." Even though you may have an elaborate business plan with specific goals, sometimes things snowball. Sometimes the transition involves doing things differently in your practice, or perhaps, it's time to retire.

Choose Your Direction

Be proactive in determining your future and the role you desire your career to play in the overall scheme of your life. Consider the following scenario.

Robin Smith is a massage therapist who has been in practice for 18 months. The majority of her work is deep-tissue and sports massage. She decides to get training in chair massage so she can diversify her practice, and because she sees it as a way to increase her visibility in the community and enlarge her clientele base. After a while, she secures a corporate account to provide chair massage once a week for Acme, Inc. employees.

All is going well and after several months, the company's director asks her to come in 2 days each week. Robin is ecstatic! She enjoys the change of pace of working part time at the company and is relieved to have a steady income source.

Soon, Acme, Inc. expands exponentially. Smith finds herself working more and more there and less and less at her own practice. A year passes, and she is in the position of needing to hire additional therapists to fulfill the massage needs at Acme, Inc. The prospect is exciting to her, yet she is also experiencing a vague sense of uneasiness. At first, she dismisses her discomfort as fear. Upon further reflection, she discovers that the uneasiness stems from the fact that, although she is very "successful" with her corporate massage, she isn't really doing much of the type of work she truly enjoys.

Points to Ponder

What are some resources that could help Robin make a decision? What would you do in this situation?

Often, changes are so subtle that you don't even notice them until something forces you to evaluate your situation and life. In this scenario, Robin easily adapted her practice to include the corporate work when it was part time. Not until she was required to make a major shift did she even question the direction her career was taking. At this point, Robin has many options. Her choice need not be an all-or-nothing proposition. The following ideas cover the major ones. Many sublevels of activities can be developed within these four career positions.

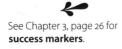

See Chapter 3, page 26 for **success markers**.

- Devote herself completely to managing the corporate account. This includes hiring and managing staff, directly working with clients, marketing the service within the corporation, and overseeing all aspects of the operation.
- Do most of the steps above and hire enough staff so she can still work on private clients 1-2 days per week.
- Manage the account, not do any chair massages, and work on private clients 2-4 days per week.
- Sell her corporate contract to another therapist, invest the money, and go back to working with private clients. She might include a clause in the sales agreement that she be retained as a consultant.

Decision-Making Pinnacles

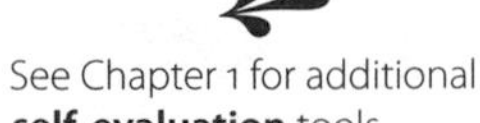

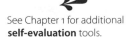

See Chapter 1 for additional **self-evaluation** tools.

It can be difficult to change career direction when you are experiencing the outward manifestations of success. Some common indicators that point to the need to re-evaluate your practice's growth may include:

- Working too many hours, yet not having enough billable hours
- Developing the practice to where there's too much work to do by yourself
- Outgrowing the physical space
- Needing additional skills to better serve your clientele
- Attempting to appeal to too many target markets
- Offering too wide a range of services
- Experiencing restlessness or vague dissatisfaction
- Being bored with the type of work you do or the clients you see
- Experiencing physical or emotional exhaustion on a frequent basis

Exploration and Evaluation

The first step in determining your best course is a thorough evaluation of your wants, needs, and values. Start this exploration process by putting aside your career. Focus on the bigger picture of your life. Are you satisfied in most areas? Are you living the life you choose, or have you acquiesced to what has come your way?

You can't make decisions based on fear and the possibility of what might happen.
—Michelle Obama

After you've identified the elements of life that are truly important to you now, examine how your career fits into that picture. How does your business support your life vision, and how does it detract from it? Once this groundwork is established, you can more easily be objective in your business direction decision-making process.

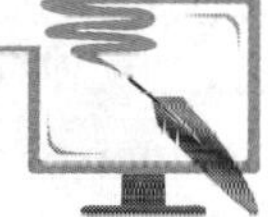

Business Evaluation

Write a business description that includes the following:

- Brief history of your practice with opening date, major achievements, and mission statement.
- Facilities description.
- Summary of services, products sold, and fees collected.
- Client overview: total number of clients, including their profiles.
- Financial statement, including the average number of sessions per week, gross income, and net profit.
- Staff and associate job descriptions.
- Activity synopsis of a typical week.

After you've composed your business description, compare it to your original business vision that you did in Chapter 1 and your career goals in Chapter 2. If you don't have a written business plan, take a few moments to remember why you chose this career and recall your aspirations. Then compare your original vision to your current status. Notice your feelings and thoughts during this process.

§6

Options

Ultimately, there are no right or wrong answers when it comes to making a choice to either stay on a path and make adjustments or to totally change. The only true factor is what is the best decision for you in terms of your overall needs, wants, and goals. Keep in mind that bigger isn't always better. Also, you don't have to pursue each of your talents or abilities. You might consider working on this process with a colleague, counselor, or coach, because it isn't always easy to see all your options by yourself, as in not seeing the forest for the trees.

Selling a Practice

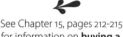

People have many reasons for selling their businesses. The standard ones are burnout, relocation, serious injury or permanent disability, the desire for a career change, death, boredom, disagreement with a business partner, lack of capital, or retirement. Just because you want (or need) a change, selling isn't the only avenue. Many alternatives exist. You can cut back your hours, find partners, incorporate other practitioners, change the business structure, get help, give the business away, sell part of it, franchise, expand, or close it (see the next section).

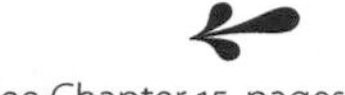

See Chapter 15, pages 212-215 for information on **buying a practice**.

The topic of selling a business is fraught with misconceptions—the biggest one being that a buyer will come out of nowhere and make the seller wealthy. Another common fallacy is that selling a business is like selling a house: while everyone needs a place to live, no one needs to buy a business. Also unlike real estate, there are generally no accepted ways to set a selling price, and you can't compare selling prices of other wellness practices. The most frequent assumption is that buyers fully appreciate the years of sacrifice it took you to build your practice; in most instances, they don't. Another major misconception is that the less information you give the buyer, the better. Nothing could be further from the truth. Uncertainty is always discounted, and buyers always pay less for less information. Also, legal ramifications can occur if you fail to disclose full information (also known as fraudulent inducement).

Most businesses are bought by individuals. Employees usually don't have the money and competitors usually only want a part of the business. In this field, you're most likely to sell your business to another practitioner who is either new to the field, new to the area, or wants to expand his target markets. Buyers usually don't fork over the asking price in one cash payment; they want the business to earn more than enough money to make the loan payments. They want a high-return, low-risk, satisfying lifestyle, and something that's affordable. Make it easy for them. Help them deal with the uncertainty. Provide understandable information, point out business strengths, answer questions, and help them answer questions they're getting from the significant people in their lives.

I realize this process may seem overwhelming and you may be uncertain if all this work is worthwhile. But if you have built up a thriving business, you owe it to yourself to attempt to sell it and recoup some of your investment of time, energy, money, and reputation.

Regardless of where you are in your practice (just starting out or nearing retirement), begin organizing your business now so it is easier to sell at any time since it takes an average of 2-4 years to sell a small business.[1] Establish a clear system for documentation of your client files and financial records. Analyze your business, and clarify your goals and business vision. Start implementing changes now: capitalize on your strengths and do whatever is necessary to eliminate (or at least abate) your limitations. The effort you invest can only enhance your overall success.

Four Ways to Leave Your Business

The four most common ways to leave your business are:

1. Transfer ownership to a family member.
2. Sell your interest to a co-worker, key employee, or all employees.
3. Sell to a third party, such as a competitor or someone interested in entering your field.
4. Liquidate by selling your assets, usually at "fire sale" prices.

Consider the following elements when deciding which method to use: minimizing risk, exercising control, achieving personal objectives, assuring payment, maximizing flexibility in structuring the deal, and fixing value. Your needs in each of these elements determine your best selling strategy.

Transfer Ownership to a Family Member

Many people prefer to keep their businesses in the family as it's a way to hand down legacy. The downsides to this method are: it simply might not be an option, it could increase family tension, and it might stir resentment from the nonfamily members in your business. The benefits include: exercising more control (particularly in terms of setting a monetary value on the business), and the repayment schedule.

Sell to a Co-Worker, Key Employee, or All Employees

This method significantly reduces your risks, and you can increase the likelihood of retaining the same quality and degree of success if you have a staff person buy into your business while you're still active. In effect, you're pre-qualifying your buyer through on-the-job training and observation. You can even establish a fund within the operation of the business to go toward the eventual purchase price. The downside is that you don't have control over the quality of services provided once you leave.

Sell to a Third Party

Selling to a third party (e.g., a competitor or someone interested in entering your field) is the preferred method when the business is too valuable to be purchased by anyone other than someone with access to a lot of capital. This is most likely to be your best avenue if you have a sole-practitioner business.

The disadvantages are that the buying party inherently has more bargaining power, you can't be certain if the buyer's style and abilities will fit well with your current clientele and staff, and you may be required to carry some (or even most) of the purchase price, which means you will still be involved in the business for 1-3 years. The benefits are that you most likely get a good price, and, if you have any staff at all, you will be giving them the opportunity for continued employment.

Liquidation

Liquidation, or simply closing down your practice, should be considered the last resort, although, sadly, it's the most common method chosen by the majority of wellness providers.

The Eight Selling Stages

The best time to sell your practice is contingent on the readiness of your business and the readiness of the marketplace. Most businesses aren't in a position to be sold because they aren't set up for a smooth transition—particularly in terms of documentation. If most businesses were to attempt to sell, they would not get a good price since owners tend to maximize after-tax cash flow and minimize profitability. They set up their business structure in terms of wages and legitimate perks in a manner which optimizes their lifestyle while doing the best they can to reduce taxes.

Figure 23.1 The Eight-Stage Selling Process

1. Review your motives for selling your business and consider the alternatives.
2. Analyze your business to determine if you're selling what buyers want.
3. Assemble an excellent team of advisors.
4. Set a selling price for your business.
5. Prepare your business for sale and make it easy to purchase.
6. Market the sale of your business.
7. Sell the business.
8. Transition the business to the new owner.

Selling a business usually takes a lot of work and time. Using a broker helps to reduce some of your direct time and energy involved, but it doesn't eliminate it.

Review Your Selling Motives and Alternatives

Reflect upon the reasons you want to sell your practice and clarify your goals. Determine which methods you will use for selling your business. The following exercise assists you in choosing the best method for you.

Choosing a Method for Selling Your Business

Take out some paper and ask yourself this set of questions for each of the four methods described in the Four Ways to Leave Your Business section:

- Why does this method appeal to me?
- What reasons make this method appropriate to me?
- What conditions need to be present for this method to be appropriate for me?
- Why might this method not be appropriate for me?

Analyze Your Business

You need to make sure your business is sellable. Put yourself in the position of a potential buyer. Why would they want to purchase your business? What exactly would they be buying? Can they work with your current clients? Analyze your business point by point to determine its scope and condition. Compile a written analysis which includes the following factors:

Company History: How long has your practice been in existence? What is the growth rate of your client base? What is your educational background?

Staff and Associates: Do you have employees? If so, what are their job descriptions and how long have they worked for you? Do you have associates? If so, what services do they provide, what financial agreements are in place, how long have they been associated with your business, and how do they fit in with the overall structure of it?

Description of the Business: Summarize your business in terms of the services offered, equipment, products, supplies, location, resale items, fee structure, client profile, position statement, competition analysis, and differential advantage.

Financial Status: Figure out the true profit of your practice. Assemble the appropriate documents such as tax returns, profit and loss statements, accounts payable, accounts receivable, and the current year's ledger.

Equipment: If you want to sell your equipment, check its condition. Are the items in good shape? Is it worthwhile to include them in the cost of the sale? Most equipment decreases in value over time, particularly electronics (e.g., telephones and computers). Items such as your treatment table may cost much more to replace at current prices.

Facilities: If the buyer will be utilizing your office space, you need to check the condition of the premises, evaluate the overall appearance, and have options ready for the transfer of real estate.

Overall Risk: This is what buyers use to determine the return they require on their investment and what affects their pricing calculation. The risk is evaluated from the point of view of not earning a return on the invested time and money or possibly losing their investment.

Strengths and Limitations: Ironically, this is the last step a seller takes in analyzing the business, yet it's the buyer's first step. After you complete a detailed analysis of your business using the above factors, note which characteristics stand out most clearly. Clarify your opportunities and drawbacks. Think about your strengths as your selling points and your limitations as part of your improvement plan. Keep in mind that your practice may be sellable, even if it isn't in shape to be sold right now. Reorganization and improvements can always be made.

Assemble Your Advisory Team

Your advisory team saves you a lot of time and eliminates some of the inherent frustration involved in selling your business. Minimally, this team includes an accountant and an attorney. Another member to consider is a financial planner. It is also helpful to get feedback from other practitioners who have sold their practices. I highly recommend working with a business broker. Brokers know how to organize the appropriate documentation, set a price, and market the sale of your business. You can hire one to handle the total selling process or as a consultant.

Set a Selling Price

Many formulae exist for the pricing of a business, although valuing and pricing is hardly an exact science due to the large number of variables. It is extremely difficult to measure certain factors such as goodwill, risk, quality of staff, the ability of the new owner to work well with current clients, and, if your practice is sold to an established wellness provider, the cost savings by eliminating duplication of efforts and reducing potential competition. Unfortunately, very few people sell their wellness practices, so we have limited role models available, and comparisons with other professions or businesses aren't necessarily valid.

Ultimately, the price a buyer pays is a subjective decision which is (hopefully) backed by objective information. The amount you receive depends on the value of the business and its affordability to the buyer. It is important that you distinguish the difference between price, value, and affordability.

Price is what someone is willing to pay.

Value is what something is worth. This figure is derived from what the business owns, what it earns, and its differential advantage. Rarely do businesses sell for what they're "worth," particularly wellness practices. This is mainly due to the high risk involved because of the personal nature of this field. Intangibles greatly influence the success of a practice, such as the marketing abilities of the owner and the clients' expectations of the types of treatments they receive.

Affordability is what the buyer is capable of paying. You may find a potential buyer who would be ideal to take over your business, agrees to your price, yet still may not purchase your business because of the terms. Thus, in many ways, what the buyer can afford depends on you.

Figure 23.2 The Six Most Common Methods for Pricing a Business

Price Based On

1. Assets
2. Capitalized earnings
3. Integrating assets and cash flow
4. Duplication cost
5. Carry back
6. Net present value of future earnings

Price based on **ASSETS** is done by determining the market value of the assets being sold and deducting the cost of liabilities to be assumed by the buyer. Assets include furniture, fixtures, equipment, supplies, inventory, client lists, leasehold improvements, accounts receivable, real estate (this isn't limited to owning property, it could include possessing a lease in a prime location), and corporate contracts. This is a fairly straightforward method.

BizPricer® Business Valuation Software

www.businessbookpress.com/catalog/s101.htm

Most service businesses are based on **CAPITALIZED EARNINGS**. To obtain this figure, first calculate the adjusted cash flow and deduct a fair wage for the new owner. This is the base figure for this method. Next, determine a fair return that a buyer should receive for investing in this business. Most buyers use a 15-20% figure for a low-risk business and a 25% or higher figure for a risky business. Convert this percentage into a multiple by dividing it by 100. Multiply the base figure by the multiple to get a selling price.

If the business has both **ASSETS AND CASH FLOW**, the first step is to determine the value of the hard assets. Then calculate the adjusted cash flow. Add those two figures together. If, as the seller, you want a full cash sale, this number is your selling price. If the business is in excellent condition or your selling terms include payments over several years, the amount you can ask for is the hard assets plus up to twice the adjusted cash flow.

Pricing your business on the **DUPLICATION COST** is done by taking the market value of assets and combining it with the cost for the number of years it would take a beginning practitioner to reach the same profit level. It can be rather tricky to determine the latter figure, particularly if you didn't market and build your practice on a consistent basis. Also, since the potential buyer is unknown, he may be excellent or abysmal at marketing.

These formulae aren't foolproof. The factors that affect the selling price vary significantly with each business. I highly recommend working with a business broker and an accountant to help you determine which method or combination of methods is best for you.

CARRY BACK is generally appropriate for small businesses. Calculate the adjusted cash flow of the business. Deduct the anticipated wages the buyer would need and the expenses required to run the business for 1 year. This figure gives you the cash available on which to set the sales amount. If you assume the loan to be a 5-year payoff, multiply the cash available by 5. You can add a reasonable down payment amount to this figure to get a total selling price.

The **NET PRESENT VALUE** method is worth considering if you've built a very strong, diversified practice which includes other practitioners, corporate contracts, concessions at a health club, or product sales. The technique involves the following steps: Adjust the company statements to show true present profit (e.g., add back in the perks you've taken); develop your business plan and project the growth for the next 5 years; calculate the profit, investments, and returns for the next 5 years; and then discount the figures to the present using a discount rate which reflects the degree of risk, as well as projected inflation. The major problems with this method are that the projections are purely speculative and the discount rate is totally arbitrary.

Calculate your selling price using all the above methods and see what the results show you. Inherent in all of these methods is the problem that they don't take into account: many practitioners buy an existing practice simply to ensure themselves of a "job." Also, your business may include intangible assets that are difficult to price. These include your credibility, heart, reputation, goodwill, and presence in the community. Many clients may stay with the new owner out of their respect and loyalty to you—given that you sell to a practitioner with the same commitment toward quality.

Another idea to consider is incorporating a contingency clause. As a result, you can ask for a higher price since you're minimizing the buyer's risk. After the down payment, the two techniques for contingent payment are: the buyer makes the additional payments only if the business meets certain expectations (e.g., at least 50% of the clients stay), or the buyer only has to pay you a set percentage of the fees received from your current clientele.

The bottom line in selling your business revolves around economics—supply and demand: Is your business saleable and are there any buyers?

Buyers will test the desirability of purchasing your business. The first test in buying a small business is how the cost returns and effort required in running the practice measure against investing their money elsewhere. The biggest test is the "justification test." The buyer must be convinced that the business can provide sufficient cash flow to repay the loan, support the business operational expenses, give a reasonable return on the down payment, and allow for reasonable wages. What a buyer can afford and what they are willing to pay more often depends on the upfront cash required than the selling price. The more favorable the terms of sale (such as no or low cash down, no security deposit, minimal interest, a lengthy repayment schedule, or contingency terms), the easier it is for you to find a buyer.

Preparing Your Business For Sale

As stated before, the single biggest mistake sellers make is not properly preparing the business for sale. Preparation involves making the requisite improvements in order to enhance the likelihood of your business selling, as well as assembling the appropriate documentation. See Figure 23.3 for the items to include in your documentation package.

Figure 23.3 Business Sale Documentation

- Opening Proposal: A one-to-four page overview of the company history, mission statement, brief business description, summary of assets, financial history, reason for sale, and pricing terms
- Samples of Marketing Materials
- Detailed Business Description
- Names of All Owners
- Copy of Lease
- Profit and Loss Statements for Past 3 Years
- Tax Returns for Past 3 Years
- Copies of Current Contracts
- Determination of Value of Leasehold Improvements
- List of Fixtures and Equipment with Replacement Value
- Value of Inventory

Marketing

Marketing the sale of your business includes the preparation, pricing, packaging, and promotion you do to bring your business and a buyer together. Accurate, organized, appealing documentation is the foundation to the successful sale of your business.

Your presentation package should include your opening proposal, samples of advertisements and promotional materials, and any other documents that highlight your success such as newspaper interviews.

The rest of the documentation should be provided to the prospective buyer only after they've signed a Letter of Intent to Purchase. Granted, this letter doesn't guarantee they will indeed buy your business, but it helps safeguard your business privacy by weeding out the less serious buyers.

The Complete Guide to Selling a Business by Fred S. Steingold

Buying and Selling a Business: How You Can Win in the Business Quadrant by Garrett Sutton

The most common marketing methods are advertising, direct mail, telemarketing, networking, and certain online platforms. Advertising is an effective technique if the potential buyers are numerous and they're easy to reach (e.g., through trade journals, newsletters, online). Direct mail works well if you can identify buyers. It is one of the best for selling a practice because you can target specific practitioners or soon-to-graduate students. Telemarketing is an avenue worth pursuing, particularly if it's done in conjunction with direct mail. Networking is an extremely effective marketing technique. The only problem is that if you do it yourself, you lose confidentiality. Most wellness providers aren't overly concerned about people discovering they're attempting to sell their practices. Although if you don't anticipate selling the business quickly, you may need to proceed cautiously to avoid losing clients. If you desire to keep the sale of your business under wraps until the last possible moment, networking should be done through an intermediary. There are also online avenues for finding buyers, but be sure to allow your broker or agent to help determine the appropriateness of these platforms.

Finding an appropriate buyer is crucial. It's to your benefit (particularly in terms of getting paid) that the buyer can easily take over and work with your clients. This can be difficult if the techniques you utilize are extremely specialized. You need a buyer whose knowledge, training, and personality is similar to yours. For instance, if you're a Trager® practitioner, it's wise to sell your practice to another Trager® practitioner—not just any touch practitioner. If you incorporate a variety of modalities, find another practitioner with diverse experience.

The Actual Sale

Once you have a potential buyer, delineate in writing both parties' expectations regarding the selling process. Keep in mind that most buyers and sellers are inexperienced and don't know what to expect.

If you don't match abilities and personalities, the buyer is less likely to retain the client base.

The next phase is to qualify the buyer. Find out where he stands financially and his sources of income. You could request a personal financial statement or a copy of the previous 3 years' tax returns. Realize that, as the seller, you're viewed as the prime source of financing, given that 75-80% of businesses are seller-financed, with the seller carrying one-half of the selling price. Another aspect of qualifying a buyer is to find out if there's a good fit between the buyer's goals and needs, and the company as it stands. The last element of qualifying a buyer is obtaining references.

After you've qualified your potential buyer, ask for a Letter of Intent to Purchase. This letter contains the names of the buyers and sellers, description of what the buyer intends to purchase, the date of offer, expiration date, price, terms, interest rate, repayment schedule, amount of deposit, closing date, and contingencies.

The next stage centers on negotiations and documentation verification. Do not be surprised if the buyer requests you sign a "non-competition" clause stating that you won't set up another practice within certain geographic limits, or requires you to refrain from promoting your business to specific target markets for a reasonable period.

Once the seller accepts the offer, she submits the rest of the documentation. The buyer then performs what is termed "due diligence." This entails examining all of the submitted information to verify its accuracy and confirm that any specified conditions are met. More negotiations may follow and the contract is drawn.

The final stage is the closing. This can be a rather stressful event, so be prepared. To ensure a smooth closing, make sure all parties understand and agree upon the terms of the sale in advance and bring copies of all important documents.

The Post-Sale

In most instances, sellers are required to continue involvement in the company for a short time after the official sale. This transition time allows for the new owner to be brought up to speed and provides the seller with the opportunity to introduce the new owner to the clients, suppliers, and staff. It may be necessary for the seller to train the new buyer, continue to work in the business for a specified time, or provide consulting services to the buyer.

Closing a Practice

Some people simply opt to close down their practices when they move or are ready to retire. It's still important to do it in a manner that honors your investment in your profession and maintains goodwill with your clients, colleagues, and companies with whom you've done business. Consult with a business advisor before making any announcements about closing, as it can take months to properly close a business. Figure 23.4 is a checklist of activities to do to help ensure a smooth transition.

> "What the caterpillar calls the end, the rest of the world calls a butterfly.
>
> —Lao Tzu

Remember, you have created a successful practice largely because of your client-centered, relationship-building skills. Therefore, at the closing of your practice, it's your final ethical responsibility to provide appropriate referrals to those clients who may be in need of ongoing care. Make a list of practitioners you know and trust, and provide it to your clients during the final weeks of your transition.

Figure 23.4 **Practice Closing Checklist**

Prior to Closing

- ❑ Meet with an advisor.
- ❑ Choose an official closing date.
- ❑ Assemble a practitioner referral list for clients.
- ❑ Notify current clients of the closing date at least 1 month in advance.
- ❑ Notify employees of the closing date (some states require a 60-day warning).
- ❑ Offer to give clients their files.
- ❑ Request closing statements from your suppliers and business accounts.
- ❑ Collect any outstanding receivables.
- ❑ Sell (or return) unused inventory.
- ❑ Terminate your office lease.
- ❑ Cancel business subscriptions or send them a change of address form.
- ❑ Notify utility companies, telephone service, and Internet provider of the date to discontinue service.
- ❑ Notify the postal service of the date to forward mail (and provide a forwarding address).

After Closing

- ❑ Store or destroy client files that weren't given to clients (rules vary by profession and state).
- ❑ Store business and employment records according to government guidelines.
- ❑ Dissolve your LLC, corporation, or partnership, and file required forms.
- ❑ Make final federal and state tax deposits.
- ❑ File final business tax forms.
- ❑ Issue final employee W-2 forms and file final W-3.
- ❑ Liquidate your assets (sell or donate to charities). Keep all receipts.
- ❑ Report the sale or exchange of business property and equipment (Form 4797).
- ❑ Contact the IRS to close your EIN account
- ❑ Cancel registrations, permits, licenses, and business names.
- ❑ Resolve financial obligations (e.g., business debts, employee payroll requirements, taxes).
- ❑ Cancel your office insurance and request a prorated refund.
- ❑ Send thank-you notes to key clients and people who've supported you.
- ❑ Notify business contacts of your status. Provide a way of contacting you (for those with whom you want to maintain contact).
- ❑ Cancel or transfer any automatic debit payments to another account.
- ❑ Close your business checking account and cancel business credit cards 3 months after the business closes.

§7 Marketing Mastery

Section 7 of *Business Mastery* explores how to master the marketing tasks that are essential to your success. Successful practitioners know who they want to work with, understand how to find those potential clients through appropriate marketing techniques, and attract the desired clients by clearly and engagingly describing what they do.

Practitioners maintain a thriving practice by being client-centered: having an inviting treatment space, using high-quality equipment, conducting thorough treatment plans, following up, and, most importantly, listening and responding to each client's unique needs. What's the best way to begin? Like building a house, it's wise to start with a foundation and build from there.

Chapter 24 provides that foundation by detailing how to identify your target markets, develop a marketing plan, and take action steps to attract new clients and build a thriving practice. The chapter also introduces a virtual toolbox of marketing concepts, such as positioning, branding, and differential advantage, along with valuable insights into how you can put them to work to grow your business.

The majority of marketing endeavors that practitioners utilize fall under the categories of promotions and community relations. **Chapter 25** provides the framework for a solid house by providing a primer of low- and no-cost marketing techniques focusing on promotions and community relations.

Chapter 26 is analogous to the furniture in the house. This chapter highlights the major marketing materials you need, along with tips on how to design and incorporate them.

Maintaining an effective online presence is like providing power to run your house. **Chapter 27** explores the key elements of designing an effective website and engaging with your community through social media and other online activities.

Think about advertising techniques as a sign on your front yard inviting people in. **Chapter 28** highlights the major print and broadcast media advertising venues. It also includes tips on content and design of display ads, with before-and-after examples.

Chapter 29 helps you to navigate the media and get them to knock on your door. It covers how to develop media relations, the steps involved in getting interviewed, how to write a press release, and the key elements in media kits.

Chapter 30 rounds out the house design by focusing on creative ways to retain clients. It explores how exceptional customer service and incentive programs foster long-term client relationships, and how you can put customer service action plans to work to enhance your business success.

Effective and consistent marketing is essential to success. The first chapters of this section explored the core marketing concepts and the major ways to get and retain clients. **Chapter 31** provides a sample marketing action plan and more than 100 specific marketing ideas to spark your creativity.

24
Marketing Fundamentals

"Marketing's job is never done. It's about perpetual motion. We must continue to innovate every day."
—Beth Comstock

Primary Marketing Principles
- The Essence of Marketing
- What Clients Want
- The Purchasing Cycle
- The Lifetime Value of a Client
- The Power of Public Opinion
- Establish Credibility
- Positioning
- Target Markets
- Competition
- Cooperation

Marketing Mix
- Promotion
- Publicity
- Advertising
- Community Relations

Develop an Innovative Marketing Plan
- Marketing Plan Components
- Marketing Assessment
- Strategic Action Plans

Getting Your First Clients
- Almost No-Cost Start-up
- Moving Forward

Key Terms

Accessibility
Advertising
Advocacy
Benefit
Branding
Community Relations
Compassion
Competition
Convenience
Cooperation
Cooperative Marketing
Courtesy
Credibility
Demographics
Differential Advantage
Efficiency
Expertise
Feature
Guarantee
Ideal Client
Image
Integrity
Lifetime Value of a Client
Loyalty
Market Research
Marketing
Marketing Mix
Marketing Plan
Niche
Positioning
Professionalism
Promotion
Psychographics
Public Opinion
Publicity
Purchasing Cycle
Reliability
Safety
Specialization
Strategic Action Plan
Synergy
Target Market
Target Market Analysis
Target Market Profile
Unique Selling Proposition (USP)
Value

The word "marketing" may trigger a wide array of thoughts and feelings ranging from tremendous excitement to fantasies of instant success, to studied disinterest, to hand-wringing dismay. Although effective marketing is the cornerstone of a flourishing practice, some practitioners shy away from any type of self-promotion as they associate it with pushy sales tactics. This avoidance may also stem from a lack of marketing knowledge or limited resources.

One of the attractions of the wellness field is its dissimilarity with the "typical" business world. But even wellness professions revolve around sales and marketing. Luckily, we rarely need to rely on traditional methods to promote ourselves. The most effective marketers focus on value-centered marketing: promoting their businesses in a way that reflects their personality, philosophy, and integrity.

Primary Marketing Principles

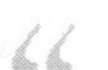

"Quality in a service or product is not what you put into it. It is what the client or customer gets out of it.

—Peter Drucker

Marketing is simply sharing information about yourself and your services with potential and current clients so they get a sense of who you are, which allows them to make an informed choice of whether to utilize your services. It isn't about coercion or pretending to be someone you're not. Simply put, marketing involves identifying your target markets, developing a marketing plan, and taking action steps to attract potential clients and retain current ones. The wide world of marketing includes promotion, advertising, community relations, and publicity. Marketing is all about empowering your clientele to value you and your services. Effective marketing involves targeting the appropriate people and informing them about the benefits of your services. The biggest mistake I see people make is overextending themselves; they try to be the practitioner for everyone. One person cannot fulfill all the needs of every client.

Marketing a service can be very different than marketing a product. For example, retailers use mass-marketing techniques such as broad-based advertising campaigns, telemarketing, and in-store promotions. Service businesses usually target a well-defined market and use a personal approach. The major portion of marketing a service business is educational in nature.

Frequently, wellness providers leave their marketing to chance. They wait for people to find them—an attitude that's generally counterproductive. (It's okay if you have an alternate source of income.) But consider why you got into this field in the first place. What good is it to desire to enhance people's wellbeing if they don't know who you are? The key is to create a marketing plan that focuses primarily on low-cost techniques that build relationships.

Very few people can afford the luxury of building their practices solely by word-of-mouth marketing. If you're very good at what you do, genuinely care about and respect your clients, and charge a reasonable rate, you will ultimately develop a strong clientele base. However, most practitioners are interested in accelerating that process, and that requires marketing savvy.

The Essence of Marketing

Marketing is about getting yourself known—building a professional reputation. The ultimate aim is to develop a thriving practice, and that means having a strong, and continually growing, clientele base.

Everything you do makes a statement about how you feel about yourself, your clients, and your practice. Thus, you're always marketing yourself—for better or worse. You may have noticed that marketing concepts and tips appear throughout most of the chapters in this book. This is because marketing isn't just about the outward activities you do, such as advertising and promotions; it also involves the way you relate to your clients, your ethics, and your professional demeanor. To attract the right clients and grow your business, your outward image must be consistent with your vision of a successful wellness professional. The more creative and natural your marketing techniques, the more successful they are, mainly because you enjoy doing them. No rule says that you can't have fun while promoting your business!

A popular phrase in this industry (and also the title of a book) is "Do what you love and the money will follow."[1] Unfortunately, most people forget about the verb in the sentence: DO.

Having a passion for what you do—and top-notch skills—aren't enough to build a thriving practice. Without a good marketing plan and consistent action steps to reach your marketing goals, it's likely your business and bank account will lag. Marketing is all about taking the right actions to attract new clients. For instance, if you don't have a full client load, invest that free time in educating people about your work or donate your services (do what you love)—then the money will truly come. Be courageous enough to do some of the practice building activities that you might not necessarily love, such as public speaking or writing articles.

Benefits vs. Features

With unfortunate frequency, we describe ourselves (and our businesses) in terms of our features. A feature isn't what attracts clients. They want to know how your services will make a difference in their wellness. A feature is a description of your service or product, (e.g., how the product was made, the training you received, the background of the practitioner and the company). A benefit is a description of how the client profits from using the services and product, how the service or product solves the client's problem, the differential advantage you provide, and the results that the client can expect.

No One Cares about Your Boat

The following story illustrates the importance of having the proper focus. I've heard variations of this story many times over the years. This version is provided by Tad Hargrave. It comes from a metaphor his colleague Bill Baren shared with him.

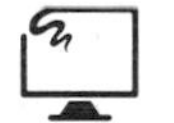

Tad Hargrave
marketingforhippies.com
Bill Baren
billbaren.com

Imagine this: your ideal client is on Island A. And she's sad because she has a problem or some unwanted symptoms. These problems keep her up at night. They frustrate her more than anything. She craves to be on Island B. On Island B are the results that she desires.

Island A		Island B
I'm unhealthy	>> **Your Boat** >>	I'm healthy
I'm poor		I've got enough money
I'm lonely		I'm in a great relationship
I'm stressed		I'm at peace

In broad strokes, it's like that. Of course, those wouldn't be very compelling in a business situation. More specific examples might be:

Island A		Island B
I'm a parent who snaps at my kids too much	>> **Your Boat** >>	I've reduced my stress level, and am more loving, calm, and centered even when my kids test me the most
I'm an athlete who needs to increase my performance but have too many injuries		I've learned how to move my body in ways that reduce the likelihood of injury, and am continuing to break my personal best records
I'm a massage therapist without enough clients		I've got enough of the kinds of clients I love

And, in this metaphor, your business is like the boat that takes them from one island to the other. Simple. This idea brings us back to the opening statement, "No one cares about your boat." Most marketing emphasizes the boat and ignores the journey that people want to take. For instance, you meet someone at a party and he asks what you do. You say, "I'm a massage therapist" or "I do this unique combination of reiki, Trager,® and shiatsu, and the work that reconnects," or "I'm a life coach." Your response seems clear enough but what if that person

§7

doesn't know what those terms mean? He might be thinking to himself, "What the heck is that? Well, don't be rude. Just nod and smile and pretend you know what she is talking about." Or what if he thinks he understands, but really doesn't, (e.g., "Oh! A yoga teacher. Right. I went to Bikram once. They help you get tight buns.").

We often assume that people hear about our boat and immediately "get it" in the way we mean it. But it's rarely the case. We also assume, often incorrectly, that people want our boat. But that's almost never true. What they want is to get off of Island A and to get to Island B. Even when people are looking for a specific treatment modality, if you dig a bit, you often find that it isn't the modality they want but the results they've come to believe it will give them.

Imagine someone has migraines for years. It's the worst. No one really knows how much he suffers and misses out on because of it. And he feels utterly lost. He is stuck on Island A with no way off. He feels helpless and hopeless. Then, one day, a friend tells him, "You should try some massage for that. It really helped me."

And immediately, his life is transformed. There's hope. His other friends tell him he's crazy and to give up on getting on this "massage boat." There is no such thing. No one gets off Island A. But, he believes. And he packs up his things and heads down to the harbor, faithful to the promise of massage and extolling it to everyone he meets; spreading the rumor of hope.

But, halfway there, he runs into a friend who asks where he's going and, upon hearing the story, says, "Oh no! Not massage. No, no, no. Migraines require structural adjustment. What you need is a chiropractor!" At first he's resistant to this but soon becomes convinced that it isn't massage he needs, it's a chiropractic adjustment. Look at how short lived his loyalty to massage was. The only reason he wants to get on your boat is because, at some level, he believes it can take him from where he is to where he wants to go. Period. If he finds another boat that can help him with his particular issues better, he will jump ship faster than you could imagine.

This is vital to understand because most wellness practitioners come from the place of, "My services can help everyone with anything! I wouldn't ever want to turn anyone away." It's as if they're trying to convince people at the harbor that their boat can take them absolutely anywhere they want to go.

But let's return to our friend with the migraine. Imagine he gets to the harbor and is overwhelmed to see dozens of boats of different modalities. But then he sees one boat named "The Migraine Cure." Guess which boat he' likely to take? He doesn't even know if the boat is massage, chiropractic, or something else—and he doesn't care.

We forget this at our own peril. We fall in love with our boats. It's understandable. It's why we do what we do. We love our modality. We've spent so much time and money learning about it. But even so, no one cares about your boat. This boat helped you tremendously. It might have saved you from drowning. But still, no one cares about your boat. Even if potential clients think they care about your boat, it's only because they've come to believe it can help them on their journey. That's it.

So, the clearer you can be about the nature of the journey you take people on, the better you're going to do. And, of course, it isn't quite so simple. You need to consider the design and aesthetic of your boat, your sailing style as a captain, the map you use, and the route you choose—those all factor into a person's choice. And the journey may not be so obvious. Perhaps your love is so fierce that they just want to be around you regardless of the modality you're using, but that's still a journey. *No one cares about your boat!*

Identify Your Ocean Journey

Think about where your career is at this point. Describe your "boat." Think about your clients and identify their "Island A" and "Island B." Next, list the ways you can you offer to get them from Island A to Island B.

What Clients Want

According to social psychologists, motivational needs range from physiological to transcendence. Many postulate that the core human needs are to avoid pain and gain pleasure. In terms of receiving wellness care, clients have many wants in addition to the desire to achieve their specific wellness goals. Dr. Joe Vitale, author of *Inspired Marketing*, states, "In short, all the marketing experts who say pain is the greatest motivator have forgotten the power of our driving force in life: Love. Our goal as marketing and business people isn't to tell people what's wrong with them or to remind them of their pain, but to help them imagine and then experience the pleasure they long to have."[2] The following are the top client concerns, not necessarily ranked in order of priority. All of these factors can profoundly impact your success, so be sure to address them in your marketing materials.

See Chapter 3, pages 50-52 for information about **motivation theories**.

Convenience: The two major aspects of convenience are location and appointments. In real estate lingo, the phrase is "It's all about location, location, location!" In terms of location, consider things such as: Are you near the majority of your target markets? Is your office easy to find? Is there ample parking? Is it accessible? Regarding appointments: Do you offer online booking? Do you have a receptionist service or front desk personnel? Do you offer evening and weekend appointments?

Accessibility: Following up on the location, is it easy for your clients to get into your office? For instance, if one of your markets is people in injury rehabilitation or seniors, are there ramps (and elevators if you aren't on the first floor)? Also, if you do hands-on work on a table, is it hydraulic? (This can be crucial if any of your clients have limited mobility or if you're really tall, you don't want clients to feel as though they have to pole vault to get on the table.)

Efficiency: Most people have busy lives and appreciate efficiency. Can people easily book appointments? Do you offer a variety of payment options? Is your check-in and check-out process smooth?

Safety: Safety is paramount! Is your office in a safe neighborhood? Is there proper lighting for evening appointments? If there are steps leading to your office, are they in good condition? Are there handrails? Is your equipment sturdy and in good condition? For instance, you don't want people to be worried about falling off a table or having it collapse under them.

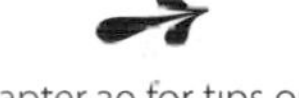

See Chapter 30 for tips on **client retention**.

Value: People want to get good value for the money they spend. Sometimes this is a bit difficult to identify with wellness care. Clients can more easily justify the time and money spent on your services if they have observable and/or quantifiable results (which is where doing treatment plans and regular assessments is crucial). Do you offer a good return on investment (ROI)? Do you do thorough intake interviews and follow-up with progress assessments? Do you also do the extra things to make your clients feel valued?

Courtesy: Keep in mind that your clients pay your bills. Treat them with respect and courtesy. Do you greet clients with a smile and handshake? Do you call them by name?

Reliability: Reliability can make or break your practice—and is one of the major complaints employers have with practitioners. Are you punctual? Is the quality of your work consistent?

Compassion: Whenever you provide wellness care, you must honor clients for who they are and have compassion for their issues and challenges. Are you able to offer comfort while maintaining boundaries? Do you take the time to listen to clients and discover their concerns and goals? Do you conduct thorough intake interviews and co-create treatment plans with your clients? Are you well-versed in the issues, options, and protocols of the major common concerns of your target markets?

Integrity: People trust you with their bodies! It's imperative that you're a person of integrity. Do you maintain a client-centered approach? Do you keep your agreements? Do you honor confidentiality?

Attention: Treat your clients like they're the center of the universe. For some people, that can be more valuable than the actual "work" you do with them. Do you review your client files before each session and make notes afterward? Are you fully present during the session? Do you attempt to accommodate clients' special requests (e.g., adjust temperature, regulate sound, play their favorite music)?

Acceptance: People crave to be accepted for who they are. Plus, so many people have body issues. Coming from a position of acceptance can be incredibly healing for your clients. Do you operate from a position of non-discrimination? Are you able to respect clients even if they don't share your beliefs or don't do what you recommend?

See Chapter 5, pages 80-82 for more on **professionalism**.

Professionalism: This covers a lot of things from your attire, business practices, attitudes, and communication skills. Also, professionalism includes maintaining a clean, safe environment, and using high quality products and supplies. Do you ensure that all of those things match the image you wish to portray?

Expertise: Clients expect you to excel in your work. Do you keep up with current research? Do you regularly take CE classes? Do you read trade journals? Do you confer with other wellness care practitioners?

Figure 24.1 **What Clients Want**

- Convenience
- Safety
- Efficiency
- Value
- Accessibility
- Courtesy
- Reliability
- Compassion
- Integrity
- Attention
- Acceptance
- Professionalism
- Expertise

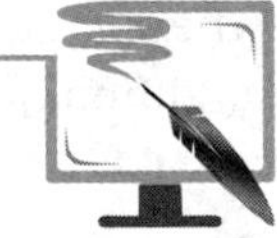

Analyze Your Ability to Meet Clients' Wants

Review the list in Figure 24.1. Identify the ways you already meet those wants. Next, highlight the other wants that you would like meet. Delineate how you could meet those wants, and create a plan of action to make it happen.

The Purchasing Cycle

> "Price is what you pay. Value is what you get.
> —Warren Buffett

Understanding the purchasing cycle, (sometimes known as the buying, marketing, or sales cycle) enhances your marketing effectiveness. Most people make decisions emotionally and then justify them rationally; the "feel-good" factor is a powerful force when it comes to people spending money. Marketers have taken this into account and made a science out of understanding the cycle that consumers go through as they make purchasing decisions. The models describing this process vary from 5-8 steps. Essentially, the purchasing cycle is a description of the patterns most people go through when contemplating utilizing your services or making purchases. The following information is adapted from the article, "7 Stages of Buying Cycle: From Awareness to Advocacy."[3]

Awareness: Awareness is the first step. This is the point where potential clients identify a problem or a need. It could also be the moment where they recognize the difference between the ideal and the reality. For instance, a potential client might be thinking, "I

Figure 24.2 The Purchasing Cycle Steps

1. Awareness
2. Information Search
3. Interest
4. Evaluation
5. Purchase
6. Support
7. Repeat/Loyalty
8. Referral/Advocacy

need to do something about this chronic tension I have in my neck." This is also the point at which potential clients recognize that your type of service or product can be a solution.

Information Search: The Information Search stage is where potential clients look for options. Most people start searches by looking through their lists of wellness providers. Brand awareness is key for potential clients at this point in their search. If they already know about your practice, their own internal search of what they already know will lead them to you. Next they ask friends, colleagues, family members, and other wellness care providers for recommendations. The third phase is external searches, such as looking through local wellness publications and conducting Internet searches (e.g., generic search engines, online wellness directories, review websites like Yelp).

> "All things being equal, people will do business with, and refer business to, those people they know, like, and trust.
> —Bob Burg

Interest: The Interest stage is where potential clients develop an increasing interest in learning more about your specific services and how you can help them achieve their goals. Reach these people by providing engaging information on your website and Social Media venues. Nurture these relationships with interesting follow-up emails. You can also directly contact prospects.

Evaluation: In the Evaluation stage, potential clients evaluate different wellness care approaches as well as specific practitioners. They weigh the information they've received from personal recommendations and external research. They evaluate different types of services as well as brands. For instance, they might ask themselves, "What are the benefits of using Service A versus Service B? What does Wellness Clinic X offer that Independent Practitioner Y doesn't?" This stage includes many factors including pricing, location, practitioner's experience, company's reputation, availability, and ease of scheduling. In the evaluation phase, potential clients have ruled out some options already and narrowed down the choices to a few contenders.

Purchase: The Purchase phase is where all your marketing comes to fruition. This is when potential clients decide with whom to entrust their wellness care. Note that past experiences and loyalty come into play at this point if a client is considering returning to a known practitioner.

Support: The Support stage is where you focus on making sure clients are getting the most out of their use of your products and services. Provide clients with self-care information and products to use between sessions. Post articles and tips on wellness care. Send clients resource links to information specific to their needs and goals. Satisfied clients become repeat clients, which drives the next stage of customer loyalty.

Loyalty: The Loyalty stage is about the long-term client relationship that provides for ongoing repeat business. Increasing loyalty has a major impact on total revenue and profitability. It's much more cost-effective to maintain an existing client than to find a new one. It's also important to identify those clients in this phase that are likely to become advocates in the next phase.

Advocacy: The Advocacy phase is about helping your best clients help you by referring new clients to you through their Social Networks and direct word-of-mouth referrals. Make it easy for clients to promote your practice, make the process rewarding, and recognize their efforts.

The Lifetime Value of a Client

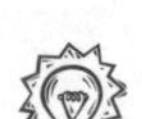

Dramatically increase the lifetime value of a client by replacing your typical clients with ideal clients.

The lifetime value of a client is the total dollar amount your typical client brings into your business. If you're just starting out, your financial forecasts are guesstimates. Eventually, you will base your forecasts on your own business history, but in the beginning, you can be more accurate if you base them on industry data.

Understanding the lifetime value of a client puts your marketing time and expenditures into perspective. The cost of actions such as the extra time you occasionally give a client, providing a free or low-cost initial consultation, placing confirmation calls, sending greeting cards and newsletters, and offering special promotions, pales next to the potential ROI. The following formula calculates this amount:

See Chapter 15, pages 194-197 for tips on how to gather **industry statistics** and estimate **a community's supply and demand.**

1. Determine how much money your average client will spend during the entire client/practitioner relationship in session fees and product sales. For example, let's say that your typical client sees you 10 times a year at $60 per session. This client works with you for 4 years and purchases $80 in products each year.
   a. Number of years: 4
   b. Sessions: $2,400 = $60 x 10 sessions x 4 years
   c. Next add the product sales: $320 = $80 x 4 years
   d. The total value per client: **$2,720**
2. Calculate the value of client referrals. For example, let's say your average client (from step 1 above) refers only 1 new client every year.
   a. **$10,880** = 4 years x $2,720
3. Determine the total **overall lifetime value of a client** by adding the final numbers from steps 1 and 2.
   a. **$13,600** = $2,720 + $10,880
   b. Keep in mind that the actual funds you directly receive from the client are $2,720, but their value to your business is much more.

Imagine how much you can increase the lifetime value if each client were to schedule 1 more session per year or purchase $20 more in products. You can exponentially increase the lifetime value of a client by creating a referral plan that encourages clients to refer people to you. For instance, if your average client referred 2 people each year (who become regular clients) then the lifetime value of each client is $24,480!

The Power of Public Opinion

Before you begin to develop your marketing plan, assess your community's opinions and perceptions about preventive wellness and alternative therapies. Are wellness services such as massage therapy, nutritional counseling, and acupuncture viewed as nonessential luxuries (fluff)? Or is your business located in an area where people are open to alternative wellness approaches and focused on healthy aging? Are there specific target markets within your community that currently work with wellness practitioners on a regular basis?

Understanding the wellness quotient of your community is crucial, because it's a lot easier to swim with the current than against it. If a high percentage of people are actively seeking alternative therapies and can afford regular preventive wellness services, your odds of success are much greater than in a community that is skeptical of alternative approaches to wellness.

Establish Credibility

One of the best methods for establishing credibility and increasing visibility is public speaking.

Unlike most other professions, wellness practitioners are judged by who they are, not just what they do. Thus, establishing credibility is essential to the long-term success of your practice and is the foundation of any successful marketing venture. People need to feel that they can trust you and your expertise to assist them in reaching their wellness goals. They need to feel that you are authentic. Authenticity traits include regularly engaging in self-evaluation activities to increase self-awareness, having integrity, operating from one's values, and being heart-centered. When I first started doing marketing workshops I titled them "Marketing from the Heart," as I believed then (and still do now), that this is the most appropriate approach to take in marketing a wellness practice.

Your level of professionalism plays a major role in the status of your credibility. Your actions must echo your words. Don't make promises, either verbally or in printed materials, that you cannot fulfill. Don't make claims that you cannot substantiate. It's better to be conservative in your offerings and exceed them, than to make grandiose proclamations and fall short.

Figure 24.3 Credibility Components

- Length of time in the field
- Testimonials and success stories
- Pictures
- Appearance and demeanor
- Guarantees
- Professional affiliations
- Communication skills
- Credentials
- Vocabulary
- Public image
- Hours of education and training

Positioning

Effective positioning of your business starts with you determining what niche you intend to fill. Prospective clients need an easy way to differentiate you from your competition; your position statement provides that information. Positioning and target markets go hand in hand. It's difficult to explain one without the other. As a matter of fact, if you have more than 1 target market (which is usually wise), and they're vastly different, you may need a separate position statement for each of those target markets. Here are several examples of successful positioning:

- When 7-Up® was developing its marketing campaign, a soda usually meant a brown-colored cola drink such as Coca-Cola® or Pepsi.® To counteract that assumption, they coined themselves the "Uncola."
- Wheaties cereal is known as the Breakfast of Champions.® They back up their position statement and reinforce their image by putting pictures of famous athletes on the front of their cereal boxes.
- Enterprise Rent-A-Car focuses on convenience to the customer with the statement "Pick Enterprise. We'll pick you up."

> "A brand is no longer what we tell the customer it is; it is what customers tell each other it is.
> —Scott Cook

Branding Your Image

A brand is a "unique sum of impressions" that can be your business' greatest asset.[4] It's derived from what your clients and the public think and believe about your business. In a marketplace crowded with talented wellness providers and discerning consumers, practitioners who develop a strong brand image have a competitive advantage. Such a brand image is rooted in clarity of purpose—as defined in your mission statement—and is reflected in consistent and concise messages that convey who you are and what you promise to deliver to clients. These messages continually broadcast to your clients what's important to you and what you value. These messages take many shapes, such as marketing programs, promotional materials, logos, business cards, everyday interactions with clients, and your office environment. For wellness providers, a strong brand most often translates into loyal clients and a steady stream of new clients. Whether clients find you through word-of-mouth or the Internet, your brand is like a trusted friend that creates an emotional connection with clients. In short, a strong brand attracts those who will bond with you and appreciate what you offer.

Create Your Brand

- Describe the image you wish to portray.
- Survey your clients and colleagues to find out how they describe you and your practice. How closely do their descriptions match the image you wish to convey?
- How do your office environment, client communications, marketing programs, promotional materials, and attire align with this image?
- What changes are needed to alter the elements that aren't in sync with your desired image?

The Differential Advantage

The next step in developing a position statement is to define your differential advantage, also known as a USP (Unique Selling Proposition). You must know how to describe what makes you different (unique) from other wellness providers in your field. No two people are exactly alike, even with the identical training.

Stay centered in your enthusiasm about your work and the results it produces. This is what attracts people to want to learn more about who you are and what you do.

Reflect upon your practice. Think about what you really do: the intention of your work, your image, the range of skills and techniques you employ, the products you use, the results your clients receive, and what your clients say about you and your work. Your differential advantage may stem from yourself, your specialization, the range of services offered, the results you commonly produce, geographic location, or a combination of factors. Remember that what usually attracts potential clients aren't the features of your practice, but how those features are going to benefit them.

Another way of differentiating yourself from other practitioners is through specialization. You may prefer to work on a particular condition or a specific clientele. Perhaps one of your greatest strengths lies in the actual service you offer. Do you have specialized knowledge? Are you the only one in your area who does a certain type of work? Do you own state-of-the-art equipment? Do you offer a greater range of services and products than most other providers?

Focus on the core problem your business solves and put out lots of content and enthusiasm, and ideas about how to solve that problem.
—Laura Fitton

One of the most significant, yet often overlooked, advantages is your actual office location. If you're situated in a large professional building, your appeal is accessibility; people can schedule appointments during breaks, before or after work, and they don't need to drive. If you do on-site work, one of your major benefits is convenience—clients don't have to go anywhere or do anything but enjoy the session. If your office has a particular ambiance (e.g., a fitness motif, a clinic setting, a retreat atmosphere), expound upon those qualities.

In most instances, the strongest factor in your differential advantage is you. What you do, and how you do it, is greatly influenced by your background, personality, education, and philosophy toward the nature of wellbeing.

Define Your Differential Advantage

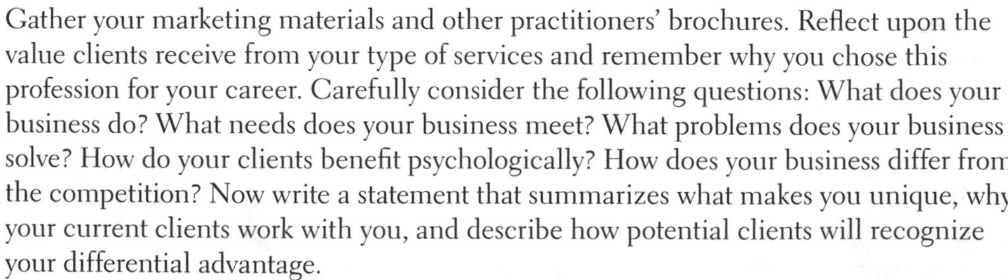

Gather your marketing materials and other practitioners' brochures. Reflect upon the value clients receive from your type of services and remember why you chose this profession for your career. Carefully consider the following questions: What does your business do? What needs does your business meet? What problems does your business solve? How do your clients benefit psychologically? How does your business differ from the competition? Now write a statement that summarizes what makes you unique, why your current clients work with you, and describe how potential clients will recognize your differential advantage.

Your Position Statement

Some people choose a position statement because it resonates with them. Others create statements to draw a specific clientele. It's best if you can do both.

To prepare for the next exercise, review your responses to the differential advantage questions and highlight the crucial facets. Combine those with your image statement to formulate your general position statement. After you finish the next section on target marketing, you may find you need to create additional position statements (one for each of the different markets).

Figure 24.4 Position Statement Examples

The following position statements illustrate the range of differential advantages: types of services, philosophy, specific clientele, and location. Position statements are similar to slogans—though not always so catchy.

Services

Some position statements are based solely upon the service(s) provided. This approach is usually taken when a practitioner has specialized knowledge, a unique service, a particularly clever slogan, or state-of-the-art equipment.

"On Pins and Needles? Try Acupuncture for Relief"

"We Use the Latest Advances in Dental Technology"

"Trained by <insert well-known name here>, Founder of <insert type here>"

Philosophy

Most wellness providers have strong beliefs about the nature of wellbeing and their particular approach to wellness. Quite often, this is the major quality that distinguishes one practitioner from another.

"We Treat You as a Whole Person"

"The Beginning of a Healthy Lifestyle"

"Combining Ancient Healing Wisdom with State-of-the-Art Technology"

Specialization

Some position statements are based on appealing to a target market. For example, you may prefer to only work with one gender or a specific age group. Maybe your focus is treating a specific condition or part of the body.

"Seniors are Our Specialty"

"Making Your Pregnancy More Comfortable"

"Giving Athletes that Competitive Edge"

"The Specialists in Head and Neck Injuries"

Office Location

Expound upon your location's accessibility, convenience, or ambiance.

"Providing All Your Wellness Needs in One Location"

"Only Twenty Minutes from Downtown, Yet a World Apart"

"Have Table, Will Travel"

Many clients are willing to pay more for a practitioner who has advanced education in a specific modality or a specific client condition.

§7

Create Your Position Statement

Write your position statement. Evaluate it in terms of the following criteria:

- Does it convey a true benefit?
- Does it differentiate you from your competition?
- Is it unique?

Target Markets

Target markets are groups of people who share similar characteristics. The whole concept of target marketing may seem very scary at first. On the surface, specialization appears to limit the pool of potential clients. Many practitioners fear that by defining a market, they will lose business or choose the wrong one. An additional concern is that other practitioners will take anybody and therefore absorb some of their business.

In most instances, however, narrowing your field actually increases your overall number of clients. Target marketing is analogous to archery: the goal is to get your arrow as close to the center as possible. The outer rings are bigger and easier to hit, but the high score comes from hitting the center. The same goes for attracting clients; you can appeal to the general masses (the outer rings), but it takes more money and time (multiple arrows) to get the same return on your marketing investment than it would if you focus on a target market (hitting the bull's-eye with 1 arrow).

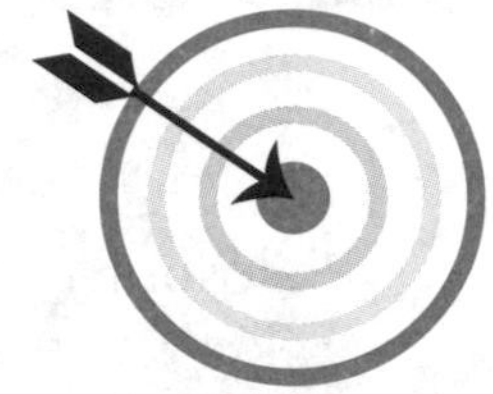

> "I cannot give you the formula for success, but I can give you the formula for failure—which is: Try to please everybody.
> —Herbert B. Swope

The purpose of choosing specific target markets is to make your practice more enjoyable, simplify your marketing, and increase the success of your promotional endeavors. The world abounds with opportunities, and it's impossible to pursue them all or attempt to be everything to everyone. You need to decide where to focus your marketing energy and resources. As a side benefit, specialization and having distinct target markets immediately reduce your competition.

Wellness is very intimate work. Think about who you want in your space. Actively seek those types of clients. This doesn't mean you must limit yourself to only working with people in your target markets. While it's fine to work with whomever wanders through the door, invest your marketing time and money toward attracting your desired target markets. Take the time to identify the qualities and characteristics of your ideal client.

Ultimately, the number of target markets you have depends mainly on the size of your practice and the scope of your knowledge. Some target markets are more productive than others. Most successful practitioners have one or two major markets and a couple of minor target markets. Working with several markets helps to avoid the potential disaster of selecting an unsuitable one. Numerous benefits abound when you aren't restricted to only one type of clientele; in particular, your skills become well-rounded by experiencing a variety of people with their own unique issues. Plus, not being restricted to just one type of clientele allows you to balance altruistic goals and financial needs. For instance, one of your passions might be working with a specific market that doesn't normally have the funds to pay for your services. If you have another target market that covers your bills, you could work with the former population for free or on a sliding scale.

Consider applying for a grant for working with a needy population.

You may also find that certain aspects of your target markets overlap, such as they all shop at the same health food store. Knowing the commonalities assists you in streamlining your marketing endeavors, as you can combine some of your activities (e.g., conducting demonstrations, posting brochures at the health food store).

Identifying Your Ideal Client

Your ideal client is a subset of your target market(s). The first step in identifying this ideal client is to write your responses to the following questions:

- How would you describe the people who use (or would use) the kind of services you provide?
- What type of person is most drawn to your practice?
- What types of people do you want to reach?
- Which groups do you most relate to or already have clients in?
- What types of services would be the most fulfilling for you to offer?
- What qualities do you want your services to exude?
- What problems, conditions, and issues do you want to address in your work?
- What type of environment do you want to work in?
- What are the characteristics of the people you prefer to have as clients?

Given your responses to the preceding questions, who would be most easily attracted to working with you? Who would you really enjoy being around?

Demographics and Psychographics

The more you know about your potential clients, the easier it is to develop an appropriate position statement and design an effective marketing campaign. The two most common means of market analysis are Demographics and Psychographics (aka. Lifestyle Factors), which describe a person in terms of objective data and personality attributes.

Figure 24.5 Demographics and Psychographics

Demographics are categorical statistics such as:

- Age
- Income Level
- Occupation
- Gender
- Geographic Location
- Education Level

Psychographics are the major determinants in whether someone becomes a client.

- Special Interest Activities
- Philosophical Beliefs and Values
- Social Factors
- Cultural Involvements
- Wellness Needs
- Wellness Goals

Connecting with the Right Clients

Some typical wellness target markets are: high-stress executives, pregnant women, athletes (in general or a specific subgroups such as triathletes, cyclists, or gymnasts), infants, children, people in self-improvement programs, pre- and postoperative recovery patients, people with disabilities, attorneys, seniors, the entertainment industry, natural disaster survivors, people in addiction recovery programs, patients of other primary care providers, small business owners, crime victims, students, animals, abuse survivors, computer operators, military personnel, restaurateurs, dancers, artists, people with specific issues such as long-term illness or injury rehabilitation, and other wellness providers.

> “We exist to serve the marketplace. The better we do that, the more profits we will make.
> —Stephen Martin

A common misconception in the wellness field is that people with money are a great target market. Affluence isn't a market, it's a demographic statistic only! Just because individuals have the means to easily pay for wellness services doesn't mean they ever avail themselves. If all the people who could afford your type of service attempted to book an appointment, you and your colleagues would have to work 24 hours a day, 7 days a week.

Still, many wellness providers fall short of their income goals. Obviously, the means isn't a determining factor. You need to discover what motivates someone to receive your services. To grow a successful business, you must identify your target markets and clearly communicate the benefits of your services in a way that attracts potential clients' attention and inspires them to schedule a session with you.

People want to feel that their unique needs are understood. So, even though we know just about anyone can benefit from complementary wellness services, we need to find a way to communicate with potential clients in terms and language that appeals to them. Your marketing becomes authentic when you choose specific target markets, identify their particular needs and wants, and focus your marketing and business operations to serve them.

Matching Needs and Benefits

So far we've explored potential target markets. Now it's time to look at how to analyze those markets. The first two steps are: describe each of your target markets in terms of their general needs, concerns, and goals; and connect specific benefits with each item.

The goal is to inspire people to find out more about your services and how those services can benefit them.

Too often we focus on the direct physical needs a client has, but often those are secondary to achieving other goals. For instance, a client sees you to help reduce pain in his lower back. While alleviating that pain is important to the client, what he really wants to do is easily pick up his grandchild. You will have a better connection with clients and they will be more committed to receiving regular treatments when you've identified the "bigger" goals. Think of this in terms of marketing. A picture of someone easily lifting a child is going to resonate more with this client than a generic photo of someone with good posture. Also, consider their desires; perhaps it isn't something they "need" but they would "like."

Below are brief descriptions of sample target markets, their concerns, and words or phrases that could address those needs. Use these examples as a springboard for analyzing your target markets. Keep in mind, the more accurately you identify the needs of your target market, the easier it is to determine the appropriate terminology.

Pregnant Women: Pregnancy is a time of great change; physically, hormonally, and emotionally. In addition to being concerned about the health of her child, the mother also contends with a changing body image, fluctuating emotions, a possible reduction of activity level, back pain, and edema.

When addressing these areas of concern, incorporate phrases such as: reduces edema; improves circulation; eases discomfort; soothes; enhances connection between mother and child; encourages relaxation; promotes a healthier pregnancy; reduces anxiety; relieves muscle tension and stiffness; enhances wellbeing; increases ease and efficiency of movement; and provides an environment for self-appreciation and nurturing.

Infants: Infants often have difficulty adjusting to being outside the womb and the birth process itself can be traumatic. They may develop sleeping problems, colic, and other ailments that can definitely benefit from complementary health services. Even though the receiver is the child, the parents are the ones to whom you must market your services. Use terms such as: soothing; nurturing; strengthens immune system; safe; gentle; fosters easier and deeper breathing; encourages sound sleep; and promotes healthy development.

Seniors: As people age they become more concerned about their overall health, mobility, and mental acuity. They may be experiencing stiffness, pain, and a lack of touch. Emphasize your benefits with terms such as these: improves blood and lymph circulation; tonifies; promotes healthier, better nourished skin; improves digestion; optimizes joint flexibility; increases range of motion; offers caring and nurturing touch; maintains health;

improves posture; reduces blood pressure; heightens capacity for clearer thinking; reduces stress; and relieves muscle tension and stiffness.

Athletes: Athletes are concerned with avoiding injuries, improving performance, and reducing downtime due to pain or injury. Accentuate benefits such as: improves circulation, flexibility, and mobility; relieves muscle soreness and chronic pain; improves endurance; speeds recovery time; tonifies; supports achieving peak performance; reduces risk of injuries; and enhances concentration.

Entrepreneurs: Your typical entrepreneur is on the go, experiences a lot of stress, must make decisions quickly, has numerous responsibilities and "job titles," and keeps a tight schedule. To appeal to this market, focus on the results and convenience. Use phrases such as: increases stamina; rejuvenates; relieves stress and tension; improves concentration and creativity; alleviates headaches; enhances sense of wellbeing; convenient; accessible; increases productivity; promotes deep relaxation; improves sleep; and provides an easy, affordable way to take care of yourself.

Wellness Providers: Caregivers often ignore their own wellbeing. They often experience fatigue and burnout, in addition to the actual physical stress of their jobs. To best reach this market, remind them that they know the importance of taking care of themselves. Use phrases like: take time for yourself; relieves tension and stiffness; balances chi; relaxed state of alertness; increases stamina; reduces injury; improves posture; enhances self-image; increases career longevity; and provides care for the caregiver.

Personal Growth: People who are actively involved in their personal growth experience this clearing physically, spiritually, and emotionally. Their self-image tends to undergo major shifts. In approaching this group, use phrases such as: tonify your body as well as your soul; soothing; reduces stress and tension; "natural adjunct" to current personal growth techniques; greater ease of emotional expression; increases self-esteem; strengthens immune system; promotes deep relaxation; encourages peak performance; and evokes a heightened awareness of the mind-body connection.

> "People don't buy what you do, they buy why you do it.
> — Simon Sinek

Target Market Profiles

A target market profile is a statement that defines your market in terms of their needs, how your services address those needs, who else caters to the target market, and where they can be found. Once you've determined those components, you can choose effective marketing methods. At this point, you may be wondering how you could possibly know this information, particularly if you're just beginning your practice or are branching out into new directions. Start by conducting market research. Read books and articles about your target market. Get feedback from wellness practitioners, as well as other businesses that cater to your desired market. Research trends online. Discover information by contacting organizations that deal with your target market and by conversing with people who train practitioners to work with that specific population. Be sure to also talk with those who are in the know—members of your target market.

Most of the information gathered in a target market analysis applies to the majority of the members of the given target market. For instance, factors such as trends, basic needs and goals, types of groups they belong to, and national publications they read, are the same for cyclists regardless of where they live. The details that vary include the specific local publications, stores, practitioners, groups, and events.

After you've completed a target market analysis (see Figure 24.6), you're ready to create a target market profile. Start with the general known facts about your target population and adjust them according to your own findings and feedback from others. If you're in practice, review your client files and integrate that data with the research results. The whole purpose of creating a profile is to assist you in developing an effective, natural, marketing plan.

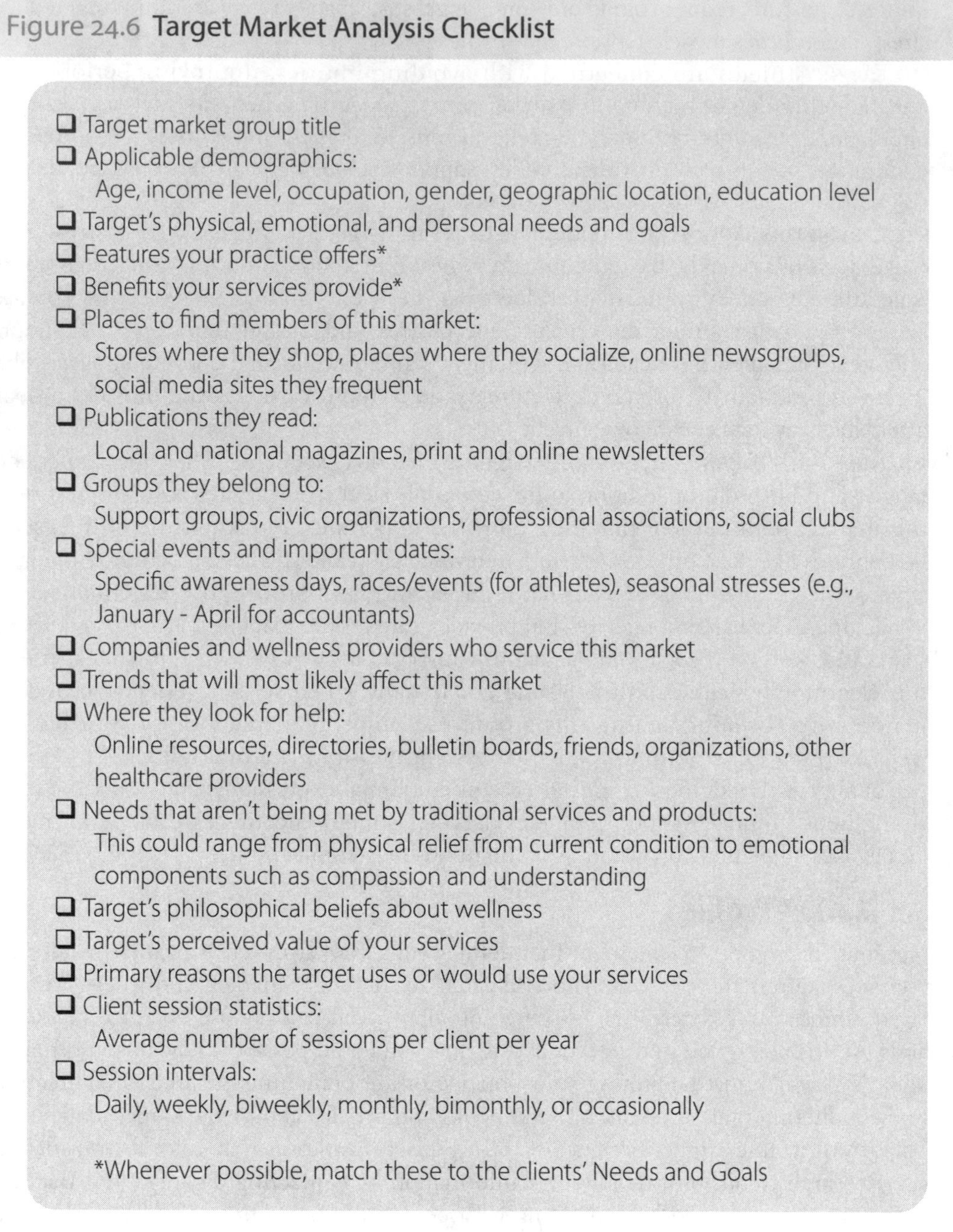

Figure 24.6 Target Market Analysis Checklist

- ❑ Target market group title
- ❑ Applicable demographics:
  Age, income level, occupation, gender, geographic location, education level
- ❑ Target's physical, emotional, and personal needs and goals
- ❑ Features your practice offers*
- ❑ Benefits your services provide*
- ❑ Places to find members of this market:
  Stores where they shop, places where they socialize, online newsgroups, social media sites they frequent
- ❑ Publications they read:
  Local and national magazines, print and online newsletters
- ❑ Groups they belong to:
  Support groups, civic organizations, professional associations, social clubs
- ❑ Special events and important dates:
  Specific awareness days, races/events (for athletes), seasonal stresses (e.g., January - April for accountants)
- ❑ Companies and wellness providers who service this market
- ❑ Trends that will most likely affect this market
- ❑ Where they look for help:
  Online resources, directories, bulletin boards, friends, organizations, other healthcare providers
- ❑ Needs that aren't being met by traditional services and products:
  This could range from physical relief from current condition to emotional components such as compassion and understanding
- ❑ Target's philosophical beliefs about wellness
- ❑ Target's perceived value of your services
- ❑ Primary reasons the target uses or would use your services
- ❑ Client session statistics:
  Average number of sessions per client per year
- ❑ Session intervals:
  Daily, weekly, biweekly, monthly, bimonthly, or occasionally

*Whenever possible, match these to the clients' Needs and Goals

Sample Target Market Profiles

The following fictitious examples include client analyses, profiles, and ideas for reaching those populations. Additional in-depth marketing techniques are explored in the following chapters.

Massage Therapy Prenatal Clients

By compiling the information from Figure 24.7, you could create this profile:

My typical prenatal client is 32 years old. She has been married at least 3 years and already has 1 child. She is under the care of a physician, keeps a healthy diet, goes to childbirth classes, exercises regularly, and gets a massage once per month. She attends cultural events such as theater or concerts at least 2 times per year and dines out at least once per week. She shops at The Bouncing Baby Boutique, buys books on child care at The Basic Book Store, *frequents Nature's Haven Health Food Store, reads the local weekly Entertainment Guide, and subscribes to Parents magazine. Her combined family income is greater than $50,000. She holds an administrative position and works through her eighth month of pregnancy. She is a strong believer in the healing arts. Her major reasons for getting massage are to: have an easy, healthy pregnancy; feel better about herself; relieve lower back pain; increase stamina; decrease edema; improve her body image; reduce stress; and enhance the overall wellbeing of herself and her baby.*

Figure 24.7 Massage Therapy Prenatal Client Analysis

- 30% are referred by childbirth educators, midwives, and health centers.
- 20% are referred by friends.
- 20% were clients before they became pregnant.
- 30% are referred from direct promotional endeavors.
- The average age range is between 28-35 years.
- The majority experience discomfort.
- They are under the care of a physician.
- 70% take health-related classes like Lamaze and exercise.
- 50% never had a professional massage before their pregnancy.
- 50% shop at The Bouncing Baby Boutique.
- The majority read the local Entertainment Guide.
- 60% are professionals or teachers
- The combined family income level is between $45,000 and $80,000.
- 70% attend at least 2 cultural events per year.
- 65% are interested in nutrition and shop at health food stores.
- 70% receive massage once per month.
- 10% receive massage once per week.
- 15% receive massage twice per month.
- The majority are more motivated to receive massage in their last trimester.

Reaching the Prenatal Market

The prenatal market can be approached in many different ways. Before investing any time or money into a promotional endeavor, check your profile to evaluate the likelihood of success. Let's say someone approaches you with an opportunity to place a listing in a promotional piece that is being mailed to "working women" within a 3-mile radius of your office. You need to obtain much more information before determining if it's worth the risk. Keeping in mind that no promotion is ever guaranteed to be successful, compare their proposed demographic and psychographic statistics with your target market profiles to see how well they match.

In developing your marketing plan, prepare for potential obstacles—especially with a target market such as pregnant women. Many other people such as a partner, physician, or even a mother may influence whether a woman receives massage. Your promotional efforts, particularly your print media such as brochures and cards, need to reassure the significant people in the pregnant woman's life. The following ideas are a starting point for reaching this market.

Design attractive promotional materials. In addition to business cards and brochures, consider creating one-sided flyers that are good for tacking on bulletin boards and making informational handouts on different topics of concern to pregnant women. Print these on your letterhead or include your name, title, address, website, and phone number at the bottom of the page. Place your promotional materials wherever pregnant women tend to frequent:

obstetricians' offices, childbirth classes, fitness centers, health food stores, maternity shops, bookstores, childbirth centers, and offices of other allied wellness professionals.

Establish your credibility and build up contacts by volunteering your services (massage or other) at organizations that serve pregnant women, such as wellness clinics, the La Leche League, and Planned Parenthood. Write articles on topics of interest to pregnant women and those around them, such as prenatal wellness care or the benefits of massage during pregnancy, and submit them to your local publications. Also, post your articles on a variety of pregnancy blogs, discussion board websites, and e-zine sites.

Regularly update your website and social media pages with your articles and include a tips section on wellness care for the expectant mother, new moms, and babies. Also, link with online sites that provide support or products to this market. Put client testimonials on your website. Include photos of some of your happy, pregnant clients (get their written permission). Keep people returning to your site by including weekly health tips, announcements, and special offers. Be sure to also list your practice on other sites which this market is likely to visit.

Give an instructional program that teaches birthing partners how to use basic massage strokes for the back, legs, and arms on their pregnant partners. Arrange speaking engagements by contacting pregnancy-related organizations, Lamaze classes, birthing centers, and midwifery associations, as well as business networking groups such as Entrepreneurial Mothers. You could even get another business to sponsor a more extensive program—and handle the promotion and cover the expenses.

Establish a strong referral network of allied professionals such as obstetricians, midwives, nutritionists, labor and delivery nurses, childbirth educators, and other wellness providers. List your name and a concise, engaging description of your practice in appropriate print and online publications. Be sure to put these listings under the heading of "Pregnancy" or "Prenatal Care," in addition to "Massage." Some recommended publications are telephone directories, local wellness publications, newsletters directed toward pregnant women, and special editions of the newspaper, such as an annual health and fitness guide.

Increase your visibility by participating in joint promotions. Some techniques are: include your brochures with mailings of other businesses that cater to pregnant women (e.g., maternity shops, baby stores); set up a booth at expositions such as baby shows, fitness fairs, and anyplace else that attracts your target market; and donate a few sessions as prizes at a major fundraising event. The list goes on....

Acupuncture Senior Clients

Given the information in Figure 24.8, the senior client profile could resemble this:

> *My typical senior client is a retired 70-year-old woman. She leads a semi-active lifestyle; walks 2 miles at least 4 times per week and swims in the summer months. She is on a fixed annual income of less than $24,000 and dines out only once or twice per month. She is a member of at least 1 senior's club and attends 4 to 5 cultural events per year. She frequents museums, libraries, and historical sites. She donates at least 3 hours of volunteer work each week and takes 1 class per year at the community college. She reads the local Senior World Monthly, gets massaged every 6 weeks, receives an acupuncture treatment every 3 weeks, occasionally shops at Nature's Haven Health Food Store, and takes 3 vacations per year. While she does work with a few wellness practitioners, she mainly uses conventional medicine for her health care. This client's major reasons for getting acupuncture are to feel better and be more energetic, enhance mobility, reduce joint inflammation, increase circulation, and relieve pain and stiffness.*

Figure 24.8 Acupuncture Senior Client Analysis

- 75% are retired.
- 80% are on a fixed annual income of $20,000 to $30,000.
- The average age range is between 65-90 years.
- 65% are women.
- The majority eat dinner before 6 p.m.
- 60% regularly volunteer for charities.
- 65% are on a modified exercise routine: walking, swimming, and golfing.
- 20% live in a "retirement" community.
- 60% own their own homes.
- 50% listen to classical music.
- 35% belong to the American Association for Retired Persons.
- The majority are concerned about their longevity and quality of life.
- 60% are on a nutritional program.
- 65% read the local Senior World Monthly publication.
- The majority have a lot of free time.
- 55% attend community theater.
- The majority experience pain, stiffness, and some restriction of movement.
- 60% have more than 1 chronic medical condition.
- 50% see a doctor at least 3 times per year.

Reaching the Senior Market

The senior market is best reached through education. Create a promotional packet that contains your brochure, and be sure it incorporates appropriate terminology and is printed in an easy-to-read, large-sized font. Also, include business cards, informational handouts, and reprints of articles on the benefits of acupuncture and Traditional Chinese Medicine for seniors. By the way, this packet is also useful to send with your letter of introduction to allied professionals.

Place your promotional material on bulletin boards at senior centers, golf courses, wellness centers, medical supply outlets, Elderhostels, community centers, libraries, gerontologists' offices, the Department of Parks and Recreation, pharmacies, bingo halls, volunteer centers, fitness clubs, and offices of allied wellness providers.

> "If a window of opportunity appears, don't pull down the shade.
>
> —Tom Peters

Establish your credibility and build contacts by volunteering your services at a local nursing home, a seniors' rights advocacy association, or even a senior center. Get your name in print by publishing an article on the benefits of acupuncture or by being interviewed by the press. You can also promote goodwill and gain publicity by donating treatments to major fundraising events.

Give presentations at wellness centers, community colleges, senior centers, nursing homes, and other groups like civic organizations that seniors tend to join. Choose the organizations you want to develop an affiliation with and mail them your promotional packet that includes a cover letter expressing your interest in presenting a lecture or demonstration.

Also, consider teaching an extended weekly class on geriatric wellness at one of the centers or colleges. Many cities have a community cable channel. Find out if they broadcast a program designed for seniors, and get yourself booked to appear on that show.

Take out listings in appropriate print and online publications. Again, be certain to also put your name under the headings of "Senior Wellness" or "Geriatric Care" in addition to "Acupuncture." Some suggested publications are healthcare directories, your local seniors' publication, newsletters directed toward seniors, and special "senior sections" in the newspapers.

Put client testimonials on your website and social media pages. Also include photos of some of your senior clients doing activities, such as stretching or playing golf (again, get written permission). Each season, post information on the suggested changes in diet, herbs, and activities. Keep people returning to your site by including weekly health tips, announcements, and special offers. Be sure to also list your practice on other sites which seniors are likely to visit.

Another effective promotional technique is setting up a booth at events that attract seniors, such as golf tournaments, garden shows, and health fairs.

You can be very creative in reaching the senior market. For example, many restaurants offer senior discounts on early dinners. You could join forces with one of those restaurants and have your cards (with or without a discount of your own) displayed on the tables at the restaurant, and, in return, you distribute the restaurant's coupons to your senior clients.

These examples are only a small segment of available options to reach the senior market. Whatever methods you choose to increase your clientele, take the time to establish credibility, allay concerns, and build rapport.

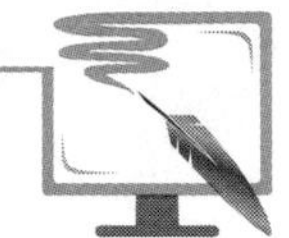

Target Market Exercise

Describe Your Current Clientele

Define your current client base and ascertain the specific markets you currently have. Complete a target market analysis for each of your major target markets. Next, write a descriptive profile for each of your target markets.

Identify New Markets

Select at least 2 target markets and complete a target market analysis and profile for each one.

Evaluate Your Markets

Examine the data from your current and desired target markets. Highlight areas of commonality. Look for traits that your clients share and see if you find patterns. Evaluate your position statement (from the exercise in the previous section): Does it appeal to your target markets? Do you need to change it or create additional position statements? If so, rewrite it now.

Evaluate Your Services

List at least 3 new services and 2 new products that you could add to your menu of offerings to increase your ability to meet your clients' goals.

Competition

A strange paradox of competition versus abundance exists in this career field. There truly are enough potential clients in the world for everyone, and yet not many practitioners have as many clients as they want. Part of the dilemma stems from the fact that the people are "potential" clients. You need to make them aware of you and the benefits of your services. It isn't as though there are limitless numbers of people anxiously waiting for you to let them know you exist; you must create the need.

> "Bicyclists race faster against each other than against a clock.
> —Norman Triplett

Understanding how competition impacts your business can help you make wise marketing decisions. Think of competition as a way of distinguishing yourself from other wellness providers. One of the most exciting facets of this industry is that practitioners usually aren't attempting to prove that they're "better" than others—but that they're different. For this reason, marketing is vital to your career. You must sell people on your services and then on you! Don't assume that you're going to attract the people who "know better," take care of themselves, and use alternative wellness services. Such people probably already have a network of wellness providers. You may need to attract clients who are exploring new modalities due to a health challenge or life change. You may also need to create new markets and possibly share an existing market.

Don't take it for granted that people know what you do because you have a certain title. Define what you do. Explain the benefits of what you offer and what sets you apart from other practitioners in your field. Every practitioner is unique and brings her experience and personality into play along with whatever techniques are employed. The power of your marketing increases with the level in which YOU are integrated into those marketing strategies.

The best way to evaluate other practitioners is to take notice of what people say about them.

The other sources of competition are the products and services that your target markets employ to meet their needs. For instance, if you're a nutritionist and one of your target markets is people who suffer from migraines, your competition can include physicians, hypnotherapists, somatic practitioners, meditation instructors, biofeedback practitioners, acupuncturists, herbalists, and pharmaceutical companies. Many factors determine how migraine sufferers choose to address this health concern, such as the severity and frequency of the migraines, the overall cost for care, knowledge of the breadth of care options, attitudes about certain wellness options, and the perceived value of your type of service.

Some people pay whatever it costs to get the care they need, and they select the method(s) based on their perceived value. Others must choose between options they can afford.

Competition Survey

Rarely is evaluating the competition a straightforward task. You need to do some footwork. It can be easy to ignore this phase since many practitioners aren't willing to challenge their preconceptions about competition. Although your ultimate success depends more on your abilities and communication skills than what your competition does, the more you know about your competition, the easier it is for you to determine the most advantageous manner to market your practice.

See Chapter 15, pages 194-195 for more tips on **scoping out the competition**.

The first step is to identify your most direct competition. Begin your research by studying local wellness directories (or go online). For example, you look through the directory and discover that 40 other practitioners are listed. Of those 40, perhaps half of them appear to provide similar services as yours. This information tells you that you have at least 20 direct competitors and 20 indirect competitors. First focus on your direct competitors. Start your research by checking out their websites. Look to see what services and products they offer, if they have other practitioners working with them, and their prices. Delve deeper to get a sense of what markets they seem to be targeting by how they describe themselves and their services, the graphics they use, and the client testimonials they highlight.

Call them and request brochures, particularly if they don't have websites. Some places to find wellness practitioners' brochures and flyers are bulletin boards at health food stores, offices of other practitioners, and bookstores. Also, check out other local publications (you may want to get several months' worth of editions) to discover if your competitors are listed in any of those publications. Ascertain who is doing what and where they're doing it. These local publications and bulletin boards may be your primary source of information about your competitors, since many wellness providers don't advertise in traditional ways.

Finally, use their services. You may discover that only a few of these people are in direct competition with you: actually offering similar services to the same market at a comparable rate.

Competition Analysis

Compile a profile on each of your major competitors.
Include the following information:

- Name
- Location
- Length of time in business
- Description of services offered
- Manner in which services are provided
- Office hours
- Fee structure
- Clientele description
- Business strengths and limitations
- Differential advantage and market position
- Methods of promotion

Analyze the information you've gathered on your competition. Look for patterns and trends. Compare it to the assessment of your own business.

- How does your business compare to the competition?
- What are the strengths your business has in comparison to the competition?
- What are the challenges your business has in comparison to the competition?
- What are some steps you can take to meet those challenges?
- How can you take your competitors' weaknesses and turn them into unique benefits of your practice?

Cooperation

Once you complete your competition analysis, you might identify some practitioners who really aren't your competition and with whom you could collaborate. Cooperative marketing often increases the success of marketing activities, reduces the risks and costs, saves time and effort, and makes those tasks more enjoyable. Pooling your resources helps you afford more imaginative, elaborate, expensive, and long-term marketing projects. These projects can include simple activities, such as you and a colleague placing each other's brochures on your front desks; to more weighty activities, such as joint advertising, co-sponsoring a fundraiser, submitting proposals to corporations for your services, sharing a booth at an expo, and giving presentations to the general public.

> "Any activity becomes creative when the doer cares about doing it right, or better.
> —John Updike

Cooperative marketing is a great way to overcome marketing reluctance. You also generate a powerful synergy as the creative process is significantly enhanced by team effort versus a "solo act." Humans tend to function better in groups. History demonstrates that people working together create greater results than can be achieved by working apart. A vivid example of this can be related to protests. An individual writing letters to government officials may have some impact, but 1 million people marching in Washington, DC is impossible to ignore. Yet, you don't need quite that magnitude of numbers to have impact, as the synergy created in collaboration is a powerful force.

The benefits of cooperative marketing extend beyond just stretching your marketing budget. Some of the most dreaded aspects of marketing become less of a chore when you don't have to do them alone. For instance, even though public speaking is one of the most effective means of promotion, many people are so uncomfortable being in front of a group, they don't schedule any speaking engagements. Presentations, seminars, and demonstrations are much less intimidating and more impactful when done by two people. It isn't necessary to do everything by yourself!

As much as most practitioners claim they don't believe in competition, very few actively share in marketing their practices. Many are unwilling to even brainstorm ideas with their colleagues for fear of someone else successfully implementing their plans. We need to alter this scarcity consciousness.

For best results, develop a working relationship with at least 3 other practitioners:

- A practitioner in your field who targets a different market.
- A practitioner who offers different services to the same target market.
- A practitioner who shares your target market.

Keep in mind that you don't need to limit mutual marketing relationships to other practitioners. You can also work with retail establishments, suppliers, and organizations.

One way to ease into working with others is to jointly plan a small scale marketing activity. You can increase the scope of your marketing alliance as you build confidence in yourself, your co-marketers, and the process. In essence, you're creating a short-term partnership, so create an alliance proposal that includes the purpose, priorities, goals, financial outlays, and interaction expectations. To give you a picture of how cooperative marketing may work, we look at several examples of marketing alliances and some creative ideas for generating new business.

See Chapter 15, pages 200-201 for tips on **working in a partnership**.

Same Service—Different Target Market

Following are examples of joint marketing ventures among wellness providers who specialize in the same method of wellness care, but work with different target markets:

Acupuncturists: one mainly works with people in recovery programs, another targets the geriatric population, the third works with people with disabilities.

Nutritionists: one targets construction workers, another works with physical therapy clients, the other works mainly with athletes.

On-site chair massage therapists: one works on hair stylists, one targets attorneys, the other works with car salespeople.

Hypnotherapists: one targets other wellness professionals, another works with abuse survivors, the third works with corporate executives.

Marketing Ideas

See Chapters 25 - 31 for specific **marketing ideas**..

Share a booth at conferences, health fairs, and expositions. Don't limit your exposure to just the traditional venues; consider participating in home shows, business expos, state and county fairs, and community art festivals.

- Advertise in local publications and also consider radio or television advertising.
- Co-write an article and submit it to your local publications.
- Contact the media to do interviews.
- Give presentations to the general public.

Different Service—Same Target Market

Some of the most effective cooperative marketing takes place when providers of different services and products focus on the same market. In this case, let your market determine who is best to join forces with for cooperative marketing. Review your target market profiles to assist you in compiling this list. The following are some examples of matching target markets with a group of allied practitioners.

- Most athletes could use the services of a massage practitioner, sports physician, personal trainer, and hypnotherapist.
- People active in personal growth might be interested in seeing a massage practitioner, Rolfing® practitioner, hypnotherapist, counselor, and aromatherapist.
- Pregnant women might assemble a wellness team consisting of a massage practitioner, midwife, gynecologist, Lamaze instructor, and nutritionist.

Extend your combined promotional efforts to include other businesses who share the same markets. Some examples are: health food stores, restaurants, educational organizations, hair salons that use natural products, bookstores, specialty clothing shops, and cultural groups.

Marketing Ideas

- Design wellness packages for businesses and special interest groups. In addition to the standard wellness providers (e.g., massage practitioners, counselors, chiropractors, physicians), consider including a vendor of ergonomic devices like chairs or pillows, a supplier of relaxation CDs and self-improvement products, a health food restaurant to supply healthy snacks, and a biofeedback specialist for stress management.
- Place cooperative advertisements in local publications. If you're in a professional building or shopping complex, get together with the business owners to do joint advertising to attract new clients to your location. You can also sponsor an open house for the public, advertising free demonstrations, music, munchies, and door prizes.
- For those who aren't conveniently located next to one another, consider sharing advertising to promote the benefits of each other's services. This might include wellness providers and related businesses. A recent advertisement in my community paper featured a chiropractic service, a massage therapist, and a bookstore.
- Sponsor an event, such as a fundraiser for a local charity or a health awareness day. You can also provide a booth for refreshments or your services for major races.
- Design a special flyer that describes the services, products, and benefits of the people involved in the cooperative venture. Another possibility is to combine your separate promotional materials into 1 packet and send a direct mailing to potential clients.
- Co-sponsor seminars on health-related topics. For example, develop a stress management workshop with a counselor, aromatherapist, and a bookstore.
- Create packages for celebrations: holidays, birthdays, "thank-goodness-tax-season-is-over," and anniversaries. For example, you could put together a Valentine's Day special that includes dinner, flowers, music, and massage for two.
- Place a display with your cards and brochures next to the cash register at a restaurant, and put coupons from the restaurant in your waiting area.

Marketing Communications for Massage Therapists by Sohnen-Moe Associates

sohnen-moe.com/products/tools/#product-marketing-communication

Same Service—Same Target Market

The best time to join forces with others in your field who target the same market is when the market is too big for you to handle yourself. For instance, this may occur when you contract to provide services for a large corporation. Depending on the size of the company, you may even need numerous practitioners. Another similar situation arises when you're working with a specialty group such as an athletic team.

Marketing Ideas

- Submit proposals to corporations for your services.
- Send direct mailings to specific groups of people.
- Give in-person or video presentations.
- Volunteer at athletic events.
- Sponsor an athletic or charitable group (e.g., underprivileged children).

Cooperative Marketing

- List at least 2 people who do similar work as you but target different markets.
- List at least 2 people in allied fields who share your market(s).
- List at least 2 people in totally different businesses who share your target market(s).
- List at least 3 marketing projects that would be a lot more fun to do with others.

Marketing Mix

Now that you've clearly defined your target markets and gained a solid understanding of marketing basics, we take a look at how to put marketing techniques to work to grow a thriving practice. These techniques can be divided into four major components: promotion, publicity, advertising, and community relations. We briefly describe these components in this section and the following chapters explore these topics in depth.

Promotion

Promotion involves the activities and materials you produce to gain visibility. The money invested is indirect (for instance, while it does cost money to print business cards; it costs nothing to distribute them). Often promotional activities are free of cost. Some of the most effective promotional techniques are: networking, generating word-of-mouth referrals, holding open houses, public speaking (this can be anything ranging from a short 15-minute talk for a local business group, to presenting workshops and giving demonstrations); writing articles for local newspapers, magazines, newsletters, and online blogs; sending your own newsletters and email blasts; and being active in social media.

"In the factory we make cosmetics, but in the stores we sell hope.

—Charles Revlon
Revlon Cosmetics

Publicity

Publicity involves building media awareness about you or your business, often in connection with a special event or milestone. Publicity lends an air of credibility to a business that advertising cannot. People are more likely to utilize your services if they read an article about you, listen to an interview with you on the radio, or watch you on television, than if they see an advertisement about your business. When a respected journalist or reporter makes a positive statement about you, it has much greater impact than if you said the same thing about yourself. Some examples of publicity are news releases, announcements, feature stories, interviews, and press conferences.

Advertising

Advertising differs from publicity and promotions in that you must pay directly for your exposure. Some forms of advertising include display ads in publications, radio and television commercials, classified ads, billboards, directories, Internet ads, and bus-stop benches. Mass media advertising has typically been avoided by wellness practitioners, mainly due to the impersonal nature and the relatively high cost.

Community Relations

Community relations are goodwill activities that create a positive public image for you and your business. Community relations increase your visibility and enhance your image, but only if it's clear you're doing the activities to serve the community and not just to build your business. You can cultivate these relations by: devoting your time and services to a charity or community organization; assembling a disaster relief team; giving presentations in public schools; sponsoring an activity for a special cause; developing a newsworthy persona outside of being a wellness provider; hosting your own radio show or public access cable show; giving free demonstrations; sponsoring a public interest program; and becoming a spokesperson for your profession.

Figure 24.9 The Bicycle Story

An acupuncturist wants to build her practice. She places a bus stop bench advertisement outside the most popular cycling shop in town. That's **advertising**.

She sponsors a cycling team (offers team members discounts on her services and free pre- and post-race mini-sessions for major local events). She prints T-shirts with her name and number for the cyclists to wear. They wear the T-shirts while riding through town carrying a banner announcing their next big race. That's **promotion** (for both the acupuncturist and the cyclists).

In their excitement, the cyclists topple 3 elderly gentlemen while riding through the park. A newspaper reporter just happens to be there and reports it. That's **publicity** (although not the best kind).

The acupuncturist gives each gentleman a 15-minute session. They're no longer in pain and harbor no bad feelings toward "her" cycling team. The gentlemen come to the race to cheer on the team. That's mastering **community relations**.

Develop An Innovative Marketing Plan

> "Learning and innovation go hand in hand. The arrogance of success is to think that what you did yesterday will be sufficient for tomorrow.
> —William Pollard

Successful marketing is based on having a clear vision for your business, defining your target markets, clarifying your differential advantage, determining your position statement, and designing a marketing plan that utilizes creative and effective strategies which reflect your values. Successful practitioners include a good mix of promotion, advertising, publicity, and community relations in their marketing plans. Marketing your business takes time and creativity—particularly with a small practice. Don't always rely on previously used methods (even if they seemed to work), especially if you're approaching the same target group. People like and respond to variety. They tire of seeing or hearing the same thing over and over again. The other reason for altering your marketing modes is to reach potential clients who may have been uninspired by your earlier endeavors. Use an assortment of approaches in an ongoing, consistent manner. Marketing never ends; it's an integral component of your business. Plan on investing at least 15% of your time in marketing to maintain your practice, and more to expand it. If you're just starting out, you may need to increase it to more than 50%.

The methods available for marketing your practice are vast (unless your specific profession has distinct precepts). You don't have to be a genius to develop a sound marketing plan, you don't have to go the traditional route, and it isn't necessary to spend a lot of money (although it's so easy to do). Developing an innovative marketing plan is crucial as marketing has greatly evolved in the last several years. What used to work might not be as effective. Consumers are much more savvy and want to be reached through creative and personal marketing methods. A lot of competition exists for where people spend their money on health and wellness. Your marketing methods need to identify what makes you unique to other practitioners in your specific field, as well as what sets your work apart from other wellness care choices.

Being innovative means reaching your target markets in a way that they don't expect. It also means being flexible in your thinking, responding quickly to change, and utilizing new technology. You gain a competitive edge by regularly reviewing your marketing plan and adapting your marketing strategies. The key to innovation is to look at what you've done (or are considering doing) and then ask yourself:

1. Is this the most effective method? If so, you might want to let it be.
2. What techniques were not as successful as desired?

3. How could you produce better results?
4. Is there another approach that could be used? If so, and you haven't seen it used, then research it. Perhaps it's not cost-effective and then again, perhaps nobody thought of it?
5. Are you utilizing appropriate technology?
6. Are there marketing ideas from other industries that you could use? If so, what characteristics made those innovative marketing campaigns impressive?

After asking yourself those questions, start revamping your marketing plan by highlighting your current marketing activities that have those same characteristics as the campaigns under number 6. Next, identify which of your current strategies could use retooling. Make a list of new strategies that you might like to try. Survey your clients on which of your current marketing endeavors stands out for them, get feedback on proposed strategies, and ask for their suggestions. The final step is to update your marketing plan.

The crucial factor for selecting a marketing venue is: Does it appeal to your target market? Many years ago I heard a speaker talk about the need to learn how to broadcast on station WIIFM (What's In It For Me?). This is particularly true in marketing. Your marketing endeavors need to convey to the recipients exactly how your company is going to help them personally.

Marketing Plan Components

Marketing plans are internal planning documents: they keep you focused and assist you in choosing the most effective ways to build and maintain a thriving practice. Marketing plans answer the following questions: Where are you now? Where do you want to be? How can you meet prospective clients? How can you determine their needs and wants? How can you convey or demonstrate your ability to assist clients in reaching their wellness goals? Figure 24.10 illustrates the major components of a marketing plan.

> "In marketing I've seen only one strategy that can't miss, and that's to market to your best customers first, your best prospects second, and the rest of the world last.
> —John Romero

Figure 24.10 Marketing Plan Outline

I. Overview
- Statement of why you're in this business
- Results you intend to create
- Summary of how you will accomplish your goals

II. Positioning
- Differential advantage
- Image

III. Target Market
- Demographics
- Psychographics
- Needs and goals

IV. Marketing
- Analysis of previous promotional activities
- Recommended changes for future plans
- Overview of competition's marketing

V. Strategic Action Plans
- Marketing mix goals and activities
- Timetables
- Budget

§7

In Lewis Carroll's classic *Alice in Wonderland*, the Cheshire cat tells Alice, "If you don't know where you're going, it doesn't matter which path you take." This applies to any type of planning—and particularly to marketing. I recommend you read all of the chapters in the Marketing Mastery section before you develop your marketing plan.

Marketing Plan Foundation

- Why are you in this business?
- What is your purpose for marketing?
- What are your priorities for marketing?
- What are your major goals for marketing?
- What are your strategies for developing and implementing your marketing plan?

Marketing Assessment

After compiling the information for the first three stages of your marketing plan, the next phase is to assess your previous promotional endeavors and those of your competitors. If you're just starting out in practice, skip this exercise and proceed to the next section. I recommend you do this assessment exercise at least once per quarter.

Marketing Assessment

- List the marketing venues you currently employ.
- How is your business perceived by your clients, colleagues, and prospective clients?
- If you offer more than 1 service, have you promoted each one?
  If no, why not?
- Have you been satisfied with the quality of your marketing efforts?
  If no, why not?
- What have been the results of your promotional activities so far (i.e., how many of your current clients resulted from which types of marketing)?
- What changes would you like to see happen?

The **Marketing Mastery** marketing plan.

A free subscription service that includes a full-year marketing plan, monthly goals and weekly activity reminders.

sohnen-moe.com/resources/marketing-mastery/

Strategic Action Plans

The final portion of the marketing plan is the design of your marketing campaign. Refer to the following chapters for specific marketing techniques. Keep in mind important dates such as holidays, clients' meaningful occasions, and seasonal events. Plan your campaigns thoroughly. Be aware that you may need separate promotional strategies for each target market. Remember to include some cooperative marketing activities into your overall marketing plan.

Implementing your marketing plan of action begins by setting up a schedule. Establish a timeline and specific deadlines for all the steps—and stay on schedule. Integrating your goals into the timelines so they follow a logical order enables you to stay within your time frame. Set realistic deadlines. As I always say, there's no such thing as a bad goal, just a bad deadline.

The next phase is to evaluate the results. If things are going as anticipated, review the rest of the plan to see if you can make any changes to further enhance the results. If you appear to be off target, identify the problems by asking yourself the following questions: Were the goals realistic? Was the timeline too ambitious? Did you need to rely upon too many outside factors? Did you expect more of a percentage increase than occurred? Were there any errors in your plan or in your calculations? Was any of your data inaccurate? Did you choose an inappropriate target market?

Once you've identified the obstacles, some possibilities for alleviating them are to change the basic goals, alter the timeline, correct the mistakes, or possibly even modify the overall strategy.

In summary, developing a top-notch marketing campaign requires creativity, clarity, and insightful analysis to design strategies, determine an annual marketing budget, and assess how well the various parts of the plan complement each other. Allot ample time to evaluate the effectiveness of your campaign during each phase. Track what works and what doesn't—and make adjustments as needed to ensure outstanding results.

Figure 24.11 Marketing Strategy Questionnaire

For each marketing strategy, ask yourself the following questions:

- Is the strategy realistic?
- Does this strategy fit into your budget?
- What are the ramifications of spending money on this strategy?
- Is this strategy unique?
- Is the market large enough to return a profit from this strategy?
- Does this strategy relate to your other strategies?
- Does this strategy accent your strengths and differences?
- Does this strategy appeal to your target markets?
- Is this strategy directed toward your target markets?
- Are people likely to respond to this strategy? If yes, why?

If your answer to any of these questions is no, alter your strategy. If your answers are all yes, it's time to put your marketing plan into action.

Getting Your First Clients

I'm often asked, "What is the best way to market my practice?" Alas, as much as I would love to give a concrete answer to that question, it's impossible. No one-size-fits-all formula works. The marketing venues you choose are best determined by your target markets. The trick to marketing success is to determine what's most important to your potential clients and communicate how you can meet their needs and goals.

When starting out, talk with everyone about your profession: family; friends; neighbors; and people in line at the grocery store, movies, and department of motor vehicles. Share your enthusiasm for your work and the results it produces. Excitement is contagious!

Decide how many sessions you want to work each week and do it. It doesn't matter if you have to give free sessions in the beginning. You need to establish your credibility and build relationships. The way to do that is to work with as many people as possible. Actually, many companies use the stratagem of giving things away to obtain long-term customers. Think about all the book, music, and DVD clubs. They lose money on their initial sales, yet they know that the lifetime value of the customer is worth it. Other large corporations bank on the reliability of this type of promotion and give away samples of their products. They're confident that once people experience the products, they'll continue to use them.

The concept of "giving to get" also holds true for wellness services. For example, if you give away 40 sessions in 1 month and only 10 of those people become regular clients (or refer you regular clients), then those 40 hours of work will bring you $136,000 over the next 4 years (based on our sample lifetime value of a client from earlier in this chapter). Not a bad investment at all!

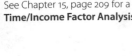

See Chapter 15, page 209 for a **Time/Income Factor Analysis**.

Estimate how much money you want to make and how many clients it takes to reach that goal. Program your mind to expect a set number of sessions, and soon you will find that those sessions are all filled with paying clients. Having said that, it's best if those free sessions are given to people who are likely to become clients, actively generate word-of-mouth referrals, are members of your target market(s), or are centers of influence.

Building a practice requires consistent marketing, business acumen, perseverance, and optimism. Many practitioners give up too soon because they don't receive enough positive feedback and rewards don't come as quickly as desired. While exceptions do exist, it takes most people 2 to 3 years to build a thriving practice. You might need to take a part-time job in the beginning to augment your income. The caveat is to make sure that at the outset of your career, you set specific parameters for when you will take the plunge into full-time practice (e.g., number of clients, amount of money saved). Otherwise, you may never make that transition.

Almost No-Cost Start-up

The four fundamental items needed to start out are business cards, a telephone, an appointment scheduler, and the ability to introduce yourself. These may be the only tools you need if you want to work part time or reside in a community where you're the only practitioner of your kind. Most practitioners need more than that.

Specialty Clothing

www.4imprint.com
www.cafepress.com
www.insideoutbodywear.com

Keep in mind that marketing a wellness practice is based on education and relationships. Make emotional connections with people. Do whatever you can to increase your visibility in your community: attend networking meetings, take classes, write articles, hold open houses, deliver talks, maintain an active online presence, and give demonstrations. Wear logo clothing with your profession or slogan emblazoned on it. Always carry your business cards with you. Volunteer in your community and get interviewed by the media. Post your business cards and brochures wherever your target markets are likely to see them.

Moving Forward

Once you have your first clients, it's time to take the steps to fill your appointment book. Marketing your practice can oftentimes appear overwhelming and arduous, yet no rule says you can't have fun while promoting your business. You can incorporate creative approaches to building your clientele. Keep in mind that the most effective means of marketing wellness services is through a personal approach. Given that the majority of people become your clients out of an experience with you, it's vital that your marketing plan include informal ways for people to get to know you and your work.

The following chapters in this section provide detailed information and examples on innovative marketing ideas.

25
Promotions and Community Relations

"Without promotion something terrible happens... Nothing!"
— P.T. Barnum

Word-of-Mouth Marketing
- Natural vs. Planned WOM
- The Direct Referral Process
- Generate Indirect Referrals

Networking
- Work Your Network
- Choose a Networking Group

Develop a Dynamic Introduction
- Self-Introduction Design

Build Professional Alliances
- Increase Public Awareness
- Develop Direct Affiliations
- Initiate Contact
- Forge Relationships
- Maintain Connections

Public Speaking
- The Public Speaking Circuit
- Successful Presentations
- Delivery

Events
- Open Houses
- Booths
- Fundraisers
- Client-Hosted Parties

Key Terms

Affiliations
Ambiance
Back-Door Approach
Booths
Buzz Marketing
Centers of Influence
Client-Hosted Parties
Connections
Direct Referral Process
Events
Front-Door Approach
Fundraisers
Grassroots Marketing
Image
Indirect Referral Process
Nervousness
Networking
Open Houses
Presentations
Professional Alliances
Public Awareness
Public Speaking
Referral
Relationships
Resources
Self-Introduction
Side-Door Approach
Sponsorship
Theme
Topic
Viral Marketing
Word-of-Mouth Marketing

Promotional techniques and tools attract the attention of potential and current clients, as well as keep you and your services favorably positioned. Community relations increase your visibility and enhance your image. A lot of overlap exists between the two, although with community relations, the focus is on serving the community (with the side benefit of it promoting your practice), whereas promotions are designed to directly build your practice. For instance, if you give a workshop on stress reduction at your local health food store, that would fall under the category of promotion; while you're providing information to help the attendees, your main focus is to build connections and hopefully gain clients. Yet if you gave a presentation on stress reduction for students at a high school, that would fall under the category of community relations; your main purpose is to help the students become healthier.

The majority of marketing endeavors that practitioners utilize fall under the categories of promotions and community relations. This chapter highlights some of the most effective techniques, with guidelines for implementation. I encourage you to experiment with some of these techniques and find the ones that produce good results for you and that you enjoy.

Word-Of-Mouth Marketing

Word-of-mouth (WOM) promotion (sometimes referred to as buzz marketing, grassroots marketing, and viral marketing) is a powerful tool. Many people claim that wellness practices are built by WOM marketing. And there are statistics to demonstrate WOM impact. In December of 2014, the Word of Mouth Marketing Association (WOMMA) unveiled third-party research that measures the total marketplace impact of WOM promotions at $6 trillion dollars, and found that the value of a WOM impression is anywhere from 5 to 200 times more valuable than a paid media impression. Also, offline WOM has twice the impact of online WOM.[1]

People prefer to receive wellness care from someone they know. The second best option is working with a professional who has been highly recommended by a friend or family member. Unfortunately, many people don't know how to foster WOM referrals. They think that offering an excellent service at a fair price is enough. Most clients have a natural inclination to share their experiences with family, friends, and colleagues, yet they can be reluctant to be forthcoming about their wellness care. Unfortunately, satisfied clients don't necessarily talk about you—at least not usually enough to fill your appointment book with new clients. In all actuality, people are more likely to talk about your business when they're unhappy. However, there are many things you can do to encourage positive word-of-mouth referrals.

The most effective way to build WOM referrals is to cultivate relationships. Developing a solid reputation and fostering goodwill is pivotal, and it's even more crucial if you reside in a small town.

See Chapter 5, page 86 for tips on **enhancing goodwill**.

Timing is critical: you get the most impact from WOM promotion within the first 2 weeks of a client working with you or within 2 weeks after a promotional launch, so be sure to emphasize your promotional activities in those first weeks. This is backed up by the WOMMA study that states about 90% of online WOM and 73% of offline WOM impact occurs within the first 2 weeks.[2]

Natural vs. Planned WOM

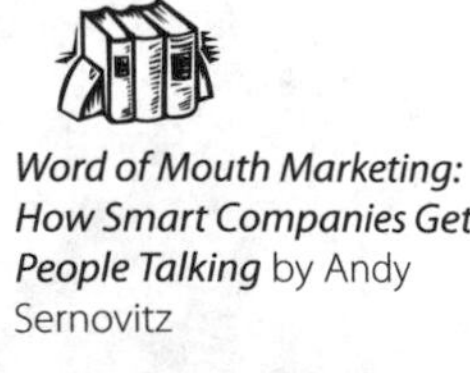

Word of Mouth Marketing: How Smart Companies Get People Talking by Andy Sernovitz

Most practitioners rely on the natural WOM that results from doing good work, genuinely caring about clients, and having a solid reputation. You can increase referrals by incorporating the tips in Chapter 30 on excellent customer service. Still, unless you have a strong network of supporters, this approach could take a long time. While you cannot control how and when you get referrals, there are many ways to generate a positive buzz about your practice.

Figure 25.1 Top 12 Tips to Generate Buzz

1. Cultivate relationships with centers of influence.
2. Recruit cheerleaders.
3. Make it easy for people to share about you (e.g., brochures, business cards, newsletters, websites, open houses).
4. Be interesting and innovative.
5. Cultivate an attitude of gratitude—thank your clients in writing or in a brief telephone call.
6. Develop a referral incentive program for current clients.
7. Stock appropriate products for clients to purchase.
8. Send regular communications (e.g., greeting cards, newsletters, wellness tips).
9. Be a source of knowledge (e.g., give presentations and demonstrations, write articles).
10. Establish a presence in your community (e.g., network, volunteer, send press releases, get interviewed).
11. Refer clients to appropriate colleagues.
12. Do a good job and pay attention to "the little things."

The Direct Referral Process

Directly asking for referrals is a common and accepted form of building any service business. If you don't tell your clients you would like their assistance, they might assume you're fully booked and aren't accepting new clients. The direct referral process consists of four major stages: request the referral, repeat the request, reward the referral, and reciprocate the referral.

Request The Referral

Talk with your most satisfied clients and enlist their support. Ask them to tell their colleagues and friends about you. Supply them with business cards, brochures, and perhaps even some discount coupons for a percentage off an initial session (see Figure 25.2).

You can also email each client a brief description of yourself and a personalized statement of how your services assisted that specific client in achieving her wellness goals. Request that the client make any desired adaptations and send the note to people who might be interested in your services.

Repeat the Request

The next time you talk with your clients, repeat the request. People don't always hear things the first time. They may have been preoccupied (or if it was right after a session, they may have been too relaxed for the request to sink in). Find out if they need more promotional materials, and ask them how you can make it easier for them to promote your practice.

Send them a thank-you note even if you haven't received any referrals. Recognize them for their intentions and support. They could be sharing information about you and passing out your cards, but you might never know it. They don't have control over whether or not the people they talk to call you to set up an appointment. Everyone likes to be acknowledged, and knowing that you appreciate their efforts can inspire them to continue referring people to you.

Reward the Referral

When you do get a referral, immediately send a thank-you note. Reward the referral with something tangible such as a free session, an add-on service, a product sample, a plant, or flowers.

Reciprocate the Referral

The last stage in the referral process is reciprocation. Whenever someone refers a client to you, go out of your way to either refer another client or customer back, use her services and products yourself, or supply her with some type of desired information.

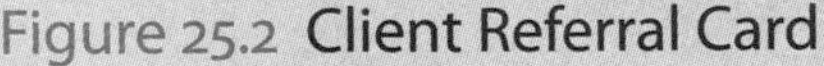

Figure 25.2 Client Referral Card

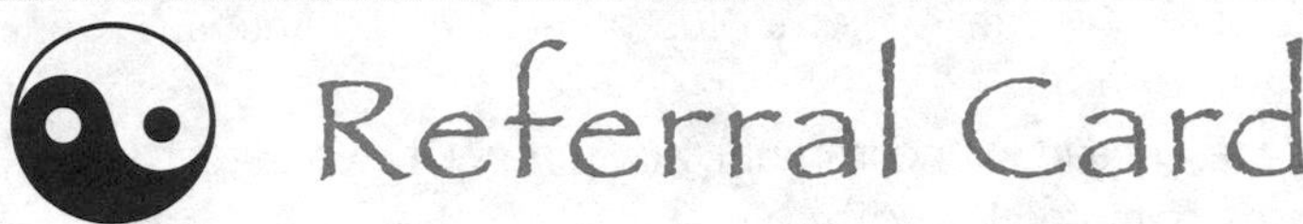

To:

From:

Give this card to a friend for $10 off their first appointment...
and get $10 off your next visit!

Mia Lan Acupuncture

518 Broadway, Suite 3, Anytown, NJ 08413
207-555-3271 ❖ www.mialan.example.com

Generate Indirect Referrals

Another option to cultivate referrals is to compile a list of referral sources (e.g., all former and current clients, colleagues, friends, family members) who value your work. Ask them to write down the names addresses, phone numbers, and email addresses of people whom they think could benefit from your services. Send those prospects a personalized letter of introduction, your brochure, and include a discount coupon or referral card. Keep track of which people respond to your letter. Contact the rest within a month. Inquire if they received the letter and ask if they would like additional information (such as articles or pamphlets), invite them to an open house or workshop, offer a free consultation, or perhaps even book a session. Another option to make this feel less like cold calling is to provide your referral sources with an email (complete with the subject line, written message, links or attachments) that they can forward to people they think would benefit from your work.

Developing a solid referral process is great for augmenting your practice as long as you don't depend on it as your major source for new clients. Ultimately, when it comes to establishing a thriving practice, you're the only one who can do it. The key is to design and implement a sound customer service plan. When it comes to WOM promotion, the most important mouth is your own!

Networking

Establishing a strong network is fundamental for success in the wellness field. Since so much of our business comes from WOM (referrals from clients, friends, and other networking associates), it's crucial to begin fostering these associations immediately!

Networking is essentially a group of interconnected or cooperating individuals who develop and share contacts, information, and support. An effective network is composed of many different types of people: individuals from whom you get information; experts whose services you utilize and can refer to others; people who keep you informed of events and opportunities; role models; those who are genuinely concerned about you, listen to you, and support you; mentors; people who actively refer potential clients to you; and centers of influence.

> "You can make more friends in two months by becoming interested in other people than you can in two years by trying to get people interested in you.
> —Dale Carnegie

Centers of influence can have a dramatic impact on your practice. These are individuals who are well known and highly respected by your target market(s). Just one word from them could inspire droves of people to flock to your roost.

You can network informally by sharing resources with the people you contact or formally by joining a networking group. The most successful networkers are those who actively support others in making connections. Networking is a perfect example of the adage: the more you give, the more you receive.

Work Your Network

Enhance your networking abilities by recognizing the vast potential for making connections for yourself and others. Whenever you meet someone, jot a few notes about them: where and when you met, who introduced you, what line of business they're in, what their interests are, and what types of resources they have. Think about the other people you know to see if it would be beneficial for them to meet each other. Even if you're unable to make any connections right away, you may do so in the future. You never know when a contact will come in handy.

Become visible in your community: attend business, civic, and social events; join professional and networking associations; take seminars and classes. Attend various types of functions so you can widen the scope of people you meet.

Custom Lanyards
www.lanyardstore.com

Follow up on leads and information with a phone call, note, or email. Take the initiative. Always thank people that help you (either by giving you their time, support, advice, leads, or contacts), even if you don't use their help or if the leads don't work out. When you're given a recommendation to utilize someone's services, tell the person who referred you. When you give out referrals, make note of who you referred to whom. Find out if the referral was successful.

Maintain contact with people in your network and stay up-to-date with what's happening. People's lives are constantly changing and so are their networking needs. Given natural attrition, add at least 2 people per month to your active network to keep it thriving. The most fundamental element in effective networking is to follow through on your commitments.

Choose a Networking Group

§7

Effective networking can be exciting, as well as financially rewarding! Be active in at least 1 business association. Numerous types of networking groups exist from monthly social clubs, to community groups such as the Chamber of Commerce, to weekly "needs and leads" business associations. Participate in functions at which you meet people to develop mutually beneficial relationships. Many people join networking groups with high hopes that many of the members will become clients. Although this can occur, most successful networkers focus on building strategic alliances and cultivating centers of influence.

See Chapter 26, pages 407-409 for information on **business cards**.

Determine which organization is best for you by assessing your needs and clarifying your purpose and goals for networking in general. Ascertain the types of contacts you desire and appraise the assets you can offer others. Delineate your purpose and goals for each specific group you're considering. You may want to become a member of one group mainly as a means for getting clients and join another association because you strongly support their goals and activities. You may decide to become part of an organization for the educational and informational opportunities, or join a club to make new friends and have fun. Sometimes one organization can meet several of your criteria.

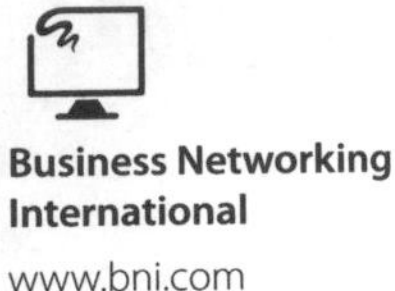

Business Networking International

www.bni.com

Figure 25.3 Networking Tips

- Wear clothes with pockets when attending networking events; one pocket holds your business cards, the other for cards you collect. Also, keep your hands as free as possible—it's extremely difficult to shake hands when you're balancing a beverage, plate of food, and a purse, smartphone, or briefcase.
- Print unique business cards that include a call to action.
- Always carry plenty of business cards and keep them in an easily accessible spot.
- Consider printing a customized lanyard and name tag.
- Wear a custom printed shirt with your name and logo.
- Arrive early to meet new people.
- Use Twitter before and during an event to connect with people.
- Clearly state what you do. After a brief conversation, people are more apt to remember an occupation than a name.
- Periodically reassess your needs, priorities, and contacts.
- Keep your contacts up to date in your smartphone or customer relationship app.
- Collect business cards. On the back of the card write the date, where you met, who introduced you, and any other specific information you want to remember.
- When you give out referrals, make note of who you referred to whom. Then find out if the referral was successful.
- Follow up initial meetings with a phone call, note, or email. Take the initiative. Everyone likes to know that people are interested in them.
- Maintain contact with people in your network. Know what is happening.
- Add at least 2 people per month to your active network.
- Join professional associations.
- Develop your own personal, professional, or educational support groups.
- Attend workshops.
- Share your resources and contacts.
- Attend community functions.
- Thank people who help you (either by giving you their time, support, advice, leads, or contacts). Be a giver and a receiver.
- Follow through on your commitments.
- Actively cultivate your current network and begin increasing it today.

Attend 1-2 meetings as a guest. Get a feel for the group. Notice whether you share any common interests and goals. Ask to see their bylaws and mission statement. If they don't have anything written, talk to several members and get feedback on their impressions of the group's purpose and philosophy. Find out the types of businesses and professions represented by the membership. Many organizations have a substantial membership fee, so do research before joining to determine if it's the right group for you.

Figure 25.4 Networking Group Checklist

Assess Your Needs and Goals

- ❑ Identify the types of support you need.
- ❑ Determine the type(s) of groups that would be in alignment.

Research Potential Groups

- ❑ What is the group's purpose (mission statement)?
- ❑ What year was it established?
- ❑ When does it meet, duration, and location?
- ❑ What are the dues and fees?
- ❑ How many total members?
- ❑ How many active members?
- ❑ What is the number of members in your field?
- ❑ What types of businesses and professions are represented?

Attend at Least Two Meetings

- ❑ Determine the group's philosophy.
- ❑ See if you share any common interests and goals.
- ❑ Decide if you're comfortable referring business to the members.

Building an Effective Network

An effective network is composed of many different types of people. List the names or titles of the people who fit into each category (some names may be repeated since people often have more than one role in your life).

- Your sources of business- and practice-related information
- People who could be centers of influence
- People who actively refer potential clients to you
- Experts whose services you use and can refer to others
- People who keep you informed of events and opportunities
- People who genuinely care about you, listen to you, and support you
- Your mentors
- Your role models

Now that you have specified the people in your current network, review the lists. Do one or two people perform most of the roles? Are there any areas that are lacking names? Are most of the people the same type? How do you feel about your network?

The next phase is to identify your needs and goals:

- List the kinds of support you would like to have right now.
- What additional types of support do you need over the next year?
- Who would you like to add to your network?
- List at least 10 goals for improving your network.

Develop a Dynamic Introduction

No matter what you do in life, your ability to introduce yourself well greatly impacts your success. Current studies claim that you only have between 4-20 seconds to make that vital first impression.[3,4] New research reveals that you only have about half a second to establish trustworthiness through your voice.[5] Frequently, people turn off many potential clients because they don't present themselves positively and professionally. They haven't taken the time to develop even a rudimentary introduction, let alone a powerful one. Because this industry thrives on WOM promotion, you must inspire others by the way you introduce yourself.

Actually, it's wise to have several exciting introductions down pat. The advantage is this: you may want to vary what you say and how you say it depending on the time parameters and the audience. Your introduction will differ if you're talking directly with one person rather than a group. Most likely you'll use different terminology when you're talking to a group of your peers rather than a business group, or even a mixed group.

For instance, in most networking groups, you're only allotted 30 seconds or less to introduce yourself. Without a prepared introduction, you probably will only say a small portion of what you wish to convey. Yet 20 seconds is ample time if your basic introduction is clear, concise, and engaging. In the article titled "The Schmooze Factor," Kathy Gruver gave this entertaining example of a creative option to work with networking groups that employ a bell or buzzer to end your introduction, "I was at an event where they forgot the bell and were just having the timing person say 'Stop.' I changed my elevator speech around in my head and planned it so the 'Stop' worked in my favor, timing it so that my last line was, 'Give me a call if you'd like your pain to' When the man said 'Stop' everyone laughed."[6]

I recommend creating a memorized 20-second and 30-second introduction. It's also wise to design a 1-minute and a 5-minute presentation in which you memorize your opening and closing lines, and have a clear outline of key points you wish to cover. Conversely, I highly discourage memorizing any presentation that's more than 30 seconds in length, since this puts too much emphasis on the words and not the relationship between you and your audience. Another problem with a memorized speech is that if you forget a word, or someone asks you a question, you may get totally thrown off track and not gracefully recover.

Self-Introduction Design

"Features" are what you do. "Benefits" are how what you do helps others.

Designing your introduction needn't be a grueling experience. You can generate and refine several introductions in less than 3 hours. Make this project more fun by getting together with several friends to work on your introductions. As a side benefit, the material you develop for your introduction(s) can be utilized in creating other promotional material, like brochures, social media profiles, and press releases.

Begin your adventure by collecting descriptive material: informational packets on your area of expertise, magazine articles, brochures from other practitioners, and promotional pieces on yourself. Go through this information and highlight the words and phrases that appeal to you.

Then, write a detailed statement of what you do. Be certain to distinguish the features from the benefits and include information from your differential advantage statement.

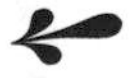

See Chapter 24, page 358 for more on the **differential advantage**.

The subsequent phase is the writing of your introduction. First, choose a specific audience and a time frame (e.g., a business networking meeting and 30-second general introduction or the introduction to a 20-minute presentation). Look over all of the material you have—the highlights from your sample promotional pieces, your business description, and your written differential advantage statement. Combine these to formulate your written introduction. Review it, replacing any passive words or phrasing with the dynamic, active, present tense.

Alleviate the habitual use of the same language patterns and vocabulary by using a thesaurus to discover different words (e.g., terms, statements, jargon, expressions). If you do this exercise with colleagues, read your introductions to each other and get feedback. Repeat this complete process for each introduction you prepare.

The final step is refining your introduction. The best way to do this is to rehearse it in front of friends (ones that are honest with you). Get their input on the content AND your delivery. If this isn't feasible, practice out loud, standing tall in front of a mirror. Use an audio recorder (video-recording is preferable), and critique the results. "All the world's a stage," and these are your lines. Keep practicing until you're very comfortable with what you say and how you say it.

Figure 25.5 Simple Yet Effective 20-30 Second Introductions

"How would you like to make your pregnancy—or that of a friend's—much more enjoyable and comfortable? This can be achieved by receiving regular massages. I'm Mary Smith, and I'm a licensed massage therapist, specializing in prenatal massage. The work I do with pregnant women assists them in improving circulation, reducing edema, enhancing muscle tone, and easing tension and fatigue. Please feel free to talk with me after the meeting. I have cards, brochures, and gift certificates available at the back table."

"Hello, I'm Kerry Billings, and I'm a chiropractor. I've been in practice since 1999 and have recently moved to Sunny Hills. My focus is on wellbeing and preventive care. I have an extensive background in Oriental philosophy and incorporate that into my approach. Please call me if you're interested in more information. I don't charge for an initial consultation. I look forward to meeting with you and assisting you in achieving optimal health."

"Do you experience a lot of stress? Is your life filled with activities—career, family, and friends? Are you involved in a fitness program? If you answered yes to any of these questions, you probably experience some form of physical discomfort—be it muscular aches and pain, fatigue, or even tension headaches. Yoga can help reduce stress, improve circulation, ease tension, and improve muscle tone. I'm Randy Harris, and I'm a certified yoga practitioner. If you would like more information on how yoga can enhance your wellbeing, please talk with me after the meeting."

Write Your Self-Introduction

Write a self-introduction. After you're done, note how you feel about yourself and your introduction. What could make your introduction more powerful? Does this inspire you to learn new modalities or get additional experience working with a specific condition? If so, add those to you career goals. Also, consider how you could adapt this introduction for other uses. Test out your new introduction with the next 3 people you see. (It's okay to tell them you are practicing for something.) Observe their reactions and then further tweak your introduction, if necessary.

Build Professional Alliances

Every day the wellness field becomes more integrated. Providers from all realms are working together—blending philosophies, as well as actual client care. You can guide the direction this takes by developing affiliations with other wellness providers. Cultivating strong professional alliances provides value for you personally, as well as for your clients.

One of the main benefits is having a diverse referral base to properly support your clients' wellbeing. Working with other practitioners provides you with a means to get away from working alone. These associations can also supply you with new clients and offer you the opportunity to participate in case management.

Professional alliances take time and commitment. Build your network of professional wellness alliances through establishing credibility, initiating contact, forging relationships, and maintaining connections. They can be best developed with a two-tiered approach. The first level is built on increasing awareness of the benefits of your specific services. The second level involves forming direct affiliations with other practitioners. It's crucial to always be working on both levels.

Increase Public Awareness

See Chapter 29 for details on getting **publicity**.

Increasing public awareness can be accomplished in many ways, from distributing educational materials to hosting elaborate media events. One of the most effective techniques is public speaking: offer to do presentations and demonstrations for professional, business, civic, and special interest organizations (such as fibromyalgia support groups). Host exhibits at health fairs and expositions. Blog or write articles for local publications. Get interviewed by the newspaper, radio, and television. Be a guest on local health-related talk shows. Find out if and when your local paper publishes a special health supplement and arrange for your interview to appear in that section.

Although these activities are geared toward increasing public awareness about the benefits of your services, they also increase your credibility and visibility. Additionally, the exposure serves to establish you as an expert.

Develop Direct Affiliations

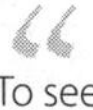

To see power as the ability to enhance others' lives expands society's narrow understanding of more traditional concepts of power.
—Pythia S. Peay

Assemble a list of people with whom you want to build alliances. Start by identifying allied providers who work with your target markets. Conduct an online search to find local providers. Ask your clients, colleagues, friends, and family for names of people for your list and why they recommend them. Determine your purpose, priorities, and goals for developing these alliances, and create an action plan. Consider how much time you want to invest, the types of professions (and how many) you want to include in your network, and the levels of interaction you desire.

Foster Professional Alliances

- List the types of service providers that could assist your clients in achieving their wellness goals.
- Match those categories with names of providers whom you currently know.
- Note which categories are lacking names and set goals to meet those types of practitioners.

Start developing affiliations by establishing credibility. Many allied providers (particularly physicians) are required to obtain layers of licensure and certification. This leads them to judge competency by the number and types of certificates hanging on a wall—so some type of professional certification is helpful. Yet pieces of paper aren't the only badges of credibility.

An interesting synergy often occurs in developing affiliations. Once the first connection is made, others occur more easily.

You can enhance your visibility and credibility by getting involved in the activities described in the previous section on increasing public awareness. In addition to those activities, you could attend meetings at which there are other practitioners, join a local wellness organization (usually sponsored by a hospital), or volunteer your services for a charitable organization.

If you aren't well versed in the language of professional healthcare providers, learn to speak it now: be aware of their philosophy, approach, and terminology. While it's fine to refer to your leg as a "calf" when talking to the general public, you're less credible if you aren't more technical while addressing other practitioners (in those instances, you might reference a specific muscle, such as the gastrocnemius). Keep in mind that not everyone shares your particular approach to wellness care. While many practitioners believe in and specialize in prevention, others (e.g., physical therapists, general physicians, surgeons) spend most of their time working with people on the remedial side of health care.

Initiate Contact

Some people prefer the front-door approach while others feel more comfortable with the side-door or even back-door method of developing affiliations. You might consider using a combination of these approaches. Regardless of the approach, be sure to emphasize how your services enhance their practices and support their clients' goals. Briefly share about your training, highlight any unique modalities or equipment you use, and provide client testimonials.

Front-Door Approach

The three most common front-door approaches are the telephone, the mail (or email), or in person. Some people feel very comfortable just walking in and introducing themselves. This is a lot easier if your office is located close to other providers. In general, though, people prefer to initiate contact with a letter or telephone call. When you know the practitioner, a phone call usually suffices.

An effective technique for generating prospective alliance partners is to send a mailing to targeted wellness professionals. Direct the emphasis of your letter to the benefits of the reader. First introduce yourself and say what you do, including your abilities and qualifications. Focus on how you can help them, their practices, and their clients. Create a separate letter for each type of practitioner you contact. For each type of provider you contact, include examples of how your services address their specific needs. (See Sample Introduction Letter, Figure 25.8.)

For instance, chiropractors see people who suffer from arthritis, back pain, fibromyalgia, migraines, injuries from sports activities, job injuries, and automobile accidents. Psychiatrists work with people experiencing pain, stress disorders, and migraines, as well as support people in personal growth and wellbeing. Obstetricians work with women experiencing back pain, edema, hormonal fluctuations, and body image issues, as well as support general mother/child wellbeing. Touch therapists work with people of all ages, providing services ranging from relaxation to injury rehabilitation.

Highlight the mutual benefits of your association. Reassure your prospective colleagues that your intent is to support and complement each other's practice, not compete for clientele. Close the letter by telling them how to contact you, and that if you don't hear from them within the next 2 weeks, you will contact them.

Enclose your promotional material and a research article that lends credence to your claim for potential benefits. You can also include a stamped, pre-printed return postcard that allows the practitioner to respond directly. After the letter has been sent, you must follow up.

Figure 25.6 Sample Reply Postcard

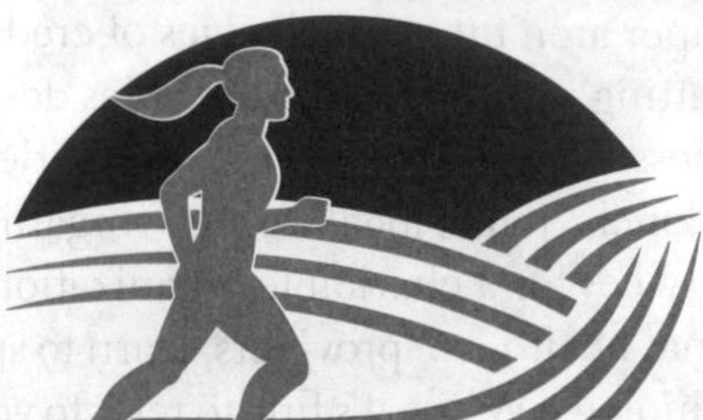

Sports Massage Clinic
3197 Bender Creek Circle
Burlington, VT 43579
802-555-5555
ginny@example.com
www.sportsmassageclinic.example.com

Yes! I am interested in pursuing a possible alliance:
❑ Please send me more information.
❑ Please call me to set up a meeting to discuss our possible alliance.
❑ Please call me to schedule my complimentary session.
The best time to reach me is: ____________________
My phone number is: ____________________

❑ I'm not interested in developing a professional alliance at this time.

Side-Door Approach

Wellness Councils of America
www.welcoa.org

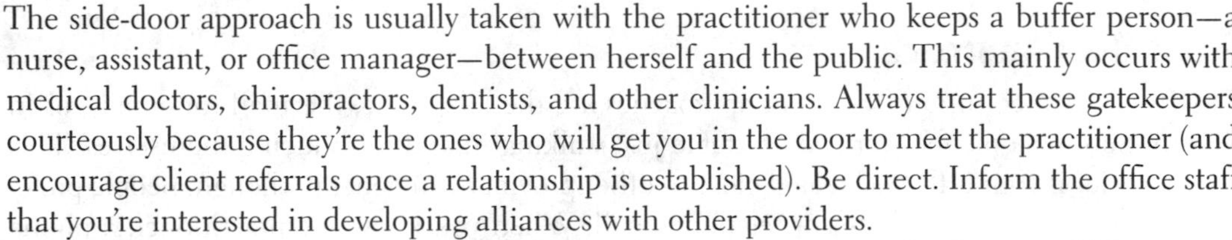

The side-door approach is usually taken with the practitioner who keeps a buffer person—a nurse, assistant, or office manager—between herself and the public. This mainly occurs with medical doctors, chiropractors, dentists, and other clinicians. Always treat these gatekeepers courteously because they're the ones who will get you in the door to meet the practitioner (and encourage client referrals once a relationship is established). Be direct. Inform the office staff that you're interested in developing alliances with other providers.

If you're unable to make an appointment with the practitioner, ask when would be a good time to drop off your brochure. When you deliver your brochure, ask the office manager if she has any questions about your services or background, and offer to demonstrate your work, for example, by teaching a 5-minute self-massage routine. Give free sessions to the provider and the staff. This is time well invested, because if you get the opportunity to demonstrate your services, and the recipient is impressed with the benefits, that person is likely to be interested in building an alliance with you. Give a certificate for the session(s), and if possible, book the appointment(s) before you leave.

See Chapter 19, pages 264-266 for **HIPAA guidelines**.

Another way to build alliances through the side door involves your current clients. When conducting intake interviews, ask your clients if they're working with other wellness providers. If so, get their permission to send a note to those providers. This could range from a simple letter of introduction informing each practitioner that you're working with their client, to a more in-depth report with a brief description of your assessment, treatment plan, and progress notes. (Note: Be sure to follow HIPAA guidelines when appropriate, and also include your promotional literature and extra business cards.)

Back-Door Approach

The back-door approach can appear to be the least threatening entrance to developing professional relationships. There are various ways to enter through the back door. You can get to know other practitioners by sponsoring a talk show on radio or cable (on which you bring wellness providers as guests) or by hosting an open house. You can also encounter practitioners by attending networking events, social engagements, professional society meetings, special interest group meetings, professional development seminars, and civic functions. Research these groups to determine which ones are most likely to attract the types of practitioners you wish to meet.

An example of attending events to develop professional alliances and get clients happened when I did a seminar tour in Australia. One of the participants in my workshop in Brisbane was a business coach. She attended my seminar for a dual purpose: to learn new information, but mainly to get new clients. Here was a perfect opportunity: she could spend 2 days getting to know many people who were obviously interested in their professional development—with the knowledge that I wouldn't be there to work with them on an ongoing basis.

Forge Relationships

Your first official meeting with a wellness provider sets the tone for the relationship. Be punctual and look professional. Ideally you will also be giving a session, so your clothing can be a little more casual. Wear what you normally would while working with a client in your facility. Business attire is appropriate if you aren't giving a session. Greet the practitioner with a handshake and smile.

Briefly share information about yourself and encourage the provider to share information about her practice. Discuss ways in which you could be of mutual benefit (including reducing the demands on her time and energy), and set goals. Confer about approaches to different situations, and determine how you would like to work together. Be certain to cover the preferred methods of future communication about shared clients. Some people favor written correspondence only, while others like to discuss cases and proactively work together to enhance clients' wellbeing.

> "No road is long with good company.
> —Turkish Proverb

While it isn't imperative that the practitioner experience your work, I strongly advise you make it happen. If she claims she is too busy, offer to do a modified session at her convenience. Also give a free session to the staff (see the previous section on initiating contact). Be upfront: tell her that it's important to experience your work firsthand to ethically feel good about making referrals to you. The converse is also true. For you to refer clients to her, you need to experience her work—or in the very least get a sense of her methodology and style, which can be done by assessing the person's demeanor, office environment, and written materials (such as intake forms and information pamphlets).

When you give her a treatment, do an intake interview (modify it if time is limited), take notes, and submit a sample of your records. This is of particular importance if you aren't a primary care provider, because it demonstrates your ability to do charting and follow-up. Before you leave this meeting schedule the next one—whether it's a telephone conversation, another session, or a more formal face-to-face meeting. Sometimes the steps to forging a relationship take several meetings to accomplish.

Maintain Connections

Maintain connections by employing customer service principles. Consider these examples:

- Send a thank-you note after your first meeting.
- If they haven't used your certificate within 3 weeks, remind them, and ask them when they would like to book the session.
- Acknowledge all referrals.
- Regularly submit typed progress reports (check with client first).
- Call about dramatic results.
- Schedule a brief meeting at least twice per year.
- Reciprocate by sending them clients.
- Leave an ample supply of your brochures and business cards for display and distribution.

- Supply them with "prescription" pads.
- Obtain a plentiful stock of their cards and brochures.
- Place monthly check-in calls (instead of asking if they've run out of brochures or cards, assume that they have, and ask how many you can bring by).

You want to make it as easy as possible for allied health providers to make referrals to you. In addition to stocking your promotional material, consider printing prescription pads with your contact information to give to the providers and their office staff.

Figure 25.7 Sample Prescription Pad

Sports Massage Clinic
3197 Bender Creek Circle
Burlington, VT 43579
802-555-5555
SportsMassage@example.com
www.SportsMassageClinic.example.com

Date:

Patient:
Address:
City: State: Zip:
Telephone:

Condition Related To:
❑ Auto Accident ❑ Work Injury ❑ Stress/Relaxation
❑ Other:

Body Areas To Be Treated:
❑ Neck ❑ Back ❑ Shoulders ❑ Legs ❑ Arms

Diagnosis Description & Codes:

Duration: ❑ 8 weeks ❑ 6 weeks ❑ 4 weeks ❑ other:
Frequency: ❑ daily ❑ 3x/week ❑ 2x/week ❑ weekly
❑ biweekly ❑ monthly ❑ other:
Medically Necessary: ❑ Yes ❑ No

Prescribing Doctor:
Doctor's Provider #:
Address:
City: State: Zip:
Telephone:

Signature:

Figure 25.8 **Sample Introduction Letter**

Mind-Body Progression

October 15, 2020

Ben Casey, Ph.D.
123 North Swan Road
Sea City, CA 90000

Dear Dr. Casey:

I was intrigued by your advertisement in the Sea City Healthy Connections Directory under "Psychotherapy." You appear dedicated to the health of the whole person. As a licensed acupuncturist and Traditional Chinese Medicine (TCM) practitioner, I also see the significance of the mind-body connection and how addressing the health of one area while excluding the other is an incomplete process.

I am interested in developing an alliance to better serve our patients. I provide a complete range of services that include general wellness, stress reduction, pain relief, injury rehabilitation, and illness prevention. Many of these were listed in your advertisement as well. I am also a master herbalist and have worked with people of varying ages.

Acupuncture and TCM, as a complement to psychological counseling, can support optimal wellbeing in powerful and beneficial ways. As an adjunct to your therapy, clients utilizing my services may find a decreased need for medication, thus lowering the possibilities of medication interactions.

As we tend to approach holistic health from different angles, I believe many of our clients could benefit from our combined services. For example, I see clients who experience emotional releases during sessions and who would benefit from professional counseling. Likewise, I'm sure you have clients who could benefit from acupuncture and TCM.

I look forward to meeting with you personally to discuss the possibilities of mutual referrals. Feel free to call my office at 555-5555. Otherwise, I'll contact you within the next two weeks to schedule a time to meet. I've enclosed my brochure and a copy of a research article on the benefits of acupuncture for mental health.

Sincerely,

James Kildare
Enclosures

721 N. Somerset Place ❖ Arcadia, CA 91077 ❖ 415-555-5555
jkildare@mind-bodyprogression.com ❖ www.mind-bodyprogression.com

§7

Public Speaking

Remember "show and tell" from grade school? This was your opportunity to share something wonderful that happened to you or to show off a favorite possession with your fellow students. Most kids look forward to show and tell. I hated it at first. My family never went anywhere exciting, and I didn't have any exotic toys. But that's when I discovered the two keys to grabbing people's attention: exude enthusiasm, and demonstrate uniqueness. Both elements are crucial. Who would have known back then that I was learning how to be a good public speaker? For most of us, show and tell was our first experience at public speaking—only it wasn't called that. It was simply sharing, and usually it was fun.

As the school years progressed, most of us had to get up in front of a class to give reports, recite poems, make speeches, and engage in debates. Often the topics were imposed on us, and it was difficult to muster much enthusiasm. It's no wonder that, as adults, most people dread public speaking. In fact, surveys show the majority of people dread public speaking more than they fear death.[7]

Public speaking isn't just about getting up in front of 25 (or even 2,500) people to give a formal presentation. It's about the ways you share information with others. These activities range from: casual encounters, such as talking with people while waiting in lines and networking at social and business functions; to informal events, such as holding open houses and giving parties; to more formal examples, such as providing free talks at civic, professional, and business meetings, doing demonstrations at public events (e.g., fairs, health expositions), facilitating workshops, and giving keynote speeches.

> "Grasp the subject, the words will follow.
> —Cato, The Elder

As in show and tell, public speaking is easy as long as you share something that excites you and can make a difference in the audience's lives. As wellness providers you've got it covered—you frequently witness profound changes in your clients! How can you NOT be enthusiastic about your work? When I was in practice, I was always talking with people about massage—whether or not I initiated the conversation. Granted, I didn't corner people in elevators (well, hardly ever), but I wanted the world to know how wonderful massage was and how it could change people's lives. It isn't necessary to become a zealot—just be open. I suggest that every day, before leaving your house, you remind yourself of all the benefits of your services, and recall at least two instances when you or one of your clients experienced a significant change. This puts your work in your conscious awareness so that you're more cognizant of appropriate instances in which to share it.

How to Prepare, Stage and Deliver Winning Presentations by Thomas Leech

Present Yourself Powerfully by Cherie Sohnen-Moe

One of the most successful ways to do "public speaking" is to talk with people whenever you're waiting in a line: share information about your services, recommend stretches, tell them about the latest product you've discovered, and offer to show them something to alleviate their pain. It may sound hokey, but if you're enthusiastic and sincere, it's the best form of education and marketing.

Educating people about your field is vital to the growth of your profession, as well as building your own practice. Start where you're most comfortable (typically casual encounters or informal events). Commit to sharing information about your services at least 5 times weekly. Once you've increased your level of comfort and confidence, you can move on to more formal presentations and demonstrations.

Semi-formal and formal presentations can be fun. They aren't limited to traditional platform speaking. Plus, you don't have to do them alone. You can ease your discomfort and make the presentation more appealing by co-leading or holding panel discussions. Actually, in this industry, the most effective presentations are informal in nature and include demonstrations and group participation. Here are some ideas for semi-formal public speaking:

- Host a weekly wellness challenge for clients (and their friends), where each week you present a new topic, show a self-care technique, facilitate a meditation, or lead a fitness routine. Follow this with a short social time afterward.

- Facilitate a wellness-oriented book club.
- Provide a stress relief brown-bag lunch presentation at corporations and schools.
- Host a monthly mini-wellness retreat where you discuss a wellness topic, do activities such as yoga and meditation, drink tea, eat healthy snacks, and listen to relaxing music. You could also charge a nominal fee and include a sampling of some of your services.
- Sponsor an allied wellness care provider brown-bag lunch series (held in the other providers' offices and you supply the lunches), where you talk about how your services would be a great adjunct to what they offer, and give a short demonstration.

The Public Speaking Circuit

Many wellness providers contend that the major catalyst for growing their practices is giving "free" talks. Even though you don't get paid for these presentations, they're a superb training ground and a great way to establish credibility, generate goodwill, and attract new clients. I recommend approaching public speaking from two points: general education and marketing. General education public speaking involves talking to anyone who will listen. While the audience might not necessarily be likely candidates for your services, you raise the consciousness level—which benefits the profession as a whole.

> "You can speak well if your tongue can deliver the message of your heart.
> —John Ford

As a marketing tool, public speaking requires finding out which groups are most likely to include members in your target markets. Utilize your public speaking time wisely by making certain that at least one-half of your formal presentations are to groups with members in your target markets. The following list contains examples of several target markets and places where they could be found (and likely sponsors of your presentations).

Figure 25.9 Sample Target Markets for Giving Presentations

- **Specific Health Concerns:** Support groups, clinics, bookstores, wellness provider's offices, and health food stores.
- **People in Recovery:** Counseling offices, treatment centers, and specialty bookstores.
- **Animals:** Veterinary clinics, pet stores, grooming centers, 4-H clubs, dog obedience classes, and county fairs.
- **Seniors:** Volunteer organizations, senior centers, civic groups, and parks.
- **Pregnant Women:** Lamaze classes, the La Leche League, baby boutiques, and Ob/Gyn offices.
- **Athletes:** Sporting events, health fairs, sporting goods stores, sports medicine facilities, and health food stores.
- **Attorneys:** Bar association meetings, law library, and legal aid department.

Getting on the public speaking circuit is easy. Contact civic clubs, professional societies, your Chamber of Commerce, business groups, and networking associations. These organizations are always on the lookout for speakers. Their members enjoy learning specific techniques that improve the quality of their lives. Indeed, any topic relating to wellbeing or stress reduction is in demand. Even bookstores frequently sponsor talks. The most common duration of these presentations is 20 minutes, but they can range up to 1 hour.

Successful Presentations

The key to successful presentations is planning. Investing the time in planning can make the difference between a powerful, flowing, fun presentation and one that's stilted and ineffective. Planning includes understanding the audience, assessing their needs and objectives, determining the presentation purpose, researching the topic, designing the presentation, and matching facilities to program requirements. Evaluate and update your information and audio-visual materials before each presentation—regardless of whether you're preparing a talk from scratch or if you're delivering the same topic for the fiftieth time.

Sample Topics

Some general ideas for wellness presentations are: Stress Management Techniques, Self-Massage, Stretches and Exercises People Can Do at Their Desks, Self-Hypnosis to Gain the Competitive Edge, Couples Massage, Acupressure, Peak Performance Through Proper Nutrition, Preventive Wellness, Infant Massage, Hydrotherapy, Nutrition, Movement, Aromatherapy, Healthy Baby Care, Common Use of Herbs, Personal Growth, and Fitness.

Here are some examples of catchy titles you could use:

- Top 10 Tips for Relaxation
- Rx for Stress Without Side Effects
- You Knead This
- Desk-ercise
- When Good Foods Go Bad
- You 2.0
- Golden Rules for a Healthy Baby
- The Power of Touch
- Reach Your Peak
- Use Pressure to Release Pressure
- Stressed is Desserts Spelled Backward – How to Manage Stress without Overeating

See the *Business Mastery Workbook* for additional **Presentation Titles**.
https://sohnen-moe.com/bm5-workbook-request/

You can also give talks on other subjects in which you have experience or training. Some of the most enjoyable "talks" are when you demonstrate your services. You could create numerous different presentations for every example given above. You can also tie in your presentation with holidays or major events and title them accordingly. Two examples are: "Stress Deduction" during tax time, and "The Gift of Touch" for the pre-holiday buying season.

Research Studies
massagetherapyfoundation.org/

Resources

Vast resources are available for ideas on presentation topics, products to sell, and handouts. Peruse your personal library and search the Internet. Check your books and magazines for topics of interest. Go to health food stores and bookstores. Research information about your specific industry, and then look at general topics such as health, wellness, fitness, stress, and complementary health care.

A Physician's Guide to Therapeutic Massage by John Yates, Ph.D.

Alternative Medicine: What Works by A. Fugh-Berman, M.D.

Presentation Design

A well-prepared presentation is more effective, increases your audience's enjoyment, and is much more fun for you to do. The following information highlights the steps involved in presentation design.

Presentation Purpose: Decide whether the focus is informative, persuasive, or a bit of both. Think about what you want your audience to take away from the presentation.

Audience Analysis: Attempt to find out ahead of time what types of people will be attending, their interests, and special needs.

Presentation Opening: In addition to your personal introduction, customary openings are stating a central idea, asking a question, or previewing the presentation.

Presentation Body: This section typically focuses on a single point with information or evidence to support the premise. Incorporate a mixture of experiential activities and audio-visual materials. Allow time for questions.

Presentation Conclusion: Summarize key points, restate the central idea, answer the opening question, or call the audience to action. Don't underestimate the importance of this step; make this as clear as possible and they will remember you. Thank the audience and your host, and remind them how they can contact you.

Delivery

In presentations, how you say something is often just as important as what you say. Most people spend the majority of their preparation on the content and very little time considering the best ways to impart that information. Power and presence are established through the mastery of body language, while the energy in your voice conveys your sincerity. The methods used to communicate information often determine whether or not the information is fully received.

Incorporate activities that involve the major senses of sight, sound, and touch. People like to feel as though they're being talked with directly—even if they're part of a large group. Some creative techniques for involving your audience are: have the audience participate in an activity such as stretching; lead a visualization exercise; ask questions and have the group raise their hands or stand up in response (e.g., How many of you get headaches? How many of you have ever received an acupuncture treatment? How many receive acupuncture regularly?); make specific reference to a participant or the group (e.g., "Since everyone here today either suffers from fibromyalgia or is close to someone who does, you know how debilitating pain can be."); request feedback; facilitate a question-and-answer format; and give a demonstration.

> "It's all right to have butterflies in your stomach. Just get them to fly in formation.
> —Dr. Ron Gilbert

The more experiential the activity, the better. When talking about touch therapies, show the group how to do some simple techniques on themselves or each other. If the group members know each other well and aren't dressed in business suits, you can organize a massage circle. If you're including information on aromatherapy, bring some essential oils for the audience to smell.

The activities need not be elaborate to be fun and effective. You can demonstrate stretches that the audience can do with you while sitting in their chairs. You can lead activities based on popular games, such as crossword puzzles and Scrabble,® and even design a wellness edition of Trivial Pursuit® or Jeopardy® that includes facts about your specific industry.

Overcome Nervousness

Some people are fortunate in that they're naturally good speakers; they feel comfortable being in front of a group, easily relate to their audiences, and can think while on their feet. Most people must develop these speaking skills.

Toastmasters International
www.toastmasters.org

The first step is to assess your attitude. Many people are hesitant to do any type of public speaking for fear of appearing inept. The beauty of doing presentations about health and wellbeing is that you intrinsically know the benefits of this work. Granted, you might not know everything about a specific topic or have an answer for every question—but audiences rarely expect that.

The second step is to increase your knowledge and experience of public speaking. Take classes (through your local community college, university, a private company, or online), read books, or join a public speaking group such as Toastmasters International.

The final step is to practice. By joining a group such as Toastmasters or even a local networking group, you get regular practice in public speaking. You can always devise ways to weave information about your services into your topics. Another practice option is to create a support group; members can meet to coach each other on presentations and do public speaking engagements together.

Everyone gets nervous. The difference between a good presenter and a poor one is that the good presenter knows how to manage her fears. Use the adrenaline that's pumping through your system to keep you alert and sustain a high energy level. Learn to translate that nervous energy into excitement for your topic.

Figure 25.10 Top 10 Tips to Alleviate Nervousness

1. Before your presentation, visualize yourself having a fabulous time; being dynamic, energetic, and connecting with the audience.
2. Take a few deep breaths and relax your body.
3. Get a touch therapy treatment prior to speaking.
4. Avoid eating a heavy meal before speaking.
5. Drink warm decaffeinated liquids (e.g., lemon tea).
6. Maintain good posture: unlock your knees and stand with equal weight on both feet.
7. Organize your notes and audio-visuals.
8. Wear comfortable clothes.
9. Find a friendly face to look at when discomfort arises.
10. Practice, practice, practice.

Events

You can promote your practice by getting involved in local events. Of the myriad possibilities, this section highlights hosting open houses, having a booth at community expositions, participating in community fundraisers, and conducting specialty parties. See figure 25.11 for overall tips for events that are open to the public.

Figure 25.11 Success Tips for Public Events

- Identify the purpose, priorities, and goals.
- Create a theme.
- Set a budget and keep to it.
- Script an outline of the event.
- Send media releases to get press coverage and interviews.
- Post announcements in online event calendar sites.
- Distribute flyers to nearby businesses and locations where your target market(s) frequent.
- Post announcements on your website and social media accounts.
- Mail personal invitations to key guests.
- Have at least one assistant during the event.
- Provide food and beverages.
- Personally greet each attendee.
- Include an educational presentation.
- Collect contact information.
- Encourage attendees to sign up for your free newsletter.
- Take pictures.
- Follow-up with attendees and the media.

Open Houses

Hosting open houses is an excellent stage for promoting your practice. Open houses provide relatively inexpensive, low stress opportunities to meet your neighbors, network with allied practitioners, introduce potential clients to your services and products, and inspire current clients to increase the amount or type of treatments they receive.

Open houses are the perfect venue to celebrate the opening of a business, an anniversary, or the achievement of a major business benchmark. They're an excellent forum for announcing a new product, new service, or new staff. You can also host focused open houses to introduce yourself and your services to a specific group, such as allied healthcare providers. The following steps help ensure a successful event.

Pre-Planning

Decide the purpose, priorities, and goals of each open house. Next, establish a budget. Then, envision the event and outline the flow of activities. If possible, create a theme, such as "Spring Rejuvenation." Incorporate an educational element, such as a presentation (e.g., stress reduction techniques, nutrition, self-massage, stretching), or a demonstration of a specific technique, product, or piece of equipment. Make sure that the educational segment's duration is under 10 minutes and perform it several times throughout the event.

Provide food and beverages. People tend to be more conversational while nibbling on a snack or sipping a drink. You may even find a local restaurant or health food store that is willing to supply these for free or at a reduced cost if you include their company's information in your promotions.

Pick a good date and time. "Good" depends on your office location and the flexibility of your intended audience. For instance, if your office is surrounded by other professional practices, and your main purpose is to network with your neighbors, perhaps an open house during lunchtime or one that takes place midweek from 4:00 to 6:00 p.m. might be most appropriate.

Compile a guest list, including general categories such as all the allied health practitioners in a half-mile radius or people with fibromyalgia.

Promotion

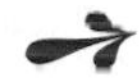

See Chapter 26, page 412 for more on **flyers**.

Design attractive flyers. Use an attention-grabbing headline, describe the planned activities, and highlight the benefits of attending. Always offer some type of freebie that everyone receives (e.g., "All guests receive a sample of XYZ product."), provide a compelling incentive for attending (e.g., "Attend our open house and receive a 50% off coupon for [insert the product or service you want to highlight]."), and offer at least 1 major door prize such as a gift, product, or service package. Also, boost attendance by mentioning that refreshments are served.

See Chapter 29, pages 462-463 for tips on **media releases**.

Personally deliver flyers to nearby offices. This is also a great opportunity to introduce yourself and network. Post them in places where your intended guests are likely to see them, such as bulletin boards in specialty stores. Email flyers to potential guests (e.g., your current client list). Send personal invitations to key guests and call them 1 week before the event if they haven't responded. Place reminder calls to all key guests several hours before the open house (e.g., "I'm really looking forward to seeing you this evening.").

If your open house is for the public, post an announcement on your website and social media pages, local media event posting sites, and perhaps even the online sites of organizations and companies where your desired guests frequent. If the open house is celebrating a momentous occasion, you can send media releases to hopefully procure an interview or even live coverage.

Event Logistics

An open house runs more smoothly and is much more enjoyable if you have assistance. If you're a sole practitioner without any staff, enlist a good friend (or two) to be responsible for the overall flow of the event, including making sure the supplies are stocked, clearing away any used dishware, selling products, and booking appointments. If you have staff, assign them specific roles. You need to focus on your guests. Be sure to personally greet each attendee. If you're leading the presentation portion of the event, have your assistant greet any newcomers and then point them out to you after your presentation, so you can greet them too.

Collect contact information from all of the guests; have a registration book or a bowl where people can put their cards (offer a stack of small forms that people can fill out if they don't have business cards).

Have someone take lots of pictures (consider hiring a professional photographer if this is a major event). Get releases from people in the photographs; print a general photo release at the top of the registration book or have a form where people can opt out.

Follow-Up

A successful open house is one that flows smoothly, the guests enjoy themselves, and you build relationships. A successful open house doesn't end after the last guest has left. Follow-up is pivotal.

See Chapter 29, pages 469-470 for **media follow-up**.

Two days after the event, send a thank-you note to everyone who attended. While this can (and should) be done through email, I urge you to mail cards to the key guests. If an attendee didn't make an appointment, set up a meeting to discuss collaboration ideas, or purchase something, consider including an additional incentive (e.g., an extra 30 minutes when they purchase an hour session, a free product when they book a session). Ideally you have another event scheduled, such as a workshop, and you can invite them to attend or interview you.

Also, contact the media. If press representatives attended the event, send a thank-you note immediately after the event and another one once the event gets published. If the media didn't show up, send a brief highlight of the event, along with a couple of photos and a testimonial from a key attendee. Inform them of your next event and encourage them to attend.

Booths

Another effective method for gaining visibility is to set up a booth at conferences, conventions, expositions, and trade shows. You can meet a lot of people at these events. Choose shows that attract your target markets. Be creative in your choices. For instance, if one of your target markets is infants, take a booth at a baby fair or even a bridal trade show. A wellness booth will stand out amongst the plethora of product vendors. Establish your community presence by being part of wellness and health expositions. Other factors to consider when selecting shows are: the targeted attendees, the cost in terms of time and money, the other companies exhibiting, and the show's past success. Find out if the expo offers sponsorship opportunities. While it does cost you more, it can be beneficial if the event is promoted well and does substantial advertising. Plus, there are often other benefits to being a sponsor, such as a larger booth or a prime location.

Trade Show Displays
www.exhibitoronline.com

Discover which shows are happening in your community by contacting your convention bureau, the Chamber of Commerce, and the sales directors at major hotels. Check specific trade journals, local business publications, and the Internet.

Make sure your booth design fits your image. You can create your own or purchase a portable display. For additional ideas, refer to the previous section on Open Houses. The following tips assist in making this a productive experience.

Figure 25.12 Making the Most of Your Booth

- Send out invitations to prospects to attend the show and pick up a free product at your booth.
- Be sure to have ample promotional materials available. You may want to print special flyers (much less expensive than brochures) for these events.
- Display your promotional materials in such a way that people will take them. This enables you to engage in a conversation with someone and not be concerned about missing potential clients.
- Although it's great to have an elaborate booth, don't let the lack of one be a deterrent. Do the best that you can within your budget. Personalize it somehow with plants, photographs, or flowers.
- Grab potential clients' attention with an eye-catching sign. If you're unable to hang it up, put it on an easel. Make sure the graphics and words are easily viewed from all sight lines.
- Provide ongoing hands-on demonstrations.
- Give away product samples.
- Set out a bowl or basket to collect business cards. Put a sign in front of the bowl stating, "Enter here for a free drawing of...." If possible, donate your services or products. If that isn't appropriate, then give a prize, such as a book, a basket of healthy goodies, or a gift certificate from a local store.
- Play a video that either demonstrates your services or gives interesting information (in an entertaining format). Be sure the program is less than 6 minutes long and looped (so it plays continuously).
- Bring necessary supplies. In addition to your promotional materials, make sure you have plenty of logistical supplies (e.g., equipment, masking tape, extension cords, pencils, paper, tissues), refreshments, and extra clothing (in case you get cold, sweaty, or spill something on yourself).
- Bring a friendly, knowledgeable person to help staff your booth. You need to take breaks. You must walk around and check out the other booths. Some of the best networking takes place between booth owners.

Fundraisers

One of the easiest ways to gain visibility and promote your practice while doing good is to donate your services for fundraising events. Target the appropriate groups according to your purpose (whether for professional advancement or personal gratification).

One idea is to choose a charity that has special meaning to you and donate a day's revenues. Send announcements to your colleagues, clients, and the media informing them of the designated day and date. Depending on the type of service you provide, you could hold this "event" in a public place (check with your local zoning and licensing board first). You can make it a regular event such as once a quarter or even once a month.

Another option is to announce to your clients that for every specified dollar amount (say $50) they donate to your favorite charity, they get a free treatment (such as a half-hour session or an adjunct service). Caution: Communicate upfront the exact services you're offering. You may qualify recipients by requiring a copy of the check and a receipt for proof. Be sure to notify the charity and even the media.

If one of your major goals is to increase your visibility in the community, donate your services to events that are attended by people in your target market or those that are highly

> "There are two ways of spreading light: to be the candle or the mirror that reflects it.
>
> —Edith Wharton

§7

publicized. For major fundraising events, make certain your donation is substantial enough to be considered one of the top prizes: this increases the likelihood of you being included in all the various types of promotions, advertising, and media coverage.

See Chapter 5, pages 85-88 for profiles of **socially responsible companies**.

Client-Hosted Parties

A party is a fun and creative way to market your services. The best way to hold this event is to have a current client sponsor a casual in-home or in-office gathering. This approach has proven extremely effective with products such as vitamins, cosmetics, designer clothing, and, of course, the most famous, Tupperware.®

This marketing strategy works because the guests feel comfortable. They're in a safe environment, the atmosphere is festive, and they can experience the services or products firsthand. I know a Rolfing® practitioner who dramatically increased her clientele through these types of parties.

You may be wondering how a party differs from an introductory demonstration given at your office. The major differences are in the sponsorship and the tone of the event. These parties tend to be small and intimate, usually 5 - 10 friends or colleagues of the sponsor.

People attend the party not only to find out more about what you have to offer, but also because their friend invited them. These people are usually more open to your presentation and more likely to become clients than strangers who come to an introductory demonstration they saw announced in the newspaper. Also, guests at the party expect to have fun and receive more personalized attention than if they were at a more formal demonstration.

Sponsorship

The first step to organizing a party is to choose an appropriate sponsor. Review your client list and pick several possibilities. The key characteristics are that the client values your work, is fairly outgoing, is reliable, and knows a lot of people.

> "Far better it is to dare mighty things, to win glorious triumphs even though checkered by failure, than to rank with those poor spirits who neither enjoy nor suffer much because they live in the gray twilight that knows neither victory nor defeat.
> —Theodore Roosevelt

Talk with your potential sponsors. Most clients eagerly agree to sponsor a party if you offer them some form of compensation either in services or products. I recommend giving the client 1 treatment just for organizing the party, and 1 treatment for every 3-4 attendees. You can also give a bonus of 1 session for every person who becomes a client. Be certain to tell the sponsor to limit the number of guests to approximately ten. If too many participate, the informal nature becomes disrupted, and you lose the power of intimacy.

Even though your sponsors may be enthusiastic about the party, it doesn't necessarily follow that they can coordinate well. Play an active role in the party's preparation and promotion. Once a client has decided to be a sponsor, set aside at least 1 hour to plan the event. Choose a date and select the format. Factors that influence the choice of format include the number of prospective guests, their background, the time allotted, and the time of year the party is scheduled to take place.

For instance, if 5 people attend, you could include more hands-on time with them than if 10 people show up. Also, if the guests are conversant with your type of services, there's no need to spend much time covering the basics—you can focus on the specific benefits or unique applications of your techniques. If the party is slated for 3 hours, you must prepare more information and activities than if the party lasts an hour.

Party Preparations

After the date has been chosen and the format selected, the sponsor creates a guest list and sends out invitations that include RSVPs. The next stages of preparation include scripting the party and rehearsing, creating appropriate handouts, assembling supplies, and supporting your sponsor.

Theme and Ambiance

Be creative by incorporating the time of year into your presentation. Make it a theme party. For example, if the party takes place close to St. Patrick's Day, you can use green paper for your handouts, and decorate accordingly. If the party occurs close to Thanksgiving, include an exercise or discussion about the things for which everyone is thankful—particularly regarding their health, and discuss ways to ensure continued good health.

Design the party in such a way that the atmosphere is lively and promotes involvement. The sponsor usually provides refreshments, and the first portion of the party is spent casually getting to know each other.

Script

When you script the party, designate time parameters for each segment. A sample 2-hour party outline might look like this: 15 minutes informal talking; 5 minutes self-introduction; 10 minutes discussion on benefits of your services and description of your work; 10 minutes group activity; 10 minutes break; 15 minutes demonstration on model; 20 minutes questions and demonstrations on guests; 10 minutes break; 15 minutes additional questions and demonstrations on guests; and 10 minutes wrap-up.

> "The secret of success is to be ready for opportunity when it comes.
> —Benjamin Disraeli

When you begin your presentation, give a brief overview of who you are, your training, and your philosophy toward your work and health. Describe your work and do a formal demonstration on a model (preferably the client who is the sponsor). Position your table, chair, or mat so that the guests can easily gather around to see you in action. Encourage people to ask you and the model questions.

If you're a touch practitioner, allow every participant the opportunity to experience your technique after you've finished the demonstration. This could be anything from a 5-minute neck session to a 3-minute hand massage—and you can do it while talking and answering questions.

If you think the group will be playful, include health-oriented games. Offer prizes for correct answers to general health questions, such as how much water the average person should drink each day, or to the first person to correctly identify a specific muscle.

Your script would include more details of the actual content to be covered in each section. After designing the outline, rehearse the presentation several times, making any necessary adjustments to the script.

Handouts

Handouts are an integral part of any successful presentation. Most people are visually oriented, so it's important to give the guests something to look at and hold. People are also more likely to remember what you said and did if they have something to refer to at home. Design 1 or more handouts that are tailored to the specific presentation or to the group. For instance, let's say the guests are all co-workers at a computer data entry company. You could create a handout that shows self-care techniques for alleviating eye strain and avoiding repetitive stress syndrome. However you design your handouts, include your name, phone number, email, social media pages, and website.

Gift Bags

Gift bags add a nice touch, and they can be assembled to match with the party's theme. Include items, such as product samples, business cards, brochures, promotional items with your logo (e.g., pens, magnets), and coupons. You could even put a special prize in 1 of the bags (e.g., a free session).

Supplies

The basic supplies needed for any presentation are: promotional materials (e.g., cards, brochures, gift certificates, appointment book); personal items (e.g., throat lozenges); and general purpose supplies such as facial tissue, name tags, markers, transparent tape, scissors, masking tape, glue, an extension cord, trash bags, a clock, writing implements, paper, and a receipt book. I always keep a small, lidded carrying box stocked with these items. Also, bring any specialized equipment or supplies needed for your specific presentation, such as handouts, table, linens, lubricant, music system, music, props, and charts.

Sponsor Support

The final element in pre-party preparation involves supporting your sponsor. Keep in contact with this person. Check in regularly to get updates on the responses to the invitations and offer any assistance in follow-up or organization of the event. Call your sponsor to find out if there are any last-minute hitches. Arrive at the party at least 1 hour ahead of time to help with any logistical needs, arrange your equipment and supplies, display your promotional materials and products, and prepare yourself. You want to be organized and centered when the guests arrive so you can concentrate on building rapport and getting to know them.

Product Sales

Depending upon the type of work you do, you may also want to display products at the party. Be sure to describe the products, their benefits, and how to use them. Do a product demonstration. If possible, use the products while working on your model.

If you intend to sell products at the party, you must be clear on your focus, and the guests should be told ahead of time so they bring a method of payment. Realize that most people have never seen some of the wonderful, professional-grade accouterments available for their wellness and relaxation, and they will enjoy the opportunity to see and test these products.

See Chapter 21, pages 311-312 for ideas on **products to sell**.

The income generated by the product sales gives you immediate compensation for your time, whereas the long-term benefits are achieved by the new clients you generate from the party. As long as you keep perspective and concentrate the majority of your presentation on hands-on work, product sales can be a profitable adjunct.

Party Follow-Up

The final activity to ensure positive results from the party is proper follow-up. Send a thank-you letter to your sponsor, mail (or email) notes to all guests thanking them for attending, and confirm any appointments that were made.

26
Marketing Materials

"If anything is worth trying at all, it's worth trying at least 10 times."
— Art Linkletter

Design Overview
- Artwork Sources

Business Cards

Brochures

Flyers and Circulars

Articles
- The Article Writing Process

Reports

Newsletters
- Ready-Made Newsletters
- Newsletter Content
- Cooperative Newsletters
- Newsletter Design
- e-Newsletter Tips

Welcome to My Office Kit

Direct Mail Materials
- Wellness Surveys
- Postcards
- Greeting Cards
- Sales Letters
- Envelopes
- Mailing Lists
- Generating Responses

Gift Certificates
- Expiration Date Debate
- Early Redemption
- Stocking Up
- Marketing Gift Certificates

Custom Gift Cards

Coupons

Personalized Gift Items

Signage

Key Terms

Articles
Brochures
Business Cards
Call to Action (CTA)
Circulars
Content Farm
Copyright
Coupons
Direct Mail
Flyers
Gift Cards
Gift Certificates
Greeting Cards
Listserv
Logos
Mailing Lists
Newsletters
Opt-In
Pay-Per-Click (PPC) Advertising
Personalized Gift Items
Postcards
Quick Response (QR) Codes
Sales Letters
Signage
Specialty Advertising
Welcome to My Office Kit
Wellness Surveys

High-quality marketing materials generate a professional image. These materials can be in a digital format, printed, or both. They range from the basic business cards and brochures, to special reports that offer solutions to your clients' health concerns, to handouts of "quick tips" to distribute at speaking engagements or post on your website. Although websites are a vital component of overall marketing, they're really in their own category and that information can be found in the next chapter.

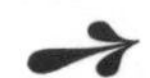

See Chapter 27, pages 430-437 for details about **websites**.

The written word is a powerful tool. Like a magnet, clearly written and compelling promotional materials can attract the interest of potential clients actively looking for a wellness practitioner. Equally important is developing a "voice" in your writing that communicates your unique personality, philosophy, and talents in a way that differentiates you from your competitors.

Figure 26.1 Marketing Materials

Must-Have Basics
- Business Cards
- Appointment Cards
- Brochures
- Stationery: letterhead and envelopes
- Greeting Cards
- Gift Certificates
- Educational Pamphlets
- Client Handouts
- Client Forms
- Newsletters
- Website

Optional
- Displays
- Signage
- Posters
- Referral Cards
- Coupons
- Personalized Gift Items
- Doorhangers
- Flyers
- Direct Mail Letters
- Articles
- Reports
- Informational Videos
- Gift Cards
- Punch Cards
- Comment Cards

Most of your printed materials are given out by you, your friends, colleagues, and clients. They can be distributed to individuals, passed out at networking meetings and events (e.g., open houses), mailed, and posted in public facilities and other businesses. Place them in health clubs, wellness centers, medical care supply shops, health food stores, offices of other wellness practitioners, bookstores, and places that the people in your target markets frequent. You can also contact organizations like Welcome Wagon to include your promotional materials in the packets they supply to newcomers.

Welcome Wagon
www.welcomewagon.com

The first time you contact the owners or managers at establishments where you want to post marketing materials, do it in person. This gives you an opportunity to introduce yourself and build rapport. Show them your materials so they can easily recognize them and hopefully point them out to their customers. After a relationship is built, it isn't necessary for you to hand-deliver the materials each time; you can mail them or have a service distribute them. It's wise to visit these establishments at least twice a year to maintain connections and deliver an appropriate gift (e.g., healthy treats, a plant) once a year.

Practitioners also send their marketing materials via email. Use broadcast emails (other than e-newsletters) sparingly; otherwise they may be perceived as spam. Reserve these to highlight special promotions or articles of major interest, such as newsworthy research findings in preventive wellness and holistic health.

Design Overview

Your visual promotional pieces reflect the character of your business. The ultimate design of your materials depends on your target markets and the image you wish to portray. These items don't all have to look identical (actually that isn't a good idea), but the colors, designs, and overall look should blend well. For your visual promotional materials to be effective, they must appeal to the clients you want to attract—which might not be the layout that you personally like the best. Keep in mind that they aren't meant for you; they must appeal to your target markets!

The Non-Designer's Design Book, 4th edition by Robin Williams

The three major choices for most of your basic marketing materials are: work with a graphic artist to design your marketing materials; purchase pre-printed materials that you can personalize by affixing an address label or inserting a panel with specific information about yourself; or order pre-formatted materials you can customize before printing.

United States Patent and Trademark Office

www.uspto.gov/trademark

International Trademark

www.wipo.int

Artwork Sources

www.massagenerd.com
www.freedigitalphotos.net
www.dreamstime.com
www.istockphoto.com

My experience in preparing my printed materials leads me to recommend leaving it to the experts by hiring a graphic artist to do the job. If cost is a concern, find an artist who is willing to barter services. Be very cautious about adopting a logo. Avoid using one unless you're certain that you want to live with that symbol for a very long time. People tend to remember logos and associate you with your logo even if you no longer use that particular symbol. It's much easier to change a business name or image and alter the design or style of stationery if it's without a logo. Wait until you're certain it's what you want. Also, check to see if anyone else has the same or similar one. Contact your Secretary of State for requisite forms to trademark your logo in your state. You can also trademark your logo on a national or international level.

You can create attractive printed marketing materials on your computer, particularly if you purchase paper products that are specifically designed for desktop publishing. You can find hundreds of full-color brochure paper complete with matching business card stock, letterhead, envelopes, postcards, and labels. Some companies also provide specialty papers to be used for newsletters, certificates, greeting cards, note cards, flyers, and signs. These paper products provide an opportunity for you to experiment without a huge outlay of money. Plus, many online companies allow you to put your information into their templates (or supply your own artwork) and they will print the items for you. Your print materials should tastefully stand out (through design, ink color, or paper color) when floating in a sea of other wellness practitioners' marketing pieces.

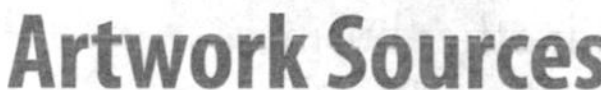

Artwork Sources

Use visuals in your marketing materials, such as clip art images, original drawings, and photographs. You can find a lot of artwork online. Be sure to follow copyright guidelines because not everything you find in an online search engine is free to use. You need to determine the reproduction rights (and royalty-free doesn't necessarily mean you can use it without payment or attribution). If you have a picture or piece of artwork (that you created or own the rights to), you can scan it into your computer and incorporate it into your layout. If you don't own a scanner, most smartphone cameras can take a good representation (if you take the photo in high definition with appropriate lighting).

§7

Business Cards

The business card can be your most effective, least costly marketing tool. Choose a card that reflects who you are and captures the essence of your practice. Always carry lots of business cards wherever you go. Keep extra cards in your car or alternate method of transportation. Be generous with your promotional materials. The whole purpose is to circulate them, not hoard them. Whenever you pass out your cards, always hand out at least 3 per person.

Remember that when it comes to cards, the beauty is in simplicity. A lot of controversy surrounds the amount and type of information to include on your card. Some people attempt to turn their business card into a brochure. Effective business cards convey the major benefits you offer in a quick glance. They should grab attention, but not be so jam-packed with information that potential clients don't feel the need to ask you questions.

The first step in designing your cards is to look at the business cards you've collected over the years (including your competitors' cards) and identify what you like and dislike. Determine the content (refer to the Define Your Differential Advantage activity) using as few words as possible. Choose an appropriate image for your target market(s) that matches your other print materials. Add color whenever possible. Print them on high-quality cardstock and consider using the back of your card for additional copy or as an appointment reminder.

See Chapter 24, page 358 for details on the **differential advantage**.

Be sure to include the basics: name, address, phone number, cell phone number, email address, website, and your business social media pages. Select an email address that ties into the name of your business or the type of work you do. Catchy and clever nicknames have their place, but not on your business cards. I highly recommend including your photo on the card, as people tend to remember faces better than names. Always proofread carefully! I'm amazed at the number of cards without phone numbers, area codes, or incorrect numbers. Have fun with your business cards! They can be uniquely shaped or have something attached to them. For instance, in the article titled, *6 Ways to Market Aromatherapy Massage,* Liz Fulcher suggests attaching a 1-milliliter sample of an aromatic oil you might use in a session.[1]

Business Cards

www.vistaprint.com
www.printbusinesscards.com

sohnen-moe.com/products/marketing-materials/#product-biz-card

If you're in school, have your business cards ready to go before you graduate. Don't worry if you don't have your office yet or haven't chosen a business name. Design a card with your name, phone number, title, and, ideally, a short benefit statement. You can print temporary cards by putting "student" on the card with your anticipated graduation date.

The two major ***faux pas*** with business cards are: not having them when you need them (which is always); and correcting information by hand.

Create Your Business Card

Think of what you want on your card as well as what is required by your profession (e.g., license number, professional notation). Look at other business cards and identify what you like and dislike. Next, sketch out your card. Does the style, color, and message convey your intention? Should you use the back for appointments?

Get feedback from colleagues and representatives from your target market(s). A fun option is to do this activity with friends or colleagues. Plus, you get immediate feedback.

Brochures

Your brochure is often the hub of your printed marketing materials. The purpose of a brochure is to inspire prospective clients to call you. Avoid the temptation to fill up every square inch with content. When developing your brochure, remember that you must establish credibility and focus on the benefits a client derives from using your services. Techniques for establishing credibility in printed materials include providing credentials, numbers, lists, specific details, research findings, testimonials, success stories, pictures, and guarantees.

Figure 26.2 Sample Business Cards

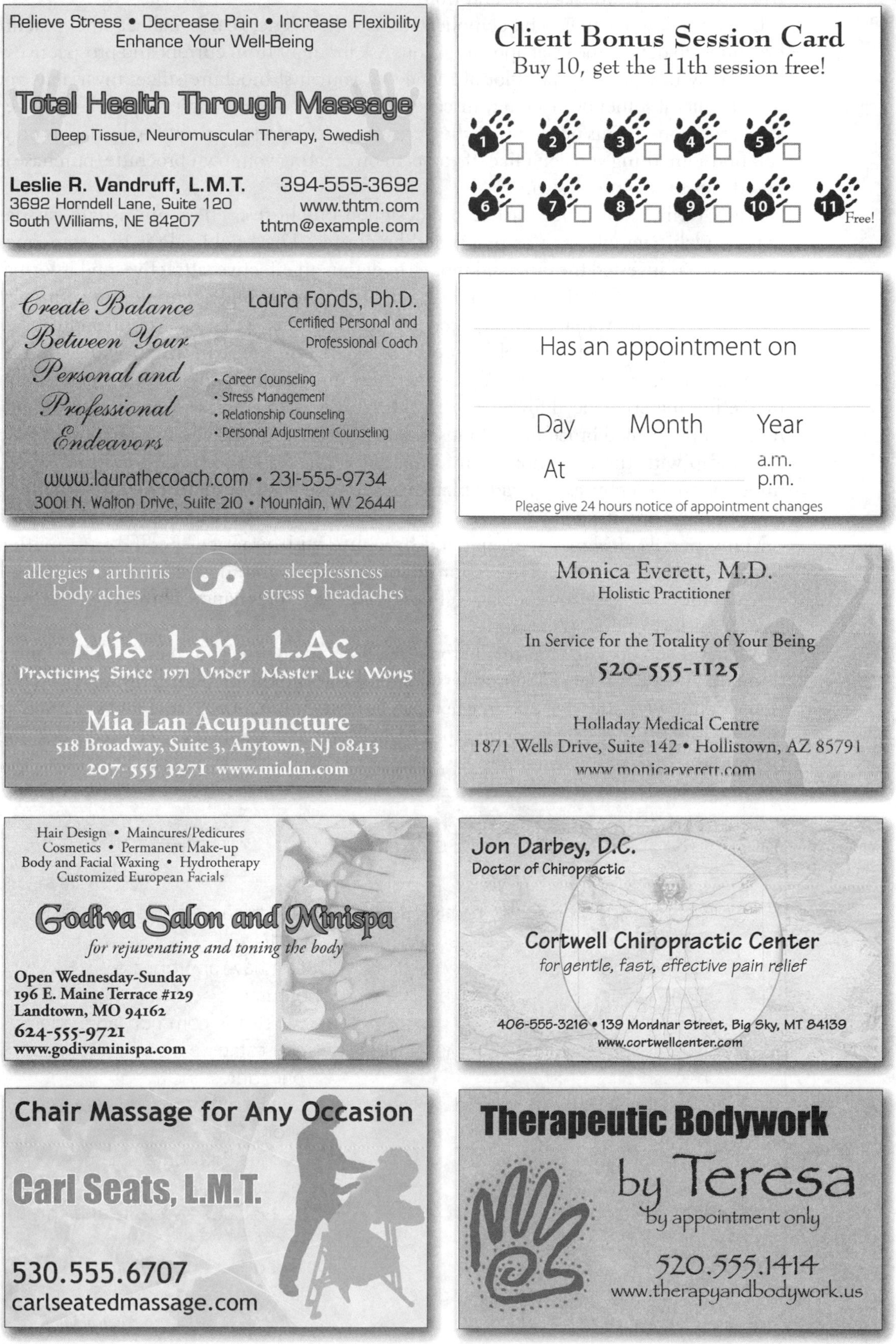

Relieve Stress • Decrease Pain • Increase Flexibility
Enhance Your Well-Being

Total Health Through Massage

Deep Tissue, Neuromuscular Therapy, Swedish

Leslie R. Vandruff, L.M.T.
3692 Horndell Lane, Suite 120
South Williams, NE 84207

394-555-3692
www.thtm.com
thtm@example.com

Client Bonus Session Card

Buy 10, get the 11th session free!

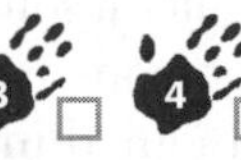
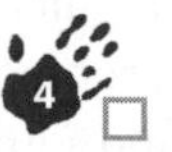
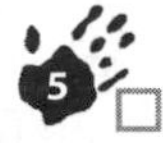
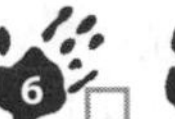

1 ☐ 2 ☐ 3 ☐ 4 ☐ 5 ☐
6 ☐ 7 ☐ 8 ☐ 9 ☐ 10 ☐ 11 Free!

Create Balance Between Your Personal and Professional Endeavors

Laura Fonds, Ph.D.
Certified Personal and Professional Coach

- Career Counseling
- Stress Management
- Relationship Counseling
- Personal Adjustment Counseling

www.laurathecoach.com • 231-555-9734
3001 N. Walton Drive, Suite 210 • Mountain, WV 26441

Has an appointment on

Day Month Year

At a.m. p.m.

Please give 24 hours notice of appointment changes

---

allergies • arthritis
body aches

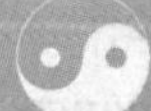

sleeplessness
stress • headaches

Mia Lan, L.Ac.

Practicing Since 1971 Under Master Lee Wong

Mia Lan Acupuncture

518 Broadway, Suite 3, Anytown, NJ 08413
207 555 3271 www.mialan.com

Monica Everett, M.D.
Holistic Practitioner

In Service for the Totality of Your Being

520-555-1125

Holladay Medical Centre
1871 Wells Drive, Suite 142 • Hollistown, AZ 85791
www.monicaeverett.com

Hair Design • Maincures/Pedicures
Cosmetics • Permanent Make-up
Body and Facial Waxing • Hydrotherapy
Customized European Facials

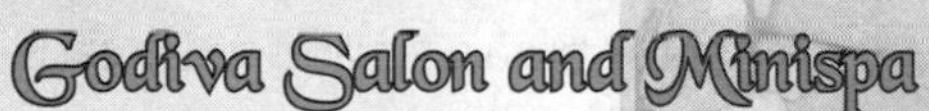

Godiva Salon and Minispa

for rejuvenating and toning the body

Open Wednesday-Sunday
196 E. Maine Terrace #129
Landtown, MO 94162
624-555-9721
www.godivaminispa.com

Jon Darbey, D.C.
Doctor of Chiropractic

Cortwell Chiropractic Center
for gentle, fast, effective pain relief

406-555-3216 • 139 Mordnar Street, Big Sky, MT 84139
www.cortwellcenter.com

Chair Massage for Any Occasion

Carl Seats, L.M.T.

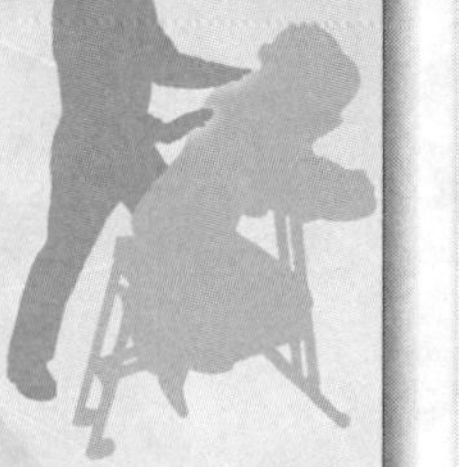

530.555.6707
carlseatedmassage.com

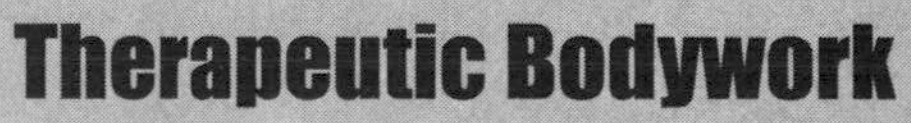

Therapeutic Bodywork

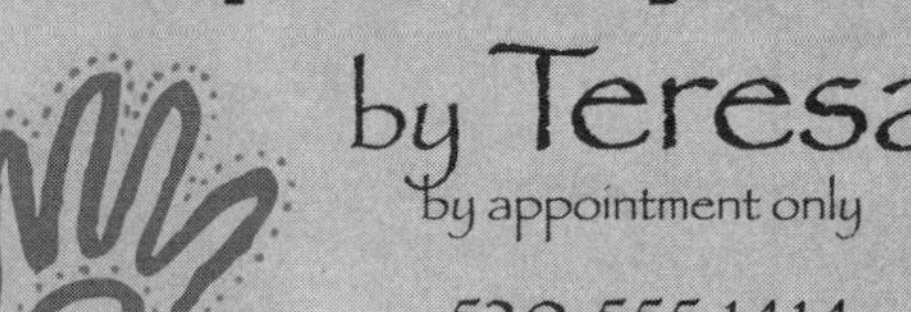

by Teresa
by appointment only

520.555.1414
www.therapyandbodywork.us

See Chapter 24, page 351 for details on **benefits and features**.

One of the key elements of an effective brochure is to include at least 1 photograph of yourself—preferably one in which you're working with a contented client. The old cliché is true, "A picture is worth a thousand words."

Brochure design can be a bit complicated. As with business cards, collect other practitioners' brochures to determine what appeals to you. Ask for input from current and prospective clients. It's usually unwise to spend a lot of money on your first brochure since, invariably, you will want to alter it somehow. You may discover that the type style doesn't work well with the paper stock, someone points out an error, the perfect way to express yourself finally dawns on you, or you find something you don't like. If you plan on creating your own brochure, purchase a book on effective brochure design.

Save money, trees, and energy by utilizing the Internet to post and send promotional materials such as announcements and newsletters.

Many wellness providers utilize pre-designed brochures. These are usually available as downloadable templates or as preprinted brochures. The bright side is that someone other than you has invested the time and money to design an effective, attractive, and informational marketing tool. Often the cost is significantly less than if you were to design your own. The problem is that they aren't personalized. Some companies will allow you to add your contact information to the back panel before printing. If not, you can affix a label or apply the information with an ink stamp. You're the most important aspect of your practice, and your marketing materials need to reflect that. One of the best ways to overcome the impersonal nature of preprinted brochures is to insert a panel with your specific information.

A stamp with the practitioner's information works well also. I used to order some great informational brochures that had a blank space on the back for such. They are usually custom designed, but are inexpensive.

Pre-Designed Brochures

sohnen-moe.com/products/marketing-materials/#product-client-ed

hemingwaymassageproducts.com
acupuncturemediaworks.com
www.bluepoppy.com

Many people design a personalized brochure with practice-specific information and purchase pre-designed brochures for client education that describe in detail the adjunct services they offer, address specific wellness issues (e.g., pregnancy, fibromyalgia, arthritis), or provide history of their profession.

Whatever you do with preprinted brochures, don't handwrite your name, address, and phone number on the back—it looks unprofessional! Ideally, run the brochures through a laser printer (some companies offer that option when you order their brochures), so it looks like you created the brochure. If that isn't an option, print labels on a complementary colored stock and affix them to the back of the brochures.

Figure 26.3 Brochure Design Criteria

- Does it easily distinguish who it's for?
- Does it identify with the target client's problem?
- Does it provide a solution to the problem?
- Does it appeal to the target client's needs?
- Does it have an interesting teaser?
- Are the main benefits listed first?
- Is it believable?
- Is it attractive?
- Is it easy to read? Does it flow?
- Are the type sizes and styles easy to read?
- Does it have sufficient white space?
- Are the type sizes and styles easy to read?
- Does it have appropriate photographs?
- Is it written in common language?
- Does it establish credibility?
- Is your address included?
- Does it include a map of your location?
- Does it include contact names and numbers?
- Does it include a website and email address?
- Does it direct the client to take action?

Figure 26.4 Sample Brochure

Let chair massage work for you!

- It increases employee effectiveness. Research reports that massage enhances alertness and helps increase employee productivity.
- ...ces work relations. Employees who ...air massage find the quality of their work relationships improve, both with each other and with customers.
- It makes a great incentive. Chair massage is a wonderful way to recognize birthdays or service anniversaries, provide rewards for good attendance or an accident-free period, or give a bonus for achieving goals or completing projects.
- It is a wellness program people actually use. Employees take advantage of chair massage because it is convenient, easy to use, and most of all, because it feels good.
- It gives employees a tool for controlling their responses to stress. When employees recognize tension and the strain it causes, they can release it before it becomes a problem.
- It reduces employee turnover. When employers invest in the well-being of their employees, the return is improved morale and loyalty.

benefits

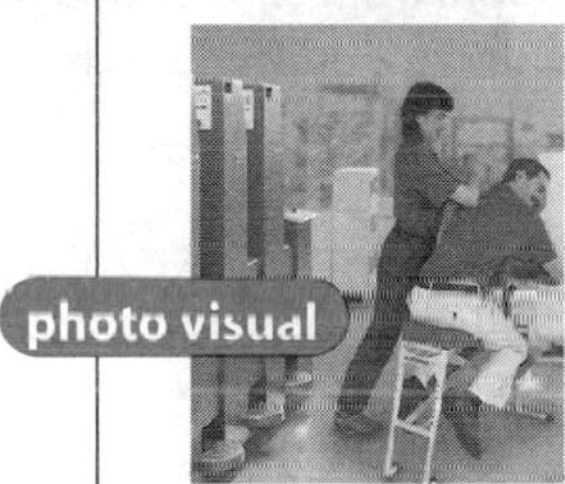

Research shows that chair massage can increase employee effectiveness and reduce turnover.

How to find out more

Your massage practitioner can meet with you to discuss implementing a program that fits your organization's needs. At that time, she or he will be happy to a... practitioner quali... and financial arrangements. If you still have questions, ask about arranging a demonstration or presentation. Experience first-hand the many benefits of chair massage.

call to action

OUTSIDE

space for personalized information

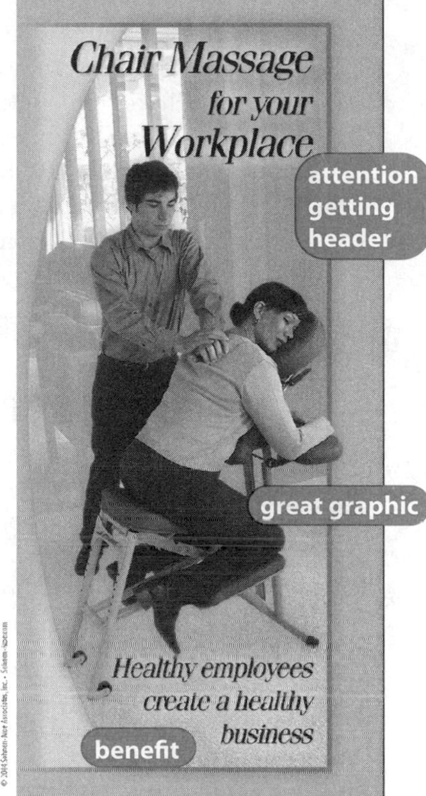

Chair Massage
for your
Workplace
attention getting header
great graphic
Healthy employees
create a healthy
business
benefit

What is chair massage?

Chair massage is a brief, stress-reducing massage ... seated in a comfortable, ...le chair. The massage chair ...titioner and can be set up ... location. Chair massage:

- ... minutes.
- Uses no oil and is applied directly through clothing.
- Is given by a massage practitioner professionally trained in effective, safe seated massage techniques.
- Addresses tension primarily in the upper body (back, neck, shoulders, scalp, arms and hands), but creates an overall sense of well-being.
- Leaves employees feeling relaxed, refreshed and ready to return to work.

descriptive text and features

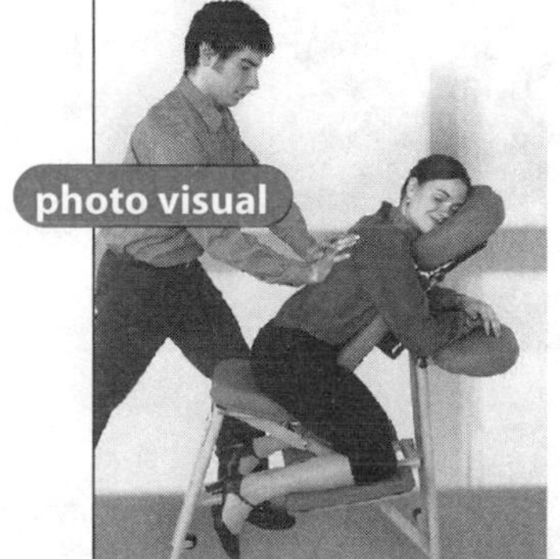

How employees will benefit

Chair massage in the workplace offers many advantages to the employee.

- Reduces muscle tension, a major contributor to chronic pain, repetitive strain injurion and low-back pain.
- Boosts alertness.
- Reduces stress.
- Increases circulation.
- Calms the nervous system.
- Provides a complete change of pace so the body and mind can relax and rejuvenate.

benefits

IS STRESS REALLY A PROBLEM?

You can't open a news... without reading about the negati... ...ects ...ess ... employees aren't ex... ...stress ...ork, other sources of stress can have ... ...verse impact on work performance.

According to *Fortune Magazine*, The American Institute of Stress estimates that stress and its consequences, such as absenteeism, burn-out and mental health conditions, cost American businesses more than $300 billion a year. In studies at the 3M Corporation ... ...versity ...ical School Touch Research Institute, chair massage recipients demonstrated a significant reduction in stress responses.

INSIDE

credibility

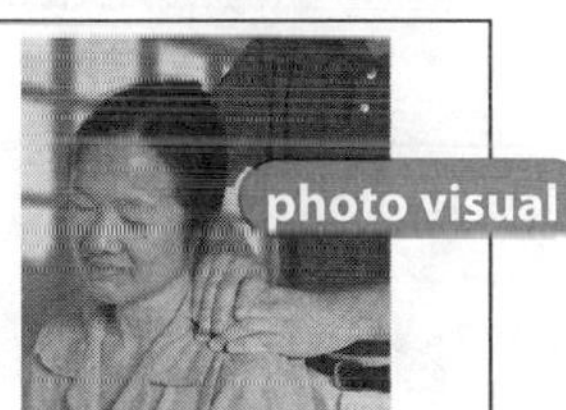

It's easy to set up and run

- Designate a coordinator. He or she will help with logistics, announcements and scheduling.
- Identify a location. A s... conference room, break...
- Give it a try! Set up a ... as a wellness program ... employee appreciation ...
- Encourage employees to use it. Make sure they know you support the program. Use it yourself and encourage your managers to do the same.

supporting information and call to action

Cost-effective? Yes!

- There is no up-front investment in equipment or facilities.
- Chair massage is flexible enough to schedule into the workday without interrupting work flow.
- Chair massage is one of ... wellness programs av...
- Chair massage lowers health care costs. Experts say up to half of all illnesses are induced by stress.

features

This sample brochure is used for illustrative purposes only with permission by Sohnen-Moe Associates. Please honor the company's copyright.

§7

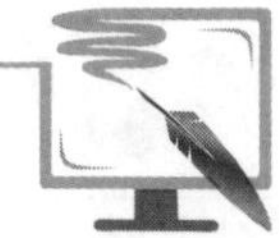

Create Your Brochure

Collect wellness practitioners' brochures. Identify what you like and dislike. Make a list of key words or phrases that inspire you. Write the content of your brochure (remember to focus on your differential advantage and the benefits you provide). Do a mock layout by sketching it or using desktop publishing software, following the tips in Figure 26.3.

Once you have a brochure draft (or perhaps a few), get feedback from colleagues and representatives from your target market(s). A fun option is to do this activity with friends or colleagues. Plus, you get immediate feedback.

Flyers and Circulars

Flyers and circulars are pamphlets designed for mass circulation about a specific event such as an open house, workshop, or a sale. They're usually printed or copied on one side so they can be posted on bulletin boards, inserted into mailings, and distributed at your colleagues' places of business. They can also be printed specifically to be used as door hangers.

One of the strongest marketing benefits of these types of promotional tools is that you determine your target (e.g., all the dentists in a 3-mile radius, people who shop at the local health food store).

Design tips include the information covered under brochures, plus the following: use an attention-grabbing headline, make it easy to respond (e.g., phone, fax, toll-free numbers), use a scannable QR code (Quick Response), and close with a call to action, such as "Call Today," or "Stop by Our Open House to Receive a Sample of Our Custom Blended Products."

Figure 26.5 Reducing Marketing Materials Printing Costs

Whether you design your own printed promotional materials or elect to utilize the services of a graphic artist, follow these tips for reducing your print media costs:

- Work with interns from local colleges.
- Barter for services.
- Get at least 3 bids.
- Use common size and weight paper for the specific type of printing.
- Use a photocopier for short print runs.
- Print samples before using expensive paper and ink.
- Use the printing services of trade and vocational schools.
- Reuse effective material (as long as it isn't being sent to the same people).
- Purchase customizable business cards, brochures, and postcards from online vendors.

Articles

Writing articles enhances your credibility and provides a venue for you to increase your connection with current and potential clients. North America is home to more than 100,000 newspapers, magazines, journals, and association newsletters. Many of these publications are quite receptive to freelance article submissions that are beneficial to their readership. Sometimes they even pay you for the articles—but even if they don't, it's great exposure! Plus, there are countless online opportunities to publish articles of varying lengths. The key to getting published is to know the publication's target market and the types of information they currently provide to their readers. Your approach should be to provide new, unusual, or important information that will benefit their readers. Also, websites that provide support for your target markets might be interested in your articles.

Article Submission Website
ezinearticles.com

You can submit articles to article sites (also referred to as article directories). These are websites with collections of articles written about different subjects. Google classifies these article sites as reference sites. Most articles are 1200-2500 words, and some article sites are particular about the type of content that is submitted. Most of the time the articles have to be informational and educational and cannot promote your business, but your bio as the author should have a live link to your website or even a link to a specific page on your website with a special offer for a service that was described in the article. There are even content farms (companies that employ people to create articles) where you can have articles written about your services, products, website, events, and even about you.

Find online article directories and websites that provide support for your target markets. Regardless of whether your articles get published by an outside source, use them as promotional tools. Post your articles on your website and in your newsletter. Some people include short articles in their blogs. Send them to current clients and make them available to prospective clients.

See Chapter 27, page 437 for details on **blogging**.

The Article Writing Process

Write articles on general wellness, the value of your particular area of expertise, or the latest innovations in your field. Start by identifying the topics that you're passionate about. If you're at a loss for topics, think about the types of questions your clients frequently ask you.

Figure 26.6 Article Development

1. **Title**: Construct a catchy title. Some people recommend starting off with a title, although I've often found that the title doesn't come to me until the article is completed.
2. **Opening**: Write an opening paragraph that grabs the readers. Briefly review the topic and explain the benefits the readers will receive by reading the article. Remember WIIFM! (What's In It For Me)
3. **Body**: Use this section to elaborate on the subject matter. Include facts, research findings, anecdotes, quotes from experts, and testimonials. Keep the paragraphs relatively short and include subheads.
4. **Conclusion**: End your article with a strong conclusion. Summarize key points, tell the readers how they can apply the information in the article to enhance their wellness, and provide a call to action.
5. **Author's Box**: Write a very brief biography that lists your credentials, expertise, other published articles or books, and contact information.

§7

> Either write something worth reading or do something worth writing about.
> —Benjamin Franklin

The steps to writing an article are similar to those when preparing for a presentation. Begin by writing a summary of what you want the readers to learn and what actions you want them to take. Next create an outline. Then write the article. After you've completed the article, set it aside for a couple of days. Then reread it and make any edits. Enlist editing assistance from friends, colleagues, and a member of the target market the article addresses. Another option is to hire a professional writer to customize an article for or about you.

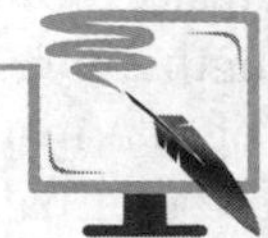

Get Your Article Published

List 5 topics that interest you and could benefit your readers. Follow these steps for each of the topics:

- Locate at least 2 publications that might be interested in the topic.
- Obtain copies of the publications to find out their format, average word count, and style.
- Request submission guidelines (usually available online).
- Send a 1-page query letter that describes your article idea and why you think it will benefit the publication's readers. Also include a brief biography that lists your credentials.

Reports

A free report is another way to build a relationship with a new client. Reports range from a one-page handout to a multi-page booklet. Give these reports to clients, and distribute them at other wellness professionals' offices, centers where your target markets congregate, health food stores, health expositions, and places where you give presentations.

Create reports on a variety of topics that address your target markets' concerns. For example, you could give new clients a report on "What to Expect After Your First [insert your specific field here] Session." Think about your client's concerns and write reports to address them (very similar to writing articles).

If you don't want to create this type of educational material, you can purchase pre-printed pamphlets that address various wellness topics. Attach a note with a few sentences introducing the report, and invite the reader to ask you any questions about the topic.

Newsletters

Newsletters are used by all kinds of organizations and businesses as an effective informational marketing tool. Newsletters provide a forum to communicate with your current and potential clients. Readers tend to pay more attention to a newsletter than an advertisement—and it's less likely to get tossed out as junk mail or spam.

Good newsletters pique the reader's interest. They balance promotional content with specific information that benefits the reader. The language tends to be more conversational in tone than a typical advertising piece or technical publication.

Most wellness providers are multitalented and clients are often unaware of the scope of services they have available. A newsletter gives you an ideal opportunity to educate your clients about your other areas of expertise.

Newsletters don't need to be an elaborate production to be effective. You can even create a simple one-page newsletter that you print on your letterhead. Publishing an e-newsletter (also known as an e-zine) is a good option, since the majority of people have access to email and the Internet. Online newsletters are eco-friendly, save you printing and postage, and get delivered immediately. Plus, you can easily update them, and add brilliant colors and pictures. Other than nominal listserv management fees, it costs very little to send out an e-newsletter to hundreds or even thousands of people.

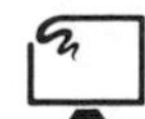

Listserv Companies

www.constantcontact.com
mailchimp.com
www.aweber.com

Before you decide upon the appropriate length, style, format, and content of your newsletter, you must first clarify your purpose and goals for your newsletter and determine how to make it attractive to your target markets.

Newsletters can be published on a set schedule (e.g., monthly, quarterly, biannually) or you can simply produce them whenever it's appropriate. Oftentimes, a business owner generates a newsletter when a change occurs in the company or something major happens within the industry.

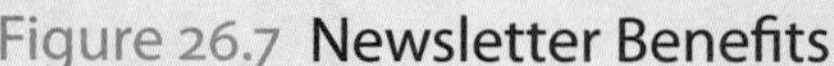

Figure 26.7 **Newsletter Benefits**

- Educate readers on the benefits of your services.
- Attract new clients.
- Encourage current clients to come in more often.
- Bring back lost clients.
- Inspire clients to try different services.
- Promote products.
- Provide information.
- Build client loyalty and improve client retention.
- Enhance credibility and improve your image.
- Increase referrals and gift certificate sales.

Ready-Made Newsletters

Several companies produce newsletters specifically for wellness providers to purchase and distribute to their clients. The advantages of buying a ready-made newsletter over designing your own are a lower overall cost and time savings. The disadvantages are that ready-made newsletters lack your personal touch and you don't have control over the content or layout. If the newsletter templates aren't sold in a kit, you have to hope the publisher gets them out in a timely manner. Also, the information may be inaccurate or dated. The good news is that most of these companies now offer online versions of their newsletters that can be easily customized.

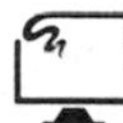

Ready-Made Newsletters

acupuncturemediaworks.com
www.massagemarketing.com
www.fitpronewsletter.com

Two ways to personalize a ready-made newsletter to maximize the benefits are: write a column for a pre-existing newsletter; or purchase a ready-made newsletter and insert a note or personalized page. If you decide to insert a page, be sure that it matches graphically in terms of overall style and typefaces. Some newsletter publishers place a blank section on the template for personalization.

Newsletter Content

The content doesn't have to be elaborate, just useful, interesting, and geared toward helping your clients find solutions to their health and wellness concerns. Include a feature article, health tips, information about special promotions, and newsworthy announcements. Your newsletter can encompass new services, changes in hours, how-to's for stretches, relaxation exercises, specific tips on self-care, technical information regarding new research, survey results and product reviews, a detailed description of one of your services, websites and toll-free numbers of interest, articles, new products, success stories about your clients (get written permission first), book reviews, cartoons (be sure to follow copyright guidelines), advertisements, specialty columns such as a question-and-answer column, a section on different wellness modalities and their specific benefits, a "what's new in…" column, poems, articles written by clients, puzzles, contests, inspirational quotes, interviews, anecdotes, letters to the editor, and discount coupons.

Gather information for your newsletter from newspapers, magazines, books, radio and television programs, documentaries, workshops, other wellness providers, and your clients. Subscribe to other wellness practitioners' e-newsletters. Note what gets your attention and what bores you. Use what you learn to create content that engages your readers and keeps them looking forward to your next edition.

It's fairly easy to obtain reprint rights of articles from existing publications. These are usually available at low or no cost. They provide variety for your readers and ease the load of material you personally generate. After you've located appropriate articles, contact the editor of each publication to ascertain their reprint policies.

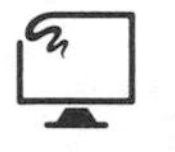

Free Articles
www.articledashboard.com

Many online article banks offer low-cost or free reprint rights. Search for articles by subject, such as "massage" or "stress" or "nutrition" or by your target market's concerns, such as "arthritis." If your newsletter is targeted to a specific market, contact the public relations department of other organizations that cater to that market. Those organizations might have articles of interest and most likely will gladly give them to you free of charge. If you're unable to get reprint rights for material that you want to include, you can directly quote a sentence or two under "fair use" regulations. Be sure to attribute the source. Getting other professionals that serve your target markets to write a regular column for your newsletter is another source of material.

Keep printed newsletter length to 4 pages or less and digital newsletters even shorter. Provide enough information to inspire someone to read it, but don't fill it with so much material that it requires a significant block of time to read. The idea is to create a newsletter that grabs your potential readers' attention so they read it immediately, and to furnish readers with just the right balance of graphically appealing and interesting material so they read it from beginning to end in one sitting.

Copyright Permissions
http://www.copyright.com

Also, leave your readers anticipating your next issue by giving them a preview. For example, "In the next issue, we describe 6 techniques for alleviating headaches," or "Next issue includes an interview with Alexa Swift, a local track star who shares how she reduced her sprint time by 10%."

Keep your newsletter straightforward and personal. Remember, it isn't a magazine or a newspaper—it's a personal communication to keep you in touch with your current clients, educate the public, and promote your practice. Newsletters keep you and your clients connected.

Cooperative Newsletters

Creating a printed newsletter from scratch can seem overwhelming and financially prohibitive. Ease the burden by teaming with wellness providers and people who provide products or services to the same target markets. Thoroughly analyze your target market so you can determine who to consider as a co-producer of your newsletter.

For example, let's say that one of your target markets is infants (technically, the infants' parents or guardians). Many professionals and companies service this market: pediatricians, baby food companies, specialty stores (e.g., clothing, toys), baby seat manufacturers, bookstores, childbirth educators, massage practitioners, acupuncturists, chiropractors, and educational companies that publish information for the parents of infants.

Another market with a multitude of attending providers is personal growth. People in this category often utilize the services of psychotherapists, counselors, and other wellness providers such as touch practitioners, nutritionists, holistic physicians, homeopaths, acupuncturists, chiropractors, herbalists, and estheticians. They may attend workshops and 12-Step meetings. They read books on personal development and spirituality. They often shop at health food stores and natural clothing shops. They're usually environmentally conscious, and are probably involved in some type of physical fitness program, such as exercise and yoga.

Don't limit yourself to the obvious. Sometimes the more unique the pairing, the more effective. For example, an on-site massage practitioner and a "quick-print" copy shop might co-produce a newsletter. They could utilize a slogan such as, "For people who don't have an extra hour." Also, your co-sponsors can be located in a different city. For example, you could team up with a baby food company or a home exercise equipment manufacturer from another locale.

> "Design is thinking made visual.
> —Saul Bass

Newsletters often center on a theme, particularly when they're a cooperative venture. Several possibilities are: a "generic" wellbeing newsletter that appeals to a specific market such as athletes, pregnant women, or stressed executives; or a newsletter that addresses specific health issues like arthritis, aging, or carpal tunnel syndrome.

Newsletter Design

Computers have allowed desktop publishing to flourish. Most people who use newsletters to promote their practices either buy pre-designed ones or create them on their computer. But even if you don't have the software, many graphic designers and print shops can produce your newsletter for you. If you plan to self-publish a printed newsletter on a regular basis, I highly recommend that you invest in a quality page-layout program such as Adobe InDesign.® Using word processing software is generally not a good idea.

If your newsletters are going to be online, most listserv email management companies such as MailChimp and Constant Contact offer a wide assortment of templates where you can easily drop in your content and it looks great.

Be certain the newsletter style and colors match your image, as well as appeal to your target markets. You can purchase pre-designed laser-printer newsletter paper from companies such as Paper Direct. These companies usually offer free downloadable layout templates. Keep in mind, your newsletter will continue to evolve, so don't worry about it being perfect from the start.

Paper
www.paperdirect.com
Online Printing Services
www.vistaprint.com

We produce a school newsletter totally in-house. We hired a graphic artist to design the basic layout so we could simply place the new information within the template. For many years we sent out a newsletter 4 times a year and changed the color of the paper with each issue. At first we printed them on our own copier; then when we had a mailing list of more than 1,000 we sent them to a printer. Now, we have almost 4,000 people on our Teachers Aide Newsletter list and it's a monthly digital publication. If you're reproducing 200 copies or less, it may be advantageous to print them on your laser printer or copier. I highly recommend digital newsletters (particularly from an environmentally conscious point of view), although you may want to have some printed copies to hand out at events or send to those clients who don't use computers.

As far as technical layout is concerned, include plenty of white space. Too much type is overwhelming and unattractive. Limit the number of different typefaces. Air out the copy by incorporating visuals such as photographs and graphics. Keep the style consistent. Simplicity is the key. Avoid using too many lines and boxes, and make certain that your graphic images don't detract from the content.

If you're printing newsletters, consider using screens (a graduated shading of ink from clear to solid): they provide visual depth and can make it appear that you've used an additional color of ink. You also want your newsletter to stand out visually and tactilely. This can be accomplished by printing it on colored paper, using textured stock, or folding it so it's a different size than most mail (e.g., magazines, #10 envelopes). Note, oddly shaped mailers often require additional postage.

Entice your potential readers to open your newsletter immediately by prominently displaying your company name and logo. If you're unsure that readers would recognize your name, highlight the newsletter's purpose or slogan. Then list the contents or use some type of teaser. Let your potential readers know why they should read your newsletter right now! If it's an e-newsletter, be sure the subject line identifies you and encourages readers to open the email.

Massage Marketing
www.massagemarketing.com

Figure 26.8 Marketing with Newsletters

by Jon Lumsden of Massage Marketing

A newsletter works in 10 different ways. You can get a lot more mileage from each issue than by just mailing copies to your existing clients. You have an effective marketing tool at your disposal, so make the most of it:

1. Mail or email your newsletter to potential clients.
2. Encourage your clients to share their issues with others.
3. Generate new business by mailing to selected professionals with a cover letter introducing your services.
4. Use it as a handout at health fairs and public presentations.
5. Leave copies with willing merchants.
6. Use as inserts in community newspapers.
7. Mail to nearby residents.
8. Use with a cover letter and mail to new neighbors with a first-visit discount.
9. Provide issues to services like Welcome Wagon.
10. Use in place of business cards.

e-Newsletter Tips

Build your subscriber list by directly inviting clients and contacts to sign up and including a sign-up form for your e-newsletter on your website. Also, whenever you attend a public event, let the group know you have an e-newsletter. Ask them to give you their business cards if they would like to subscribe. It also works well to offer a giveaway, such as a discount coupon or special report for those who sign up.

You can send newsletters to subscribers and post them on your website. Create a separate subscribers' email list so that you can easily send out your newsletters to your list.

Include your complete contact information, website address, and attach an email subject line that clearly identifies your newsletter so it won't be automatically deleted. This also reduces the chances of your email being flagged as spam.

Make sure your e-newsletter is "opt-in," which means asking clients or associates first before adding them to your email list. Simply put, you need permission to market to clients on the Internet. Anything else is spam. You also need to include an unsubscribe option. Consider automating your e-newsletter distribution and list management with a communication company.

If you're looking for a good way to get published in other places on the Internet, put a blurb at the bottom of your newsletter that says people are free to use the material from your e-newsletter as long as they give you credit and include a link to your site.

Client Educational Materials Notebook

Research websites, magazines, and companies that have articles, reports, or handouts that address your clients' concerns. Compile a list of those sites, the types of information, and the links. Identify the requirements for sharing with your clients. For instance, some might allow you to freely duplicate the information, others might require permission, some might charge a fee, and some might only allow you to provide a link. Put printouts of the various materials into a notebook that has topic tags (this can be displayed in your office for clients to peruse before sessions). Additional Idea: This compilation can provide you with content for your newsletters; you could write a short review of 1 item in each of your newsletters.

Welcome To My Office Kit

Welcome kits help solidify the professional relationship. Ideally, send a "Welcome to My Office" kit as soon as clients book their first session. Items to include in this kit are: a personalized welcome letter; your specific practice brochure; a pamphlet describing (in friendly language) what clients can expect from your services, what they need to do to prepare for the session, your policies and your procedures; several business cards; client intake and health history forms; a sample gift certificate; your recent newsletter; a map to your office (if it's not already on the back of your brochure); and other promotional materials (e.g., a copy of a published interview). This may sound like a lot of material, but the few dollars it costs to assemble and mail this kit demonstrates your professionalism and concern about your clients, and helps develop rapport.

You could do something similar with a digital kit (saved as a PDF), but it most likely won't have the same impact. Digital kits are handy when you don't have enough time to mail a kit. If you only send a digital kit, hand clients an adapted version of it at their first appointment. Remove the client intake and health history forms if they've filled them out online.

Direct Mail Materials

Direct mail promotions are simple, inexpensive, and highly effective marketing tools. According to the Direct Marketing Association, 65% of consumers from all ages have purchased something from a direct mail piece.[2] Even with the popularity of email blasts, physical mail still ranks as an effective marketing tool.

Some of the most compelling statistics are as follows:[3]

- Direct-mail marketing yields, on average, a 13-to-1 return on investment ratio.
- 79% of households say they read or scan direct-mail ads.
- 39% of customers say they try a business for the first time because of direct-mail advertising.
- 56% of customers find print marketing to be the most trustworthy type of marketing.
- 48% of people retain direct mail for future reference.

Direct mail pieces are great for introducing yourself to potential clients, as well as keeping in touch with current ones. They range from a formal letter of introduction to announcements to surveys. (See Figure 26.9 for a sample survey.) These materials are personalized, and you can address specific needs in a friendly, low-pressure manner.

§7

Many local printers, and online companies such as VistaPrint,® can print and mail your direct mail pieces. Some companies even have templates to help you design your marketing materials, and others offer design services.

See Chapter 27, pages 444-446 for details on **pay-per-click marketing and pre-testing**.

Direct mail and digital mail can work hand-in-hand. For instance, before paying to print and mail a promotion, pre-test it for conversion using an inexpensive pay-per-click campaign.

Wellness Surveys

Sending a wellness survey to potential clients can attract interest in your services and open the door to new business. It also works well to invite potential clients to educational events in connection with a survey. This can be a very effective way to introduce the benefits of your service, build trust, and foster new client relationships. Be sure to offer a free gift or discount as an incentive and send a thank-you for participating in the survey.

Postcards

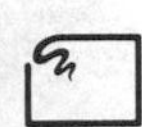

Design, Print, Address, and Mail Postcards

www.postcardmania.com

Postcards are a fast, easy, and inexpensive method of reminding clients of follow-ups and appointments, sending announcements, or just saying hello. According to the U.S. Postal Service, almost 60% of households read postcards.[4] They're also a good technique for generating new clients. Postcards can be sent 1 at a time, in a mass mailing, or used as part of a promotional advertising campaign. They encourage people to take action quickly and are most effective when the action required is free (e.g., "Visit our website for the top 10 things you can do to improve your health today," "Call for a free wellness update today"), or includes an upgrade in services, such as "Book your next private yoga appointment by March 31st and receive a pass for 2 free group classes."

Greeting Cards

Greeting Cards

www.cordialgreetings.com
sohnen-moe.com/products/marketing-materials/

Greeting Cards are an excellent tool for connecting with clients, networking associates, and referring professionals. They can be used to wish people good tidings, as well as encourage client retention. Keep a variety of cards on hand so that you can quickly send one when it's appropriate. If you need to make a special effort to buy a card, then you might not do it. Here are some ideas for when to send a greeting card:

- Reaffirm the professional relationship. After a client's first visit, state that you look forward to working with her to achieve her wellness goals.
- Thank-you for referrals.
- Keeping in touch.
- Special occasions such as birthdays and anniversaries of their first appointment.
- Milestones reached in their work with you, their profession, or personal achievements.
- Inspire clients to return.

Sales Letters

A sales letter is a direct mail marketing piece to generate business. Keep sales letters short (one page) and succinct. As most people's mailboxes are overflowing with form letters and marketing pitches, tailor each letter to a specific individual within a target market. Do your homework and find out as much specific information as possible. Add your special touch. Consider signing your letter in an ink that's a different color than the type. The key elements to success are a great design (see Figure 26.10), an excellent mailing list, and follow-up.

Figure 26.9 **Prospecting Survey**

Westside Wellness Center
6000 N. Windy Way • Fairbanks, AK 99710
907-555-5555 • www.westsidewellness.com

Susan Izensnow
1900 Frostbite Circle
Fairbanks, AK 99711

15 April 2020

Dear Ms. Izensnow:
We realize that your wellbeing is a high priority. Your opinion of chiropractic care is important to us, and finding out how you feel assists us in meeting your expectations. Please return this survey and we will send you a free booklet titled, ***Ten Things You Can Do Today to Increase Your Vitality and Longevity***.

Are you currently under chiropractic care? ❑ Yes ❑ No
If yes, how often?

❑ On a regular schedule
❑ On an as-needed basis
❑ Weekly
❑ Biweekly
❑ Monthly
❑ 6 times a year
❑ 4 times a year
❑ Less than 2 times a year

If you're currently under chiropractic care, please describe what you like best about it:

What you like least about it:

If you don't receive chiropractic care, please check which of these reasons apply:

❑ Too expensive
❑ My insurance won't cover it
❑ My insurance limit is up
❑ I don't have the time
❑ Other:
❑ Treatment has concluded
❑ Uncertain of the benefits
❑ Not a convenient location
❑ Hours not convenient

If you were to utilize chiropractic care, which of these features would be most important to you?

❑ Working with the same physician each time
❑ Flexible office hours, including evenings and Saturdays
❑ Other:
❑ A guarantee of satisfaction
❑ Honoring insurance claims

Thank you very much for your time in filling out this form. Return this survey today and receive your free booklet.

Sincerely,

Thomas Moore, D.C.

P.S. If we receive your survey in the next 10 days, we will also send you a complimentary registration for one of our upcoming seminars.

§7

Figure 26.10 **Sales Letter Design Tips**

- Use an eye-catching headline.
- Highlight the benefits immediately.
- Use your prospect's name.
- Clarify why you have selected the recipient to receive your letter.
- Build rapport and develop credibility.
- Keep it short.
- Use sincere, friendly language.
- Include powerful words such as "new," "free," "save," and "now."
- Provide a guarantee.
- Offer incentives.
- Include testimonials. Always use a full name. If possible, include a company name, title, and location.
- Include a time limit or expiration date.
- State your offer in clear, simple terms.
- Provide step-by-step instructions so your readers know how to respond.
- Close with a call to action.
- Use a postscript (P.S.) at the end of the letter. It's the most-often read part of any letter (along with the headline).
- Use bold type to emphasize key points.
- Print the letter on high-quality paper.
- Enclose a response card or an invitation.

Envelopes

Your envelope needs to motivate readers to open it and see what's inside. Printing teaser copy or an illustration on the outside helps. Also, a large or irregularly shaped envelope stands out from regular mail. If you're sending letters to general consumers (current and prospective clients), use a first-class stamp instead of metered or bulk mail to increase the odds of your letter getting opened. You increase the odds even more if you hand write the recipient's name and address.

Figure 26.11 **Direct Mail Envelope**

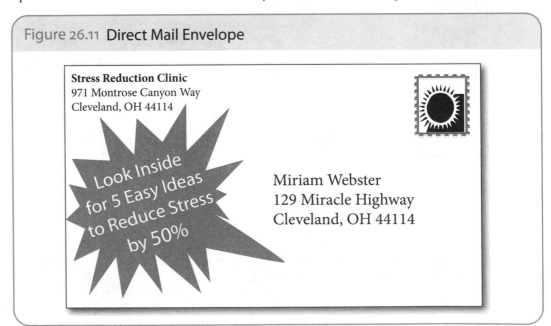

Mailing Lists

You can develop your own internal mailing list by starting with your client list, and adding information from business cards you collect (at networking events and your public speaking functions) and leads generated leads from Internet marketing. You can also purchase lists through a broker, contact organizations and associations that serve your target markets (they often share their lists for a nominal charge or free), and sometimes you can obtain the addresses of new residents for free through the utility companies

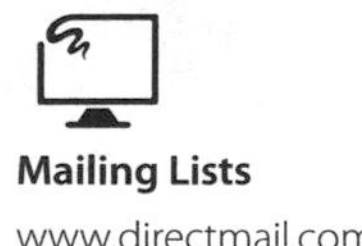

Mailing Lists
www.directmail.com

Generating Responses

Some incentives that inspire people to respond to direct mail are: free merchandise or service; free demonstration; free literature such as a newsletter, catalog, or handout; technical assistance; discount coupon; free training; and a free consultation.

Response cards are very effective for generating leads and come in two major categories: Business Reply Cards (postpaid) and Courtesy Reply Cards (not postpaid). Postpaid cards get the best response (free is usually better). Keep the information clear, concise, and engaging. Restate your offer, and include an incentive for a quick reply. Use check-off boxes with different options—the less amount of time and energy the recipient has to expend, the more likely they'll respond. Perhaps include "Maybe" along with "Yes" and "No" options. Put your name, address, phone number, and website on the bottom. If possible, print the recipient's name on the top of the card.

An alternative to mass mailing is to send out 1 letter each day to prospective clients and other wellness providers with whom you wish to develop alliances.

Follow-up is crucial. You can greatly increase your direct mail letter response by following up the mailing with a telephone call.

Gift Certificates

Gift certificates provide a surge of income into your practice and offer an easy way for clients to share your services with their family, friends, and colleagues. They can also be both a marketing tool to generate new clients and a goodwill promotion when given as presents or donated to charities. They are a tool to increase your client base, so it's in your best interest that they get redeemed. The true profit is generated not from the certificate sale but from subsequent sessions that the new client books. Each person who uses a gift certificate can become a regular client. Thus, the initial certificate (whether purchased or given as a promotion) can launch a wonderful business relationship and bring in thousands of dollars in fees.

See Chapter 24, page 356 for the **lifetime value of a client**.

Gift certificates can be in a digital format where they can be purchased and downloaded from your website, or you can have pre-printed versions available at your office. I suggest using both formats. In today's time-pressed and hectic world, gift certificates for wellness services are growing in popularity. Many clients appreciate the convenience of this gift-giving option, and are enthusiastic about this unique and thoughtful way to support the wellbeing of others.

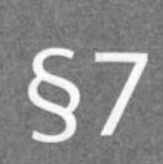

Gift certificates can be for a specific service or a dollar amount. Some people prefer to give a gift certificate that doesn't have a dollar amount listed. The challenge to that option is if the certificate isn't redeemed quickly and your prices go up, then you "lose" money. If this is a concern for you, consider putting that money into an interest-bearing account (to make up for any fee increases) and transfer the money into your checking account when the certificate is redeemed. You could also put a note on the certificate that says something like, "Prices are subject to change, and recipient may be responsible to pay the difference." I don't advocate this option as I would rather have the opportunity to transform a one-time gift recipient into a regular client.

Figure 26.12 **Sample Gift Certificate**

A Gift of Relaxation and Health

OUTSIDE

great graphic

Gift Certificate for Massage (or whatever the certificate will be for - or just leave this line off)

To: ______________________ From: ______________________

This certificate entitles you to: ______________________

INSIDE

For Your Appointment Contact:
Your Name / Business Name Address (optional)
Phone Website and/or Email (recommended)

personalized information

Directions to your place of business, indication of your specialties or business motto (optional)

Policies such as '24 hour cancellation required,' or expiration date

Expiration Date Debate

Many states have strict regulations concerning gift certificates: some don't allow expiration dates, some dictate how far they may be postdated, and several require that if the certificates aren't redeemed within a certain period of time, then the money must be deposited with the state. You can put an expiration date on gift certificates when they're used as promotions (no money has been exchanged), such as donating certificates to a charity auction.

Some people advocate increasing one's revenue stream by aggressively selling gift certificates with very short expiration terms. Often the majority of certificates expire before being redeemed, and the practitioner receives the income without having to perform any services. While this scam might appear tempting, consider the long-term consequences of this and the ill will that this might generate.

For most people, a gift certificate is a significant investment. Your gift certificate sales will dramatically increase if you develop a system that allays concerns about purchasing something that might not be used. People feel more comfortable purchasing certificates that either have a flexible expiration date or no expiration date. Another approach is for the certificate to revert to the purchaser if not used by the expiration date.

Some practitioners put a reasonably short expiration date on their gift certificates (such as 3 or 6 months) to encourage people to come in soon, yet always extend the date upon request. Others charge a token reactivation fee to extend the expiration.

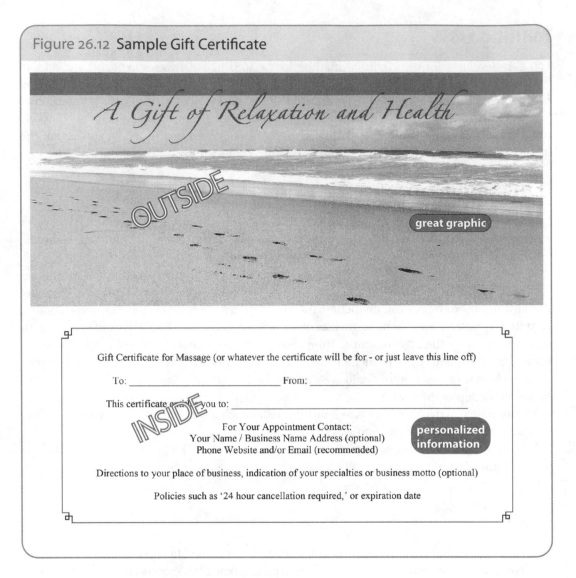

Regulations about Gift Certificates

www.ncsl.org/research/financial-services-and-commerce/gift-cards-and-certificates-statutes-and-legis.aspx

In one of my workshops, a massage therapist shared the following method for successfully integrating gift certificate sales:

Whenever he sells a gift certificate, he posts who bought the certificate and the name and contact information of the intended recipient (if this is unknown at the time the certificate is bought, he checks back with the purchaser in a month or so). His gift certificates include a 6-month expiration. One month prior to the expiration, he calls the recipient to give notice that a session needs to be booked before the certificate expires. After 6 months elapse without redemption, and he cannot contact the recipient or the recipient doesn't schedule an appointment, he contacts the original purchaser and tells her that the gift certificate reverts to her use. He sells a lot of gift certificates and has a redemption rate in the high 90th percentile! His clients feel comfortable about purchasing gift certificates from him because they don't have to worry about the certificates (and their money) going to waste.

Points to Ponder:

What are the potential drawbacks to this approach? What are the potential legal and ethical consequences of not redeeming an expired certificate?

Early Redemption

The sooner your gift certificates get redeemed, the better. Print an encouraging phrase on the bottom of the certificate to assist in early redemption, such as:

- Take Time Out for Yourself Today
- Enhance Your Wellbeing Right Now
- Relax and Revitalize Today

Another idea is to offer incentives for early redemption, such as:

- Book your appointment within 2 weeks and receive a free paraffin dip for your hands.
- Use this gift certificate within 1 month and receive an extra 15 minutes.
- Redeem this certificate within 1 month and receive a 15% discount on all self-care supplies.

Stocking Up

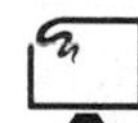

Gift Certificate Templates

sohnen-moe.com/products/marketing-materials/#product-gift-cert

You can purchase ready-made gift certificates or design and print your own. The major benefits of purchasing ready-made certificates are a lower initial investment of time and money and the variety of design options. Most of these certificates are printed in full color on high-quality paper and are available in a wide range of styles (some generic and others for specific events, such as birthdays).

If you're in a solo practice and sell a large quantity of certificates, then you might consider printing your own. You can customize the certificates with your contact information (e.g., name, address, phone number, website, list of your services). If you choose this route, the certificate design can match the style and color palette of your letterhead, business cards, and brochures. You can also purchase gift certificate templates and print them as needed. There are some very attractive gift certificates printed on cardstock and bordered in foil (silver, gold, or copper) with a matching foil-lined envelope. Regardless of whether you purchase certificates or make your own, be sure they convey your desired image.

Key information to include on a gift certificate is the recipient's name, the giver's name, and a description of the services to be provided (or the dollar amount). Other useful items to add are the certificate number, date of issue, the name of the practitioner who issued the certificate (particularly for a multi-practitioner office), and (if you insist) an expiration date. If you custom-print your certificates, include your contact information. If you purchase ready-made certificates, put your business card in the envelope or attach it to the certificate (some certificates are slit so you can easily attach your card).

Marketing Gift Certificates

Gift Certificate Envelopes and Holders

www.bayleysboxes.com

Some work settings lend themselves to a high volume of gift certificate sales. Upscale salons and day spas are a prime example, since gift certificates for services and products are commonplace in these settings. Yet relatively few practicing wellness practitioners actively promote gift certificate sales—they typically make them available only to current clients. The certificates are an afterthought. Usually the only action a practitioner takes is a special holiday promotion, reminding clients that they can give the gift of health. Don't be limited to seasonal sales; gift certificate sales can be an integral part of a year-round marketing program.

At the very least, insert a sample gift certificate in your welcome kit and prominently display one in your waiting area (framed and either on a stand or hung on the wall). Hang a poster about gift certificates on your doors, bathroom walls, and treatment spaces. Mention your gift certificates in all your promotional materials, particularly brochures, flyers, website, and advertisements. If you distribute a newsletter, print a notice about gift certificate sales in every issue. Tactful, tasteful reminders about gift certificate availability are always appreciated.

Always keep a stack of gift certificates handy (be certain to display a sample one) whenever you're involved in an activity associated with your practice, such as public speaking events, open houses, and exposition booths.

While gift certificate sales are excellent tools for increasing revenue, keep in mind that the true profit is generated not from the sale of the certificate but from the subsequent sessions that the new client books.

The majority of gift certificates get sold in December. Here are some fun display ideas:

- Place a gift certificate against a candle and wrap them both with a bright ribbon.
- Attach a gift certificate to a "holiday" plant.
- Put a certificate in a beautiful box.
- Put a ribbon around a number of certificates (let's say 10) attaching a colorful note that says something like "Gifts for Others" and then wrap some certificates (perhaps 2) and attach another colorful note that says "And I get this!"
- Purchase small bottles of holiday-themed essential oils and attach a gift certificate with a ribbon.
- Purchase miniature dreidels and chocolate Hanukkah gelt and place some of each in a mesh bag, tie with a light blue ribbon and attach a gift certificate.
- Kwanzaa candle colors are green, red, and black. Get one of each, tie them with a colorful piece of material and attach a gift certificate.
- Attach a gift certificate to a large, plastic-wrapped candy cane.

Also, sell your certificates to businesses to use as incentives or rewards. Many companies regularly reward customers, clients, and employees with substantial gifts. For example, real estate agencies and title companies usually give gifts to their clients upon closing. Purchasing a home can be extremely stressful, so wellness care makes an excellent gift alternative to the customary houseplant or kitchen accessory.

Another option to increase your gift certificate sales is to offer free gift certificates (for services or products) to cross-promoting partners to use as incentives. They can make a similar offer for their customers who purchase gift certificates (or some other incentive program). A bookstore could be a great co-marketing partner. You could offer a $10 book gift certificate for every 2 wellness certificates purchased. The bookstore could offer a 15-minute mini-service certificate for every $75 worth of book certificates purchased. The certificates don't need to be of equal value as long as the total exchange is equitable. For instance, you could give the bookstore 10 certificates for mini-sessions (let's say at a value of $30 each) or 5 full-session certificates to be used in whatever type of promotion the bookstore chooses, and, in return, the bookstore would give you thirty $10 book gift certificates.

Custom Gift Cards

Custom gift cards are similar to gift certificates. They can infuse additional revenue and establish your brand identity. Plus, these plastic cards are reloadable and reusable. You can personalize each gift card when you sell them, if you have the right equipment.

You can create fun marketing campaigns with gift cards, such as a self-mailer with a snap-out card, a postcard with the card affixed, and keytags (good for loyalty programs).

Here are some statistics from studies about the use and effectiveness of gift cards:[5]

- More than $100 billion is spent on gift cards annually in the United States.
- 93% of U.S. consumers purchase or receive a gift card annually.
- Consumers spend an average of a little over $200 per year on gift cards.
- 72% of customers will spend more than the value of their card.
- On average, the recipient will spend 20% more than the gift card value.
- 90% of gift cards are used within the first 60 days.
- 83% of corporations use prepaid gift cards for employee incentives.

Gift Card Suppliers
www.plasticresource.com
ecardsystems.com
www.customgiftcards.com

Coupons

Coupons encourage people to try new services and products. They help generate new clients and prompt current clients to return. Some people don't use them because they think they're somehow demeaning, yet, according to a research study, 80% of consumers surveyed admit feeling smart when they use a coupon.[6] The bottom line is that coupons are extremely effective when used correctly. While free is always best in the consumer's eye, it isn't the only option. Still, the discount needs to be enough to provide impetus. For instance, $5 dollars off a $75 session most likely won't produce a huge influx of new clients (although it would certainly make current clients happy). Coupon campaigns are more successful when you offer a dollar amount off rather than a percentage discount (e.g., $10 off a $100 purchase, rather than 10% off all orders of $100 dollars), unless the discount is 50% or higher.

Another option that works for many practitioners is to offer a short session for free (e.g., a 30-minute massage) that can be upgraded for a fee to a full session. Coupons can also be used to promote ancillary services or products. For instance, a coupon could state, "Bring this coupon to your next session and get a FREE 6-ounce container of The World's Best Aloe Vera Ointment."

Coupons are easily printed from your computer, so they can be customized. If you don't have a color printer, use a jazzy paper or purchase special laser printer stock that's designed to be used as coupons or mini-certificates. This paper is usually heavier, has borders and is perforated. When you print coupons in small batches, you can include a short expiration date. Unlike gift certificates, coupons can have an expiration date without any legal concerns since the client doesn't purchase the coupon. Since many shoppers prefer digital coupons, include QR codes on your printed coupons to make them work with a mobile device.

§7

Personalized Gift Items

Personalized gift items—also known as premiums and specialty advertising—provide a daily reminder of your business while either being passed around from person to person, landing on a refrigerator, or being seen on handy items. The variety of these items is amazing. You can get almost anything personalized with your company name or logo! Some typical gift items in this category are erasers, magnets, pens, pencils, note pads, letter openers, stress balls, bookmarks, bumper stickers, calendars, mugs, visors, nail files, aromatherapy eye pillows, sports bottles,

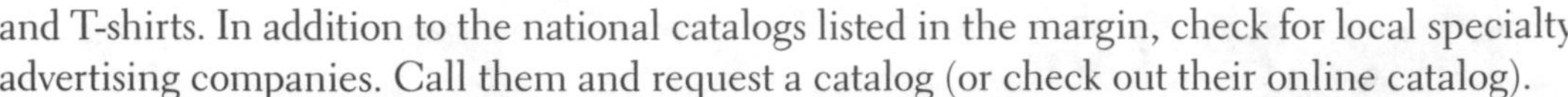

and T-shirts. In addition to the national catalogs listed in the margin, check for local specialty advertising companies. Call them and request a catalog (or check out their online catalog).

Premium Sales

www.bestimpressions.com
www.4imprint.com
www.amsterdamprinting.com
www.wethinkpromos.com

Specialty advertising items can be worthwhile in any business. They're fun promotional tools and often quite inexpensive. For wellness providers, the main focus of premiums is to develop relationships with prospective or current clients. In most instances, the perceived monetary value of the item isn't as important as its use, so select items that the recipients want or need. Choose items that either directly remind your clients of you (or your specific services) or are of definite interest (or benefit) to the people in your target markets. The key elements to print on these items are your company's name, phone number, and website.

You can distribute these as gifts at special events or whenever a new client comes in for an initial visit. Include them in your mailings or hand them out whenever you're so inclined.

See Chapter 21, pages 311-312 for tips on using **product samples as gift items**.

Gift items can also be used as incentives (e.g., offer a free tote bag with every $50 spent on products). An inexpensive idea for a beneficial personalized gift item is to print labels and affix them to water bottles (just don't cover the original product label). You can inexpensively purchase bottled water by the case. Most print shops have specialty labels in different colors, shapes, and designs (e.g., golf balls, hearts, stars) that you can imprint with your name, phone number, address, and website. Every time your clients come in for an appointment, greet them with a smile, a handshake, and a water bottle. If they drink all the water before they leave, offer to refill it from your water cooler.

Signage

Most landlords require some type of signage. Your office sign creates an important first impression: it welcomes clients, introduces potential clients to your business, and reinforces your company's image and brand. In addition to identifying your business, some signs can be easily changed to highlight special offers or to catch people's attention with an inspiring or humorous statement.

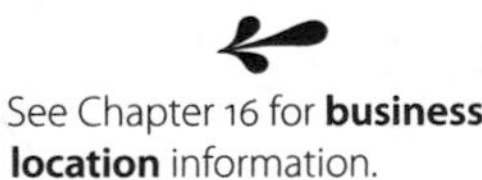

See Chapter 16 for **business location** information.

Signs can be a powerful marketing tool to generate new clients, particularly if your building is in a high-traffic area. If your sign is prominently displayed and attractive, people who pass by your location on a regular basis are more likely to look you up when they need your type of service.

Office signage is often very expensive, so take the time to research options. Check out the signs used by surrounding businesses as well as other businesses that offer services similar to yours. Note what attracts you and what you don't like. Also, review your lease for specific requirements and restrictions. After you've done some initial research, sketch out your ideas. Finally, work with a reputable sign company to make the actual sign. Before finalizing the contract, have the sign company create paper mockups so you can test them out for readability (from a variety of angles and distances) and overall attractiveness.

27
Online Presence

"The Internet has turned what used to be a controlled, one-way message into a real-time dialogue with millions."
—Danielle Sacks

Website Savvy
- Planning
- On-Page SEO
- Hosting Services
- Content
- Creative Design
- Marketing Perspective
- Drive Traffic to Your Website

Blogs

Videos

Social Media Marketing
- Social Media as SEO
- Posting Schedule
- Increase Engagement
- Reusing Content
- Multiple Social Sites
- Personal vs Businesss Use

Online Advertising
- Customer Personas
- Elements of an Online Ad

Key Terms

AdWords
Algorithm
Backlink
Banner Advertising
Blog
Business Page
Call to Action (CTA)
Conversion
Crosslink
Data-Mining
Engagement
Facebook
Forum
Friend
Funnel
Google+
Hashtags
Home Page
Hosting
Instagram
Internet Service Provider (ISP)
Keyword
Landing Page
Lead Capture
Lead Magnet
Link
LinkedIn
Listicle
Listserv
Metadata
Meta-Tagging
Newsfeed
Online Advertising
On-Page SEO
Opt-In
Pay-Per-Click (PPC)
Persona
Pinterest
Portmanteau
Post
Ranking
Scalable
Search Engine Marketing (SEM)
Search Engine Optimization (SEO)
Server-Side Scripting
Social Media
Social Media Optimization (SMO)
Traffic
Twitter
URL
Vlog
Webmaster
Website
Website Page Fold
YouTube
Yelp

The Internet offers a wealth of resources for growing your business. Today, the key is integration and "keep-in-touch marketing," marketing that builds strong, lasting relationships on or off the Internet. From websites to blogs, from email newsletters to online discussion groups, to social media, these web-based marketing tools make it easy to connect with thousands of people with a minimum investment. You really maximize all the benefits when you have a full sales process combining all your offline marketing and print materials with your online marketing efforts. Most people remember to include their social media icons, website, blog, and newsletter links on their printed materials, window signs, company letterhead, and invoices. But, do you have your address and phone number, website, blog, newsletter, and social page links in your automated email signature for every outgoing email? How about listing your upcoming live event or workshop on your social pages? During the live event are you snapping photos and tweeting about them with special event hashtags?

> "If you make customers unhappy in the physical world, they might each tell six friends. If you make customers unhappy on the Internet, they can each tell 6,000 friends.
> —Jeff Bezos

We live in a digital age, so marrying the offline with the online experience can really boost the results for business. There also has to be integration between the offline purchase and getting clients back online to leave a review, make a recommendation, and continue to stay connected, so you can leverage their excitement to develop a whole tribe of raving followers on your blog, social media pages, newsletter subscribers, and website.

According to Michael Port, author of *Book Yourself Solid*, "If you're not online, you're out of line."[1] As the landscape of Internet marketing is vast, this section provides valuable insights and resources to help you understand the toolbox known as online marketing and how to incorporate the sales process into what is commonly known as a sales funnel. It's a funnel because you use leads from social media, live events, and customer referrals, to direct them to your website. Once there, you exchange their name and email for a piece of valuable relevant information, and continue to follow up with automatically preset emails.

This chapter walks you through the sales funnel process and demonstrates how it works to help automate the marketing side of your business. It also provide the practical know-how to evaluate what online tools are best suited to your business. For a more in-depth orientation, plan to read several of the recommended books and online sources, or attend a seminar with a local Internet marketing expert.

Website Savvy

You have a couple of options when it comes to building a website. Various website companies and organizations offer what is called pre-designed or template sites. These are very easy to use, cost effective, and are a popular option for practitioners who are working from home or just starting out, yet there are 6 major limitations:

1. These types of sites don't allow for very much customization and typically don't work well with additional programs like online scheduling and some payment gateways. The plus side is some of them offer these programs as premium monthly services.
2. As your practice grows, and if you want to create a more custom-built website, none of the formatting is yours and most of the content and images won't be transferrable unless you provided it. Some of the template website companies will offer to put the content in a transferrable file for you but it won't have any of the coding for the website itself.
3. Any search engine optimization (SEO) done with images, blogging, articles, backlinks, and social media will always link to their company website address (not yours), so all SEO effort must be started over when you build your own website.
4. Some template sites offer to purchase the URL for you and then they own it, or will transfer the URL to you for a fee. Confirm with the company that you own your URL address.
5. Most don't offer lead capture or list building options without additional fees. Have you ever heard the saying the "money is in the list"? That means that as you start to build a clientele, you will want to create a database of ways to connect with them on a regular

How to Use the Internet to Advertise, Promote and Market Your Business or Website with Little or No Money by Bruce C. Brown

Social MisAlignments: The Chiropractor's Guide to Marketing Online by Stephanie Beck and building relationships with your clients and potential clients. You want an easy and effective way to connect with any visitor on your website.

basis. Your website is one of the best traffic magnets when it comes to capturing emails and building relationships with your clients and potential clients. You want an easy and effective way to connect with any visitor on your website.

6. Not all template sites include hosting fees. Read all the fine print.

The advantages of template website companies are that they're what is known as drag and drop websites; this means they're very user friendly and don't require any special coding. Most template sites offer preformatted pages, allow you to choose from a variety of colors, typically have images that are suited for your business, and some also provide sample written content. Another advantage is your website can be live within 24 hours. Note, while some companies offer a limited FREE website like www.wix.com and www.wordpress.com, be sure you read the fine print, as you'll most likely need to upgrade to their monthly paid services to have all the features you may need.

Check with your professional associations to see if they offer FREE websites for their members.

These template sites are extremely cost effective and efficient, especially if your operating budget is limited to get started. Each has various monthly plans that can range from free to $800 a month, depending on the features you need. Building your own website would be a better way to go in the long run if you have a little larger budget for a one-time fee of $1,000 to $2,500, and can afford around $150.00 a month for SEO and hosting fees. Seriously consider having a website built for you if your short term plan (within the first 3 years) is to expand your practice to include retail or add on other practitioners, spa technicians, and services.

Consider the following analogy: Even though all massage therapists are taught the same basic strokes, if I pay for a one-hour massage from 10 randomly selected therapists, my results may vary a little depending on the skill level and experience. It also varies if I pay for a deep tissue versus a relaxation massage. Each therapist will provide what I paid for, but how it's provided and how I feel afterwards will vary. The same can happen with website creation. When you evaluate and compare various website companies or individuals, the first thing you need to realize is that not all websites are created equally. Website programmers, designers, and graphic artists can all build you a website. Some have specialized training for on-page SEO and a small number have a strong marketing background or copywriting skills. Remember to ask about their skill level and know what you're asking them to provide. Not every website builder includes on-page SEO, and almost all of them charge more for copywriting or content creation. The 5 elements to good website design are: planning, on-page SEO, content, creative design, and marketing.

Website Templates

www.ocoos.com
www.websitebuildertop10.com
www.templatemonster.com
www.acupuncture-websites.com
www.yogisites.com
imatrix.com
www.massage-therapy-websites.com

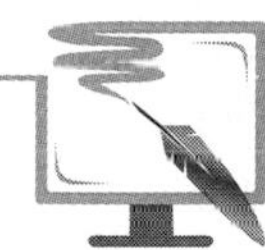

Website Vendor Comparison

Compare and contrast 3-5 websites offering pre-design (check to see if your professional associations offer this). Items to consider are: base cost, cost for extras (e.g., online scheduling, email, SEO package, URL ownership, web hosting, transfer of information), ease of use, support available, time frames to start, images available, and number of allowed pages. Next, do the same comparison for contracting someone to custom build your site. Finally, compare both lists.

Planning

Planning is critical, whether you use a template site or build your own. Start with an end in mind. What is it you want every visitor to know when they visit your page? What action do you want them to take? Any website designer should start by asking you to define the general purpose of the website so she is clear on the functionality and the number of pages needed. It helps both of you if you already have the action plan and target audience for each of the

§7

individual pages of your site. Start with the home page and work your way through each page. This helps your designer to offer the best design that is user friendly and will help get you the results you want. Most websites can be built and go live within 2 weeks if the goals are clear and the information is organized at the start. Many website designs realistically take 3-4 weeks only because most people don't know what they want or what's possible. The cost will most likely be higher if you want a project completed within a short time frame. Note, some designers are strategists (offer several ideas and options or offer other suggestions of things that worked well for other clients), while others are implementers (will only build exactly what you requested).

> "Websites promote you 24/7. No employee will do that.
> —Paul Cookson

Keep in mind, not every person who clicks on your website is ready to make a purchase or book a service. Your clients have plenty of options. Sometimes people want to learn more about you or your services before they're ready to book an appointment. Therefore, it's good to offer some way to connect with them while they're visiting your website so that you can continue to connect with them once they leave. This technique of lead capture (also referred to as an opt-in form), means a visitor enters their name and email in exchange for access to some piece of information, discount coupon, report, checklist, training video, ebook, podcast, webinar, live event, or other promotional kit that would pique their interest. Other ways to get this done are to have them subscribe to your email list, newsletter, or blog. This allows you to cultivate your relationship by continuing to offer them valuable information. Always include offers of your products and services so that when they're ready to make that decision, they have an easy way to do so.

On-Page SEO

Search Engine Optimization, or SEO, is a process of maximizing the highest number of visitors to your website by ensuring that your website appears at the top of the search results list, generally on page 1 of most search engines. All search engines such as Google, Bing, Yelp, and Yahoo, and even social sites like Facebook, Pinterest, Google+, YouTube, Twitter, LinkedIn, Vine, and SlideShare, have primary search results where content on specific pages of your website or social business profiles are listed and ranked based on what the search engines consider most relevant to users. The kind of content that's searched on your website and social profiles include blog posts, links to articles, videos, newsletters, images (with the right meta-tagging or descriptions), social media updates, and audio recordings, and all can be linked back to your website and are part of SEO services.

The mission statement of the number one search engine company (Google) is simple: To organize the world's information and make it universally accessible and useful.[2] Their objective is that every time anyone enters words into a search field, they find exactly what they are looking for the first time. Therefore, the words entered into the search fields are continuously being identified and matched by the search engine to specific types of websites. The algorithm is constantly modified as more and more people search every day. Thus, if a person enters a word like massage, the search engines have matched that general term with people who are searching for information about massage schools to become a massage therapist, large national massage therapy franchise chains, or, unfortunately, adult entertainment, and therefore those websites will generally be listed first.

Every website that is hosted and live on the Internet is indexed by the search engines based on the keywords used in the title and content of your website. Although massage may seem like a keyword to use, think about what kind of websites came up in the search; massage schools, national massage chains, and adult entertainment businesses that have invested a lot of money to receive a high ranking for that term. Therefore, unless you plan on opening a massage school, running an adult entertainment facility, or have the thousands of dollars to compete with the national chains, using a general keyword like massage would not be good for your practice because you may never be able to rank on page 1 for that particular term.

Consider the following scenario:

Stephanie's television finally quit working and she decided to replace it with a flat screen TV. She started out by entering "flat screen TV" in the search field. She was inundated with various ads to sell her flat screens, LED, Plasma, brands, sizes, etc. It was so confusing. She soon realized she didn't know the difference between LED and Plasma or what options she wanted (e.g., HD, bluetooth), so she refined her search to learn more about the differences. She also asked her friends on social media what they had or recommended, and specifically researched reviews for Samsung plasma TVs. After seeing the reviews and getting feedback from friends, she was ready to purchase and entered "Best price on Samsung Plasma 62" TV in San Diego." This gave her many local options.

Points to Ponder

As a TV store owner, would it be best to use a term like "flat screen TV San Diego" or "best price plasma TV San Diego"? Which do you think is more likely to lead to purchases? Do you see why it's important to have reviews of your products and services? Why is it important to have friends and clients recommend, like, comment, and share on your social pages?

You need keyword research and on-page SEO for a website to be indexed properly and attract the right type of clients to your practice. On-page SEO for your website refers to optimizing all images on your website, headers, pages, titles, and more. Some website designers don't invest the time in meta-tagging images for social shares and optimizing pages, especially if they know the clients don't plan on continuing to provide content or invest time in ongoing SEO services. The initial on-page SEO does help to get the website indexed by the search engines, but in most cases without properly identifying the visitors' needs, choosing the best words to rank, and continuing to invest in ongoing SEO services, the website will most likely never increase in ranking. So, unless you specifically pay for on-page SEO or keyword research, it won't be included in the basic website package.

> "One of the Internet's strengths is its ability to help consumers find the right needle in a digital haystack of data.
> —Jared Sandberg

Most website companies (either template or independent developers) will offer an SEO package upgrade. Ask about social share features and keyword research. Some of the packages are designed for mass use, meaning they provide generalized ranking for local businesses that may not be your ideal target audience. You may end up with clients, but they aren't your preferred type of clients. Most "mass" market packages are inexpensive and good, and some of them even work fairly quickly. However, you might not be happy with the long-term results because they aren't producing your ideal client. Still, this is a good option when you first get started and aren't sure what type of clients are going to be your best clients.

Identifying Keywords

Make a list of words that you feel are keywords from your profession. Enter each word into a search engine and note what you find. What comes up may surprise you. Keep experimenting with general term as well as specific phrases until you hit on the keywords that bring up exactly what you would be looking for if you were a client interested in your type of services.

Hosting Services

A webhost provides the online "space" and resources to operate your website. You can work through your Internet Service Provider (ISP) or another hosting company for these services. Choosing the right web hosting company ensures the smooth sailing of your website, and avoids unexpected bouts of downtime that may result in clients perceiving you as unreliable or unresponsive. A good starting point is to ask people you know, who have websites, for their recommendations.

Website hosting services generally cost from $5 to $150 per month. Annual contracts may offer a reduced fee. The difference in fees depends on the additional services you select, such as server-side scripting (which programs the behavior of the server), databases, online "storefronts," SEO services, and the number of different websites and email accounts you require. Multiple email accounts are normal for a website: "webmaster," "service," "sales," and "info" are common generic accounts. Other factors that impact cost are uptime guarantees (i.e., how often the service becomes unavailable), site development assistance, levels of technical support, secure hosting services, and site backup services.

Content

> Marketing is telling the world you're a rock star. Content marketing is showing the world you are one.
> —Robert Rose

The content on your pages helps the search engines identify the type of visitor to bring to your pages. While several template sites provide content you can use, sometimes "canned" content that is used on hundreds of websites isn't the best option. You want to use the keywords that have been identified by thorough keyword research of your target audience. Next, you need to craft the content so the keywords flow naturally on the pages of your website. Other factors to consider are what's acceptable by the FDA, what's legal, and what's ethical. That means understanding your city, county, state, and federal guidelines. If you hire someone to write content for you, or use pre-written content from a template site, keep in mind ignorance is not a defense if any wild claims are made. You are still liable for what is said about your practice. Make sure that the writer is aware of your specific regulations and how your clients think.

Most people write the content themselves in order to save money. If you do this, remember to write it from the client's perspective. The content has to be centered on connecting with the visitors so they feel like you understand their problems. Avoid focusing on what your practice does. This type of writing takes a certain amount of finesse and artistry. Sometimes you can save money by creating it yourself, then sending it to an expert in content development for editing. Editing and rewriting can sometimes cost you a lot less than having an expert write it in the first place, however this can be the most time consuming part of website development and why some websites can take 3-7 weeks. Most developers require all the content before starting the project, and won't build out one page at a time.

Creative Design

Web Design Tips
www.webpagesthatsuck.com

Most people are visual buyers, so creative design is critical, as it's the finishing touch, the icing on the cake, so to speak. It's best if you can find a good marketer to help you with both the content and creative design, but most of the time people hire a graphic artist for this job. Graphic artists are excellent at creating something visually engaging but may lack training on the SEO to produce engagement (e.g., subscriptions, sales, appointments). Yet, creative design is where most people invest the majority of their time, money, and effort. We think that something has to look "pretty" to make people want to do business with us. But the truth is, if you have defined your plan and functionality effectively, crafted your content with the right keywords, and have all your pages with the correct SEO from a marketing perspective, it doesn't have to be "pretty" to produce numbers.

You will inevitably win more clients with a clean, basic website that's extremely user-friendly and has content that makes the visitors feel like you understand their problems. So, invest your time into keywords, content, and making the experience extremely easy to do business with you. Ideally, work with a graphic artist who is flexible, can take direction, and can provide you with what you want–more clients (not just to make it look pretty). Most of what a graphic artist creates doesn't get ranked by the search engines. Therefore, you still need an SEO developer to assist with ways to get your pages ranked. Ultimately, the pages on your website are a waste of money if they don't result in increased clientele.

Figure 27.1 Elements of Website Design

Good
- Eye appeal, pleasing color scheme
- Clear and easy-to-use navigation
- Accessible by the visually or manually impaired
- High information value
- Quick-loading graphics
- Easy-to-find contact information
- Balance of content and white space
- Easy to find scheduling and purchasing information

Poor
- Clutter
- Poor navigation
- Lack of contrast
- Flash or animated graphics
- Ugly background images
- Sound files
- Slow-to-load pages
- Black background color

Figure 27.2 Make Your Site Inviting

- Use catchy heading (you only have 5 seconds to capture a visitor's attention).
- Use appropriate meta-description and meta-keyword tags on each page.
- Don't try any "tricks" to get higher placement in search engines.
- Match the Page Title with the page's main heading.
- Use main keywords in the title, filename, and near the top of the document.
- Your homepage should load quickly, grab attention, and provide a clear roadmap.
- Create a section for electronic news releases and media materials (e.g., include announcements about workshops, open houses, and special promotions).
- Include highlights on new developments and research findings in your field.
- Include general interest information on holistic health and wellness.
- Include links to non-competitive wellness professionals and organizations.
- Post success stories and testimonials (be sure to obtain client's permission).
- Offer discounts for online purchase of products and gift certificates.
- Promote online appointment scheduling by offering package deals.
- Provide a way for visitors to give you feedback (e.g., a "Contact Me" form, direct email link, or a survey).

Marketing Perspective

Online Marketing Tips
website101.com

Marketing perspective is a combination of all the items previously discussed. It's important to understand what makes a good headline, sub-headline, and what are the "hooks" to use to connect with visitors in a way that makes them want to do business with you. Knowing where the best place is to capture the eye, which colors perform the best, what needs to go above the fold of a website page (the portion of the webpage that's visible without scrolling), and where to put the images and videos so they show up on all types of devices (e.g., laptop, tablet, smartphone), is a combination of content creation and creative design. Keep in mind, making something look pretty to you, may not be the best marketing strategy for your clients–it needs to be attractive to your target market. A well-trained, experienced marketing consultant can assist you with your outline and formulate a solid strategy for each of your pages. Some marketers are also really good copywriters, so they can help you with your content creation. Others may have experience working with graphic artists and website designers, so they can help manage this project for you. Be aware that a good website programmer is often not a good marketer, as these are two different skillsets.

Drive Traffic to Your Website

Unfortunately, unlike the premise of the movie *Field of Dreams*, where an Iowa farmer hears a mysterious voice saying, "If you build it, he will come," just designing a great website isn't enough to attract a lot of visitors. You need to take action to attract people to visit your site.

Figure 27.3 Website Marketing Tips

- Print your website address on all your promotional materials (e.g., business cards, brochures, flyers, newsletters).
- List your website on professional directories for your field (e.g., acufinder.com).
- Send press releases to local media about your website.
- Notify your Chamber of Commerce and Visitor's Bureau about your special events.
- Post your address with regional website directories and city sites (usually the listing is free but a charge is assessed if you want a direct link to your site).
- Crosslink your site with other wellness practitioners' websites and affiliated sites (i.e., provide reciprocal links). For example, if you specialize in working with fibromyalgia, link up with some of the online fibromyalgia support groups and resource organizations.
- Purchase advertising on sites that you feel would be a likely place for your target market(s) to visit.

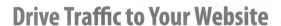

Research Complementary Websites

Compile a list of sites that you feel would attract your target market(s). Determine the types and costs for advertising on those sites. For example, if you work with pre- and post-natal clients, you could investigate places such as, baby stores, ob/gyn practices, day care centers, maternity shops, Lamaze classes, and other parent/baby classes.

Search Engine Directories

Search engine directory listings are another way of driving traffic back to your website and are considered a service of SEO. Most of these directories are general in scope and list websites across a wide range of categories, regions, and languages. However, some directories are focused on a particular niche and restricted by regions or occupations. When you first launch a website, you will often receive messages to list your business on their website to get traffic.

The most important thing to keep in mind when utilizing directory listings to gain traffic is that you need to be certain to list your business address exactly the same every time, and that it matches exactly the same on your website and social media pages. For instance, if street is abbreviated as "St." on your website, it MUST be abbreviated with a period on every listing. Computers are meticulous when it comes to matching data. Think of it as a highway of information that's rolling along and it comes to a gated community. In order to pass through, it must have the correct information. If the code says you must have 9002 A St. and you have 9002 A Street, even though as humans we know it is the same address, computers don't see it that way and won't allow traffic to continue.

List your URL

www.scrubtheweb.com/addurl.html

www.google.com/webmasters/tools/submit-url (requires account login)

The second most important part is to complete every field available on a directory site. For instance, many review sites or Google listings allow you to upload photos and include descriptions about your products and services, so be sure to complete each stage.

Blogs

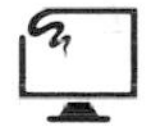

Technorati

technorati.com

Copywriting Tips

www.copyblogger.com

Blogging is a world unto itself. This form of Internet website, a portmanteau of web and log, first emerged in the mid 1990s. Technorati, a recognized authority on what's happening on the World Wide Web, tracks over 100 million blogs. A blog is a regularly updated website that contains postings in chronological order. In essence, it's a running commentary on a topic that the blogger knows, likes, or is passionate about.

A blog can attract new clients and keep you connected with colleagues who share your interest in holistic wellness. The secret to blogging is building relationships. Think of it as a dynamic conversation that connects those who have information of value to share.

Blogs have been rated as the 5th most trusted source for accurate online information.[3] Nearly 40% of US companies use blogs for marketing purposes and companies that blog have 55% more website visitors.[4] Companies who blog receive 97% more links to their website and get 67% more leads per month than those that don't.[5] Plus, blogging is an effective way to keep the search engines directing traffic to your website on a regular basis.

Many people don't feel comfortable with the thought of blogging, yet it can be one of the best lead magnets when done right. One of the most common fears reported by practitioners is that they don't know what to write about. A great way to overcome this is to start by making a list of topics or questions you had about your offerings before you chose to become a practitioner. Think back to why you first chose to receive a session. How did you feel afterwards? What were some of the benefits? If you aren't good at typing, use the voice memo on your phone and then download one of the mobile APPs that convert voice to text automatically. Think of it as interviewing yourself, how would you respond or what would you say to one of those questions? I bet you would easily be able to share your story or talk about that experience for 5-10 minutes. Most of us will use 250-500 words during that time. A blog post only needs to be 500-1200 words total. By answering common questions or sharing your own personal experience you could easily have several blog posts to get you started. One style of popular blogging is to write a "listicle," which is an article presented in the form of a bullet point or numbered format. For example: "10 Ways to Start Your Day Happy" or "5 Methods for Quick Relaxation." These types of articles are not only popular, but are easy to write and quick to read, so are often chosen over other formats.

What is really great is that by sharing your own personal experience and describing or talking about it from the client's point of view, you'll most likely use keywords that attract other people who are looking for that same type of experience. (Be sure to provide keyword metatags for your blogs.) Once you start working with a variety of clients, you'll have ample topics because your clients will undoubtedly keep you in stock with questions that can be generalized and used as blog topics for future posts. Note, maintain client confidentiality and HIPAA compliancy by not sharing specific details regarding a client or mentioning a client's name publicly (even if the client gives you permission).

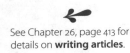

See Chapter 26, page 413 for details on **writing articles**.

Some key activities to increase linking on your blog include: listing blogs you like; commenting on others' blog posts; posting ideas, articles, resources, and links from other bloggers and the Internet; and posting a thank-you message when someone gives you a link.

Videos

Videos, in general, are a great way to promote your practice. They're personal and engaging, and highly popular. You can make instructional videos where you teach your clients ways they can take care of themselves, interview interesting people (including yourself and clients), showcase new products and techniques, or repost other's videos (get permission first). You can also do a vlog (a video-recorded blog). These videos can be placed on your website, as well as your social media pages, such as YouTube, Pinterest, Instagram, and Facebook.

You can also advertise on other people's videos.

Keep most of your videos under 2 minutes in length. Speak in a natural voice and avoid distracting noises. If you're a good editor, you can add some special visual effects and introductory music. Be sure to include some type of call to action (e.g., invite viewers to visit your website, subscribe to your blog, post a comment, schedule an appointment), and incorporate keywords into your scripts. When you upload the video, title it, write a good description, add relevant keywords and tags, and include your contact information. Announce your video by writing a blog about it, tweeting a link, or posting it on Facebook.

Besides YouTube, many other social networks like Facebook, Twitter, and Pinterest have added a video feature that allows users to upload directly to their platforms rather than sharing a link from another site (like YouTube, Vine, or Vimeo). The directly uploaded videos often get more play with the algorithms and have prime featured space on newsfeeds. For instance, a video uploaded directly on Facebook has more real estate space in their newsfeeds than a video link shared from another source. Therefore, there are some advantages to uploading the video directly onto each social site to avoid losing any SEO value.

Social Media Marketing

According to a Nielsen survey, people trust social media sites more than branded sites.[6] People expect companies to brag about themselves on their websites and have the best testimonials on them. As a result, people will search for businesses using social media, as they feel it provides a more balanced and objective perspective. In fact, this same survey cites that 46% of online users count on social media when making a purchase decision.

Social Media Videos

www.youtube.com/user/srbsolution

Social media is more than a passing fad; it is definitively here to stay. Social media APPS and channels of distribution may evolve, but the concept of social media is now big business and part of all of our lives. Social media isn't limited to the major platforms such as Facebook, Twitter, Pinterest, Snapchat, Instagram, Google+, LinkedIn, YouTube, Foursquare, Swarm, Vine, Meetup, Flickr, or one of the other wildly popular social sites.

Social media also includes newsgroups, listservs, and forums that serve your target market. According to web etiquette and group rules, it isn't appropriate to directly promote yourself in these types of venues. However, it's fine to list your website address or blog address as part of your signature line when you make posts that add value to the discussion topic. Posts that convey unique insights and useful information are appreciated and position you as a trusted and knowledgeable expert in your field.

Social media platforms are great avenues to connect with current clients and potential new clients, build lasting relationships, generate leads, increase your mailing list, gather referrals, send people to your website, and build your brand awareness. Social media sites aren't like eBay or craigslist. In general, people aren't logging onto them to seek out products and services to make a purchase. While users do buy from these platforms, the purpose is, first and foremost, to be connected.

Think of social media sites as rented or leased space, similar to the website template sites discussed earlier. Since you don't own the space, you can't control how the content is seen or when users see it. The best thing to do is to use these social media sites as lead finders to get visitors to click through to something you do own as quickly as possible. For instance, at least 2 times a week, give your followers opportunities to join your email or newsletter list. Share links to your blog posts so they can go from a social media site to your website and then subscribe to your blog updates. You control the content on your websites, and once you have them on your email or newsletter list, you can control when that information is shared with them, regardless if they're on social media.

> "Social media is one area of business where you don't need to outspend your competitors in order to beat them.
>
> —Hal Stokes

Profile: Nancy Triplett

Nancy Triplett is a massage therapist and educator since 2000. She states, "I've used social media for a long time for various projects and manage quite a few pages for others. A few years ago, I was going through a rough time in my life, and really focused on what made me happy and brought me joy. The answer, in a nutshell, was to inspire and be inspired. Facebook was new to me then, but I kept thinking about (and actually posting) inspirational thoughts on my own personal page. I saw a news show that highlighted a local minister with a Facebook page that posted bible verses each day. From all that, I created the "Daily Dose of Inspiration" and still maintain it to this day. I thought 30 or so of my friends would like it…today I have around 8,000 followers from all over the world! I did it for myself at a time I really needed it, and it spoke to many!" www.facebook.com/dailydoseofinspiration.

Social Media as SEO

Most people don't consider social media to be a form of SEO services. Yet, when applied with the right strategy, your postings or updates will be listed on page 1 for particular keywords if your updates have enough likes, shares, and comments. Strategically, it makes sense to include the keywords you want to rank as hashtags, or naturally in your sentences, when you make your updates on social sites. Using keywords in every update is not realistic; however, you could make it part of your strategy to include keywords in your updates at least once a week. An example of a keyword might be "Massage Therapist [your city name]."

Most social experts agree that Pinterest is soon catching up to the likes of YouTube as one of the fastest growing social platforms to be used as a search engine. YouTube is the 2nd largest search engine and the 3rd most visited website worldwide, behind only Google and Facebook respectively.[7] As of April 2014, Pinterest announced it reached 1 billion "Place Pins" on its site. You can also create Rich Pins that include extra information embedded in the Pin itself. There are 6 types of Rich Pins: movie, recipe, article, product, APP, and place. Imagine having images of your services that have a rich pin embedded with your location, directions, and phone number. You could also have images of your retail products that directly takes the user from Pinterest to the shopping cart on your website.

Hashtags

Hashtags are metadata tags used on social networks that allow users to create communities of people interested in the same topic by making it easier for them to find and share information related to it. In her article, "How One Little Symbol (#) Gets You More Clients," Stephanie Beck says,[8]

> *Although Twitter was the pioneer and leader in using hashtags, other platforms such as Instagram (owned by Facebook), Pinterest, Tumblr, Vine, Google+, Flickr, and as recent as June 2013, Facebook added the hashtag option for their users. But social media platforms weren't the ones to invent the usage of hashtags. Actually, Stowe Boyd was the first person to use the word in 2007 to track topics on online forums.*

Hashtags are important because people use the hashtag symbol (#) before a relevant keyword or phrase (no spaces) to categorize updates and help them show more easily in the search fields on the social platforms. Clicking on a hashtagged word in any message shows you all other updates marked with that keyword.

A great strategy for using hashtags is to include them in all your updates. You can create a specific hashtag word for upcoming events, product names, specific services, contests, recipes, favorite books, and more! For most social platforms using 2 or more hashtags per update is recommended, the only exception is Instagram, where 5-15 hashtags are common per update. Be aware that you only want to use hashtags that are relevant to your topic. For example, during a major world event like the Olympics, many times #SummerOlympics will be trending on Twitter. You only want to use #SummerOlympics in your updates if it's relevant to what you are sharing. Don't try to "game" the system by using hashtagged words to gain views because the social media algorithm will hurt you if people report your updates as irrelevant.[9]

> "Content is King but engagement is Queen, and the lady rules the house!
> —Mari Smith

Do your research before creating a new hashtag or a special word around an event, product, or service. Go to a social media site and enter the hashtagged word into the search field to see what kind of updates are associated with it. You can also go to www.hashtags.org where you can enter any creative words you are considering using and it will give you historical data on that word, along with statistics on how many updates include that word across all the social media networks (including the forums).

Have you ever seen a hashtag and wondered what it meant? Most social networks limit the number of characters to no more than 13, but not all of them use this regulation. As a result, sometimes words get abbreviated and it can be tricky to figure out what they mean. You can go to www.Tagdef.com and enter any hashtag and it will provide the definition of what that hashtag means, all the different listings of updates, and where it was used. Another great source for researching hashtags is www.trendsmap.com. Enter your zip code or a region of the world and it brings up the hashtags that are trending on Twitter for that region or area within the last 7 days.

Posting Schedule

Given how much time is spent on the Internet and social media platforms, you need to consider how to utilize your time effectively without having to spend all day on it! Most business owners shy away from social media because of a misconception that it will take too much time to be effective, when the opposite is actually true. You need to re-evaluate your time if you are spending more than 30 minutes a day on social media for your practice, (i.e., actual posting, replying, liking, commenting, checking the social influencer pages daily). Organizing your updates and formulating your social marketing plan should take about another 4 hours per month. This is an excellent investment of time in something that can be such a powerful lead generating and relationship building tool.

According to a 2015 study by Global Webindex,[10] the amount of time spent each day on the Internet continues to increase. The total hours spent online via PCs, laptops, mobiles, and tablets has increased from 5.5 hours in 2012 to 6.15 hours in 2014. One of the reasons attributed

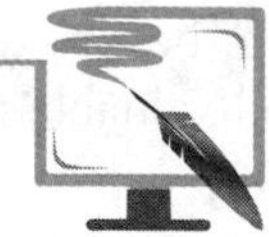

Research Hashtags

1. Create a hashtag using your company name, product, or service, and research it as follows:
   - Enter it into www.hashtag.org. Write down any updates and how it was used (if any).
   - Go to www.trendsmap.com, enter the zip code of your target audience, and record the trending hashtags for that area. Note any keywords or phrases that could be used by your target audience.
   - Enter the #hashtagged word or phrase into the search field of the social media platform you plan on using. Summarize the messages that contain the word or phrase. Are any of the messages relevant to how you want to use the hashtagged word in your update?
2. Given the above research, describe why you would or wouldn't use the hashtag.

> "Social media is a contact sport.
> —Margaret Molloy

to this rise is the increased time spent on social networks, which increased from a daily average of 1.61 hours in 2012 to 1.72 hours in 2014. It may seem like some of your clients are constantly on social media, but the fact is out of the 864 million active users on Facebook daily, the 400 million tweets sent daily on Twitter, or the 6 billion hours of video watched each month on YouTube, the average person is only spending approximately 10-20 minutes at a time on social media. Unfortunately, you don't know which 20 minutes they are going to use it. The likelihood that your followers will see your updates is very small if you only update once a day or twice a week. Consider how far down in the newsfeed you scroll when you use social media. Chances are it isn't very far. Well, if you post at 8am in the morning but your fans don't log in until 10 am, or noon, or 7pm at night, do you think they will actually see your post from 8am? Not unless that follower is highly engaged with your page or opts to have your posts appear at the top of their newsfeeds. This is why sharing an update 3 times a day, 7 days a week is effective, and increases the percentages of your fans and friends of your fans actually seeing your updates, and engaging with them.

Social Media Management Tools

Often, the ideal times for your target readers to view your posts aren't times when you're available to post. Consider using a service that automates your social media posts. If you only use Facebook as your social network, then use the free scheduling tool provided by the network. If you use multiple social networks for your business, then utilize programs that allow you to schedule for multiple social networks at one time. These are great time savers because you can schedule several days or up to 9 months in advance. Remember, you still need to log in a couple of time a day to answer questions, like other comments from non-competing pages, and share updates from their pages. You can also link your notifications to your phone or email, so you'll be alerted whenever someone is interactive.

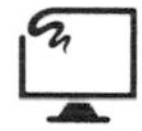

Scheduling Tools

hootsuite.com
www.socialoomph.com
www.amplifieied.com
meetedgar.com

§7

Increase Engagement

All social media sites measure the amount of engagement each user gets. Engagement refers to the number of times your update is liked, loved, commented on, shared, and followed. Each social site has a different spin on what they call it. For instance, on Facebook you can like, share, or comment on any public update from any user. On Twitter you can favorite, comment, or retweet an update. On Pinterest you can love a pin or re-pin it to one of your boards. Those users with the highest engagement get their updates listed first in the newsfeeds of their fans.

Because you want people to be engaged with the information you are sharing, be sure you are sharing relevant or educational information that your followers would find valuable the majority of the time.

Social sites are about building relationships. Think of it as having one-on-one conversations. The conversation wouldn't last very long if you met someone for the first time and all you did was talk about your practice, your hours, and what kind of services you offered, and never asked that person a question, or shared something about yourself, or offered to help. Limit your promotional content to a maximum of 30% of your posts. Offer helpful tips, share information (e.g., recipes, a stretching video, an inspiring quote), or ask a question. Have fun with your interactions and offer a variety of ways for people to engage with you.

Diligently evaluate which updates get more interaction. Increase your engagement by posting regularly and quickly responding to questions or comments. Keep posts short, colorful, and helpful. Be real, candid, and let people see your human side. Keep the content interesting, familiar, inspiring, and share-worthy. Before you schedule anything to be shared ask yourself these questions:

Does this make my potential clients feel more connected to my business?
Does it make them feel emotionally supported or recognized?
Does this update give them an opportunity to socialize or improve their personal life?

Social Influencers

In addition to posting on your own pages, regularly visit the pages of your specific social influencers. Social influencers are people or companies with lots of friends and are active on several pages. They can also be people who might not engage often, but when they do, they almost always cause more people to engage as well. They can be celebrities or centers of influence for you specific target markets. For instance, social influencers on a global scale would include people such as Oprah, Dr. Oz, Ellen DeGeneres, and Ashton Kutcher. They have a huge public following whenever they like, comment, or follow. Refer back to the the activity from Chapter 25 where you identified your potential Centers of Influence. Make sure you like their pages and follow them on the different social media outlets.

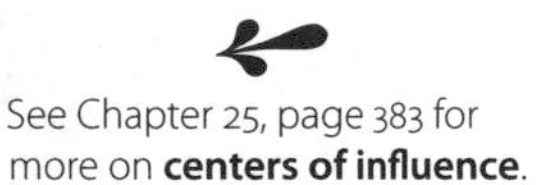

See Chapter 25, page 383 for more on **centers of influence**.

What matters most is the amount of social engagement a person or company gets. They don't necessarily need to have a huge following to have a lot of influence on a business. Let's say that a local yoga studio has 500 "active" Facebook fans, and every time it posts it gets 100+ comments, shares, and likes. If you know that your clients like yoga, it would be wise to be active on that page. You would also want that page to be active on yours or share posts from your page, because every time they like something of yours, it gets you more engagement from their fans. Plus, those updates from pages that already have high social engagement, are shown first in newsfeeds. By sharing from highly engaged pages, you're potentially increasing placement in your fans newsfeeds; at least those fans that Facebook has already pre-determined like yoga.

Reusing Content

One of the most frequently asked questions is, "Can I use the same content on multiple social sites?" The answer is yes and no. Each social media site has a special language or tone unique to their users, and your content should be adapted appropriately. Let's use the topic of donuts as an example, and the ways you can modify your content on the various social media platforms. For instance, on Pinterest you would share your favorite donut recipe. Twitter is a more present status, and you might tweet "Hey! I'm eating a donut." Facebook is a more casual and personal type of share such as, "I like donuts." LinkedIn uses a more professional tone where you might share, "I want to work at a donut shop." A Meetup post could be, "Join us for Donut Tuesdays!" The topic is still donuts in each example, but in order to maximize your time and get the best results, make sure your updates and conversations match how the users are utilizing that particular social platform.

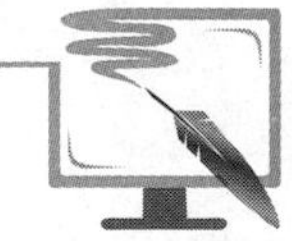

Create Posts

Think of a product or service that you will be featuring in your business. Create 5 informational or educational posts for Twitter, Facebook, LinkedIn, and Google+ on a topic that's related to the benefits of your product or service. For example, if you offer massage, create updates that support the benefits of massage (e.g., reducing stress, relieving pain, improving sleep). Get feedback from colleagues and people in your target markets, and make appropriate changes to your posts.

Multiple Social Sites

Each social media platform has its own approach, and some people are naturally attracted to different sites. There are definite advantages to having business pages on different sites. For instance, most Twitter users dislike Facebook. They might have a profile on both, but the reality is they'll typically choose 1 social site to log in daily. Therefore, most of the time you won't have the same fans on Facebook that you do on Twitter, LinkedIn, Google+, or any other social network.

Which one do you start with? The best answer is start with the social site where the majority of your clients and potential clients are hanging out. If you don't know where that is, ask them. You can also research the statistics on specific social sites: find out what they promote, and what they say about the average demographics of their users. At the time of this edition, Facebook is by far the most popular and generally used by most people.

> "Social media is about sociology and psychology more than technology.
> —Brian Solis

Although each platform has a unique style or way the users communicate, the following 6 psychological[11] reasons are why users love social media platforms:

- They want or need to connect with others.
- They need emotional support, validation, or recognition.
- They want to have fun or be entertained.
- They are bored or looking to procrastinate.
- They use social media to organize their personal or social life.
- They want to connect with family or friends with whom they've lost touch.

Personal vs. Business Use

Separate your personal use of social media sites from your business use by creating a business page. People appreciate authenticity, and it's a big turn off if you establish yourself as a "friend" (person) but mainly present content as a business. Users relate to and engage with business owners that they know and feel they can trust. While it's great to put a face to your business and be personal, always keep in mind whether you are a team of 1 or 21, you are a business person. Plus, many of the social sites offer business accounts great features that personal accounts can't access.

You must exercise caution with social media, and carefully consider what is being shared at all times. Even if you have a separate business page, people can still find your personal page (either purposefully or by accident), especially if your business name is also your personal name. Your business persona trumps your personal persona. Make sure that your personal page is tasteful, utilize privacy settings when available, and avoid making posts or uploading pictures and videos that you wouldn't want your clients to see.

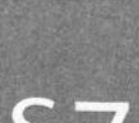

Online Advertising

Whether you're a new wellness practitioner or experienced business owner, it's no small task to gain a working knowledge of Internet advertising. Many practitioners shy away from online advertising because of the perceived cost barriers and complex landscape. In many cases this is a wise move, but not always. Sometimes a closer look can reveal affordable and cost-effective ways to increase traffic to your website and bookings from new clients. For group practices with an ample advertising budget and an Internet savvy business owner, online advertising often amounts to a cost-effective way to boost profits.

Sites to List Yourself

www.acufinder.com

Online advertising venues include search engine marketing (SEM), search engine optimization (SEO), email marketing, local online advertising, online video marketing, banner advertising, mobile advertising, and social media optimization (SMO) strategies.

Pay-per-click advertising (PPC) is one of the most common SEM methods. PPC charges the advertiser only when a person clicks on a text ad or a visual product-based ad that leads to that advertiser's website. PPC allows advertisers to sign up and bid on specific keywords—relevant to the particular goods or services available on their website. While this type of advertising is scalable and cost-efficient, it's an art and requires both financial and marketing savvy.

Facebook Marketing: 25 Best Strategies on Using Facebook for Advertising, Business and Making Money Online by Kenneth Lewis

Online Advertising: Market Like a Pro and Explode Your Business! by Online Business Buddy

Search engine optimization 2016: Learn SEO with Smart Internet Marketing Strategies by Adam Clarke

Ultimate Guide to Google AdWords: How to Access 1 Billion People in 10 Minutes by Perry Marshall, Mike Rhodes, and Bryan Todd

You may want to visit Google (www.google.com) and click on "Advertising" to get a picture of how Google AdSense and Google AdWords work. As Google is the top search engine, it's a worthwhile starting point. In short, Google AdSense automatically delivers text and image ads directly to individuals' websites; Google AdWords lets you generate text ads that accompany specific search engine results.

There are also online directories where you can list your business. Some are a combination of directory and social media platform, such as Yelp. With an average of 142 million users per month, Yelp allows business owners to maintain an account listing for free, or opt for the paid services that include advertising.

Customer Personas

Whether you choose Google Adwords, special directory listings, or social media ads, the rules of marketing haven't changed in over a decade. The perfect ad is creating the right message that is seen by the right people and at the right time. That sounds like a simple task and yet 90% of all failed online ad campaigns are because most business owners have the wrong target audience with the wrong message or offer.

Focus your message on one particular area or niche for each ad, and identify your customer persona. Shape your advertising content to make prospective clients feel like you are speaking directly to their heart, to the point where they ask themselves "Are they reading my thoughts?" or "That is exactly what I was looking for." The better you know your ideal client's personal habits, likes, hobbies, and interests, the better job of targeting you can do with your headline, image, and offer. It helps to give your customer persona a name and describe them as if you were talking about a real individual. This makes it easier to select specific demographics you want to advertise to online, especially when advertising on the social media sites. Each of the social networks is a huge data-mining program that tracks every user's interest every time a user likes, comments, or shares about a particular topic or business page. Facebook in particular is a master at matching businesses up with users who are most likely to purchase their products!

See Chapter 24, pages 360-367 for details on **target markets** and **your ideal client**.

Use Facebook to find out what interests your fans or the fans of non-competitive pages that you believe would be potential clients for you. For instance, a yoga studio, smoothie bar, or gym might have the same type of customers who would also like your type of services. If you have a Facebook page with fans, then use your own Facebook page title to do the search. If you don't have a Facebook business page yet, you can substitute any non-competitive Facebook business page name. In the search field on Facebook, type in the phrase; "Fans of

[Your Business Page Name]." Check the list to see which fans have the most influence, who has the most mutual friends, where they work, and how many other pages besides yours they have liked. This information provides a good indication of how much time they spend on Facebook. Next, type in the phrase; "Favorite interests of fans of [Your Business Page Name]." Look for interests that you also like, that you can use to make a personal connection with them. Then, type in "Favorite pages of fans of [Your Business Page Name]." Get creative with the different searches. Facebook will start to prompt you with other questions like "Pages liked by people who like [Your Business Page Name]" or "Pages liked by people who live near [Your Business Page Name]." Notice how they are engaging with those pages and read through their comments, as this will help you build on the customer persona and help you identify the mindset of your perfect client.

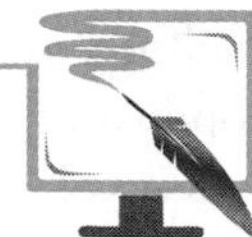

Facebook Data-Mining Strategies

Use these search phrases on Facebook to discover more about your ideal client:
- "Fans of [Your Business Page Name]"
- "Favorite interests of fans of [Your Business Page Name]"
- "Favorite pages of fans of [Your Business Page Name]"
- "Pages liked by people who like [Your Business Page Name]"
- "Pages liked by people who live near [Your Business Page Name]"

What interests, needs, and concerns did you to identify? What are the commonalities? How will this information change what you do in your online marketing?

Elements of an Online Ad

Online ads have a headline, image, and sometimes a description, depending on the platform and type of ad you are running. Typically, two of the components that are the most influential in catching the consumer eyes are the headline and the image. The best converting headlines have been questions that relate directly to your perfect customer persona's needs, wants, or desires. Avoid sounding like a brand looking to promote and more like a human looking to connect. Make the headline sound like you are a person who cares and is speaking directly to the person on the other side of the ad (not a group of people). The more personal you are with your ad copy, the better response you should receive.

The image is also important. When your social media ads are directed to your followers, it's best to use a photo of yourself in the ad because those people are familiar with you. It's best to use a different image if you're targeting all new people on social media. Note, online photo ads that generally get the best results are babies, pets, and faces of beautiful women. Humor can also be a great marketing tool to draw new fans. Quality images that provoke a laugh are good when using an ad campaign to build followers. Make sure your image tells a story, and the story you tell makes a connection to your perfect client persona.

The last part of any ad is the Call to Action (CTA). Given that your headline should relate to your target audience's need, want, or desire, your CTA should offer a solution to fulfill that need, want, or desire. Sometimes I see where an ad is targeting the right group of people with the right message but the offer or promise in the ad doesn't match what the offer is on the website or landing page. Ensure that the messages in your ads are congruent with wherever you take them next in the sales process.

Most online ads work best if the person can complete the task online (e.g., purchase a product, schedule an appointment). If you try to use online ads to make the phone ring for appointments, you're introducing a twist in the road for your potential clients. People generally won't stop what they're doing online to make a phone call, so consider this when you are mapping out your sales process for online ads. The offer has to be really compelling for users to abandon their online activities.

Testing Ad Effectiveness

Testing is going to be your most effective tool for successful campaigns. And because it's digital, you can adapt or change your message quickly, unlike traditional print advertising. Traditional print marketing, like newspaper ads, magazine ads, postcard mailings, or sales flyers, can cost up to thousands of dollars, and you can't modify anything on the mailer or ad without investing more money and running it again. You're gambling that the headline, image, and offer are going to connect to a certain percentage of those folks, if they even open and read it. Even if you have your own mailing list and print flyers in your office to add to invoices or hand out at your reception counter, that's still a few hundred dollars of "testing" your message to see if it works.

See Chapter 28, pages 448-455 for details on **print advertising**.

With digital ads, you have data within 24 hours of launching a campaign and you can make any changes in an instant. You can design a campaign using 3-5 different messages for a very nominal amount. Digital advertising eliminates the risk for a lot less investment. Once you have a proven message that converts with your targeted audience, this can actually assist you to refine your print and broadcast advertising for better conversions. Test your target audience, your ad copy, the images, the CTA, and the landing page. As you test each element, be sure to test one component at a time so you know what worked and what didn't. Remember, this is a marathon and not a race, and not everyone wins the big trophy their first time out. But, if you follow the right guidelines and test to find the right message to the right person at the right time, then even when you're testing, you can have success from the start.

28 Print and Broadcast Advertising

"Creative without strategy is called 'art.' Creative with strategy is called 'advertising.'"
—Jef I. Richards

Print Advertising
- Display Ads
- Classified Ads
- Directories

Broadcast Advertising
- Radio
- Television

Key Terms

Advertising
Advertorial
Broadcast Advertising
Classified Ads
Content
Design
Directories
Display Ads
Headline
Live Reads
Market Share
Print Advertising
What's In It For Me (WIIFM)

Advertising is gaining public notice for your business through means that require direct payment. Some forms of advertising include: display ads in publications; radio and television commercials; classified ads; billboards; directories; Internet ads; and bus-stop benches. Mass media advertising has typically been avoided by wellness providers, mainly due to the impersonal nature and the relatively high cost, yet, it's becoming more commonplace to hear ads on the radio, see billboards on the roads, and even encounter television ads promoting wellness and complementary health care.

> "You can have brilliant ideas, but if you can't get them across, your ideas won't get you anywhere.
> —Lee Iacocca

In the classic book, *Principles of Advertising*, Daniel Starch laid out the following:[1]

> *The functions of an advertisement are fivefold: To attract attention (the advertisement must be seen); to arouse interest (the advertisement must be read); to create conviction (the advertisement must be believed); to produce a response (the advertisement must be acted upon); and to impress the memory (the advertisement, in most instances, must be remembered).*

Your advertising venues contribute to your overall image; choose them carefully. Advertising is best used when your target market meets one or more of these criteria: your target is a mass market, your product or service is purchased frequently, the competition is high, or your goal is to quickly create awareness of a new service or product. Keep in mind, you can amplify paid advertising's impact by 15% when it's tied into a word-of-mouth marketing campaign.[2]

See Chapter 25, pages 380-382 for details on **word-of-mouth marketing**.

The two essential elements for successful advertising are consistency and quality. Quality relates to the ad's style, wording, and visual impact. Statistics reveal that an ad needs to be seen at least 3 times before it's noticed and up to 20 times before it inspires the prospect to take action.[3] Marketing professionals often refer to the "Rule of Seven" that states that prospects needs to hear the advertiser's message at least 7 times before they'll take action to buy that product or service.[4] While the suggested number of times a person must be exposed to an advertising message to achieve effective frequency varies greatly, the conclusion is that it works better to place a smaller (or shorter) ad on a regular basis than to do a big splashy ad one time only.

See Chapter 27, pages 444-446 for details on **online advertising**.

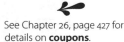

The steps in designing effective advertising are: identify your target market, grab the prospect's attention, highlight your differential advantage, list the benefits, state your offer, request a response, and provide a means of contact.

Test the conversion rate of your message through economical, online advertising methods, before investing a lot of money in any type of print, radio, or television advertising.

Print Advertising

Approximately half of all money spent on advertising in the U.S. is in print.[5] Of all the advertising venues, print advertising in newspapers, magazines, trade journals, and specialty publications, is the most preferred by wellness providers. Contact various print publications and request an advertiser's media kit. These kits contain rates for display and classified ads, demographic statistics, and a sample of the publication. Compare rates and evaluate the best venues to reach your target audience.

Display Ads

Display ads can have a strong impact. The major drawback is that they need to be large and attractive to catch a reader's attention. Here are some of the most common types of print display ads:

See Chapter 26, page 427 for details on **coupons**.

Sales Ad: The focus is on benefits and encouraging readers to book a session or buy products.

Advertorial: Combination of a sales ad packed with information written in a story format or a FAQ (Frequently Asked Questions).

Coupon: Special offers to attract new clients.

Business Card: Provides basic contact information.

Content

Creating ad copy can be difficult. Most people think they should start with the headline. Unless you're struck by a bolt of advertising genius (hey, it could happen!), begin by making a list of your benefits, and determine the offer you want to make. Save the headline composition for last. Next, write the body copy. Don't skimp on information. Studies show ads with more copy draw better than those with less. According to Demian Farnworth; "The fundamental premise behind long copy is 'The more you tell, the more you sell.' Ads that are long on facts and benefits will convert well."[6] Then again, don't pack so much in that it requires a microscope to decipher the text.

In many ways, the headline is the most critical element of an ad. People's choice of whether to read or ignore your ad is often based on the headline's impact. Five times as many people read the headlines as read the text. According to Cahners Advertising Research Report,[7] ads with benefits in the headlines and copy are 2-3 times more likely to be remembered than ads that don't stress benefits.

> "We have always said that advertising is just the icing on the cake. It is not the cake.
> —Meg Whitman

Figure 28.1 **Exciting Headline Styles**

News: Use words such as "New," "Presenting," or "Announcing."
Instruction/Advice: Use words such as "How to," "Why," "Which," "You," "This," and "Discover."
Testimonial: Utilize strong quotes from satisfied clients.
Compelling Offer: Use words such as "Free" and "Limited Offer."
Curiosity: Ask questions to inspire readers to want to know more, such as "Do you feel (want, need, desire)?"
Claim: Relay a success story.
Command: Tell the readers exactly what you want them to do, such as "Get a Massage Today!"

Design

I strongly suggest you work with a professional to graphically design display ads. In addition to the content, you have to consider the artistic aspects, such as typefaces and font sizes, ad dimensions, orientation (vertical or horizontal), and color. Most publications and advertising venues have professional graphics departments and will offer to create the ad for you for little to no additional fee (you will still supply the content).

Most ads in magazines are full-color, yet other types of publications still print in only 1 or 2 colors. The online article, *10 Tips to Successful Advertising*, explains how color plays a crucial role in drawing the eye and attracting attention.[8] Statistics from the Colour Marketing Group have found that color increases brand recognition by up to 80% and that color ads are read up to 43% more than similar ads in black and white. Color can also account for up to 85% of the reason people decide to buy.[9] Color improves readership by 40%, learning from 55% to 78%, and comprehension by 73%.[10]

Figure 28.2 Display Ad Tips

- Include an attention-grabbing, benefits-oriented headline.
- If you use a photo, put the headline below it.
- Have the subhead elaborate the headline benefit.
- Incorporate a strong visual image.
- Photographs attract more readers than drawings. Before and after pictures are also quite persuasive.
- Identify your target markets.
- Personalize the ad to an individual reader.
- Keep the body text paragraphs short and visually attractive.
- Use language that's geared toward your target market.
- Include powerful words such as "new," "free," "save," and "now."
- Provide a guarantee.
- Offer incentives.
- Broadcast on station WIIFM (What's In It For Me).
- Back up benefits with key features.
- Demonstrate credibility and reliability.
- Include testimonials.
- State your offer in clear, simple terms.
- Compel readers to take action.
- If you're selling a product, make it easy to respond: include a phone number, fax number, and other ways to contact you such as email or website; provide an order form; and offer to take credit cards.
- Include your logo, location, and phone number.
- Border your ad—it makes small ads look bigger. Don't limit yourself to plain, straight-lined boxes, but avoid overly ornate designs.
- Make the layout attractive and inviting.
- Use color whenever possible.

> "Simplicity is the ultimate sophistication.
> —Leonardo da Vinci

Figure 28.3 Sample Salon and Mini-Spa Display Ad

BEFORE

Godiva Salon and Minispa

• Bridal, Cosmetics and Hair Design • Body and Facial Waxing
• Customized European Facials • Hydrotherapy
• Manicures and Pedicures • Permanent Make-up

In Service Since 1979
196 E. Maine Terrace #129
Landtown, MO 94162

624-555-9721
www.godivaminispa.com

Problems
- **No interesting, attention-grabbing header**
- **No benefits listed, only features**
- **Meaningless use of graphic**
- **No call to action**
- **Boring layout**

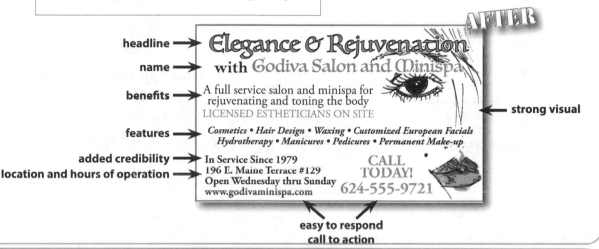

Figure 28.4 Sample Massage Display Ad

BEFORE

Total Health Through Massage

•Neuromuscular Therapy •Swedish Massage
•Subtle Body Energy Work •Deep Tissue

Leslie R. Vandruff
Licensed Massage Therapist

Call For Appointment
394-555-3692

Introductory Offer!
$30 an hour

Positives
- **Call to action**
- **Incentive**
- **Clear name and title**

Problems
- **Too many fonts**
- **No significant graphic**
- **No list of benefits**

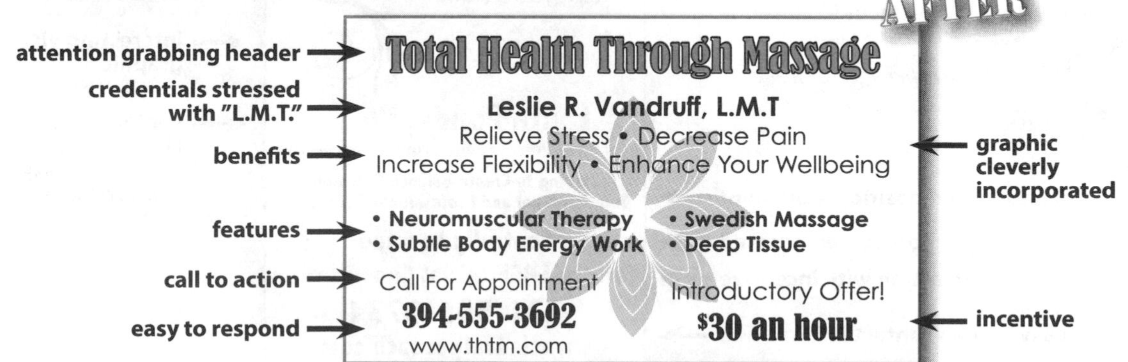

§7

Figure 28.5 Sample Acupuncture Display Ad

BEFORE

Liberate Your Life Energy With
Mia Lan Acupuncture

Acupuncture frees inhibited energy and aligns your chi for a beautiful life. It releases discomfort from:

- allergies
- arthritis
- stress
- body aches
- headaches
- sleeplessness

Call for appointment today
555-3271

Mia Lan, L.Ac.
Practicing Since 1971
Under Master Lee Wong

AFTER

LIBERATE YOUR
LIFE ENERGY WITH
MIA LAN ACUPUNCTURE

Acupuncture frees inhibited energy and aligns your chi for a beautiful life. It relaeases discomfort from:

allergies
stress
sleeplessness

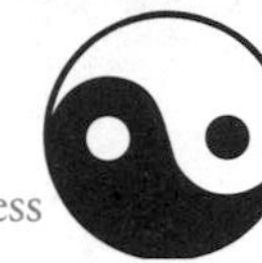

body aches
arthritis
headaches

Call for Appointment Today
207-555-3271
www.mialan.com

MIA LAN, L.AC.
PRACTICING SINCE 1971
UNDER MASTER LEE WONG

Both have:

- **Attention-getting header**
- **Interesting graphic**
- **Benefits described**
- **Credibility enhanced**
- **Features added**
- **Call to action**
- **Easy-to-read contact information**

layout flows better

Figure 28.6 Sample Counseling Display Ad

BEFORE

Dr. Laura Fonds
Ph.D.
Certified Personal And Professional Coach

231-555-9734

Career Counseling
Stress Management
Relationship Counseling
Personal Adjustment Counseling

...for a better way of life

Problems

- **No intriguing header**
- **No benefits listed**
- **Only lists number, no call to action**
- **Too much blank space, layout can be more effectively used**
- **Features OK, but is cold feeling**
- **Tag line–what qualifies better?**

AFTER

Discover Your Life Mission! ← **attention getting header**

Eliminate Self-Sabotage! ← **benefits described clearly**

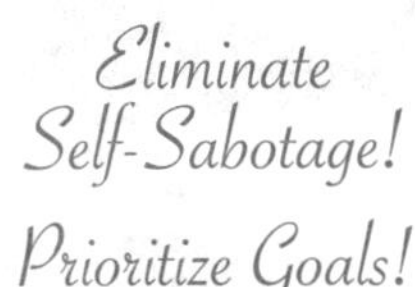

Prioritize Goals! ← **interesting visual graphic**

Laura Fonds, Ph.D. ← **contact person clearly noted, with credibility supported using Ph.D.**
Certified Personal and Professional Coach

features and position statement → **Serving to Create Balance Between Your Personal and Professional Endeavors**

convenience noted → **Centrally Located**

call to action with incentive → **Call for FREE Initial Consultation**

easy to read contact information → **231-555-9734**
www.laurathecoach.com

Figure 28.7 Sample Chiropractic Display Ad

BEFORE

PAIN?

Jon Darbey, D.C.

Mossler Graduate
Board Certified in Acupressure
Board Certified in Physiotherapy
Certified by the National Board of Chiropractors
Team Chiropractor for Univ. of LN Football Team
ACA & AAC Member
Certified for Court Approved Disability and Impairment Ratings

If you're in pain and looking for fast, gentle results from a chiropractic physician you can depend on, call Dr. Jon Darbey. Gentleness in chiropractic may be a new concept to you as it was to me before I began my six years of training necessary for our doctorate degrees. During my studies, I learned how light pressure at precise locations can bring relief to pain. Don' t let your fear of pain stop you from receiving chiropractic treatment.

Gentle Chiropractic For:

Back Pain	Neck Pain
Painful Joints	Hip Pain
Headaches	Cold Hands/Feet
Arm/Leg Pain	Fibromyalgia

CALL DR. DARBEY

555-3216

Cortwell Medical Ctr, 139 Mordnar St.
(North of 5th)

Positives
- **Interesting 3-D effect with "PAIN?"**
- **Photo as visual with clear name**
- **Call to action**
- **Purpose and features listed**
- **Location explained for convenience**

Problems
- **Too much unneccessary info in story text**
- **Started with "If"**
- **Font at call to action hard to read**
- **Too much text in credentials under his name**
- **Layout a bit funky due to no header at story text**

interesting 3-D effect with "PAIN?" ↓

attention getting header ↓

photo as visual →

name and credibility →

benefits listed →

call to action →

phone and website bold and clear →

features given →

location explained for convenience →

AFTER

PAIN?

Jon Darbey, D.C.

Call Us Today for a FREE Consultation

(406) 555-3216

cortchiro.com

Cortwell Medical Centre
139 Mordnar St.
(North of 5th)

Gentle Chiropractic For Fast, Effective Pain Relief

with Cortwell Chiropractic

Cortwell Chiropractic offers gentle, personalized care for individuals suffering from work, automobile, sports, or personal injuries.

We specialize in the treatment and prevention of discomfort for the:

- shoulder
- head
- back
- hands
- neck
- feet

New Patients Welcome
Most Insurance Plans Accepted
Same Day Appointments Available
Convenient Office Hours
In Service Since 1979

Classified Ads

Classified ads can be a productive form of advertising for wellness providers. A classified ad is a concise, engaging description of your practice or an announcement that is placed in a specific section of a publication. Classified ads are generally much less expensive than display ads—and you don't need to employ a commercial artist.

The major advantage of a classified ad is inherent in its definition. People look at those ads because they're interested in what's offered. Contrast this with display advertising in which you have to grab the reader's attention.

A catchy headline is still required for your ad to stand out. Other ways to increase the visibility of your ad are to put the headline in bold capital letters, bold the whole ad, include some type of graphic design, add color, or box the ad. Follow the same general design tips as for display advertising.

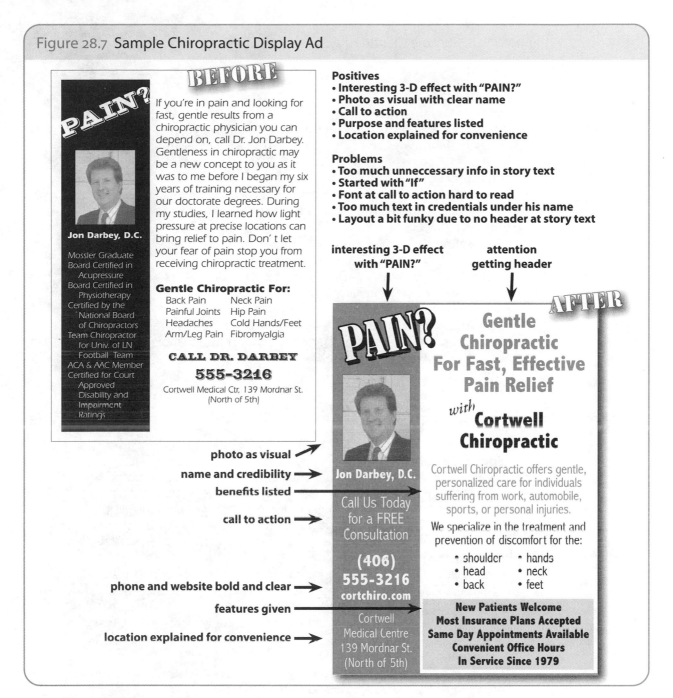

Place listings in online and print business directories, consumer telephone directories, trade journals, local publications, newsletters, and special interest books.

Figure 28.8 **Sample Classified Ads**

To Gain Leads

Sports Massage Therapy

SPORTS CHAMPIONS! Keep your competitive edge with therapeutic sports massage! Visit www.CompetetiveEdge.com for a FREE Health Tips for Athletes pamphlet. Or call 394-555-5555.

Chiropractic

BACK & NECK PAIN? FREE consultation. Call Cortwell Chiropractic Center for gentle, personalized chiropractic care. 555-5555, 139 Mordnar St. Ask for our FREE pamphlet on Tips for a Supple Spine. www.CortwellChiropractic.com

Counseling

FEELING OUT OF SYNC? Create balance between your personal and professional endeavors. Call Dr. Laura Fonds for a FREE initial consultation. 231-555-5555 www.CreateBalance.com

Acupuncture

FREE Acupuncture information pack. Release discomfort from allergies, headaches, stress, sleeplessness, arthritis, body aches, and more. 555-3271 www.MiaLanAcupuncture.com

Nutrition

FREE Information on how to achieve optimal health! Go online or call for your FREE copy of our Healthy Living Guide. 555-9643 www.NutritionNow.com

To Gain Clients

Sports Massage Therapy

SPORTS CHAMPIONS! Keep your competitive edge! Therapeutic sports massage increases your performance, relaxes muscle spasms and strains, reduces injury, and speeds up rehabilitation! We can travel to you! Call for a FREE Health Tips for Athletes pamphlet or for appointment. 394-555-5555 www.CompetetiveEdge.com

Chiropractic

BACK & NECK PAIN? Do you suffer from a work, auto, sports, or personal injury? Call Cortwell Chiropractic Center for a FREE consultation. Gentle, personalized chiropractic care releases pain from your shoulder, back, neck, head, hands, and feet. Most insurance accepted. Convenient office hours. 555-5555, 139 Mordnar St., Big Sky. www.CortwellChiropractic.com

Counseling

FEELING OUT OF SYNC? Create balance between your personal and professional endeavors! Discover your life mission! Eliminate self-sabotage! Prioritize goals! Call Laura Fonds, Ph.D., for FREE initial consultation. 231-555-5555 www.CreateBalance.com

Acupuncture

Acupuncture frees inhibited energy and aligns your chi for a beautiful life. Release discomfort from allergies, stress, headaches, sleeplessness, arthritis, body aches, and more. Call Mia Lan Acupuncture for more info or for a FREE consultation. Downtown location. 555-3271 www.MiaLanAcupuncture.com

Nutrition

Do you want to achieve OPTIMAL HEALTH? We can assist you in feeling strong, energetic, and enlivened. Call Tracy Smith, N.D., for an appointment or to receive a FREE copy of our Healthy Living Guide. 555-9643. Also visit our informative website www.NutritionNow.com.

Directories

Specialty directories provide year-round visibility to every person in your community (as well as worldwide with online directories). Directories are extensively utilized by the public for locating services. Check the subject headings offered before listing your services in a particular directory to make sure the directory fits your image and is targeted to your markets. Look to see how other wellness providers list their practices. Find out if you can add a heading if none really fit.

You needn't be overly concerned about an enhanced listing (additional lines of information) or a display ad if you live in a city where there are only a few people who provide your specific services. Then again, it could be a great opportunity for you to stand out. If you decide not to place a display ad, consider purchasing an enhanced listing, using a second color or placing a border around it. Put your listing under the most logical category if you can only afford one listing; otherwise list under each applicable category.

> "The greatest thing to be achieved in advertising, in my opinion, is believability, and nothing is more believable than the product itself.
> —Leo Burnett

Broadcast Advertising

Broadcast media, such as radio and television, reaches a wider audience than print advertising and has immediate impact. Unfortunately, you need to repeat the ad frequently because of the likelihood listeners or viewers won't be paying attention when your ad plays or they might not be in a position to write down your name or number.

Radio

Wellness providers are utilizing radio advertising more and more each day. The most common reasons to advertise on the radio are to herald the opening of a new business, introduce new staff members, announce new services or products, and invite the public to attend special events (e.g., workshops, open houses). Radio is still a personal medium and people respond well to it. According to the Nielsen Report,[11] 77% of U.S. adults listen to AM/FM radio, with the average listener spending almost 2 hours per day tuned in to the radio.

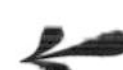

See Chapter 24, pages 361 for details on **demographics**.

The U.S. has more than 10,000 radio stations, including Internet radio stations. There might even be some that you aren't aware of that actually reach your target markets. Research the various stations to ascertain their demographics and rates. Radio advertising is a relatively inexpensive form of broadcast advertising. Radio ads are usually sold in packages of 30-second spots, and are by the day, hour, or program. The cost is based on the station's total number of listeners and market share. Depending on where you live, your cost to run an ad for a week could be several hundred dollars to thousands of dollars.

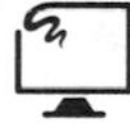

Radio station search engine
radio-locator.com

In addition to the cost to run the ad, you must figure in the cost to produce the ad. Radio stations will often offer to create your ad at no cost. The two major types of spots are produced commercials and live reads (the host reads from a script). The concerns about having the station create your ad are that the quality might be inconsistent and you can only use that ad on their channel(s). You can get a professional radio ad made for less than $1000.

§7

Live reads are usually preferable as they're more personal, listeners tend to pay more attention to them than traditional commercials, and they appear more credible (it may be their favorite deejay reading your ad). If you opt for the live read option, be sure to provide all hosts with a free session (or product). If the hosts enjoy your session or product, they might add their experience to the script (which actually gives you more air time than you pay for).

You can dramatically increase the effectiveness of radio advertising by using it in combination with another type of marketing activity.

An option to traditional advertising is to sponsor a radio show or public service announcement. In return for sponsorship (which could be in dollars or services), your name gets mentioned during the show. For example: "The Monday Morning Alternative Music Hour is brought to you by Cortwell Chiropractic Center." Many radio stations offer prize packages to their listeners. Donate your services as part of a prize package and you receive a lot of free airplay. For example, a massage therapist in Tucson offered 1 massage for the Mother's Day Package the station was giving away. Her name (which is unusual—so it's easy to remember) was mentioned several times an hour for 2 weeks! This is an example of a shrewd investment: minimal cost—extremely high return.

Figure 28.9 **Tips for Radio Advertising**

- Identify your service or product immediately.
- Highlight a benefit within the first few seconds.
- Mention your name at least 5 times within a 30-second spot.
- Keep to 1 topic or theme.
- Use appropriate background music or sound effects.
- Develop a radio persona.
- Capitalize on timely events, headline news, weather, holidays, and seasons.
- Be sincere.
- Develop a jingle.
- Make a compelling offer that includes a call to action.

Television

Television is a powerful advertising vehicle. It reaches more people than any other single medium. According to the Nielsen Report, the average American watches more than 5 hours of television every day.[12] Although most local television ads are designed to encourage the public to visit a location, such as a restaurant or a store, it's becoming more commonplace to see ads for wellness providers.

While nationwide coverage is extremely expensive, local advertising is more affordable due to the abundance of cable networks and non-affiliated stations. A commercial on a local cable company might be as low as $100 per month, whereas an ad in a prime time slot could cost from $1,000 to $10,000 per month (and a 30-second ad played during the Super Bowl costs millions). In terms of placement, if one of your target markets is stockbrokers, running your ad on any station in the morning isn't going to net you high results (their attention is on Wall Street).

A major benefit to working with local television stations is that they often allow you to advertise on specific shows. The advantage of working with a local cable company is that the cost of a commercial is generally less expensive, but those ads are usually sold in packages where you have no guarantee of when and where your commercial will air.

Consumers rate the value of your services and products on the production quality of your commercial. You can damage your reputation if your commercial looks cheap or hokey. Like radio, some television stations will offer to create a commercial for you at little or no cost—particularly if you sign up for an extended contract. But just as in radio, the caveats are that you have limited quality control and you can only run the ad on their stations or networks.

29
Publicity

"A good PR story is infinitely more effective than a front page ad."
—Richard Branson

Developing Media Relationships
- Make a Personal Connection
- Become the Expert
- Be Newsworthy
- Identify Your Hook

How to Contact the Media
- Telephone
- Email
- Mail
- Faxes
- In Person

Press Releases
- Press Release Components

The Media Kit
- Pitch Letters
- Fact Sheets
- Biographies
- Photographs
- Event Stat Sheets

Getting Interviewed
- Print Coverage
- Airtime

Planning Your Publicity Campaign

Post Coverage Follow-Up
- Acknowledgments
- Evaluations
- Capitalize on Coverage

Key Terms

Airtime
Coverage
Feature Story
Interview
Media Exposure
Media Hook
Media Kit
News Program
Newsworthy
Pitch
Pitch Letter
Podcast
Press Conference
Press Release
Public Service Announcement (PSA)
Publicity
Talk Show
Vlog

Publicity is free media exposure for your practice. It's a powerful tool for any business, yet few people take advantage of this cost-effective way to gain visibility. Some examples of publicity are news releases, announcements, feature stories, interviews, and press conferences. Publicity differs from advertising in that you don't pay for the exposure (although some media outlets do give news exposure preference to advertisers).

Publicity lends an air of credibility to a business that advertising cannot. People are more likely to utilize your services if they read an article about you, listen to an interview with you on the radio, or watch you on television, than if they see an advertisement about your business. It has much greater impact when a respected journalist or reporter makes a positive statement about you, than if you said the same thing about yourself.

Take a moment to reflect upon an interview you've read about a local businessperson. What were your impressions? Did you feel a connection with the person? Would you experience the same things by seeing that person's advertisement? Many people I know have increased their businesses significantly through their publicity efforts. Also, most wellness providers can't afford to place an advertisement that covers the same page space or airtime as an interview. Even if an interview doesn't generate a lot of direct business, you can still use it by framing a reprint on your wall, posting it on your website, and including it your marketing packets.

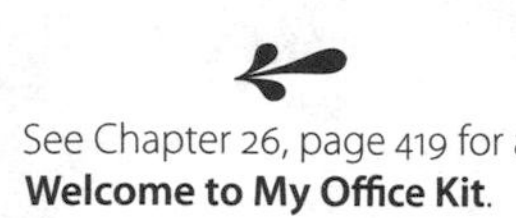

See Chapter 26, page 419 for a **Welcome to My Office Kit**.

Developing Media Relationships

Publicity is a powerful marketing tool; to get it, you must supply interesting, factual, and newsworthy information to media outlets such as radio, television, newspapers, neighborhood weeklies, magazines, newsletters, and specialty publications. While it's the media's job to inform the public about interesting people and events, they're flooded with press releases and media kits. Although most media writers publish 1 story per day, 44% of them get pitched a minimum of twenty times per day.[1] You need to capture their attention. To get free publicity, you need to market yourself to the media. You must provide evidence that coverage of you or your business will benefit their readers, listeners, or viewers. Media representatives tend to take interest in things that are new, have magnitude, contain an element of human interest, or are beneficial to the community.

Familiarize the media with your business. Send out short press releases on major business changes and events. The more often they see your name, the more recognizable you become (as long as the notices are relevant so that you aren't viewed as a nuisance). Your investment of a little time can reap great rewards.

Make a Personal Connection

Ideally, make a personal connection before pitching your story. Network with local media professionals at community events, conferences, and trade shows. You can send them direct emails responding to their recent pieces, and comment on their blog posts and social media pages. Make sure your correspondence is sincere and relevant. Avoid spamming the media! You can highlight one of their stories in your blog and send them a link to that blog. One of the best ways to establish relationships with the media is to follow them on Twitter. Allison Stadd says,[2]

> *Almost 60% have a Twitter account. So follow them, and engage in conversations about day-to-day life, a TV show they're live tweeting, a sports event, or their daily coffee shop visit.*

Also, grab their attention by marking their tweets as favorites and retweeting their tweets.

Become the Expert

Another idea for developing relationships with the media is to become the "expert in the field" who they reference as an information source. It's gratifying when someone from the media calls you for information or your opinion, even when the article isn't directly about you. Facilitate this by sending a note listing your areas of expertise and contact information (your name, business name, address, phone numbers, email, and website) to the editors and reporters of local publications, and to producers and hosts of radio and television shows.

Be Newsworthy

You increase your odds of being interviewed if you offer something newsworthy. But what makes an event newsworthy? That all depends upon the specific media. This is why you must research the different media outlets in terms of their target markets and the types of articles they write or shows they produce that relate to you. For example, does the newspaper often run interviews of local businesspeople? If so, what types of business owners have been featured? Is there a segment on a television news program that highlights healthy things to do? Are there any specialty publications or shows aimed at people who would be interested in your services?

> "My philosophy is that not only are you responsible for your life, but doing the best at this moment puts you in the best place for the next moment.
> —Oprah Winfrey

Some ideas for creating a newsworthy image include staging events, such as free demonstrations or "massage-a-thons;" disseminating information that is unique or useful to the general public, such as announcing a new wellness product or describing techniques to alleviate headache pain; forming a wellness group to study specific health-related topics; sponsoring a sports team by donating your services for pre- and post-events, and offering reduced rates for regular sessions; adopting a charitable cause; connecting with a celebrity; and giving an annual award or scholarship.

It's easier to get publicity if it's in an area that the media already covers. Ride the coattails of a national trend. Note upcoming events that will most likely generate publicity, such as charity events, tournaments, and expositions. Find a way to connect with these activities either by volunteering, becoming a sponsor, or donating your services. Then send media kits. Check the newspaper for headlines that can be related to your services. Once you develop an interesting angle, call the newspaper and offer your comments. Let them know you're available as a source for future related articles. Follow up this phone call with a letter, including your business card and a brochure.

Identify Your Hook

Generate ideas for capturing the media's attention by thinking about what makes you unique. This is your "hook" (also known as your attention-grabbing value proposition). In addition to your actual work, consider other aspects, such as how long you've been in practice, your location, your training, the equipment and products you use, the types of clients you work with, and any recent changes you've made to your practice (see Figure 29.1).

Identify Your Hooks

Make a list of your potential media hooks. Think about what makes you stand out from others in your field or what you are working on now that will set you apart in the future. After you've compiled this list, add to it other hooks that you would like to have and make a plan of action to accomplish those goals.

Figure 29.1 **Media Hooks**

- Your unique features or benefits
- Launching new services or products
- Special events: grand opening, relocation, anniversary, milestones
- You can prove you do it better than your competition
- Receiving an award
- Your credentials
- Your cost is lower
- Process you use to get results
- Result is better, faster, cheaper, etc.
- Length of time in business
- Experience in this field
- First person in the field in your city
- Testimonials from satisfied customers/clients
- Your successes with special needs groups
- Your volunteer contributions to the community
- Your mission
- Your market
- Your image
- Obstacles you've overcome
- Tie into something that has status
- Piggyback onto something that is already happening
- Consistent image
- You're the expert

How to Contact the Media

Mail, telephone, fax, email, and personal delivery are all useful means to approach the media. The method chosen depends on the newsworthiness of your materials and the media representative's interest in them. Some prefer to talk with you first and others defer until they've seen your press release or media kit. Some won't ever talk to you, but might post an announcement about you. When you're confirming the media contact's name, address, phone number, and email address, you can ask how the contact prefers to receive information.

Persistence pays!

Don't alienate the media by not playing according to their rules. Also, don't hesitate to ask them what their rules are—although most of them follow certain guidelines, everyone has their own peculiarities and preferences. The most important thing to remember is to be patient, polite, and courteous.

Telephone

The media has to be contacted by telephone at some point, either to make an initial contact or a follow-up call. Always find out first if the journalist/producer/host is free to talk. Then be brief and straight to the point. Find out which is preferred: talking about the story over the phone or sending (or resubmitting) written materials first. Also, ask if they prefer to be called on their business landline or mobile phone. When making an initial contact, you're more likely to generate interest if your story has several potential angles. (See Figure 29.2 for sample scripts.)

Figure 29.2 Sample Telephone Scripts

Initial Phone Call

"Good morning, I'm Liza Montoya from Healing Touch Massage. Is this a good time to talk? I sent you an email about my participation in a fundraiser for the upcoming Health Awareness Week. I'm offering free demonstrations on self-massage techniques as well as donating 5 gift certificates for massages. Stress is the leading cause of illness, and massage is one of the best methods for reducing stress. I think your [readers/listeners/viewers] could greatly benefit by becoming more aware of the steps they can take to reduce stress and learning some simple self-massage techniques."

Follow-up to Media Kit Interview Pitch

"Good afternoon, this is Liza Montoya from Healing Touch Massage. Is this a good time to talk? I'm calling about the media kit you requested I send, highlighting the Health Awareness Week fundraiser in which I'm participating. Health Awareness Week is approaching quickly and I was just wondering if there is any other information I can send you about myself or the fundraiser?"

Subsequent Follow-up to Interview Pitch Letter

"Good afternoon, this is Liza Montoya from Healing Touch Massage. Is this a good time to talk? We spoke several weeks ago about you interviewing me. You seemed very interested, particularly after you received my materials. We were going to discuss Asian therapies, including techniques to relieve pain, such as headaches. Since we last talked, an article about ways to destress your life appeared in Prevention magazine. Taking personal responsibility for your wellbeing is a hot topic, and I can provide information that fits in well."

Additional Point if Contacting the Print Media

"If you cannot do a feature, I would be willing to submit a written article."

Email

Email is becoming the preferred method for communicating with the media. Many news outlets prefer to receive electronic press releases. In addition to being environmentally sound, a major benefit is that an emailed press release won't need to be retyped, so a harried reporter with space to fill might choose to publish your release out of convenience. One or two photos can usually be sent as JPEG attachments without a problem.

Avoid emailing media kits that contain lots of attachments. Large files might bounce or end up in the spam folder. Send media kits as PDFs or include a link to a reputable online file hosting system like Dropbox. You can also offer to send photos and videos upon request. Always include links to your website where you should have photos and videos available as well.

§7

Mail

Mailing materials used to be the most common method to approaching the media. The major problem is the plethora of mail they receive. If you choose this method, call to confirm receipt of your press release or media kit within 2 days after it should have arrived. Send the materials to a specific person. If you cannot get the name, address it to the relevant department, such as city desk editor, calendar editor, or evening news producer.

Another suggestion for obtaining feedback is to include a stamped, self-addressed reply postcard. List the following questions: Are you planning to use this information? If so, when? Do you want more information? If so, what? Would you be interested in receiving materials of a similar nature in the future? Comments?

Faxes

For events that you would like covered, remind the newspapers, radio, and TV stations the day before or the morning of the event.

While FAXed materials are acceptable, many people don't like to receive unsolicited FAXes. Plus, they never look as nice as materials printed on your letterhead or email (and most systems transmit via efax anyway).

In Person

Deliver your publicity materials in person to the media outlets that are the most significant to you. The receptionist usually takes the materials and passes the materials to the reporter/editor/host. If you're lucky and can talk with the right person, be brief and to the point. Don't expect the person to conduct the interview right then.

Press Releases

Press releases play an integral part in effective public relations. To get a mention in the media, such as a listing in the calendar of events, a press release suffices. Actually, most news outlets now offer online Events Calendars where you can post your events yourself for free. Sometimes these listings are limited to free events, but others allow you to post workshops and classes that require participants to pay.

Keep it simple and short if you want to announce a new location, additional staff, or an award. Some publications have a special section that highlights individuals and businesses in terms of being new, a change in status, relocation, staff additions, employee promotions, and awards. These usually run 20 words or less. Don't make it too wordy, lest you run the risk of the editor omitting crucial data. Send a photograph along with the press release.

Your chances of capturing a media representative's interest in what you're doing are greatly increased if the press release can be quickly assessed. Presentation is crucial with press releases. If sending them through the mail, type them (double-spaced) on high-quality paper, preferably letterhead. Make certain they conform to the preferred format standards of source information: the release date, a headline, the body, and the conclusion. Keep your wording clear and conversational. Avoid using jargon.

Press Release Distribution

www.prnewswire.com

One-page press releases work best. If it's more than 1 page, follow these guidelines: type "(more)" at the bottom of each page—except on the last page: type "End" or "30" or "###" after the final paragraph on the last page; and staple the pages together. After you've typed your press release, double-check to make sure that you included important dates, times, locations, and contact numbers. Then proofread, proofread, and proofread again.

Many news outlets prefer to receive electronic press releases. This way they don't have to retype the information. Find out the preferred format, and submit it in that manner.

Time the sending of your releases so they're appropriately received. Some publications have a deadline date of several months before printing. Daily newspapers prefer lead time of at least 1 week in advance of the date you want the announcement to appear.

Be sure to send a quick thank-you to the appropriate editors when your press releases get published.

Press Release Components

Source Information: Name, company, address, phone number, email, and website. Put this in the top left-hand corner of the page.

Release Date: If the story or announcement can be printed as soon as it's received, type "For Immediate Release." If you want it posted on a specific date, type "For Release, Monday, October 7th." In general, it's best to have press releases that state "For Immediate Release." Otherwise you take the chance of the media representative putting it aside and forgetting about it. If printing it, place the release date below the source information and to the right side of the page (otherwise just put it on the top).

Headline: This is a succinct summary of the content of the release. Word it in such a way that you put the information that would capture your reader's attention first, without making it sound like hype. Always type the headline in bold capital letters. Two examples of headlines are: "FREE WORKSHOP ON INFANT MASSAGE" and "MELISSA BLUMENTHAL, NATIONALLY RENOWNED SPORTS PSYCHOLOGIST, HAS JOINED TOUCH, INC." Place the headline below the release date and center it between margins.

Body: This contains the details about the release. The first paragraph should be a concise statement, expressing the crucial features first. Cover who, what, where, when, why, and how. Use separate paragraphs for additional information or supplemental material. Write it in the "inverted pyramid style," as newspapers refer to it. That means placing the most important information at the top, as they usually cut from the bottom up. It's wise to use a multiple paragraph composition for the body because the space allotted for news stories and press releases constantly varies. This way, if they have extra space, and you've provided them ample material, they will use it. Conversely, if their space is limited, it's easy for them to locate and use the vital information.

Conclusion: A separate paragraph indicating the action you want the reader, listener, or viewer to take as a result of reading or hearing your story or announcement. You might type, "Call 555-5555 for more information" or "Stop by our Grand Opening on Saturday, October 12th from 10 a.m. to 2 p.m." Also, include a link to an online copy of the actual press release on your website, as well as links to any related information.

Writing Effective News Releases: How to Get Free Publicity for Yourself, Your Business, or Your Organization by Catherine V. McIntyre

Impact: How to Get Noticed, Motivate Millions, and Make a Difference in a Noisy World by Ken McArthur

I See Your Name Everywhere: Leverage the Power of the Media to Grow Your Fame, Wealth and Success by Pam Lontos and Andrea Brunais

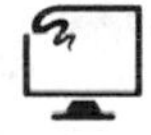

Marketing Communications for Massage Therapists by Sohnen-Moe Associates

sohnen-moe.com/products/tools/#product-marketing-communication

Figure 29.3 **Press Release Layout**

Release Date

Source Information
- Practitioner's Name
- Company Name
- Phone numbers
- Email
- Website

HEADLINE

Body
Supplemental Information
Conclusion

###

§7

The Media Kit

Send a media kit if you want to be interviewed in print or on the air. Wellness providers mainly get interviewed as a feature segment, but if you're requesting an interview in connection with an event, it can become news coverage. Media kit components include: a cover letter; a press release (optional); a fact sheet; a photograph; a biography; a brochure; a business card; and supplemental information such as articles written about you or similar businesses, pamphlets stating the benefits of your services, video clips, and a listing of previous media coverage. If your hook entails involvement with another event, include a summary sheet on the event.

> "The influence on others must proceed from one's own person. To produce such an influence, one's words must have power, and this they can only have if they are based on something real, just as the flame depends on its fuel.
> —The I Ching

Papers can easily get misfiled, so it's wise to include identification such as company name, subject matter, contact person, and telephone number on each piece of material. Ideally, put the information in a folder and enclose it in a 9" x 12" envelope, labelled "Media Kit." Then mail it or hand-deliver it. You can also send an electronic media kit, but make sure to get permission from the intended recipient or it will most likely get trashed—particularly if it includes attachments. People are leery about opening attachments from unknown sources due to the plethora of computer viruses.

Pitch Letters

The purpose of this cover letter is to grab the media representative's attention so he reads the rest of the material in your media kit. State who you are, your hook, what you're sending, and ask for action. Ideally, this letter contains 100 words, but never more than 250 words (see Figure 29.4).

Fact Sheets

Ensure accuracy by always including a one-page fact sheet that includes important, concise information. I use the following 5 categories: history, founder, credentials/certifications, awards, and today.

History: Encompasses the technical information about the company, such as what the practitioner does, a mission statement, and length of time in business.

Founder: Contains information on the wellness provider's professional background. Some practitioners may wish to combine the history and founder categories.

Credentials/Certifications: Lists licenses (with their numbers), certifications, and specialty credentials.

Awards: Lists honors received.

Today: Provides a bit more information on the practice and lists statistics such as the number of current clients, type of work the practitioner has done recently, hours, and any new announcements.

Biographies

This is a short biography of you and your practice. Keep it more conversational in tone than the fact sheet and include the following: your philosophy, a description of the types of people you work with, the modalities you use, and special equipment and products you incorporate. Keep the length to 1 page. Some people omit the biography if their brochures contain this information.

Figure 29.4 **Sample Print Media Pitch Letter**

Healing Touch Massage
321 W. Prickly Pear Way
Needles, CA 92363
619-555-5555 • www.HealingTouchMassage.com

April 4, 2020

Alice Adams
The Desert Daily
111 Arid Lane
Needles, CA 92364

Dear Ms. Adams,
People of all ages are constantly looking for new ways to feel and look better. This search has contributed to a multibillion dollar health-food and vitamin industry. Instead of focusing on the newest, flashiest product to emerge in the marketplace, I'd like to propose an alternative viewpoint.

Massage is one of the best methods to reduce stress and improve circulation. It provides recipients with an easy, affordable manner in which to feel good. Touch has been around since the beginning of time; therapeutic touch has been around for thousands of years.

My name is Liza Montoya. I'm a licensed massage therapist, in practice for six years. I specialize in Asian therapies, such as acupressure and shiatsu. I find that many people are fascinated by this approach to wellbeing. I believe your readers would benefit by increasing their awareness of wellness alternatives. I could also provide them with information on specific pressure points they can work on themselves to relieve pain, such as headaches. If we do this as an interview, I could also arrange for you to watch a session or receive a treatment. This would provide you with a more direct experience of the work.

I've enclosed my brochure, some information on shiatsu, a fact sheet, a copy of an interview in which I was featured, and a photograph.

I will call you next week to see if you're interested. I look forward to talking with you soon.

Sincerely,

Liza Montoya
Enclosures

Photographs

Photographs convey a visual representation of who you are. Get professional publicity photos taken by a photographer. These should be kept current and updated every 2-5 years. Digital photographs should be sent in high resolution format (for print) and low resolution (for online publication). Also, keep a stock of color and black-and-white prints on hand. Affix your name, phone number, and a caption on the back of the photograph. If you're being profiled or listed under announcements, the publications often use the photo you send. Reporters usually bring along a photographer when they conduct in-depth interviews.

Event Stat Sheets

Stat sheets are one-page summaries that outline the event or company background (e.g., mission statement, inception date), highlight activities, and list important dates and the contact information for the main sponsors.

Assemble Your Media Kit

Assemble a media kit for yourself (digital and print). Be sure to include all the components listed in this chapter. If you don't have professional photographs, make an appointment to get them shot (selfies are not professional looking). Create a cover letter template that can be easily adapted. Having these items on hand can give you the advantage when an opportunity suddenly becomes available and you're able to provide the kit immediately, while someone else may need to scramble to collect these items at the last minute.

Getting Interviewed

Some claim there's no such thing as bad publicity, but that isn't true. A poor interview can damage your reputation, but you can recover from it. However, if you're being interviewed because you were caught doing something wrong, then an interview can destroy your practice.

Never underestimate the power of the written word. It's often easier to get a reporter's interest for a print interview than a live interview. Also, print interviews are easier for you to recycle. Radio and television interviews are great fun and can significantly enhance your public image. At the very least, you'll be more recognizable to the general public after a television appearance. Also, consider being a guest on a podcast or a vlog that your target markets highly regard. While these forums aren't necessarily viewed on the same level as a major magazine or television news show, they can actually be more beneficial in promoting your business.

There's no such thing as "off the record."

Prepare yourself well in advance of the interview. Clarify your purpose, priorities, and goals. Envision how you would like the interview to go. Identify the key points you want to cover and practice saying them. Anticipate questions (even the difficult or uncomfortable ones) and prepare responses. Make a list of resources that can corroborate any claims you make.

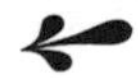

See Chapter 25, pages 394-397 for details on **public speaking**.

Rehearse your interviews with a friend or colleague. This helps you clarify your responses so you won't fumble for words during the interview, ultimately increasing your overall comfort and confidence. Also, have your coach toss in a few questions of her own, just to help prepare you for responding to unexpected or ill-informed inquiries (particularly if it's a call-in show).

Print Coverage

Research all of the publications you would like to interview you. Familiarize yourself with their styles, the types of articles they run, and the people profiled. Most publications have several departments, often with different editors. Some of the most common departments of interest for wellness providers are: business, education, events calendar, features, health, community outlook, news, and sports. Find out the names of editors and reporters for each department so you can send your publicity materials to the appropriate people. Plan your publicity campaign well in advance. Some publications, particularly magazines, have a long lead time between getting material and having it printed.

If the publication is unable or unwilling to write an article about you, ascertain the article submission guidelines and write the article yourself.

Call the person in charge of the section in which you would like coverage. Find out the deadlines and preferred submission format. Be prepared to convey the essence of your story in 30 seconds. Then make certain that your media kit or press release is in the reporter's hands within 24 hours of your call. Place a follow-up call to confirm the material was received, and ask if the reporter needs any other information from you.

Guest editorials are spots for either individuals or representatives from a group to offer their opinions on major controversial issues. This is a good forum to educate the public about wellness concerns—particularly if something has occurred within your community that doesn't support alternative care.

Most reporters do their interviews on location (e.g., your office, your home) or at the media outlet. Occasionally they'll meet you in a public place. At the end of the interview, give the reporter a copy of your fact sheet to ensure that the vital information (e.g., names, numbers, statistics) gets correctly conveyed.

Airtime

The major types of available air time are news programs, short features, talk shows, special programs, and public service announcements (PSAs). Although PSAs are usually reserved for nonprofit organizations, you can get a PSA broadcast if it provides information that benefits the community.

Observe various programs to determine which ones would be the most suitable for your message. Cable television offers more opportunities than commercial stations (you can even produce or host your own show).

Get the following information for each show: program title; focus; day and time aired; and the producer's and host's name. Call the station to find out who would be the appropriate recipient of your proposal. As with print coverage, when talking with the producer or host, ask about preferences for being approached, deadlines, and how much time you should allow to elapse before following up. Give a 30-second highlight of your story and make certain that all follow-up materials are received within 24 hours.

Once you're slotted to appear on a TV or radio program, watch or listen to the show at least once beforehand. This is imperative for television shows so you can see what the set looks like from the audience's perspective. It also affords you the opportunity to notice the style of clothing the host wears, the positioning of the chairs, and whether the cameras tend to do full-length body shots or mainly head and shoulder shots. Note the backdrop color so you don't wear similar-colored clothing—or else you will fade into the background. Watch the host's interviewing style: Is there active participation in the discussions? Do questions encourage lengthy responses or does the host tend to dominate the show?

Many talk-show hosts ask the guest to submit a list of suggested questions. While this may seem intimidating, it's a great opportunity for you to shape the program. It gives you the power to ensure coverage of the most salient points about yourself, your business, and your profession. It also solidifies the message you wish to convey.

Find out well in advance the directions to the studio, determine how long it takes to get there, and verify the time you need to arrive (which is earlier than the actual taping time). If it's a television show, find out if the studio plans to provide you with a hair and makeup artist. Ask when the show will be aired, if they provide a copy of the interview, and when you will receive it. If the station can't or won't provide a copy, arrange to have someone record the interview when it runs.

When you go to the interview, bring a fact sheet, any other supporting material, and (if previously requested) a copy of the suggested questions. Before taping, find out how the interviewer prefers to be addressed. If it's a television show, ask if you should look at the camera or the host.

Bring a jacket or an extra shirt should you spill something, or the pattern clashes with the host's attire.

When appearing on television wear rich, dark colors, other than blue. Avoid all white or "busy" patterns like checks, intricate designs, or broad stripes. Jewelry should be simple and not flashy or dangling. Keep in mind that scarves tend to bring energy up to your face. Wear shoes that are darker than your hemline. Women: Apply makeup a bit heavier than normal and make sure your lipstick has a matte finish and matches the color of the inside of your lip. Men should also wear powder to reduce glare.

Programs to Target

News Programs: Getting coverage on your local news program may be the most difficult because reporters tend to cover hard news. The most likely angle to demonstrate newsworthiness is related to emergency situations, such as volunteering your services at an event that's already scheduled to be covered (e.g., providing free stress reduction sessions to firefighters during a record-breaking fire season).

Short Features: These segments last less than 10 minutes and are often included within a news program. Increase your odds of coverage by tying in your business with another soft news event, such as a health awareness week, the Great American Smokeout, or a sporting event.

Present Yourself Powerfully by Cherie Sohnen-Moe

sohnen-moe.com/products/tools/#product-present-yourself-powerfully

Talk Shows: Talk shows and live interview shows are excellent forums for introducing the public to your business and the benefits of your services. It's usually much easier to get coverage on a talk show than to arrange for a feature interview. Hosts are always looking for interesting guests. Some shows include audience interaction. As a wellness provider, you have an abundance of information to share with the public. Plus, if the show is on television, you can give a demonstration. I know of a massage therapist who managed to give a demonstration on the radio. He brought in a massage chair to the station and worked on the deejays while they were on the air. They relayed their experiences (along with their oohs and aahs of relaxation) to the audience while the therapist described what he was doing and the benefits of massage. The station's phone lines were ringing off the hook.

Special Programs: These programs are devoted to your specific business, profession, or area of expertise. They last from 15 to 60 minutes. Usually you're the sole guest, but occasionally a producer chooses a program topic and slates several interviewees. Panels are another option for theme-centered shows.

Planning Your Publicity Campaign

Research media outlets and design your public relations plan at least 6 months in advance to get the best results. Timing is critical. Sometimes publications have deadlines months before the distribution date. In some instances it may take you months, even years, to get coverage. The disadvantage of utilizing publicity to build your practice is the lack of control. You can never be certain if or when you will get coverage, or if the coverage will portray you the way you desire. Coordinate activities to follow up your media coverage. Arrange workshops, introductory seminars, and open houses to take place within 3 weeks and then 2 months after a scheduled publicity coverage. If possible, mention these events in your interview.

Identify Media Outlets

Make a list of media outlets in your area that could provide you with media coverage. Review their websites for an updated list of the contacts, the types of coverage available, and their submission requirements. Fill out the following information for each venue:

Print	• Publication Title • Department • Department Editor/Reporter • Contact Information • Notes
Radio	• Program Title • Station • Reporter/Host/Producer • Contact Information • Notes
Television	• Program Title • Station • Reporter/Host/Producer • Contact Information • Notes

Post Coverage Follow-Up

The actual interview isn't the final stage in getting publicity. You need to acknowledge the interviewer, build rapport to encourage future media coverage, evaluate your performance, and find ways to capitalize on the coverage.

Acknowledgments

Acknowledgment is a vital element in building rapport. The greater your level of rapport, the more likely your next story will get the attention it deserves. Send thank-you notes immediately following an interview.

Print Media Contacts

Send an initial thank-you note to the print media journalist who interviewed you. Once an interview is published, send another follow-up. This time go into a bit more detail about one or two specific things (e.g., "I really appreciate the way you captured my philosophy by…."). You can also suggest a follow-up interview if there was an important issue that wasn't mentioned. Close the note by inviting the reporter to feel free to contact you in the future about this subject or similar topics. Also send a thank-you note to the reporter's editor.

Airtime Media Contacts

Send an initial thank-you note to both the host/reporter and producer for radio, television, or Internet interviews. Once the interview is aired, send another follow-up note. This time when you close the note, suggest additional topics and areas of your expertise that could be explored on future shows.

Evaluations

Review the steps you took to get coverage so that you can identify ways to make improvements or simplify the process. Read the print interview to see if it captured your intended message. If not, brainstorm ways to help ensure that your key points get accurately conveyed. Watch the video and listen to the audio recording of your interview. Assess your strengths and challenges. Note how well and thoroughly you responded to the questions, your demeanor, and any changes you want to make for future appearances.

Capitalize on Coverage

The key to effective publicity is to not simply bask in the glory of your interview being printed or aired. There are many actions you can take to increase the likelihood of your interview being noticed, as well as ways to recycle interviews to garner even more exposure.

> "Publicity can be terrible. But only if you don't have any.
> —Jane Russell

Send announcements about your upcoming interview to your clients, contacts, colleagues, family, and friends. Ask them to share it with their contacts. Post announcements on your website, blog, and social media sites. Put up signs in your office announcing the interview.

Notify people once an interview has run. Send out email blasts, post an announcement on your online venues, and put up a sign in your office. Ideally, get permission to reuse the actual interview (either as a reprint or an embedded digital file). If this isn't available, summarize the interview and provide a direct link to the interview on the media outlet website. If you obtain reprint rights, you can also include print interviews in your newsletters and as supplemental materials with future pitches to other media outlets.

Create a section on your website titled "Media" or "Press Room." Reporters sometimes visit websites to learn more about people before committing to write a story or to do an interview. They also may refer to this section for additional details. Include the following:

- Biography
- Fact Sheet
- Photographs (hi- and lo-resolution)
- Press Releases
- Articles written by and about you (with permission)
- List of all Media Appearances

Create a flyer with a list of your media interviews (along with links) and include the flyer in your Welcome to My Office Kits. Include a reprint (or summary if it was recorded) of your most recent interview in the kits.

Add an announcement to your email signature file that highlights the interview, with a phrase such as, "Featured in the October 1 edition of the Boston Globe." Include a link if the interview is available online (either in print or a recording).

Whatever you do, don't let your media coverage simply fade away.

30
Client Retention

"If you work just for money, you'll never make it, but if you love what you're doing and you always put the customer first, success will be yours."

—Ray Kroc

Beyond Customer Service
- Customer Service Levels
- Customer Service Action Plans

Prevent No-Shows

Incentive Programs
- Membership Programs

Rebook Clients
- Session Completion Protocol
- Post Session Follow-Up

Transition Practicum Clients

Recapture Lost Clientele
- Why Practitioners Lose Clients
- Tools to Determine Why Clients Leave
- Reconnect

Key Terms

Client-Centered
Client Comment Cards
Client Retention
Customer Service
Incentive Programs
Membership Programs
No-Shows
Proactive
Professionalism
Psychological Needs
Relationship-Based Marketing

A thriving practice consists of a strong base of clients who receive your services regularly, as well as a steady stream of new clients. Unfortunately, many practitioners become so focused on efforts to attract new clients that they overlook simple ways to enhance client retention. It's easy to understand how this can happen—new clients are vital to growing a business. However, this is only half of the success formula; retaining existing clients is the other half.

Many studies have been done on customer retention. One of the most common statistics is that on the average it costs 6 times as much money and takes 3 times the effort getting a new client as retaining a current one. Here are some of the highlights from the article, *50 Facts about Customer Experience,*[1] that summarizes many studies on the customer experience:

- It costs 6-7 times more to acquire a new customer than retain an existing one. – Bain & Company
- The probability of selling to an existing customer is 60-70%. The probability of selling to a new prospect is 5-20%. – *Marketing Metrics*
- A 2% increase in customer retention has the same effect as decreasing costs by 10%. – *Leading on the Edge of Chaos*, Emmet Murphy & Mark Murphy
- For every customer complaint there are 26 other unhappy customers who have remained silent. – *Lee Resource*
- 96% of unhappy customers don't complain, however 91% of those will simply leave and never come back. – *1st Financial Training Services*
- A dissatisfied customer will tell between 9-15 people about their experience. Around 13% of dissatisfied customers tell more than 20 people. – *White House Office of Consumer Affairs*
- It takes 12 positive experiences to make up for 1 unresolved negative experience. – "Understanding Customers" by Ruby Newell-Legner

> "Selling to people who actually want to hear from you is more effective than interrupting strangers who don't.
> —Seth Godin

The good news is that you can easily master the art of retaining valued clients with a minimal investment of time and effort. The trick is that the effort must be consistent to succeed. In the article, *Sixty Eight Percent Is Yours To Keep,*[2] Diane Helbig discusses how to keep clients. She states,

> *Make sure they feel valued. Appreciate them and communicate that appreciation. Don't assume your clients know that you value them. You have to tell them. Communication is a huge part of customer service. Too often we are so focused on gaining new clients that we forget to pay attention to our current clients.*

This chapter highlights time-tested ways to enhance your customer service so you can avoid the mistake of under-emphasizing client retention.

Beyond Customer Service

The core of client retention is a solid customer service plan. At the heart of all top-notch customer service plans is one thing—a consistent, careful, and creative effort to build strong relationships with clients. In marketing lingo, this is referred to as relationship-based marketing, and it involves truly caring about how you can best serve your clients' needs. In essence you become your clients' partner in wellness. It isn't about convincing or selling; it's about listening, planning, educating, and being proactive. It means going the extra mile to attune to your clients' needs and taking the time to express your appreciation for their business.

If you have staff, make sure they understand the importance of customer service. Communicate your required levels of customer service and set an example by your behavior. Provide ongoing training in documentation, treatment protocols, and product knowledge. Motivate your staff by acknowledging them when they meet or exceed your required standards.

Customer Service Levels

As in any business, levels of customer service in the wellness field can vary. To give you a picture of these levels, the following is a brief description of minimal customer service, good customer service, and exceptional customer service.

Minimal Customer Service

For wellness providers, minimal customer service means that you care about your clients, they feel comfortable and safe, your actions are professional, and you meet reasonable requests. Refrain from talking too much about yourself and keep conversations client-oriented.

Facilitate Clients' Achieving Their Treatment Goal

Establishing trust and credibility encourages people to commit to working with you on a regular basis and following through on their wellness goals. Concentrate on addressing clients' major goals; if you're a somatic practitioner, focus on the specific requested areas or incorporate other modalities. Keep accurate client files, customize each session, stay focused during sessions, and be prompt and prepared. Do good work, be a good listener, and respect clients.

> "Quality is meeting customer expectations at a competitive price.
>
> —Thad Barrington

Use High-Quality Products

Purchase reliable, sturdy equipment that can safely accommodate a wide variety of clients. For instance, a massage therapist would purchase side or length extensions if the table is too small for some clients, and use a variety of lubricants and skin care products. Keep an ample supply of clean linens and accessories such as sheets, gowns, bolsters, blankets, pillows, towels, and tissues. Maintain a wide selection of music.

Run Your Practice in a Manner That Demonstrates Your Concern

Be prepared. Greet clients cheerfully with a smile and a handshake. Speak professionally and clearly, and utilize good listening skills. Have water for clients to drink before, during, and after their sessions. Share information and resources. Send thank-you notes for referrals. Adhere to a code of ethics. Have an appointment schedule available. Return calls within 24 hours and make confirmation calls (or send confirmation emails or texts, with permission). Send appointment reminders when sessions are more than 1 month apart and call new clients within 2 days after their initial session. Inspire trust and keep confidences. Be enthusiastic about every meeting—whether it's the first or fiftieth.

Good Customer Service

Good customer service includes all of the activities under "Minimal Customer Service" plus going the extra step to meet requests. For example, a client shows up for an appointment experiencing a headache. A baseline customer service response would be to focus attention on that condition. Good customer service would include utilizing modalities, equipment, or products that aren't necessarily part of your usual routine, and possibly lengthening the duration of the session if necessary (and appropriate) until the headache is reduced.

§7

Take a Client-Centered Approach

Conduct thorough intake interviews with regular follow-up assessments. Creating treatment plans is the cornerstone to client retention and compliance. Encourage clients to identify their long-term and short-term wellness goals, and then develop a treatment plan together. By doing this, you identify their needs, clarify your role, and determine what other services they might need. Your role here is to educate clients on their options, and they choose how to proceed. It's crucial to list the long-term goals as well as the immediate ones: when they've achieved the desired results of the immediate goals, you're still there to work with them on the next phase of their wellness.

Respond to requests, such as those regarding specific techniques, pressure, or sequence. Provide referrals to other practitioners who offer other services to help clients achieve their goals. Demonstrate self-care techniques (e.g., stretches) and provide handouts. Review client files prior to appointments.

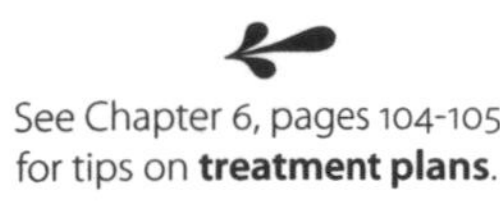

See Chapter 6, pages 104-105 for tips on **treatment plans**.

Make Your Office Environment Comfortable and Inviting

Furnish the waiting area with comfortable furniture and a beverage station. Install a dimmer control for the lighting and a way to manage the temperature in the session room. Provide a space for clients to put their belongings (e.g., shelf, hook), use clients' favorite types of products, and play their preferred style of music. If you're a somatic practitioner, use flannel sheets in the winter, have an oversized step stool near the table (if it's not hydraulic), towel off oil if necessary (ideally, provide access to a shower on premises), and allow clients a few minutes to just lie there before having to get up.

Exceptional Customer Service

Exceptional customer service requires that you be proactive—anticipating what your clients want—and making those services available. Zappos is an online shopping site that's well-known for its amazing customer service (see Figure 30.1 for their core values). One of the major themes in the book, *Delivering Happiness: A Path to Profits, Passion, and Purpose*,[3] by Zappos CEO Toby Hsieh, is to use the element of surprise as a business strategy. You must know your clients well to be proactive. This involves taking the time to ask clients about their preferences and thinking ahead about what they might want. When you provide what they need before they know it, your clients appreciate your extra attention and think the world of you.

Exceptional customer service incorporates all the activities listed in the previous sections, plus the following: communication, session-oriented activities, practice management, and support activities.

Figure 30.1 Zappos Core Values[4]

1. Deliver WOW Through Service
2. Embrace and Drive Change
3. Create Fun and A Little Weirdness
4. Be Adventurous, Creative, and Open-Minded
5. Pursue Growth and Learning
6. Build Open and Honest Relationships With Communication
7. Build a Positive Team and Family Spirit
8. Do More With Less
9. Be Passionate and Determined
10. Be Humble

Elevate the Therapeutic Relationship to a Wellness Partnership with Clients

Always review client charts before the session. Before you do any hands-on work, update their long-term treatment plans and set specific goals for current sessions. Depending on the type of work you do, consider taking before and after photographs to visually document progress. Take the time to research potentially effective techniques or other recommended services for specific client conditions, and prepare handouts of resources and referrals of other wellness providers. Place a check-in call the day after the first session and whenever clients experience dramatic changes from your work.

Do regular evaluation follow-ups. Some practitioners send clients a document titled Report of Findings (ROF). The first section of the ROF usually contains a summary of the client's concerns and goals, and the practitioner's observations and assessment. The second section contains an explanation of the treatment plan, the estimated number of sessions, the cost, and the number of sessions before re-evaluation (maximum of 10 sessions). Send this initial ROF after the first or second visit. During the re-evaluation interview, note the progress, changes, and what didn't change. Update the treatment goals and plan with the client, and set a date for the next re-evaluation. Write up another ROF and send it to the client.

Take a Proactive Approach to Communications

Practice active listening and encourage feedback. Recognize that some clients may have difficulties at times in clearly expressing their needs. Be prepared to act as a communication coach.

> "Mastery is not something that strikes in an instant, like a thunderbolt, but a gathering power that moves steadily through time, like weather.
> —John Gardner

Pamper Your Clients

Pamper your clients with state-of-the-art equipment. For somatic practitioners, this could include items such as a hydraulic table, ergonomic positioning cushions, and a luxuriously padded face cradle. Use fine linens, heated booties and mittens, and specialty products (e.g., aromatherapy, sports creams, custom-blended oils, personalized skin care formulations, customized herbal formulations). Provide an assortment of beverages such as juices, herbal teas, and personal bottles of filtered water (with your sticker attached to the bottles). Warm any equipment if it's cold outside. Somatic practitioners could have hot packs ready and prepare a warm foot bath. If the weather is warm, be sure that the room temperature is mild and the lights are dimmed. Somatic practitioners can also offer clients a cool foot bath and a chilled eye pillow in the summer.

Design a Luxurious Office Environment

Furnish your office comfortably, including a private area where clients can put their belongings. Appeal to your clients' senses by hanging beautiful artwork, and calm them with soothing sounds from an in-room water fountain and a premium sound system.

Raise the Bar in Your Practice Management Activities

Incorporate excellent customer service into the day-to-day running of your practice. Make it convenient for clients to book sessions. Ideally, offer online scheduling or have a receptionist. Return phone calls within 2 hours. Provide insurance billing (if it's within your scope of practice). If you know a client prefers a specific time slot, do your best to keep it available. Undergo semi-annual peer review, and have your clients evaluate your services annually. Review all client files monthly; look for trends, note if several people are making similar requests, and initiate appropriate changes.

Make Your Clients Feel Special

Offer a free treatment, product, or adjunct service on special occasions such as birthdays. Send an anniversary card from their first appointment with you. Give clients something for every referral—either a sample product, a 15-minute session, or a free adjunct service (e.g., a paraffin treatment). Ask clients to give you feedback either verbally or on a comment card. Invite clients to test a new product or service before you offer it to the general public. Offer incentives (see Figure 30.4) and freebies. Post published newspaper or magazine articles about your clients' achievements in your office and on your website (with their permission, of course, so as not to violate confidentiality).

Support Client's Wellbeing Outside of Sessions

Stock books and products that can be beneficial to clients—particularly items that aren't readily available at local emporiums: books on stretching, wellness, carpal tunnel syndrome, workplace ergonomics, and self-massage; stretching equipment such as exercise balls and bands; herbs and poultices; self-care tools such as rollers and eye pillows; specialty lotions, and sports creams; skin care products; and aromatherapy supplies. Keep in touch by sending clients announcements, newsletters, newspaper or magazine clippings, and website links on topics in which they've expressed interest. Post articles and tips on your website and social media pages. Hold events such as monthly open houses, demonstrations, and free workshops for clients and their guests.

Customer Service Action Plans

Customer service action plans grow and evolve throughout your career. The first step in developing a plan is to create a customer service mission statement. It might help to ask yourself what you want clients to say about your level of customer service. If you've been in practice for a while, also survey your current clients for feedback on the items they deem important.

Client Comment Cards

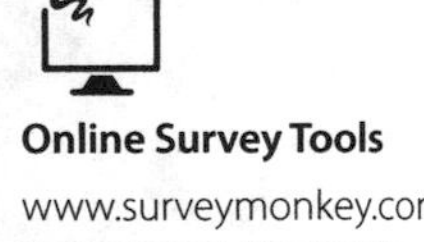

Online Survey Tools

www.surveymonkey.com
www.sogosurvey.com
www.alchemer.com

Client comment cards are a great tool for obtaining feedback on how your clients feel about you and your practice. These cards make it safe and convenient for clients to share suggestions, compliments, or complaints. They're easy to produce and usually cost-effective. Most people complete comment cards—whether it's for the offered premium, the opportunity to vent, or simply because they want to assist you in improving your practice. This can easily be done with an online survey tool. You can also mail these cards to clients' homes. If you decide to print and mail them, use high-quality cardstock, make sure the type is large enough to read, and include your name (or someone else in your office) on the return address. Print them as postage-paid response cards to make it convenient for clients to send their comments to you. The next best option is to put a "Client Comment" drop box near your office exit. Increase the effectiveness of your surveys by creating an attention-grabbing headline. Mainly ask questions for which the responses can be checked off or filled in with a rating. Include the option for comments after each question or group of questions. Close with at least 1 open-ended question.

Customer service techniques are only powerful if your clients are aware of them. You could implement major changes, but if your clients aren't directly informed, they might never notice. The major caveat to customer service actions is: Never implement a customer service activity that you aren't willing to consistently continue. Once your clients become accustomed to a

Figure 30.2 10 Phrases for Poor Customer Service

1. "I don't do that."
2. "Can you call back later?"
3. "That's not my problem."
4. "It's against policy."
5. "You don't understand."
6. "What do you expect me to do about it?"
7. "Let me put you on hold."
8. "I'll get around to it."
9. "No one's ever complained before."
10. "Make it quick."

Develop a Customer Service Action Plan

- Draft your customer service mission statement.
- Outline your goals and list the actions you commit to take.
- Answer the following questions for each activity:
  1. Is this important to my clients?
  2. How will this add value for my clients?
  3. Is this the best use of my time and resources?
  4. Is this something I can do consistently?
  5. How will my clients know about these actions?

certain level of treatment, they expect it and are offended if you're remiss. Ultimately, the key to going beyond customer service is to inspire your clients to move from a space of client satisfaction to one of client enthusiasm. Ideally, this results in "glowing reviews" that naturally translate into word-of-mouth referrals.

Prevent No-Shows

The client retention process begins before you actually see a client for the first time. This is where the pre-interview comes into play. Whenever new clients book an appointment, take the time to make them comfortable. Ascertain if they have any concerns or questions, and address them. Get them involved from the beginning. Find out what they need and explain how your specific abilities can support them (or refer them to an appropriate allied professional). Developing this type of connection dramatically increases the likelihood that clients will keep their appointments.

How you word things can have a powerful effect. In the article, *Make Your Appointments Stick*,[5] Irene Diamond suggests to change the name of "Cancellation Policy" to "Rescheduling Policy." She says,

> *This plants the seed in your client's mind that it's assumed she isn't cancelling altogether and will just rebook for another time or day.*

Remember, just because a new or returning client schedules a session, doesn't mean he will show up. You can reduce the number of no-shows by incorporating the tips in Figure 30.3 into your office procedures.

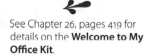

See Chapter 26, pages 419 for details on the **Welcome to My Office Kit**.

Figure 30.3 Tips to Reduce No-Shows

- Send a Welcome to My Office Kit before the client's first visit (preferably immediately after the session is booked).
- Confirm appointments by calling or texting clients the day before their sessions, emailing reminders, or both. Include a reference to why they're coming in.
- Give clients an appointment reminder card to take home. Include your rescheduling policy on this card.
- Give clients a copy of their treatment plan.
- If applicable, offer home assignments or a list of wellness tips that are designed to assist clients in attaining their goals.

If you follow these steps, you will minimize the no-show factor and won't be so disconcerted if the occasional last-minute cancellation or no-show occurs. I've found that when this has happened to me—it was perfect. Either I wanted to do something else anyway or another client would call wanting to come in right away (and fill the vacant appointment slot).

Incentive Programs

Incentive plans serve to reward loyal clients and create a way to increase the session frequency for others who simply can't afford to receive treatments as often as desired. The ideas in Figure 30.4 are geared to spark your creativity. Adapt them for your specific needs and desired results.

Figure 30.4 Top 10 Incentive Ideas

1. Offer prepaid package discounts such as: purchase 3 sessions and receive a 10% discount; 7 sessions qualifies for a 20% discount; purchase 8 sessions and receive 2 for free.
2. Present clients with a Frequent Buyer Card. This can be done in 2 ways: clients receive a free session after seeing you for a set number of sessions, (e.g., "Buy 10, Get Your 11th Session Free!"); or give a free session for a specific number of sessions a client receives within a certain period of time (e.g., "Receive 5 Treatments in 2 Months and Your 6th Treatment is Free!").
3. Provide a certificate for 50% off the client's next session whenever a client refers a new client.
4. Send an "I Enjoyed Working with You" packet after a client's first visit. Send a greeting card that states it was a pleasure working with her and that you look forward to helping her achieve her wellness goals. Include a coupon for a free adjunct service or product to be used with her next appointment.
5. Give clients a half-hour session certificate for every referral.
6. Give clients an adjunct service for every referral.
7. Have clients sponsor a demonstration party—and thus receive at least 1 free session, with the potential for many more.
8. Offer holiday specials. For example, a somatic practitioner could allow clients to purchase half-hour certificates at half price with every full-hour session they purchase. These half-hour certificates can be combined for full sessions or given as gifts.
9. Give a free mini-session for birthdays or special occasions.
10. Offer a 2-for-1 Valentine's Day special.

Your incentive program need not be limited to your hands-on work. For all the previous examples you can substitute products, adjunct services, and seminar registrations.

These incentive suggestions serve a dual purpose—they acknowledge your current clients, and many of the ideas provide a means to inspire referrals from your clients. It's wonderful to combine client retention techniques with your other promotional endeavors. However, don't rely on your clients to build your practice. It isn't their responsibility. They may be uncomfortable telling others about your services—many consider their wellness an extremely private matter.

Membership Programs

Many practitioners are implementing membership programs similar to those offered at many wellness care franchises and gyms. The major advantages that an individual or small business has is that the type of work can be specialized and customized. The major drawback is that when people sign up with a chain, they have access to a lot of practitioners and various locations.

The essential elements are that clients commit to a contract (usually 6 months or 1 year). A fixed monthly fee is automatically deducted from their checking account or charged to their credit card. The fee for this is at a reduced rate from your standard fee. The benefits for clients is that it encourages them to take care of their wellness on a regular basis, they get a reduced rate on their initial session, and they can get discounts on additional services and products because of their membership. The benefits for practitioners is that it guarantees a certain amount of cash flow each month.

Rebook Clients

The rebooking process is a natural extension of your session. People rebook when they feel comfortable with you, value your services, and are confident that they will get their desired results. I can count on 1 hand the clients that weren't regulars throughout my career as a massage practitioner and a rebirther. I took the position that I would work with clients until their goals were accomplished, which, in massage, can be a lifetime commitment! I attracted the clients who felt the same way. The exceptions were if I knew in advance that I would only work with them once or twice (e.g., they were visiting from out of town).

The situation is similar in my coaching practice. Occasionally, someone sets up a one-time appointment to discuss specific concerns or questions, but most of my clients work with me until they've reached the next level in their business. The rest consult with me when they need it, such as once a quarter or even once a year. Some of these client relationships have continued for decades!

If you do thorough intake interviews in which your clients identify their long-term and short-term wellness goals, and you develop a treatment plan together, then you already know if they want to book and approximately how often. Sometimes practitioners feel awkward asking when a client wants to return. Avoid saying, "Would you like to book another session?" A better way to phrase the question is, "When would you like your next session?"

Session Completion Protocol

Your session doesn't really end until your client walks out the door. After the technical one-on-one work is done (e.g., the massage is over, the nutritional consultation is conducted, the movement instruction is finished), it's time to do the session completion protocol. Briefly review what occurred in the session, highlight some of the client's major goals, share what to expect over the next few days, assign homework, give the client an opportunity to ask questions, make any necessary referrals, and schedule the next appointment. Give the client several of your cards and brochures, a copy of his treatment plan (or offer to email it later), and any appropriate educational handouts.

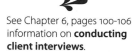

See Chapter 6, pages 100-106 information on **conducting client interviews**.

If you don't follow a session completion protocol, I still recommend asking the client, "When would you like to schedule another session?" If the client appears hesitant, suggest he calls you back when he has his appointment book handy. Don't be pushy. Tell him that you hope to hear from him soon and send him off with the appropriate educational and marketing materials.

Figure 30.5 Rebooking Materials

- Welcome to My Office Kit
- Appointment Book
- Appointment Reminder Card
- Client Treatment Plan Copy
- Brochures
- Business Cards
- "I Enjoyed Working with You" Packet
- Frequent Buyer Cards
- Greeting Cards and Postcards
- Newsletters
- Coupons
- Client Comment Cards
- Client Survey Letters
- Educational Handouts

Post Session Follow-Up

Follow the action items defined in the Exceptional Customer Service section, such as placing a check-in call the day after the first session and whenever a client experiences dramatic changes from your work. A couple of days later, send an "I Enjoyed Working with You" packet or postcard. If the client still doesn't rebook, follow the steps in the section on how to reconnect with past clients.

"There are no traffic jams along the extra mile.
—Roger Staubach

Transition Practicum Clients

You can jump-start your practice by building business with clients you worked with while in school. Keep in mind that it can be a shock for clients to make the transition from paying nothing or a nominal fee to your standard rate. Upon graduation, you may lose many clients if they're abruptly required to double or triple that amount. Ease this transition by offering them

Figure 30.6 Sample Transition Letter

Essential Wellness
123 Broadway Tucson, AZ 85710 ❖ 520-555-5555
essentialwellness@example.com ❖ www.essentialwellness.com

December 14, 2020

Susan Mountain
1212 Winding Way
Tucson, AZ 85750

Dear Susan,
I greatly appreciate your confidence in me and the support you've given me throughout my schooling. I've really enjoyed working with you in the school clinic. My educational program is complete and I've received my state license. My rate for new clients is $65 for a one-hour session. Because I value your longstanding support, I'm pleased to extend you the following special rates: For the next three months, your rate will only be $35 per session; the following three months, your rate will be $50 per session. Thereafter, the rate will be $65 per session. This special rate takes effect upon receipt of this letter.

Wishing you health and happiness,

Marie Everbody

a lower rate that gradually increases over time until they're at the standard rate. You never know, they may offer to pay your standard rate immediately.

Shortly before you open your practice, send a thank-you letter to your practicum clients to formalize your new status as a credentialed wellness practitioner, and offer the special transition program. See Figure 30.6 for a sample letter to help you transition practicum clients to your standard rate in a gracious and businesslike manner. Your clients will most likely appreciate your professionalism and special consideration, and choose to schedule ongoing sessions.

Recapture Lost Clientele

At this point you may be thinking, "It's time to increase my effectiveness and work smarter by incorporating a customer service plan and a client retention program for active and new clients." Excellent plan, but what about those inactive clients—the ones you haven't seen in months or perhaps even years? You may still retrieve your "lost" clients and renew your therapeutic relationships.

Every practice experiences an ebb and flow of clients, yet many wellness providers work under the false assumption that if a client doesn't return within 3 months, then that client is lost forever. Another potentially hazardous belief for practitioners is that as long as they continue attracting new clients, it's okay to become complacent with customer service and accept a higher attrition rate.

> "To keep a lamp burning we have to keep putting oil in it.
> —Mother Teresa

Why Practitioners Lose Clients

The reasons we lose clients are numerous and may have nothing to do with us. Clients relocate, their financial situation shifts, their lifestyles change, their schedules become so filled that it's difficult to book sessions, or the treatment series reaches its natural conclusion. Then again, it may have to do with your particular kind of work, something you said or did (or didn't), your office environment, or your business management.

The Results from Your Work

In some cases, clients may not return because they received what they intended from your work. For example, if the focus of your work is pain relief, once a client no longer experiences pain, he probably won't return (unless you have a long-term treatment plan in place that addresses the secondary wellness goals).

Another reason for losing clients is that they may not have received what was wanted or needed. For instance, a client says he wants a lot of work done on his feet, yet you spend very little time there. Perhaps clients weren't asked for regular feedback, so they went elsewhere without stating complaints or preferences. Maybe the work was too challenging. Or maybe these clients are simply experimenting with other types of wellness services.

Professionalism

Lack of professionalism can lead to a loss of clients. Practitioners sometimes cross boundaries or inadvertently offend clients. Do you talk too much during sessions? Do you break confidentiality by talking about other clients? Do you greet your clients appropriately, with direct eye contact and a handshake? Do you wear appropriate attire, maintain good hygiene, and avoid wearing strong perfumes or scents that may cause discomfort to those sensitive to or allergic to scents? Do you follow up on commitments, such as researching topics and sending materials? Do you schedule ample time to see clients and regroup between sessions? Do you return phone calls within 24 hours? Is your office clean and your equipment in good condition? You also may lose a client because the receptionist or another wellness provider in the office was curt, mishandled the client's records, or made an error when scheduling appointments.

> "An error gracefully acknowledged is a victory won.
> —Caroline L. Gascoigne

Convenience and Comfort

Lack of convenience or comfort are reasons for clients not to return. Your office may not be conveniently located for your target market. There may be scheduling difficulties due to either your hours of operation being inconducive to a client's schedule, or because a client opted to be more spontaneous rather than planning in advance for a session (and was never able to book on short notice). There may be accessibility concerns for people with physical challenges, such as those who may have difficulty climbing stairs. Even though you may do great work, you could lose clients to another wellness provider who has better equipment, supplies, accessories, or products than you do (e.g., a hydraulic table, an aromatherapy diffuser, hydrotherapy equipment, warm linens, organic skin care products, a full herbal pharmacy). Or there may be visual, auditory, or olfactory disturbances associated with your office setting that prevent clients from returning, such as being located next to a perfumery, a music studio, a day care center, or a psychotherapist who specializes in anger release.

> "Your most unhappy customers are your greatest source of learning.
>
> —Bill Gates

Finances

Financial interactions can be a source of miscommunication. There could be billing problems (particularly when it comes to insurance reimbursement). Be sure to keep track of package deals and gift certificate redemption. Be extremely careful of your wording and tone when questioning clients about their accounts, otherwise you could easily offend them. Another reason clients don't return is their financial situation may have changed and they can no longer afford your services.

Psychological Needs

A psychological component exists regardless of the main reason people schedule treatments (e.g., general wellness care, pain relief, stress reduction, relaxation, sports performance, a specific health condition). For most people, wellness services are also a way for them to honor themselves, give themselves a reward, or provide a time of nurturing that's just for them. It's their opportunity to be the center of the universe. If you aren't giving your full attention to your clients, you may lose them. For instance, if you allow your mind to drift during a session for too long or too often, your client will notice the lack of connection. Do you leave your own troubles at the door? Also, if you answer the phone while working, you're essentially communicating to the client that she isn't very important. I've actually heard of several instances where a practitioner was texting with one hand during a session! Don't let this be the reason your clients leave.

Tools to Determine Why Clients Leave

The first step in analyzing the possibilities behind your clients not returning is to perform a self-inventory to evaluate your communication skills, your professional demeanor, and your office operations. Identify the specific actions you take to provide excellent customer service and pinpoint the areas for potential miscommunication or problems. (You can also hire a colleague or business coach to analyze your practice.) This is a good time to consider what proactive efforts you can take in your practice for continued improvement. Don't be misled by the "If it ain't broke, don't fix it" philosophy. There's always room for improvement. Also, part of realizing how you may have lost clients is a valuable key to keep those current ones from leaving.

Survey Clients

The best source for information about your practice is your current clients. Send them a short client survey. Inform them you're evaluating your practice and ways to enhance your service, and would appreciate their feedback on the following questions:

- Why do they continue receiving treatments from you?
- What do they like about you and your practice?
- What are their suggestions for improvement or added convenience?

You could also assemble a focus group of current and previous clients. The purpose of a focus group is to elicit honest feedback. Ideally, the group size is about 8 people and is led by an outside facilitator. You can be present to welcome the group and return at the close of the meeting. The facilitator is crucial to keeping the dialogue on track and providing an atmosphere of trust and confidentiality. When you invite people to attend, tell them that you're looking for ways to improve your practice and would appreciate their input. You will fill the group faster if you provide some type of compensation and a meal or snack. Make a list of questions for the facilitator to ask (refer to your self-analysis).

> "The trouble with most of us is that we would rather be ruined by praise than saved by criticism.
> —Norman Vincent Peale

The feedback you receive may offer insight into why some of your clients left and thus assist you in making necessary changes. Even if you're unable to renew many of your previous clients, these changes will help you avoid losing any more.

Another idea that helps you discover why clients don't return is to send a personal letter to your inactive clients (see Figure 30.7). You can easily adapt this to an online survey and include a coupon code or attach a coupon to the survey. This type of letter also serves as a way of renewing relationships.

Reconnect

You need to grab your clients' attention to inspire them to return. Mail or email a note, postcard, or letter with an incentive. For instance, you could send a $10 discount coupon or offer a free adjunct service with their next appointment. A little reminder like that or a phone call might be enough to encourage them to rebook.

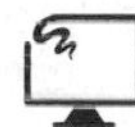

Greeting Cards
www.cordialgreetings.com
sohnen-moe.com/products/marketing-materials/

Then again, it may take several interactions to inspire a client to return. You can maintain connections using some of the techniques that you employ for keeping current clients and enlisting new ones: email open slots at the beginning of the week, post available appointments for the day on Twitter or Facebook, send newsletters, give birthday discounts, provide a special offer, promote a new product or service, hold open houses, give presentations, and create a special maintenance program and encourage previous clients to participate.

If your client surveys pointed out problem areas that you were unaware of, you could send a note to your inactive clients saying you want to touch base to let them know about some changes you're making in your practice (e.g., a new location, extended hours, additional services, updated treatment program assessment). You could also invite previous clients to come in for a free in-depth assessment and treatment plan (this is particularly effective if you weren't doing thorough treatment plans previously).

Remember, it's never too late to reconnect with a lapsed client. Sometimes people get overwhelmed with life and forget to take time for themselves. Others haven't made a commitment to receive regular wellness care. In either case, they may appreciate your follow-up. It can be the ticket to their return.

Figure 30.7 **Inactive Client Survey**

The Relax Depot
954 Miramond Way • Grand Junction, CO 81501
970-555-9712 • Fax: 970-555-9713
www.relaxdepot.com • ccross@relaxdepot.com

February 2, 2025

Phyllis Forgotten
123 Prodigal Way
Anytown, CO 81506

Dear Phyllis,
Hello! It has been a while since I've seen you. You are a valued client and your satisfaction is important to me. I aspire to establish and maintain good client relationships. Your feedback and suggestions will help me to better serve you and my other clients. Would you please take a moment to answer a few questions? Please be honest, as I desire accurate information.

What did you like about your sessions?

Did you feel that your needs and goals were met?

What are the main reasons you haven't had a session lately?

If you could change anything about our work together, what would it be?

What would encourage you to return?

Please rate my services on the following, using a scale of 1-10 where 1 is the lowest score and 10 the highest:
___ Professional competence (e.g., the scope of services offered, your confidence in my abilities).
___ Session quality (e.g., the manner in which services are provided, communication, compassion).
___ Ambiance (e.g., room temperature, comfort of equipment, lighting, music).
___ Overall customer service (e.g., scheduling, attention, providing educational materials, follow-up).
___ Competitive pricing (e.g., are the results you receive from my services comparable to what you pay for other services, products, medications, or supplements that address those same concerns?).

Please return this to me by using the enclosed self-addressed, stamped envelope. Your answers are confidential. Thank you for your time. Enclosed is a $10 coupon toward a session to be redeemed by you or a friend.

Sincerely,

Chris Cross

Enclosure

P.S. I am holding an open house on Friday, March 13 from 4-7 p.m. I will be demonstrating several self-relaxation techniques as well as displaying some nifty new equipment and products. I hope to see you there!

31
Marketing in Action

"Do what you do so well that they will want to see it again and bring their friends."

—Walt Disney

A marketing action plan is just one component of a full marketing plan. It's a summary of the goals and activities to do on a daily, weekly, monthly, and annual basis. Refer to your full marketing plan where you group your activities by the type of goals. Plan to invest at least 15% of your time in marketing activities to maintain your practice. You may need to spend 2-3 times this amount of time to successfully grow your practice. The sample marketing action plan in Figure 31.1 is based on 8 hours of marketing per week.

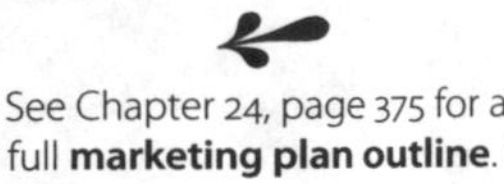

See Chapter 24, page 375 for a full **marketing plan outline**.

Figure 31.1 Sample Practice Building Marketing Action Plan

Daily

- Give clients samples, premiums, educational materials, and discount coupons for friends.
- Confirm the next day's appointments.
- Place 3 phone calls to prospective clients, and follow-up calls to current clients.
- Demonstrate or incorporate at least 1 product per session.
- Review client files prior to each session.

Weekly

- Distribute 75 business cards, 50 brochures, and 25 flyers.
- Call 1 allied wellness provider to initiate an affiliation or to follow up.
- Spend at least 1 hour working on a long-term project.
- Contact 1 group regarding a future speaking engagement.
- Send birthday cards and notes to clients.
- Spend at least 1 hour on social media.

Monthly

- Spend at least 2 hours reviewing your marketing plan and doing research.
- Choose a "letter" from the the Marketing Ideas A to Z list to spark your creativity.
- Meet with a business support group.
- Send 2 letters of introduction to allied wellness providers.
- Meet with 2 allied wellness providers.
- Attend 2 networking functions.
- Give at least 1 presentation.
- Send a newsletter to clients, colleagues, and prospects.
- Send out press releases about your public speaking engagements.
- Work with the media: send press releases and kits, do appropriate follow-up.

Quarterly

- Hold 1 open house, do a "party," or sponsor an event.
- Update client educational materials and rearrange the product display area.
- Donate services to your favorite charity.
- Offer some type of special promotion, and do a cooperative marketing project.
- Read at least 1 practice-building or professional development book.
- Get interviewed by the paper, radio, television, or a specialty publication.
- Tabulate information from Client Comment Cards and make necessary changes.

Annually

- Participate in at least 2 trade shows, fairs, or expos.
- Send out a client survey.
- Attend at least 1 practice-building or professional development workshop.

Marketing Ideas from A to Z

The following list of marketing ideas is included to spark your creativity in developing your marketing goals. Some of them are highlights of activities that you can find more details about in the previous chapters in this section. Marketing truly can be fun! Hopefully these ideas inspire you.

A

- **Acknowledgments**: Always thank the person, company, or organization that refers a client to you. Make sure to acknowledge others when they've been helpful—either in writing or with a small token of appreciation.
- **Advice Column**: Write an advice column regarding your field for a local or online publication. Not only is this educational, it builds your credibility by demonstrating your degree of expertise.
- **Anniversary Announcements**: Stick a label on your outgoing mail and create a digital decal for your online correspondence announcing how many years you've been in business.
- **Announcements**: Inexpensive promotional tools to enhance your visibility and keep you connected. Send to your current clients and select prospective clients to announce special offers, speaking engagements, and changes that occur in your practice.
- **Articles**: Write articles for magazines, newspapers, trade journals, in-house publications, and newsletters published by other organizations.
- **Auctions**: Donating services/products for silent and not-so-silent auctions provides you with free exposure and support for your community.

B

- **Bags**: Imprint cloth bags with your company name, logo, and position statement. Many people reuse bags, so your information gets seen repeatedly.
- **Banners**: Used at a booth or special event, they can include your name, slogan, or logo.
- **Billboard Advertising**: Seen by many people and is a good way of informing the public about you and your services. Look for high-traffic locations such as well-traveled main streets and intersections. Keep your copy short and to the point.
- **Breakfasts**: Speak at local business "breakfast" clubs. Having breakfast with potential networking associates is a great way to start your day.
- **Brochures**: Detailed information about you, your services, philosophy, mission statement, benefits, and specific techniques.
- **Business Birthday Promotion**: Send out announcements on the anniversary of your business stating something like, "It's our birthday and **you** get the presents!" Give them a goodie bag or a spin on a prize wheel. The gifts can be things like inexpensive items you purchase at a discount store or coupons for adjunct services.

C

- **Canvassing**: Take brochures, cards, or flyers to area businesses letting them know you're there, who you are, and what you can do for them. Distribute information to your target markets.
- **Celebrations**: Celebrate milestones (e.g., opening, moving, anniversary, 100th client), and invite your clients, colleagues, neighboring businesses, and prospective clients to celebrate with you. Provide refreshments, music, and fun.
- **Classified Ads**: There are many possible places to put ads such as newspapers, trade journals, magazines, local business and health newsletters, school PTO newsletters, and event programs (e.g., tournaments, concerts, fundraisers).
- **Client Appreciation Day/Month**: Host an event to honor your current clients that provides an opportunity for their friends and family to get to know you, and receive a "mini" session, gift, or educational material.
- **Clothing**: Imprint clothing (e.g., shirts, jackets) with your logo and business name.
- **Columnists**: Contact local columnists to write stories or a series of articles on health-related issues; propose an interview or provide information to them.
- **Comment Cards**: Give your clients the opportunity to voice their opinions about you and your company. Include one in your Welcome Kit, stack them in the waiting area, and mail them to all your clients at least once a year.
- **Conferences**: Attending or participating in service- or product-related conferences is another form of marketing and public exposure. Again, use that booth you designed to your best advantage.
- **Connections with Others**: Let related businesses know you will display signs and have information available in your office if they do the same for you.
- **Consultations**: A free consultation gives you the opportunity to demonstrate your expertise, answer questions, and hand out information. Also, offer free services for local special events.
- **Contests**: People love to play games! Contests bring attention to your business and add names to your mailing list. It's best to get people to come to your business to enter, but you can also include a sign-up on your website to capture email addresses.
- **Coupon Books or Card Packs**: Coupons are given to and compiled by companies and mailed to target markets; participants share in the mailing or distribution costs.
- **Coupons**: Terrific for marketing to prospective clients (e.g., 50% off the first visit) and rewarding loyal ones (one free session after each 10 visits). Coupons don't cheapen your practice if they're tastefully done. Many wellness providers offer introductory specials.

D

- **Demonstrations**: Allow prospective clients to experience firsthand your services and products.
- **Direct Calling**: Speaking directly with potential clients, other professionals, networking associates, and your clients, adds the personal touch to your marketing strategy.
- **Direct Mail**: Postcards, flyers, catalogs, notices, and announcements are inexpensive methods of staying in communication with your clients.
- **Direct Referrals**: Referring clients directly to other professionals is one of the strongest threads in networking and is usually reciprocal.
- **Directories**: Take out listings in appropriate directories. Publish a directory of local allied wellness providers to be given away at major events, mailed out in promotional campaigns, and distributed to other wellness providers.
- **Discount Sales**: Giving a discount can help a prospective client decide to try your services and products. Used for rewards, introductions, and referrals.
- **Donate Services to Charities**: Donating an hour a week to a community cause or charity creates goodwill and word-of-mouth marketing.

E

- **Educational Press Releases**: Each time you complete a workshop or attend a conference, send a notice to local publications. If you include links to research articles or prominent stories regarding the training or event, your press release is more likely to be thought of as newsworthy.
- **Emergencies**: Coordinate an emergency response team of wellness providers to be ready during tough times like floods, hurricanes, fires, or blizzards.
- **Expos and Health Fairs**: Participating in these events is an excellent venue for networking: gives you exposure to other professionals in your field as well as their products and services; provides an opportunity to meet potential clients; and makes use of that booth you created.

F

- **Flea Markets**: This is a place where you can reach large numbers of people while demonstrating your products and services.
- **Flyers**: Announce upcoming events, sales, and changes in service; whatever is happening with your business that the public needs to know about. In addition to posting them around town, email them to prospective clients.
- **Food Drives**: Offer to put client names into a drawing for a free session (or even multiple sessions) with every 2 cans of food they bring to your office.
- **Free of Charge**: Once in awhile, do something free of charge for your clients; perhaps a modality such as a hot pack, or upon seeing they're enjoying having their feet rubbed, let them know and give them an extra 5 minutes.
- **Frequent Buyer Cards**: Offer an exclusive discount on products or services to frequent clients. Give a free session or product after a set number of sessions (e.g., "Your 11th session is free!") or dollar amount of purchases.

G

- **Gift Certificates**: Wonderful way for clients to share their experience with others and a great marketing tool for you. Keep in mind that the profit isn't generated from the sale of the certificate but from the subsequent sessions.
- **Gifts**: Instead of always giving candy or food as gifts, help enrich someone's mind with a book, an inspirational bookmark or card, or a mug with a meaningful message. Establish goodwill and loyalty by giving small gifts to employees for work well done or for when they go that extra mile for you.
- **Golf Resorts**: Post a sign offering a free session to members who have made a verifiable hole-in-one.
- **Grand Openings**: This is a "grand" way of letting people know who you are, where you are, and what you're all about.
- **Greeting Cards**: These are a good method of connecting with clients, networking associates, and referring professionals, just to wish them good tidings.
- **Grocery Store Displays**: Set up a display in a health food store where people buy products related to your services (i.e., essential oils if you are an aromatherapist).

H

- **Health Clubs**: Submit a proposal for the health club to purchase gift certificates to give as incentives to new members who pay in full upon initiation or when members reach a milestone goal.
- **Holidays**: Decorate your office to match the holiday, offer special discounts for holidays, and give specialty gifts (e.g., cinnamon-scented oil for Thanksgiving, sports bottles for the Summer Solstice).

I

- **Introductory Letters**: Send letters to allied wellness providers to develop mutual referrals. Send at least 2 letters each week until you've amassed your desired network.
- **Introductory Seminars**: The focus is introducing your services or products to prospective clients. Having introductory prices available helps fence-sitters make a move in your direction.
- **Invitations**: These communications can be hand-delivered, verbal, mailed, or emailed. Invite people to see your facilities, come to a free demonstration, or call for information.

J

- **Jazz Festival**: Offer a reduced rate on your services to the performers at your local jazz festival in exchange for advertisements in their programs and event promotion.
- **Jingle**: Create a catchy tune and phrase that easily identifies your company (this is particularly for radio and television advertising).

K

- **Keynote Speeches**: Advise your professional associations and community organizations that you're available as a keynote speaker.
- **Kiosks**: Post promotional materials on kiosks at malls, colleges, and pavilions. Check for regulations first.
- **Kudos**: Frame and display any press, complimentary letters, and awards where they can be seen. This allows others to see your dedication and service to your profession. If you have too many to display at once, rotate them regularly.

L

- **Lectures**: Giving lectures on your service or products provides credibility to you as a professional, educates the public, and becomes a vehicle for sales.
- **Little Things**: Make doing little things for clients (e.g., providing beverages, playing their favorite music), a matter of business policy. These little things help establish client loyalty.
- **Location**: This is an important component to the success of a business. A poor location can break a business even if your service and products are good. If you're in an area that is inconvenient or unsafe, people will seek out other providers.
- **Logo**: A graphic representation of your business that helps people quickly recognize your company.

M

- **Mailing Lists**: Keep accurate lists of clients, prospects, practitioners, networking associates, and companies or individuals in related fields.
- **Meet Your Neighbors**: Visit local businesses within walking distance. Introduce yourself and get to know the owners or managers. If they don't have time to talk, offer to meet for coffee. Leave them with several business cards and brochures, and send a follow-up note about how nice it was to meet them. You could also hold an open house just for your business neighbors.
- **Memberships**: Join professional associations, business groups, and service organizations.
- **Mistakes**: We all make them, and the best way to handle them is with no excuses—just plain honesty. Create a "goof gift" to give to clients when you or a staff member makes a mistake.

N

- **Networking**: Join networking organizations, community organizations, clubs; and participate in community special events. Networking is a great way to establish trust and build professional relationships.

- **Newsletters**: Used as a consistent marketing tool, they establish your expertise and educate the public. Newsletters can also be sent to other health professionals and potential clients for marketing purposes. Another idea is to write articles or place ads in others' newsletters.
- **Newspaper:** Submit opinion pieces, articles, letters to the editor, press releases, and calendar listings. Get a newspaper reporter to interview you. Also place display and classified ads.

O

- **Open Houses**: Hold quarterly and special holiday open houses for colleagues, businesses in your community, prospects, and clients.
- **Order Forms for Product Sales**: Have these available for quick, impulse sales as well as for those who like to ponder. The elements to successful product sales are quality, availability, and convenience.

P

- **Package Deals**: Putting together packages for services and products that save clients money can improve sales without increasing marketing costs.
- **Pamphlets**: Handouts with detailed informative about specific services or techniques, or information about a specific population (their needs, what you can offer them, and wellness tips).
- **Park or Street Bench Advertising**: Place ads on benches that are seen by your target markets (e.g., in front of stores they patronize).
- **Personalized Gift Items**: Also known as premiums and specialty advertising. Keep an assortment of inexpensive, fun, useful items to give away.
- **Postcards**: Fast, easy, and inexpensive method of reminding clients of follow-ups, appointments, announcements, or just saying hello. Also a good technique for generating new clients.
- **Presentations**: Offer to give free presentations; promote health and your practice while supporting your community.
- **Professional Journals**: These publications can be a good place to advertise, as well as an outlet to write articles and make yourself known. Writing adds to your credibility as a professional.
- **Public Service Announcements** (PSAs): Send PSAs to print media and broadcast stations to announce any free lectures, community service projects, or free informational publications you offer.
- **Public Service Tie-In**: Sponsor events such as the blood donor mobile unit, police fingerprint unit for children, or fire department home safety seminars.
- **Public Speaking**: Give talks at business associations, clubs, and public service organizations. Join an organization like Toastmasters to learn platform-speaking.

Q

- **Qualify**: Design your marketing materials so that they actually pre-screen clients.
- **Quotes**: Use quotes from people who are prominent within your target market.

R

- **Radio**: Take an ad, sponsor a program, become a guest speaker on local talk shows, or host a wellness talk show.
- **Raffles and Prizes**: Providing services or products for special event raffles and prizes helps in getting your name out to the public.
- **Referral Cards**: These cards encourage clients to promote your practice. Distribute them liberally.
- **Referral Networks**: Essential as a marketing tool; not only benefits you but provides the opportunity for you to assist others with their growth and prosperity.
- **Rewards, Incentives, and Gifts**: Submit proposals for companies to offer your services for customer or employee rewards. They could offer certificates for sales incentives, to honor employees of the month, to use as premiums with their customers, and to give as holiday gifts for employees (it's certainly classier than a gift certificate for a frozen turkey).

S

- **Scholarships**: Sponsor an academic or sports scholarship for children, young adults, or members of your target markets.
- **Scripts**: Providing your employees with scripts for various circumstances helps guide them in representing your business to its optimum and aids in deterring the disasters "winging it" can create.
- **Seminars**: Establish yourself as an authority in your field, lend credibility, provide a catalyst for your services and products, and educate the public.
- **Sign Language**: Learn to communicate in sign language so you can offer services to the hearing impaired.
- **Signature Services**: Develop your own signature service, product, or technique, and give it a name. Use it in your marketing campaigns to help establish the uniqueness of your practice.
- **Signs (Indoors)**: Hang signs and posters announcing specials. Emphasize services such as "Gift Certificates Available."
- **Signs (Outdoors)**: Your sign should be clear and large enough to be easily seen and quickly identifiable. Include your logo if economically feasible.
- **Social Media**: Maintain an active presence on your social media pages as well as specialty forums that address your clients' needs and concerns.
- **Special Events**: Encourage publicity by sponsoring (or participating in) local events or holding unusual events at your place of business.
- **Special Promos and Displays**: Boost marketing efforts with "in-store" displays featuring your products, cards, brochures, and flyers that explain your services and benefits. Attract business by providing discount flyers that can be redeemed at the time of the appointment.
- **Sponsor an Athletic Team**: Print T-shirts with your name and logo for the team to wear; show up at the games to support your team; and display a sign in your office that says, "Proud sponsor of the ABC Cycling Team!"
- **Sponsor an Event or Community Activity**: Involves your business in the community and helps you meet potential clients.
- **Sporting Events**: Volunteer your services at local sporting events, Senior and Special Olympics.
- **Statement Stuffers**: Include information about specific products or services whenever you send out statements to clients. You can also place your brochure in other people's billing statements (just make sure they go to your target markets).
- **Surveys and Questionnaires**: Great way to get the "pulse" of your clients and discover what you're doing right and what needs to be changed: find out what clients want, like, dislike, and their opinion of your services.

T

- **Television**: Become a guest on local television shows. Place commercials that demonstrate your services or products and their benefits—fully utilize the dynamics of music, words, and pictures.
- **Testimonials**: Nothing hits home like personal accounts of the success of your products and services; use in marketing tools, advertising, and seminars. Always use full names and if possible the title, company, and city.
- **Theme Festival**: Band together with nearby businesses and hold a gala event such as "Spring Festival" or "Winter Warm-Ups."

- **Theme Week**: Devote a week to a particular activity (e.g., Mobility Week), and set up activities centering on mobility issues. Coordinate with your local government to sponsor city-wide events.
- **Trade Directory**: Advertise in local print or online trade directories. They're usually the first place people look when they want your specific service and/or products.
- **Trainings**: Training other professionals establishes your credibility and expertise. They range from an evening class to a weeklong intensive training.

U

- **Umbrellas**: If you live in a rainy city, purchase a stock of umbrellas with your logo imprinted on them to loan or give to clients who forget their own.
- **Uniforms**: Create a unique, professional image by putting your logo, position statement, or favorite design on clothing.

V

- **Vacation Nights**: Sponsor a "health" vacation with guest speakers, activities, drawings, and show slides (e.g., spa destinations, great places to hike and boat).
- **Valentine's Day**: Create a promotion just for your services and another promotion with another practitioner or business. Promote this with email blasts, flyers, and signs.
- **Vehicles**: Paint your car, affix a sign, or wrap it to provide great coverage as you go through your day; draws attention as it's unusual to see unique, eye-catching things on cars.
- **Videos/DVDs**: A unique method of presenting and demonstrating your services and products which can be left with other professionals for marketing; have clients view them while waiting to see you; use as part of a proposal for a corporate contract; and show as an educational tool for the public. You can also embed videos on your website.
- **VIPs**: Turn your customers into VIPs. Give them the opportunity to avail themselves of special sales and promotions.

W

- **Website**: Design a website that's inviting and involves viewers. Also, be sure that it's optimized for search engines and mobile use.
- **Welcome to My Office Kit**: Send a kit to new clients as soon as they book their first appointment. Include several business cards, brochure, pertinent information, product samples, and educational or promotional materials on the benefits of your services or products. This can be a physical kit or a digital kit, depending on your marketing preferences.
- **Welcome Wagon**: This organization greets new residents in specific neighborhoods and delivers gifts and coupons from local businesses.
- **Window and Storefront Displays**: Create an inviting display showing your services or products; make it colorful and catchy to grab the public's attention, and change it frequently. These can also be created at related businesses, not just your own. Some malls even rent "Window Display" areas in front of vacant stores or have special display alcoves.
- **Word-of-Mouth**: One of the most powerful resources for business; satisfied and dissatisfied clients talk and talk and talk....
- **Workshops**: Conduct workshops or classes in your area. Advertise in newspapers and local magazines, mail flyers, hang posters, announce them on your website, and do email blasts. Do free lectures which you can advertise at no cost by sending out PSAs to print media and radio stations.
- **Writing Articles**: Good method of demonstrating knowledge in your field, educating the public, and making yourself known.

X

- **X Marks the Spot**: Hold a contest during an event where the person who can correctly identify the most major meridian points (or whatever anatomical structures are appropriate to your practice) wins a prize.
- **X-Rays**: If you're a chiropractor or dentist, offer free x-rays as part of the initial visit.

Y

- **Yellow Pages**: Still used extensively by the public for locating services, both in print and online. Place your listing under the most logical category if you can only afford one listing; otherwise list under each applicable category.
- **Yelp**: Make sure your listing with Yelp is accurate and consider advertising. Also, if you have a high Yelp rating, be sure to promote that in your other marketing endeavors.
- **YouTube**: Create short demonstrations of your services, offer tips, or interview experts.

Z

- **Zodiac**: Create special promotions based on the different signs of the zodiac. You can also do this for Chinese astrology.
- **Zoological Society**: Sponsor an animal or event at your local zoo. Sponsorships are often published in the society's newsletters, and if the contribution is significant, the zoo might even place a plaque (with your name) on its premises.
- **ZZZ**: Create a "sleep-better" promotion that includes educational material regarding how your services support quality sleep, create a special signature service, and sell sleep-related products.

Epilogue

10 Best Ways to Guarantee Failure

Ever wonder how the most successful practitioners seem to magically attract new clients and build a thriving practice? What is their secret? Although each success story is unique in its own way, strategic plans, business savvy, a knack for marketing, and dedication are common themes.

One thing is for sure, if you follow the 10 activities listed below, you are guaranteed to fail. Maybe a little tongue-in-cheek tour of these fatal errors will illustrate why the most successful practitioners, as highlighted throughout *Business Mastery*, follow a very different path to success.

1. Open an office next to a martial arts studio or a violin instructor

So what if your clients have to park four blocks away, fend off the stray animals that congregate by your front door, and walk up a flight of rickety stairs to get to your office, not to mention the peculiar noises that crescendo at the oddest times. Who cares about a little inconvenience and a few unpleasantries?

In the wellness field, location is everything. A tranquil and comfortable setting works wonders to help your clients relax and best enjoy the benefits of your sessions. Carefully evaluate the surrounding area and business setting. Look for locations where the adjacent businesses complement what you do (or at least don't detract from your work). You don't wield much control over what new businesses open after you're set up, although you could request a provision in your lease agreement that certain types of businesses not be allowed.

Image also plays a crucial role in your success. Create a comfortable and safe indoor and outdoor space so clients want to return. Aim for a clean, organized, quiet, and private office space. Create an office environment as comfortable as possible for yourself and your clients. Also, look for ways to differentiate yourself from other practitioners (e.g., a decorative fountain for soothing sounds of water, flannel sheets in winter, an assortment of juices and filtered water).

2. Be a chatty Cathy

Talk nonstop about yourself. Don't listen to your clients' concerns. In fact, purposely eliminate addressing a health concern that they point out needs extra attention. Ignore information offered about clients' personal lives, and when brought up, interrupt with a story about how good or bad YOUR day was. When meeting someone new, babble on before you're even asked about how you got into the field and drone on about every technique you utilize in your sessions.

All successful practitioners have highly developed listening skills. This means treating clients as though they're the center of the universe. It also means paying attention to nonverbal as well as verbal communication. Ask open-ended questions, not just ones that require Yes or No responses. Also, though it may seem natural to talk about yourself, limit self-disclosure and continue to bring any conversation back to the client in the room. Encourage your clients to share their wellness goals with you. Develop treatment plans jointly with them. This helps to clarify the type of work required, set boundaries, and ensure your clients' unique needs are met. It also greatly boosts client retention.

Many people become either tongue-tied or drone on forever when asked what it is they do. Script a carefully prepared 30-second introduction about who you are and what you do. This isn't meant to be a sales pitch. Keep it simple, honest, and dynamic. Include a few benefits of the work you do and something that expresses who you are. By having this memorized introduction, you're free to focus on listening to the other person.

3. Stay at home and wait for the universe to support you

After all, many wise leaders have claimed that if you do what you love, money will flow to you. And if it's meant to be, it will happen.

Karmic laws may rule, but belief without action brings only a fraction of the potential results. The key word in the phrase, "Do what you love and money will flow to you," is the word "do." Creatively planned effort with sincere intention will reap many future returns. If you're doing what you love, tell others and this becomes marketing in the truest form. If you're in the building phase of your practice, work with as many people as possible. Do demonstrations, donate your services for worthy events, and offer your services to people in need. Loving what you do will become obvious to those who receive your work and may inspire clients' word-of-mouth referrals to you. But these are just the beginning. It doesn't take a lot of effort, but consistent, disciplined, and conscious attempts to reach out to existing and new clients are required.

4. Don't return phone calls

Assume that if a current or potential client really wants to talk with you or book a session, he'll call back. It's also okay to answer the phone while in session with a client. Your client won't mind you taking a few minutes of the time she's paid for so you can talk to someone else.

Since the phone is one of your primary communication links to customers, it's imperative that you establish times during the day to return phone calls. Usually when people call to schedule a session, they want it as soon as possible. If you wait too long to call back, the opportunity to connect may be lost. Return all phone calls within 24 hours or sooner. Keep necessary supplies, appointment scheduler, and information close to the telephone so that you won't keep anyone hanging while you're fumbling for them. Greet callers courteously and enthusiastically.

It's inappropriate to answer the telephone while working with a client. That client has paid for your undivided attention during a specified amount of hands-on time. If need be, utilize an appointment service to book sessions, employ a receptionist, or use online booking software. Whichever method you choose, make certain that the phone can't be heard in the treatment room.

5. Toss receipts

It's such a hassle, and I pay for almost everything online, so why bother, right?

Consider being a "receipt cop" a part of doing business. It's a way to increase your net income by offsetting gross income from paying clients. Most practitioners keep track of the bigger items (usually paid with a check or credit card) such as equipment, telephone, stationery, advertising, office supplies, dues, and rent. But those little cash expenses add up, such as: meals, taxi fares, and tips while at a convention; bottled water or juice bought while doing work at a corporate account; and gasoline or mileage expenses for business use of your car.

Keep a copy of checks, money orders, or credit card payments for tax records. Sometimes you can't get a receipt for cash purchases (particularly from vending machines), so keep a cash journal that documents the type of business activity you were doing while making the purchase and the details about the actual purchase (i.e., item description, place purchased, date, amount). Financial management is crucial for long-term success.

6. Be late for appointments

Time is relative (ask Einstein). The session can't begin without you anyway. Also, people are always glad to have some unexpected free time to contemplate their navel. Besides, it isn't as if clients never keep you waiting. What's a few minutes?

Without a doubt, lateness conveys the attitude that your time is more important than your client's time. It clearly registers as disrespect. If you arrive at the same time as your client, you're late. Being timely means allowing ample time to review client charts, set up your room, and get centered. Schedule yourself wisely so that you work at a comfortable pace and allot time for breaks. Timeliness is an admirable quality, especially given the personal nature of this field.

7. Assume that the whole world is your market

Attempt to make everyone your client. After all, everybody benefits from your work. If you narrow your market, you might starve to death. Place display ads, business cards, and brochures everywhere, and hope that your phone rings off the hook.

It's true that almost anyone can benefit from wellness care, but to work smarter—not harder, it's vital to focus your promotional efforts on several target markets. Decide whom you would like to work with and pursue those markets. Many opportunities exist in this world, and it's impossible to follow them all or be everything to everyone. Given that, like most practitioners, you have limited marketing resources, so it's important to know where to focus your time and money. This doesn't mean that you must refuse to work with people who don't fit your target market profile, just that you don't randomly expend your resources.

8. Never think twice about exiting clients

Once they walk out the door, forget they exist. Keep looking for more clients. You don't want to get bored by working on the same people all of the time.

Client retention is the foundation of a stable, thriving practice. It costs 6 times more to go after a new client than to retain an existing one. Pay attention to nurturing current clients. Build rapport by showing interest in your clients' ongoing wellbeing. Work with clients to create effective treatment plans and customize your sessions. Continue your customer service through appropriate follow-up. Some ways to show concern are: check in with clients the day after their session; send special occasion cards for events such as birthdays and anniversaries; make confirmation calls; and gather information, referrals, or resources for topics of concern to your clients.

9. Be a lone ranger

Become as isolated as you can. Don't share any of your ideas because someone might steal them and become successful. Don't bother with continuing education, because your original training meets the local requirements (and you're such a wonderful healer that you don't need to learn anything else).

Even though we see clients, the work of most wellness practitioners is rather solitary. Rarely do practitioners work in an environment that involves case management or discussions with peers. It's vital for your personal wellbeing as well as your business success to establish a support system. Meet with colleagues on a regular basis, choose advisors, attend networking functions, and get involved with local health-oriented activities. Seek opportunities to engage in cooperative marketing ventures.

Continuing your education is another aspect of involvement in your profession. Stay on the cutting edge of technical knowledge as well as professional development skills. Two side benefits of attending workshops are meeting other like-minded people and renewing your enthusiasm for your work.

10. Never receive any somatic wellness treatments

You don't have time to get worked on. Besides, nobody does your style of work, which is your favorite, or if they do, they certainly aren't as good as you. What you want is for clients to knock down your door, asking for your work. If you keep this up, you'll be making all sorts of money.

Think about how much you use your body. Walk your talk. Receive regular wellness treatments so you can stay healthy and strong. It's the only way to realistically sustain a long-term practice and your wellbeing. This can be difficult, particularly for those of you who live in isolated areas. But if you don't receive regular treatments, how can you ethically encourage others to do the same?

I wish you great success in all you do!

~Cherie

Glossary

Accounts Payable: The amounts one owes another person or business.

Accounts Receivable: The amounts owed to one by another person or business.

Acting As If: A method to increase goal-setting success by creating the "feeling" of having achieved the goal.

Active Listening: A communication technique where the listener provides feedback by rephrasing what the speaker said, nodding, and using sound to assure the speaker that she is being heard and understood.

Adjusted Cash Flow: When pricing a business for sale, it includes the company's earnings after expenses, and additions or subtractions for such items as the owner's salary and discretionary expenses that most likely won't be incurred by the new owner.

Advertising: Gaining public notice through means that require direct payment.

Advertorial: A combination of a sales ad written in a story format of FAQ format.

Advocacy: Recommendation or support of a cause.

AdWords: An online advertising program owned by Google that allows you to generate ads that are based on specific search engine results and which direct people to your website.

Affirmations: Positive phrases you repeat to yourself that describe how you want to be.

Airtime: The time allocated to a particular program, item, topic, or type of material on radio or television.

Algorithm: A set of steps that are followed in order to solve a mathematical problem or to complete a computer process.

Ambiance: A place's character and atmosphere.

Analgesics: A drug or topical application acting to relieve pain.

App: A software application specifically designed to be downloaded to mobile devices.

Arbitration (Binding): This form of dispute resolution takes place out of court. All parties in the dispute select an impartial third party (arbitrator), agree in advance to comply with the arbitrator's award, and participate in a hearing where evidence and testimonies are presented. The arbitrator's decision is usually final, and courts rarely reexamine it.

Arbitration (Nonbinding): The settling of disputes between two parties by an impartial third party, whose decision may be contested in a court of law.

Assets: The total resources of an individual or business both tangible and intangible. These may include cash in the bank, inventory, goodwill, accounts receivable, and equipment.

Attitude: A feeling, disposition, or expression of a positive or negative evaluation of people, objects, events, activities, or ideas.

Autonomy: The ability to make one's own decisions.

Back-Door Approach: Utilizing an indirect means of meeting prospective alliances.

Backlink: A hyperlink that links from a web page, back to your own web page or website.

Baking: The method of creating a treatment that includes using a product in a session and sending the client home with that product.

Balance Sheet: A statement of a company's assets, liabilities, and net equity as of a given point in time.

Banner Advertising: Website advertising that's image-based rather than text-based.

Barrier: A circumstance, belief, or obstacle that hinders movement, progress, or access.

Barter: The action or system of exchanging goods or services without using money.

Behavioral Theory: A scientific approach that limits the study of psychology to measurable or observable behavior.

Belief: Trust, faith, or confidence in someone or something.

Benefit: A description of how the client profits from using the services and product offered.

Bigotry: Intolerance of any creed, belief, or opinion that differs from one's own.

Blog: A website that contains postings in chronological order on topics that a blogger knows, likes, or is passionate about.

Body Language: Nonverbal communication in which people reveal clues to unspoken intentions or feelings through their physical behaviors, such as posture, gestures, facial expressions, and eye movements.

Booth: A space rented to participate in conventions, conferences, expos, and/or trade shows for the purpose of promotion.

Boredom Syndrome: A condition characterized by ennui that is spiralling downward.

Bottom Line: The final total of an account, balance sheet, or other financial document.

Boundaries: Borders or limits that separate people from their environment and from other people; personal comfort zones that enable a person to maintain a sense of comfort and safety. These can be tangible or intangible.

Brand: The unique sum of impressions about your business.

Breach of Contract: Failure to live up to the terms of a contract. The failure may provoke a lawsuit, in which an aggrieved party asks a court to award financial compensation.

Breakeven Analysis: The formula to determine when your business will be able to cover all expenses and begin making a profit.

Broadcast Advertising: Advertising utilizing airways such as radio or television and reaches a wider audience than print advertising.

Brochure: A pamphlet or leaflet containing pictures and information about a product or service.

Budget: An estimate of income and expenditures for a set period of time.

Bundling: Combining products together with other products or gift certificates.

Burnout: A psychological term that refers to long-term physical or emotional exhaustion.

Business Associate: According to HIPAA, a person or entity that performs functions or activities that involve the use or disclosure of protected health information on behalf of, or provides services to, a covered entity.

Business Feasibility: An evaluation of a proposed business endeavor to determine if it is technically possible, if the costs are obtainable, and if a profit will result.

Business Interruption Insurance: Covers a person if their business has to close because of fire or other insurable causes.

Business License: Allows one the privilege of doing business in one's city and/or county.

Business Page: A type of Facebook page that is a public profile created by businesses, organizations, and anyone seeking to promote themselves publicly through social media.

Business Plan: A written document that describes in detail how a business is going to achieve its goals from a marketing, financial, and operational viewpoint.
Buzz Marketing: A Word-of-Mouth marketing that is the interaction of consumers and users of a product or service which serve to amplify the original marketing message.
C Corporation: Under U.S. federal income tax law, refers to any corporation that is taxed separately from its owners.
Call to Action (CTA): Words that urge the reader, listener, or viewer of a sales promotion message to take an immediate action, such as "Write Now," "Call Now," or "Click Here" (on Internet).
CAM: Complementary and Alternative Medicine.
Camaraderie: Mutual trust and friendship among people.
Capital: The net worth of a business; the difference between assets and liabilities.
Capitalized Earnings: A method of determining the value of a business by taking the adjusted cash flow and multiplying it by a capitalization rate.
Care Coordination: The deliberate organization of patient care activities between two or more participants (including the patient) involved in a patient's care to facilitate the appropriate delivery of health care services.
Carry Back: A provision that allows an individual or a business to use a net operating loss in one year to offset a profit in one or more previous years.
Case Management: A collaborative process of assessment, planning, facilitation, care coordination, evaluation, and advocacy for options and services to meet an individual's and family's comprehensive health needs.
Cash Flow Projection: A report that details the estimated income and expenses over a specific period of time (e.g., each month for the next year).
Centers of Influence: People or organizations that are well known and highly respected by your target market(s). Recommendations from these sources can boost your credibility and bring you clients.
Certification: A voluntary regulatory method that offers the use of vocational titles to distinguish professional services.
Chronological Résumé: A résumé that highlights work history and experience.
Classified Ads: A concise, engaging description of a business placed in a directory under an appropriate heading.
Clearing Techniques: Various techniques (e.g., psychotherapy, yoga, martial arts, meditation, bodywork/massage) that aim to empower people to realize their deepest desires and to achieve career successes.
Client Base: List of current and inactive clients.
Client Compliance: A client's agreement to adhere to instructions for home care and treatment plans.
Client Retention: The percentage of customer relationships that, once established, a business maintains on a long-term basis.
Client-Centered: The principle that practitioners always act in the best interest of the client.
Closed-Ended Questions: A question format that limits respondents with a list of answer choices from which they must choose, such as yes or no.
Closure Stage: The last stage of a client interview, where the practitioner gives a brief overview of the session, highlights client's major goals, assigns homework, allows the client to ask questions, and schedules the next appointment.
Cloud Technology: A model for delivering information technology services in which resources are retrieved from the Internet through web-based tools and applications, rather than a direct connection to a server.
Code of Ethics: Operating principles and behavioral guidelines that members of a profession are expected to uphold.
Cognitive Theory: A branch of psychology concerned with mental processes in respect to the internal events occurring between sensory stimulation and the overt expression of behavior.
Collage: A visual depiction of an ideal utilizing pictures and words.
Combination Résumé: A résumé that combines the work history and experience with talents, abilities, and potential.
Common Law Rules: Generally accepted rules based on local custom, tradition, or usage.
Communication: The act or process of using words, sounds, signs, or behaviors to effectively and efficiently express or exchange information or to express ideas, thoughts, and feelings to someone else.
Community Relations: Goodwill activities that create a positive public image for you and your business.
Compassion: Sympathetic concern for the sufferings or misfortunes of others.
Compensation Package: The combination of a salary and benefits that an employer provides to an employee.
Competence: The ability to do something successfully or efficiently.
Competition: Rivalry between two or more businesses striving for the same market.
Confidence: A feeling of self-assurance arising from one's appreciation of one's own abilities or qualities.
Confidentiality: The client's guarantee that what occurs in the therapeutic setting remains private and protected.
Conflict: A state of disharmony between incompatible or opposing persons, ideas, or interests; a clash.
Conflict Management: The process of limiting negative aspects of conflict while increasing the positive aspects of conflict.
Conflict of Interest: The potential to be impartial because a person has a duty to more than one person or organization.
Confrontation: The act of facing and dealing with a problematic situation.
Content Farm: Company that employs people to create articles on a variety of topics.
Contingency Clause: A condition or action that must be met in order for a contract to become binding.
Contract: A written or spoken agreement, especially one concerning employment, sales, or tenancy, that is intended to be enforceable by law.
Contraindications: Any physical, mental, or emotional conditions a client has that may cause a particular intervention or treatment to be detrimental or unsafe.
Conversion: The proportion of people viewing an advertisement and going on to buy the product, click on a link, etc.
Cooperative Marketing: Working with another business to reach the same target markets, or working with similar businesses to reach different markets.
Copyright: Ownership of intellectual property (e.g., literary, musical, artistic).
Copywriting: The art and science of writing copy (words used on web pages, ads, promotional materials, etc.) that convinces prospective customers to take action.
Corporate Culture: The values and behaviors that contribute to an organization's unique social and psychological environment.
Cost of Living Adjustment: The percentage change based on the difference of the current year's average cost of the basic necessities of life, including food, shelter, and clothing, with the previous year.
Countertransference: Transference occurring in the direction from practitioner to client.
Cover Letter: A letter that is sent with a résumé to establish rapport, communicate interest in the position, and convey skills and experience.
Creative Visualization: A mental technique that uses the imagination to create success and make dreams and goals come true.
Credibility: The quality of being trusted and believed in.
Credit Score: A statistically derived numeric expression of a person's creditworthiness that's used by lenders to assess the likelihood that a person will repay his debts.
Credit Terms: Various methods of allowing someone to pay at some distant date, rather than when services or goods are received.
Cross link: A link between two sites that allows users to reference sites with content similar to what they're already viewing.
CPT Codes: Current Procedural Terminology Codes. Medical codes defined that indicate the type of services performed during a session to improve function.

Customer Service: The act of taking care of the customer's needs by providing and delivering professional, helpful, high quality service and assistance before, during, and after the customer's requirements are met.

Database: A collection of information that is organized so that it can easily be accessed, managed, and updated.

Data-Mining: A process that turns raw data into useful information. By using software to look for patterns in large batches of data, businesses can learn more about their customers and develop more effective marketing strategies, as well as increase sales and decrease costs.

DBA: Doing Business As (also referred to as a Fictitious Name Certificate).

Deduction: Any item or expenditure subtracted from gross income to reduce the amount of income subject to tax.

Defense Mechanism: Psychological strategy of relating to the world that is developed unconsciously to protect one from shame, anxiety, and other emotionally painful experiences that one is unable to handle.

Delegate: To entrust an act or responsibility to someone else.

Demeanor: The way in which a person behaves toward others, including body language.

Demographics: Categorical statistics such as age, gender, income level, occupation, location, and educational level.

Depreciation: A tax term that describes an asset's loss in value of over time.

Diagnosis: The identification of the underlying cause, etiology, pathology, or nature of a set of signs and/or symptoms.

Differential Advantage: Unique benefits or characteristics of a firm, product, or program that set it apart and above its competitors.

Direct Mail: Simple, inexpensive, and highly effective marketing tools such as postcards, greeting cards, surveys, and sales letters.

Direct Referral Process: A 4-stage process that includes requesting the referral, repeating the referral, rewarding the referral, and reciprocating the referral.

Directory: A publication listing individuals or organizations alphabetically or thematically with details such as names, addresses, emails, URLs, and telephone numbers.

Disbursement: The act of paying out funds.

Display Ad: A graphic print advertisement utilized to gain public notice for a business (e.g., sales ads, coupons, business cards).

Dissonance: Lack of agreement; inconsistency.

Distributor: An agent who supplies goods to stores and other businesses that sell to consumers.

Documentation: Recordkeeping of client files for the purpose of IRS supporting information; information on clients' progress; and information necessary for insurance reimbursement.

Domain Name: An Internet address for a business.

Drawing Account: An account used primarily by sole propriators and partnerships to track money that owners withdraw from a business.

Dual Relationship: The overlapping of professional and social roles and interactions between two people.

Due Diligence: The process of gathering information to confirm material facts in a business transaction.

Duplication Cost: Determining the selling price of a business by taking the market value of assets and combining it with the cost for the number of years it would take a buyer to reach the same profit level.

Empathy: The action of understanding, being sensitive to, and identifying with another's situation, feelings, thoughts, and motives.

Employee: A person who works for another in return for financial or other compensation, with rights and duties.

EIN: Employer Identification Number.

Employment Kit: A folder that contains documentation for employment (résumés, cover letters, references, diplomas, licenses, certifications, and other relevant items).

Employment Benefit: Non-cash compensation (e.g., vacation, sick days, insurance, training).

Engagement: A state of being involved and/or committed.

Equity: The monetary value of a property or business beyond any amounts owed on it in debt (e.g., mortgages, claims, liens).

Ergonomics: A science that deals with designing and arranging things so that people can use them easily and safely.

Estimated Taxes: The amount of taxes paid to the government based on the total amount of taxes expected to be due at the end of a specific period (e.g., month, quarter, year).

Ethical Decision-Making Model: A 6-step process: identify the problem, identify potential issues, review your profession's code of ethics and relevant laws, evaluate potential courses, obtain consultation, and determine the best course of action.

Ethical Dilemma: A situation in which two or more duties, rights, or a combination of duties and rights are in conflict. As a result, regardless of what action is taken, something of value will be compromised.

Etiquette: A code of behavior that delineates expectations for social behavior.

Executive Summary: A portion of a business plan that consists of the plan highlights.

Exit Interview: After a treatment session, the steps include: overview what took place, assign homework, review long-term treatment plan, make referrals if necessary, and re-schedule the client. Also, a survey conducted with an individual who is separating from an organization.

Exploration Stage: The second stage of a client interview, where the practitioner reviews the client's history, assesses the client, and determines the treatment plan.

Facebook: A social networking website that allows registered users to create profiles, upload photos and videos, post messages, and keep in touch with friends, family, and colleagues.

Feature: A description of your service or product.

Feature Story: An article about a person or event that's usually presented as a human interest story.

FICA: Federal Insurance Contributions Act. A U.S. federal payroll tax imposed on both employees and employers to fund Social Security and Medicare.

FUTA: Federal Unemployment Tax Act.

Feedback: The transmission of evaluative or corrective information about an action, event, or process.

Feng Shui: In Chinese thought, a system of laws considered to govern spatial arrangement and orientation in relation to the flow of energy (qi, chi, or ki).

Financial Analysis: A portion of a business plan that consists of statements about the income potential, fees, current financial status, and financial forecast.

401(K): A retirement savings plan sponsored by an employer. The employee decides the amount to invest and the employer matches the amount (usually up to 3% of the employee's salary).

Forum: A medium (as a newspaper or online service) of open discussion or expression of ideas.

Franchise: A type of license that a party (franchisee) acquires, allowing access to a business's (the franchisor) proprietary knowledge, processes, and trademarks in order to sell a product or provide a service under the business's name.

Friend: Someone who is added to a social network such as Facebook. The person may or may not be a known friend in real life.

Front-Door Approach: Using the telephone, mail, email, and/or in-person approaches to generate prospective alliance partners.

Fundraiser: A charity event to raise money for a certain person or group.

Functional Résumé: A résumé that highlights talents, abilities, and potential.

Funnel: Using leads from social media, live events, and customer referrals to direct people to a website. Once there, names and emails are exchanged for a piece of valuable information, and follow-up is continued with automated preset emails.

General Liability Insurance: This type of insurance covers any negligence resulting in injury to clients, employees, or the general public while on their premises.

Goal: The object of a person's ambition or effort; an aim or desired result.

Goodwill: Benevolence, friendly disposition, cheerful consent, willingness, and readiness.

Google+: Google's version of social networking that delivers functionality and many features similar to those of Facebook.

Grants: Money provided to people who fall within the parameters of special interest groups, either as the business owner or the market one plans to serve.

Grassroots Marketing: Word-of-Mouth Marketing that targets a small group to help spread a message to a larger group.

Gratuity: A gift of money, over and above payment due for service (see Tips).

Grievance Protocol: A plan that's put in place for the purpose of steps to follow should an employee have an issue in the workplace.

Gross Income: An individual's total personal income before taxes or deductions; a company's revenue minus cost of goods sold. Also called "gross profit."

Guarantee: A formal promise or assurance that certain conditions will be fulfilled.

Habit: An acquired behavior pattern regularly followed until it's almost involuntary.

Hashtag: A type of label or metadata tag used on social networks, created by placing a hash character (#) in front of a relevant word or unspaced phrase.

Headline: A heading at the top of an article (or page in a newspaper or magazine) that serves to grab the attention of the reader to read the article or ad.

HIPAA: Health Insurance Portability and Accountability Act. A U.S. law designed to protect patients' personal health information.

High Priority Activities: Activities that produce the majority of results (see Pareto Principle).

HMO: A Health Maintenance Organization. A type of Managed Care Organization that provides healthcare services for a fixed fee to subscribers in a specific geographic area.

Home Page: The introductory page of a website, typically serving as a table of contents for the site or a web page set as the default or startup page on a browser.

Honesty: The facet of moral character based on being fair, truthful, and sincere.

Hospice: Palliative care designed for people in the final phase of a terminal illness that focuses on comfort and quality of life, rather than cure.

Hosting: A company that provides hardware and other services to store, maintain, and provide Internet connection to websites.

HTML: HyperText Markup Language.

Image: The impression projected to the world that's a combination of one's appearance, conduct, verbal communication, body language, business policies, and facility.

Incentive Program: A plan that rewards loyal clients and creates a way to increase session frequency for others who might not be able to receive services as often as desired.

Income: Money received for work performed or through investments.

Income Tax: A government levy imposed on individuals or businesses that varies with the personal income or business profits.

Independent Contractor: A person who contracts to do work for another according to his own processes and methods; the contractor isn't subject to another's control except for what is specified in a mutually binding agreement.

Indications: Suggestions that a certain treatment would be beneficial to a client.

Informed Consent: The process of getting a client's permission before proceeding with a healthcare treatment. The client must have a clear understanding of the procedures, alternative approaches, benefits, and potential consequences. This information must be presented in a form that the client can understand and consent must be given without coercion.

Initiation Stage: The first stage of a client interview where the practitioner introduces herself, establishes rapport, discusses the client's general issues and expectations, describes services, reviews policies, and explains procedures.

Inner Critic: The negative internal voice.

Inquiry Letter: A letter that is sent along with a résumé to a company that hasn't posted a job opening. Its purpose is to introduce, share unique talents and qualifications, and establish interest in offering a position should one become available.

Insurance Claim: A formal request to an insurance company asking for a payment based on the terms of the insurance policy. Insurance claims are reviewed by the company for their validity and then paid out to the insured or requesting party (on behalf of the insured) once approved.

Intake Form: A form that asks for a client's personal and medical information.

Intake Interview: An initial interview with a client to go over the intake form, discuss policies and procedures, clarify boundaries, determine a course of treatment, and answer questions.

Integrity: The quality or state of being complete; unbroken condition; wholeness; honesty; and sincerity.

ICD-10-CM: International Classification of Diseases-Tenth Revision-Clinical Modification Code Book.

Internet Service Provider (ISP): A company that provides access to the Internet and other related services such as website building and virtual hosting.

Interpersonal Skills: The abilities enabling a person to interact positively and work effectively with others.

Inventory: A complete list of items such as property, goods in stock, or the contents of a building.

IRA: Individual Retirement Account. A retirement plan that allows tax-free contributions to an account. Taxes are levied when the money is withdrawn.

Key Business Indicators: A set of quantifiable measures that a person, company, or industry uses to gauge or compare performance in terms of meeting their strategic and operational goals.

Keystoning: The method of marking up merchandise to an amount that is double the wholesale price.

Keyword: An informative word used in an information retrieval system to indicate the content of a document.

Landing Page: A destination web page that's distinct from your main website, usually created to guide people to a specific offer.

Laws: Codified rules of conduct set forth by a society, generally based on shared ethical or moral principles.

Lawsuit: An action brought before a court of law by one party against another.

Lead Capture: A web form with the purpose of acquiring the name and email address of the visitor.

Lead Magnet: Anything that an Internet marketer offers prospective customers in exchange for getting their email addresses.

Learning Environment: Refers to the diverse physical locations, contexts, and cultures in which students learn.

Lease: A contract by which one party conveys land, property, services, etc., to another for a specified time, usually in return for a periodic payment.

Ledger: A book of financial transactions.

Legal Entity: A legal construct that allows a group of people to act as if they are a single person.

Legal Status: The standing, state, or condition of an entity in the eyes of the law.

Liabilities: Current and long-term debts an individual or business owes.

Liability Insurance: Covers costs of injuries that occur to business related visitors on your property.

Licensure: The most restrictive form of regulation, yet it provides the greatest level of public protection. Licensing programs typically involve the completion of a prescribed educational program, passing an examination, and adherance to a code of ethics or professional conduct.

Limited Liability Company (LLC): A business structure that combines the pass-through taxation of a partnership or sole proprietorship with the limited liability of a corporation.

Link: A reference to another document or website. It usually appears in a different color and is underlined for easy access, and when clicked, will take a person to the referenced site.

LinkedIn: A social networking website for business professionals. It allows you to share work-related information and maintain an online list of professional contacts.

Liquidation: The selling of assets, especially to pay off debt.

Listening: Giving the speaker your full attention by taking the time to understand and interpret the information being spoken.

Listicle: An article structured in the form of a list, typically having some additional content relating to each item.

Listserv: An electronic "mailing list" service that delivers messages to subscribers.
Logistics: The management of day-to-day tasks associated with running a business.
Logo: Abbreviation of the word logotype. A graphic mark, emblem, icon, or symbol commonly used by businesses.
Malpractice Liability Insurance: Protects against claims due to a loss, damage, or injury incurred by one's clients as a result of improper, negligent, or incompetent treatment.
Managed Care Organization (MCO): An entity that manages costs by contracting with providers who agree to charge predetermined fees. They are administered by a gatekeeper; a physician who oversees the services supplied by the organization.
Market Research: The systematic gathering and interpretation of information about individuals and trends.
Market Share: The specific percentage of total industry sales of a particular product achieved by a single company over a specific time period.
Marketing: Sharing information about yourself and your services with potential and current clients so they get a sense of who you are, so they can make an informed choice of whether to utilize your services.
Marketing Plan: A portion of a business plan that outlines marketing goals for promotions, advertising, publicity, and community relations.
Maslow's Hierarchy of Needs: A famous theory of motivation originally developed by Abraham Maslow that's based on the idea that motivation depends on human needs being met in a certain order.
Mastermind Group: A focused group setting where the individuals in the group create specific goals for their business/career and provide each other with support and inspiration for achieving those goals.
Media Hook: An aspect or trait that makes one unique or able to stand out when attempting to grab the media's attention.
Media Kit: A public relations tool designed to procure coverage. It contains promotional material and associated information about a person, firm, product, conference, seminar, program, or event.
Mediation: A common form of dispute resolution where a third party (mediator) works with disputants to agree on a fair result. It's less costly and less time consuming over the long term and can be the way to finding innovative, mutually beneficial solutions. However, mediation doesn't always result in a settlement.
Membership Program: A plan in which clients commit to a contract of some length, such as 6 months or a year, and a fixed monthly fee is automatically deducted from their checking account or credit card.
Mental Contrasting: Moving back and forth in thought between dreaming about goals and visualizing the possible obstacles that may be encountered in reality.
Mentor: A professional relationship in which a more experienced person shares information, skills, and insights with a less experienced person to provide encouragement and support.
Merchandising: The activity of selling goods or services by displaying them attractively.
Metadata: Data that serves to provide context or additional information about other data.
Meta-Tagging: A special HTML tag that is used to store information about a web page (e.g., page description, keywords) but isn't displayed in a web browser. Many search engines use the information stored in meta tags when they index web pages.
Mind Mapping Technique: A visual representation of hierarchical information that includes a central idea surrounded by connected branches of associated topics.
Mismanagement: The process or practice of managing ineptly, incompetently, or dishonestly.
Mission Statement: A portion of a business plan that conveys the essence of a business: why it exists and what values underpin everything that's done.
Morals: Standards by which behaviors and character traits are judged as right or wrong.
Motivation: The reason(s) one has for acting or behaving in a particular way.
Multi-Discipline: The combination of several professional roles to create a unique, blended career.
Multidisciplinary Team: The combination of several professional roles where wellness practitioners work in tandem with medical doctors or physical therapists for the treatment of clients.
Negative Conditioning: Allowing past mistakes, incompletions, and failures to obstruct the creation and accomplishment of new goals.
Negligence: Failure to behave with the level of care that falls below the legal standards of behavior established to protect others against unreasonable risk of harm.
Negotiation: Mutual discussion and arrangement of the terms in a transaction or agreement.
Net Present Value: The difference between the estimated value of future cash flows from an investment and the amount of investment.
Net Profit: The amount of the gross profit minus operating expenses and all other expenses; referred to as "the bottom line."
Networking: A group of interconnected or cooperating individuals who develop and share contacts, information, and support.
Newsfeed: A list of updates on your Facebook home page, including updates on people in your friend's list, as well as advertisements based on your own preferences as mined by the Facebook algorithm.
Newsletter: A publication issued periodically to the members of a society, business, or organization.
Newsworthy: Something of sufficient interest or importance to the public to warrant reporting in the media.
Niche: Subset; position.
Noise: The interference of the transfer of information.
Occupational License: This license allows one to work in a specific industry as long as one complies with that profession's regulations.
OSHA: Occupational Safety and Health Administration.
Office Logistics: Planning, execution, and control of the procurement, movement, and stationing of personnel, materials, and other resources to achieve the objectives of a business.
Online Discussion Forum: A website that provides an exchange of information between people about a particular topic. It may be monitored to keep content appropriate.
On-Page SEO: Refers to factors that have an effect on your website or web page listing in natural search results. These factors are controlled by you or by coding on your page. Examples of on-page optimization include actual HTML code, meta tags, keyword placement, and keyword density.
Open House: A time of inviting members of the public to visit a place or institution, usually for the purpose of promotion.
Open-Ended Question: A question phrased in such a manner that the client has to give an answer that isn't a simple "yes" or "no."
Opt-In: Express permission by a customer or a recipient of mail, email, or other direct messages to allow a marketer to send merchandise, information, or more messages such as a newsletter. After the opt-in, the marketer continues sending the material or messages until the recipient chooses to opt out.
Outline Technique: A technique for writing goals which utilizes a list of priorities and then list the goals under each one.
Overhead: The business expenses required to operate on an ongoing basis, regardless of the actual number of clients.
Owner's Statement: A business plan section that describes the business and the owner.
Pareto Principle: The belief that 80% of one's results (output) are produced by 20% of one's activities (input); and, conversely, 20% of one's results are produced by 80% of one's activities.
Partnership: A legal relationship between two or more persons in which each agrees to furnish a part of the capital and labor for a business enterprise, and by which each shares a fixed proportion of profits and losses.
Partnership Insurance: Protects one against lawsuits arising from actions or omissions by any of one's business partners.

Pay-Per-Click Advertising (PPCA): An Internet advertising model used to direct traffic to websites, where advertisers pay the publisher (typically a website owner) when the ad is clicked; the amount spent to get an advertisement clicked.

Peer Support Group: A group of practitioners whose main goal is to listen to each other in a manner that provides support for the many challenges that arise during the course of dealing with clients.

Perception: The ability to see, hear, or become aware of something through the senses.

Perfectionist: A person that refuses to accept any standard short of perfection.

Performance Review: An annual or semi-annual review of an employee's overall contributions to the company.

Persona: The collection of web pages visited, ads clicked on, pictures, and other browsing history of a person or group of people for the purpose of targeted marketing.

Personal Disability Insurance: Safeguards one from loss of income if one cannot work due to illness or injury.

Personal Injury Insurance: Covers an injury occurring in an automobile, at home, in a business space, or in a space that is covered by some sort of liability insurance.

Personal Service Corporation (PSC): A corporation in which the business owners are service professionals.

Personalized Gift Items: Items printed with a promotional message to be given away to serve as reminders; also known as Specialty Advertising.

Petty Cash Fund: Cash on hand to pay for incidental business expenses.

Picture Board: A technique for visualizing goals in which pictures and words are pinned to a bulletin board.

Pinterest: A social networking website that allows you to organize and share ideas with others in a visual format.

Pitch Letter: A letter intended to grab the media representative's attention so that the rest of the material in the Media Kit is read.

Planning and Zoning Permits: These permits are issued after a location has been assessed and shows that the business operation conforms with area plans, has proper zoning, and has adequate parking.

Planning Stage: The third stage in the client interview where the practitioner and client work together to create a long-term treatment plan.

Podcast: An audio program (usually talk), subscribed to and downloaded over the Internet.

Point-of-Sale (POS) Displays: Merchandise holders placed near the checkout counter; also known as point-of purchase or POP.

Policy: A statement of intent that defines expectations and is implemented as a procedure or protocol.

Policy Manual: A formalized human resources document that presents a broad overview of standard operating policies for an organization.

Portmanteau: A word or morpheme whose form and meaning are derived from a blending of two or more distinct forms (as smog from smoke and fog).

Power Differential: The role difference between a practitioner and client, in which the client is vulnerable and the practitioner has more power by virtue of training and experience.

Prepaid Package Plan: An offering for the client to purchase a bulk of services at a discounted price. It's intended to encourage clients to book more often and infuse extra income into one's bank account.

Preferred Provider Organization (PPO): A type of MCO that contracts with a group of preferred providers to deliver healthcare services to members. PPO members are free to choose any physician or hospital for services, but they receive more benefits if they choose a preferred provider.

Presence: The state of being somewhere; the ability to project a sense of ease, poise, or self-assurance.

Presentation: A demonstration or lecture of educational or promotional information to a group or audience.

Press Conference: A meeting organized for the purpose of distributing information to the media and answering reporter's questions.

Press Release: An announcement of an event, performance, or other newsworthy item that's issued to the media.

Preventive Wellness: A practice that focuses on the health of individuals, communities, and defined populations. Its goal is to protect, promote, and maintain health and well-being, and to prevent disease, disability, and death.

Primary Care Provider (PCP): A doctor who provides health care at a basic, rather than specialized, level for people making an initial approach for treatment.

Principles: An individual's rules or laws of behavior that enable her to behave with integrity.

Print Advertising: Gaining public notice for a business through the printed word (e.g., magazines, newspapers).

Priorities: In goal setting, general areas of concern.

Private Practice: A business designation for a practitioner who is self-employed.

Pro Bono Work: Work undertaken for the public good without charge, often to support charities or those with low incomes.

Proactive: Creating or controlling a situation by causing something to happen rather than responding to it after it has happened.

Procedure Manual: A written explanation of the step-by-step sequence of activities or courses of action that must be followed to correctly perform a task.

Procrastination: Put off intentionally and habitually.

Professional Credentials: Regulatory methods that establish professionalism to the public. The four types are: licensure, certification, registration, and title protection.

Professional Development: The advancement of skills or expertise to succeed in a particular profession, especially through continued education.

Professional Limited Liability Company (PLLC): An LLC for licensed service and wellness professionals. It's similar to an LLC, except that the articles of the company may have to be approved by one's professional licensing board. Requirements vary from state to state.

Professionalism: The behaviors and qualities that mark an individual as reliable, competent, trustworthy, and polished.

Profit: The surplus remaining after all the expenses are subtracted from the total revenue received.

Profit and Loss Statement: Reflects how much a company earned or lost over a specific period of time, as well as the costs and expenses associated with the earnings.

Promotions: Activities and materials produced to gain visibility. The money invested is indirect.

Protocol: A formal, established plan of therapeutic treatment or procedures.

Psychoanalytic Theory: The theory of personality developed by Sigmund Freud that focuses on repression and unconscious forces.

Psychographics: Lifestyle factors such as beliefs, values, social factors, cultural involvements, wellness needs and goals, and special interest activities.

Public Opinion: The collective opinion of many people.

Public Service Announcement (PSA): Message in the public interest disseminated by the media without charge, with the objective of raising awareness, or changing public attitudes and behavior toward a social issue.

Public Speaking: Giving a formal presentation for the purpose of education or promotion for a product or service (*see* presentation).

Publicity: The notice or attention given to someone or something by the media.

Purchasing Cycle: The pattern most people go through when contemplating utilizing services or making purchases.

Purchasing Power: Actively supporting businesses aligned with your values while boycotting companies that oppose them.

Purpose: A direction or theme utilized when setting goals.

Ranking: The placement of a website or web page within a search engine.

Rapport: A harmonious relationship marked by trust, openness, and mutual understanding.

Reciprocal Link: A mutual link between two websites.

Referral: An act of directing someone to a source for help, information, or further action.

Reflective Feedback: A communication method in which the essence of a message is captured and relayed back by rephrasing what the other person said, rather than repeating it verbatim.

Reframing: Changing the conceptual and/or emotional viewpoint in relation to which a situation is experienced and placing it in a different frame that fits the "facts" of a concrete situation equally well, thereby changing its entire meaning.

Registration: A regulatory method where a government agency keeps track of practitioners by informational recordkeeping. These types of programs may entail title protection and practice exclusivity.

Regulations: Rules or directives made and maintained by an authority.

Relationship-Based Marketing: The core of effective customer service, It involves truly caring about how you can best serve your clients' needs.

Reliability: Being able to count on someone or something; dependability.

Reputation: The beliefs or opinions that are held about someone or something.

Research Capacity: The ability to carry out research by defining a problem, setting objectives and priorities, conducting sound scientific research, and identifying solutions.

Research Literacy: The ability to find, read, evaluate, and apply relevant findings.

Respect: A feeling of deep admiration for someone or something elicited by their abilities, qualities, or achievements.

Responsibility: The state of being accountable for something within one's power; the ability to respond.

Résumé: A document (demonstrating skills, knowledge, and credentials) sent to a potential employer to secure an interview.

Retailing: The act of purchasing products at wholesale and reselling them for profit.

Reticular Activating System (RAS): A diffuse network of nerve pathways in the brainstem connecting the spinal cord, cerebrum, and cerebellum, and mediating the overall level of consciousness.

Retirement Plan: A savings plan for the future when one ceases working.

Return on Investment (ROI): A profitability metric that evaluates the performance of a business. To calculate ROI, the benefit of an investment is divided by the cost of the investment, and the result is expressed as a percentage or a ratio.

Risk Assessment: A portion of a business plan that demonstrates one's ability to anticipate and manage risks.

Risk-Taking: The act or fact of doing something that involves danger or potential loss in order to achieve a goal.

S Corporation: A closely held corporation that elects to be taxed under Subchapter S of Chapter 1 of the Internal Revenue Code. Most S Corporations don't pay federal income taxes.

Safety Protocol: A plan that's put in place, with instructions on how an employee should handle a safety issue.

Salary: A fixed regular payment, made by an employer to an employee, that's typically paid on a monthly or biweekly basis, but is often expressed as an annual sum.

SBA: Small Business Administration. Created in 1953 as an independent agency of the U.S. Federal Government to aid, counsel, provide loan assistance, and protect the interests of small business concerns.

SBA Loan: A loan issued by the SBA that offers several types of funding, from guaranteeing up to 85% of a commercial bank loan to directly loaning money.

Scalable: Hardware or software that can expand to support increasing workloads. This capability allows computer equipment and software programs to grow over time, rather than needing to be replaced.

Scarcity Consciousness: Focusing upon what you don't have in a way that all your subsequent interactions with your world are based upon that fundamental experience of "not-having."

Scientific Method: A method of research that consists of observing a sequence of actions, creating a hypothesis about the observation, using the hypothesis to predict an outcome, and setting up an experiment to see if the prediction is correct. This method must be repeatable, observable, and measurable.

Scope of Practice: The where, when, and how a practitioner may provide services or function as a professional.

Search Engine Marketing (SEM): A form of Internet marketing that involves the promotion of websites by increasing their visibility in search engine results pages primarily through paid advertising.

Search Engine Optimization (SEO): A process of maximizing the highest number of visitors to a website by ensuring that the website appears high or at the top of the list of results when a user enters those words into a search engine.

Self-Care: A habit of self-renewal that helps a caregiver to stay energized and manage stress, thus enabling one to stay at her professional best.

Self-Employed: Working for oneself as a freelancer, independent contractor, or owner of a business, rather than an employer.

Self-Employment Tax: This is a Social Security and Medicare tax primarily for individuals who work for themselves.

Self-Evaluation: The act of looking at your progress, development, and learning to determine what has improved and what areas still need improvement.

Self-Management: Taking responsibility for one's own behavior and well-being.

Self-Motivation: The initiative to undertake or continue a task or activity without another's prodding or supervision.

Seniority: Staff members who have been employed for the most amount of time or hold the highest rank.

Sentence Completions: A clearing process designed to elicit conscious and unconscious thoughts, attitudes, beliefs, and feelings so they can be recognized and released.

Server-Side Scripting: A technique used in web development that involves creating a single template page with scripts that produce a customized response for each visitor's request to the website.

Sexual Misconduct: A continuum of behavior from sexual impropriety to sexual violation. Sexual misconduct occurs when the fiduciary aspect of a therapeutic relationship is compromised, and is the result of the disregard of ethics, boundaries, and genuine care for the client.

Shareholders' Equity: The amount owners invested in a company's stock, plus or minus the company's earnings or losses since inception.

Shelf Talkers: Signs or clips that draw attention to a product.

Side-Door Approach: Most often utilized when a prospective alliance has a buffer person such as a nurse, assistant, or office manager. Side-door approaches utilize calling, emailing, mailing, and/or in person contact with this gatekeeper.

Sliding Fee Scale: A fee structure that allows people who cannot afford a full fee to pay a lower one, usually based upon income.

SMARTER Goals: An acronym for Specific, Measurable, Achievable, Realistic, Timelined, Enthusiastic, and Rewarding.

SOAP Charting: A commonly used process of documenting a client's session (Subjective, Objective, Assessment, Plan).

Social Cognition: A sub-topic of social psychology that focuses on how people process, store, and apply information about other people and social situations. It focuses on the role that cognitive processes play in our social interactions.

Social Learning: Process in which individuals observe the behavior of others and its consequences, and modify their own behavior accordingly.

Social Media: The collective of online communication channels dedicated to community-based input, interaction, content-sharing, and collaboration.

Social Media Optimization (SMO): The process of increasing the awareness of a product, brand, or event by using a number of social media outlets and communities to generate viral publicity.

Social Responsibility: The principle that holds that a business has a responsibility to refrain from unethical behavior that may bring harm to the community, and a responsibility to give back to society.

Sole Proprietorship: The simplest designation under which one can operate a business. It refers to a person who owns the business and is personally responsible for its debts.

Sponsorship: A person or organization that pays the cost of an activity or event in return for the right to advertise during the activity or event and/or receive some type of compensation.

Strategic Planning: A systematic process of envisioning a desired future, and translating this vision into broadly defined goals and a sequence of steps to achieve them.

Stress: A reaction to a stimulus that impacts one's physical or mental balance.

Stress Management: Any technique or routine developed to help someone cope with or lessen the physical and emotional effects of everyday life pressure.

Subcontracting: Paying someone else to do a task for which you have been paid.

Success: The accomplishment of an aim or a purpose. A process that involves setting and achieving goals.

Supervision: The process of working with a more experienced practitioner or counselor for the purpose of dealing with day-to-day challenges, ethical dilemmas, and setting boundaries.

Supply and Demand: The amount of a commodity, product, or service available and the desire of buyers for it, considered as factors for regulating its price.

Support System: Various groups for the purpose of receiving advice and exchanging ideas. The major categories of support systems are supervision, peer support groups, mentors, advisors, Mastermind groups, and online discussion forums.

Synergy: The interaction or cooperation of two or more organizations, substances, or agents to produce a combined effect greater than the sum of their separate effects.

Target Market: A specific group of people who share similar characteristics.

Tax Credits: An incentive that allows taxpayers to subtract the amount of the credit from the total tax amount owed.

Teamwork: The combined action of a group of people, especially when effective and efficient.

Termination: The act of dismissing an employee, or the employee breaking ties with the company.

Therapeutic Relationship: The relationship between a healthcare professional and a client.

Tickler File: A collection of date-labeled file folders organized in a way that allows time-sensitive documents to be filed according to the future date on which each document needs action.

Time Management: The act or process of planning and exercising conscious control over the amount of time spent on specific activities, especially to increase effectiveness, efficiency, or productivity.

Tips: *See* gratuity

Title Protection: The lowest regulation level. Only those who satisfy certain requirements may use the relevant prescribed title. Practitioners aren't required to register or notify the state. Thus, anyone may engage in the particular practice, but only those who satisfy the prescribed requirements may use the specific title.

Tracking: Documenting items to identify trends such as marketing activities, client profiles, appointment bookings, and income levels.

Trade Name: The official name under which a company does business, (*see* also, DBA.)

Trademark: The registration of your trade name, logo, and description.

Traffic: The amount of data sent and received by visitors to a website.

Transaction Privilege Tax License: A license issued by the State Department of Revenue that allows one to sell items, and collect and remit state sales taxes.

Transference: A normal psychological phenomenon characterized by unconscious redirection of feelings from client to practitioner.

Transition: Change; transformation; to make or become different.

Trauma: A serious injury or shock to the body, as from violence or an accident. An emotional wound or shock that creates substantial, lasting harm.

Treatment Plan: Blueprint to follow while working with any specific client. The plan is based upon all the information gathered in the interview and the session; including goals, indications, contraindications, treatment frequency, specific modalities to be used, homework, and possible referrals to other wellness providers.

Trends: A general direction in which something is developing or changing.

Trigger: An experience that sets off a traumatic memory. The trigger itself may not be traumatic, including things such as a person, place, sound, image, smell, body position, or vocal tone.

Twitter: A social networking, microblogging service that allows registered members to broadcast short posts called tweets.

URL (Uniform Resource Locater): A generic term for all types of names and addresses that refer to objects on the World Wide Web. The term "web address" is a synonym for a URL that uses the HTTP or HTTPS protocol.

Undercapitalization: When a company has insufficient capital to conduct normal business operations and pay creditors.

USP: Unique Selling Proposition.

Value-Added Service: A service added at little or no cost to promote one's business.

Values: Beliefs about what is intrinsically worthwhile or desirable, rather than what is right or correct.

Variance: An exception to a rule.

Viral Marketing: Word-of-Mouth marketing techniques that use pre-existing social networks to produce increases in brand awareness or to achieve other marketing objectives such as product sales.

Vlog: A video blog or video log, posted on the Internet, that documents a person's life, thoughts, opinions, and interests.

Webmaster: A person who maintains a particular website.

Website: A set of interconnected webpages, usually including a homepage, generally located on the same server, and prepared and maintained as a collection of information by a person, group, or organization.

Website Page Fold: The portion of the webpage that's visible without scrolling.

Welcome to My Office Kit: Information assembled for a first-time client. May include items such as a welcome letter, brochure, business card, intake form, preparation for appointment information, policies, and other promotional items.

WIIFM (What's In It For Me): An "urban slang" expression which means what are the advantages to me personally.

WOOP: Wish, outcome, obstacle, plan.

Word-of-Mouth Marketing (WOMM): A business act that earns customer referrals or recommendations through social interaction.

Workers' Compensation Insurance: This type of insurance is required by law when one has employees. It covers all of the costs that would be required to pay for any injury to an employee.

Yelp: A website and mobile app that publishes crowd-sourced reviews about local businesses.

YouTube: A video sharing service that allows users to watch videos posted by other users and upload videos of their own. These videos can also be posted or shared on other websites.

Zoning Ordinance: Written regulations and laws that define how property in specific geographic area can be used (residential or commercial), and might include other requirements, such as height, parking, and signage.

Zoning Variance: An exception to the zoning ordinance (sometimes referred to as a "special exemption" permit), usually granted by a separate board not including the planning commission or city council.

Endnotes

Chapter 1

1. Rachel Naomi Remen, M.D., "In the Service of Life," *Noetic Sciences Review,* Spring 1996.

Chapter 2

1. Gerard J. Tortora and Bryan Derrickson, *Principles of Anatomy & Physiology, 14th Edition* (Hoboken, NJ: Wiley, 2014), 485-487.

Chapter 3

1. Tom Peters, *Thriving on Chaos: Handbook for a Management Revolution* (Harper Perennial, 1991).
2. Jim Lundy, *Lead, Follow, or Get Out of the Way* (The Berkley Publishing Group, 1986).
3. Shawn Achor, "Happily Orange After," *Training Magazine,* January/February 2014, 114-120.
4. "The World Happiness Report 2013," UN Sustainable Development Solutions Network, <http://unsdsn.org/resources/publications/world-happiness-report-2013/>.
5. Roy Saunderson, "If You're Happy and You Know It…," *Training Magazine,* Jan/Feb 2014, 142-143.
6. Shawn Achor, "The Happiness Dividend," Harvard Business Review, June 23, 2011.
7. Ron Dalrymple, *The Inner Manager: Mastering Business, Home and Self* (Celestial Gifts Publishing, 1987).
8. Barbara Fredrickson et al., "Open Hearts Build Lives: Positive Emotions, Induced Through Loving-Kindness Meditation, Build Consequential Personal Resources," *Journal of Personality and Social Psychology* (2008) Nov; 95(5): 1045–1062, doi:10.1037/a0013262.
9. Ann Hawkins, "Journal to Retrain Your Inner Critic," *MASSAGE Magazine,* February 2015, 64-67.
10. Eliza Bergeson, "Procrastination and The Art of Inner Feng Shui," July 28, 2011, <http://www.elizabergeson.com/articles/procrastination-and-feng-shui-2/154/>.
11. C Diane Ealy, Ph.d., *The Woman's Book of Creativity* (Beyond Words Publishing, Inc., 1995) 89.
12. Remez Sasson, "Creative Visualization - Part One, From Imagination to Reality - Attracting Success with Mind Power," *Success Consciousness,* <http://www.successconsciousness.com/index_000008.htm>.
13. Eric Finzi and Norman E. Rosenthal, "Treatment of depression with onabotulinumtoxinA: A randomized, double-blind, placebo controlled trial," *Journal of Psychiatric Research* 52, 2014, 1-6.
14. Louise Hay, *Experience Your Good Now! Learning to Use Affirmations* (HayHouse, July 22, 2014).
15. Michael J. Losier, *The Law of Attraction: The Science of Attracting More of What You Want and Less of What You Don't* (Michael J. Losier Enterprises, 2006).
16. *What the Bleep Do We Know!?* Directed by Mark Vincente. (Captured Light & Lord of the Wind Films, LLC, 2004).
17. David Neal, Wendy Wood, and Jeffrey Quinn, "Habits—A Repeat Performance," *Current Directions in Psychological Science* vol. 15 no. 4, August 2006, 198-202, <http://cdp.sagepub.com/content/15/4/198.abstract>.
18. Ealy 241-245.

19. Rob Reuteman, "Accentuate the Negative," *Entrepreneur,* February 2015, 44-45.
20. Kristen Tammaro-Sparks, "How Much Time In Between Client Sessions Is Enough?" July 30, 2014, <http://relaxationbusinesscoaching.com/much-time-between-client-sessions-enough/>.
21. Faith Popcorn and Lys Marigold, *Clicking: 17 Trends That Drive Your Business—And Your Life* (New York: HarperCollins Publishing, Inc.,1997).

Chapter 4

1. Randall S. Hansen, Ph.D., "The 10-Step Plan to Career Change: How to Successfully Change Careers," *Quintessential Careers,* <http://www.quintcareers.com/career-change/>.
2. Jean Shea, "Learning shouldn't end when you walk out of massage school with a certificate in hand," *MASSAGE Magazine,* December 2013, 43.
3. A.T. Ferrell-Torry and O.J. Glick, "The use of therapeutic massage as a nursing intervention to modify anxiety and the perception of cancer pain," *Cancer Nurse,* April 1993,93-101.
4. C.M. Olney, "The effect of therapeutic back massage in hypertensive persons: a preliminary study," *Biological Research for Nursing,* October 2005, 98-105.
5. Les Kertay, "Ethical considerations for bodyworkers who counsel," *MASSAGE Magazine,* July/August 1998.
6. Napoleon Hill, *Think & Grow Rich* (Fawcett Crest Books, 1960), 168-169.

Chapter 5

1. Kenneth Blanchard and Norman Peale, *The Power of Ethical Management,* (William Morrow, 1988).
2. Thomas J. Peters, "Ethics is an everyday, lifetime endeavor," *The Arizona Daily Star,* September 26, 1989.
3. Merriam-Webster Dictionary, s.v. "integrity," <http://www.merriam-webster.com/dictionary/integrity>.
4. Adam Grant, *Give and Take: A Revolutionary Approach to Success* (Penguin Group, 2013).
5. Michelle Blake, "The Value of Sharing Your Values," *Massage & Bodywork,* May/June 2012, 53-59.

Chapter 6

1. J.S. Uleman, S.A. Saribay, & C.M.Gonzalez, "Spontaneous inferences, implicit impressions, and implicit theories," Annual Review of Psychology 59, (2008), 329–360. doi:10.1146/annurev.psych.59.103006.093707.
2. Andrew Young and Vicki Bruce, "Special Issue: Person Perception 25 years after Bruce and Young (1986)," *British Journal of Psychology,* Volume 102, Issue 4, November 2011, 959–974.
3. Marshall B. Rosenberg, *Nonviolent Communication: A Language of Life: Create Your Life, Your Relationships, and Your World in Harmony with Your Values* (PuddleDancer Press, 2003), 96.
4. *Oxford English Dictionary,* <http://www.oed.com/>.
5. Tracey Smith and Mary Tague-Busler, *The Key to Survival: Interpersonal Communication,* Fourth Edition (Waveland Press, 2007), 67.
6. Diana L. Thompson, *Hands Heal: Communication, Documentation, and Insurance Billing for Manual Therapists,* third edition (Lippincott Williams & Wilkins, 2006), 74.

Chapter 7

1. Tainya Clarke et al., "Trends in the Use of Complementary Health Approaches Among Adults: United States, 2002-2012," *National Health Statistics Reports* 79, National Center for Health Statistics, 2015, <http://www.cdc.gov/nchs/data/nhsr/nhsr079.pdf>.
2. Clarke *et al., Trends,* Table 1.
3. Richard Nahin *et al.,* "Costs of complementary and alternative medicine (CAM) and frequency of visits to CAM practitioners: United States, 2007," *National Health Statistics Reports* no 18, National Center for Health Statistics, July 30, 2009, <http://www.cdc.gov/nchs/data/nhsr/nhsr018.pdf>.
4. "Massage Therapy Fast Facts," *Associated Bodywork & Massage Professionals,* <http://www.massagetherapy.com/_content/images/Media/Factsheet1.pdf>.
5. "2015 Massage Profession Research Report," *American Massage Therapy Association.*
6. Douglas Helmer, Ph.D. and David Lemke, *The Massage Therapy Career Focus Workbook,* <http://www.massageresource.com/book/massage-therapy-career-focus-workbook-01.php>.

7. Heidi Smith Luedtke, "The Benefits of a Blended Career," *Massage & Bodywork*, July/August 2012.
8. Ben Benjamin, Ph.D. and Cherie Sohnen-Moe, *The Ethics of Touch* (SMA Press, January 2014), 211.
9. "Independent Contract (Self-Employed) or Employee?" *Internal Revenue Service*, <http://www.irs.gov/Businesses/Small-Businesses-&-Self-Employed/Independent-Contractor-Self-Employed-or-Employee>.
10. "Small Business Facts," *Small Business Administration*, <https://www.sba.gov/sites/default/files/Business-Survival.pdf>.

Chapter 8

1. "ISPA 2014 U.S. Spa Industry Study," *International SPA Association*, <http://www.experienceispa.com/media/facts-stats/>.
2. Tracy Stapp Herold, "Rocket-fueled growth," *Entrepreneur*, February 2015, 96-110.
3. Benjamin and Sohnen-Moe, *The Ethics of Touch*, 225.
4. "ISPA 2011 U.S. Spa Industry Report," *International SPA Association*, 35.
5. Spa Glossary, s.v. "spa," <http://www.spafinder.com/spaguide/spa101/glossary.htm#S>.
6. Duane Wells, "Drenched in History: Taking the Waters in Bath," March 11, 2013, <http://theduanewells.com/2013/03/drenched-in-history-taking-the-waters-in-bath/>.
7. Jon Marcus, "Trendspotting: More Men Heading to the Spa," *The Boston Globe*, February 28, 2015,<https://www.bostonglobe.com/lifestyle/travel/2015/02/28/trendspotting-more-men-heading-spa/4bGdTPJHdDU2Ly7fj8LVNO/story.html>.
8. H. Barry Waldman, D.D.S., M.P.H., Ph.D and Steven P. Perlman, D.D.S., Msc.D., "Patient-centric practices-no matter the size!" *AGD Impact*, November 2006, 32

Chapter 9

1. "Competencies for Optimal Practices in Integrated Environments," *Academic Consortium for Complementary and Alternative Health Care* (ACCAHC), <http://www.accahc.org/competencies>.
2. Benjamin and Sohnen-Moe, *The Ethics of Touch*, 227-229.
3. Benjamin and Sohnen-Moe, *The Ethics of Touch*, 232-233.

Chapter 10

1. Benjamin and Sohnen-Moe, *The Ethics of Touch*, 219.

Chapter 11

1. "Closer Look: Wellness ROI," *International Foundation of Employee Benefit Plans*, 2012, <https://www.ifebp.org/bookstore/Pages/wellnessroi.aspx>.
2. Jean Ives, "Massage Is In Business," *Massage Therapy Journal*, (Spring 2004).

Chapter 12

1. Dan Baker, Cathy Greenberg, and Collins Hemingway, *What Happy Companies Know: How the Science of Happiness Can Change Your Company for the Better* (Pearson Education, Inc., 2006), 202.
2. Baker and Greenberg, *What Happy Companies Know*, 197.
3. Andrew Klappholz, "Taking Notes in the Job Interview," *The Ladders*, August 23, 2010, <http://www.theladders.com/career-advice/taking-notes-in-job-interview?fromSearch=true&start=&contentSearchKeyword=Taking%20notes%20in%20the%20Job%20Interview>.

Chapter 14

1. "Consumer Price Index Overview," *Bureau of Labor Statistics*, <http://www.bls.gov/cpi/cpiovrvw.htm>.
2. "Cost-of-Living Adjustments," Social Security Administration, <http://www.ssa.gov/OACT/cola/colaseries.html>.

Chapter 15

1. Nina Kaufman, "Top Ten Legal Pitfalls That Can Sink Your Small Business Success," *Special Advisory*, <http://www.greatbusinesslawresources.com/>.

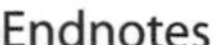

2. Laura McCamy, "Want to Start a Business? Here is What it Will Cost," *Intuit*, September 29, 2014, <http://quickbooks.intuit.com/r/business-planning/start-costs-industry>.
3. Dharmesh Shah, "How To Pick a Company Name: Tips From the Trenches," *OnStartups*, March 22, 2010, <http://onstartups.com/tabid/3339/bid/12156/How-To-Pick-A-Company-Name-Tips-From-The-Trenches.aspx>.
4. Jenny Hogan, "How To Raise Your Session Fees," *MASSAGE Magazine*, May 2010.
5. "Health Care Franchises," *Entrepreneur*, <http://www.entrepreneur.com/franchises/categories/hlth.html>.

Chapter 16

1. Dale Willerton, "Negotiate Your Massage Clinic's Commercial Lease," *MASSAGE Magazine*, June 2, 2009, <http://www.massagemag.com/negotiate-your-massage-clinics-commercial-lease-5013/>.

Chapter 17

1. David M. Anderson, "Deadly Sins," *Entrepreneur*, August 2001.

Chapter 18

1. "Case Study: Delane's Natural Nail Care," *Small Business Technology Institute*, San Jose, CA.
2. Sarah Cafiero, "How To Run A Paperless Massage Therapy Practice," *Sohnen-Moe Associates Blog*, September 10, 2012, <http://blog.sohnen-moe.com/how-to-run-a-paperless-massage-therapy-practice/>.

Chapter 19

1. "Understanding Health Information Privacy," *US Department of Health and Human Services*, <http://www.hhs.gov/ocr/privacy/hipaa/understanding/>.
2. Julie Bryant, "HIPAA hysteria," *Atlanta Business Chronicle*, December 2, 2002, <http://www.bizjournals.com/atlanta/stories/2002/12/02/focus1.html>.
3. "Health Information Privacy," *US Department of Health and Human Services*, <http://www.hhs.gov/ocr/privacy/hipaa/understanding/coveredentities/businessassociates.html>.
4. Greg Neely, "Are You Compliant? What the Latest HIPAA Rules Mean for Massage Therapists," *MASSAGE Magazine*, February 2015, 42-44.
5. "Frequently Asked Questions about Section 2706," *Integrative Healthcare Policy Consortium*, <http://www.ihpc.org/wp-content/uploads/section-2706-faq.pdf>.

Chapter 20

1. Suze Orman, *The 9 Steps to Financial Freedom* (Crown Publishers, Inc., 1998).
2. Vicki Robin, Joe Dominguez, and Monique Tilford, *Your Money or Your Life: 9 Steps to Transforming Your Relationship with Money and Achieving Financial Independence* (Penguin books, 2008).
3. "How long should I keep records?" IRS, June 30, 2015, <http://www.irs.gov/Businesses/Small-Businesses-&-Self-Employed/How-long-should-I-keep-records>.
4. Benjamin and Sohnen-Moe, *The Ethics of Touch*, 242-243.
5. Bernard B. Kamoroff, *475 Tax Deductions For Businesses & Self-Employed* (Taylor Trade Publishing, 2013), ix.
6. "Modern Trade and Barter," IRTA, <http://www.irta.com/index.php/about/modern-trade-barter>.
7. Enrique De Argaez, "Selecting a Barter Exchange," *Internet World Stats*, <http://www.internetworldstats.com/articles/art074.htm>.

Chapter 21

1. Anita Shannon, "How can offering retail products benefit my clients and help me to be recognized as a health care specialist?" *MASSAGE Magazine*, August 2011, 22.
2. Merriam-Webster Dictionary, s.v. "merchandising," <http://www.merriam-webster.com/dictionary/merchandising>.
3. Phyllis Hanton, "Holiday Spa Treatments: A Festive Touch," *MASSAGE Magazine*, December 2014, 22-25

Chapter 22

1. Benjamin and Sohnen-Moe, *The Ethics of Touch*, 211.

2. "How much is your employee ACTUALLY costing you?" *The Onin Group*, <http://www.oningroup.com/employee-cost.html>.

Chapter 23

1. Debbie Allen, "5 Mistakes to Avoid When Selling Your Small Business," *About Money*, <http://retail.about.com/od/exitstrategies/a/selling_mistake.htm>.

Chapter 24

1. Marsha Sinetar, *Do What You Love and the Money Will Follow* (Dell Publishing, 1987).
2. Joe Vitale, "The Greatest Motivator Isn't What You Think—or, What I Learned from Drew Barrymore and Adam Sandler on Valentine's Day," *Mr.Fire Blog*, (2005), <http://www.mrfire.com/article-archives/recent-articles/the-greatest-motivator.html>.
3. Greg Marlin, "7 Stages of Buying Cycle: From Awareness to Advocacy," *Marketing.AI*, <http://marketing.ai/7-stages-of-buying-cycle.html>.
4. David A. Aaker, *Managing Brand Equity* (The Free Press, 1991), 14.

Chapter 25

1. Brad Fay, "Return on Word of Mouth," *Word of Mouth Marketing Association*, (December 2014), 18.
2. Brad Fay, 19.
3. J.S. Uleman, S.A. Saribay, and C.M. Gonzalez, "Spontaneous inferences, implicit impressions, and implicit theories," *Annual Review of Psychology* 59, (2008): 329–360, doi:10.1146/annurev.psych.59.103006.093707.
4. Andrew Young and Vicki Bruce, "Special Issue: Person Perception 25 years after Bruce and Young (1986)," *British Journal of Psychology* Volume 102, Issue 4, (November 2011): 959–974.
5. Phil McAleer, Alexander Todorov, and Pascal Belin, "How Do You Say 'Hello'? Personality Impressions from Brief Novel Voices," *PLoSOne*, March 12, 2014, doi:10.1371/journal.pone.0090779.
6. Kathy Gruver, "The Schmooze Factor," ABMP *Massage & Bodywork*, Sep/Oct 2012: 99.
7. James McCroskey, "Communication Apprehension: What Have We Learned in the Last Four Decades" *Human Communication. A Publication of the Pacific and Asian Communication Association* Vol. 12, No. 2: 157 - 171.

Chapter 26

1. Liz Fulcher, "6 Ways to Market Aromatherapy Massage," *MASSAGE Magazine*, May 2013, 29.
2. Laurie Beasley, "Why Direct Mail Still Yields the Lowest Cost-Per-Lead and Highest Conversion Rate," *Online Marketing Institute*, June 13, 2013, <http://www.onlinemarketinginstitute.org/blog/2013/06/why-direct-mail-still-yields-the-lowest-cost-per-lead-and-highest-conversion-rate/>.
3. Brian Morris, "Print Marketing Statistics You Should Know," September 9, 2014, <http://expandedramblings.com/index.php/10-print-marketing-statistics-know/2/>.
4. John Mazzone; and Samie Rehman, "The Household Diary Study: Mail Use & Attitudes in FY 2012," USPS, May 2013, 39-46, 144-145, <https://about.usps.com/studying-americans-mail-use/household-diary/2012/fullreport-pdf/USPS_HDS_FY12_Screen.pdf>.
5. "Gift Card Statistics," *GiftCards.com*, <http://partners.giftcards.com/statistics>.
6. "Coupon Statistics," *I Love Coupon Month*, <http://www.ilovecouponmonth.com/statistics/>.

Chapter 27

1. Michael Port, *Book Yourself Solid: The Fastest, Easiest, and Most Reliable System of Getting More Clients Than You Can Handle Even if You Hate Marketing and Selling* (John Wiley & Sons, Inc., 2006), 159.
2. "Company Overview," Google, <http://www.google.com/about/company/>.
3. Pam Dyer, "Blogs Influence Consumer Spending More Than Social Networks," *Pamorama*, March 14, 2013, <http://pamorama.net/2013/03/14/blogs-influence-consumer-spending-more-than-social-networks/#.UUlWiVfp_Xt>.
4. "Blogging for Business Marketing Kit," *Hubspot, Inc.*, 2015, <http://offers.hubspot.com/blogging-kit>.
5. Olivia Allen, "6 Stats You Should Know About Business Blogging in 2015," *Hubspot*, March 11, 2015, <http://blog.hubspot.com/marketing/business-blogging-in-2015>.

6. "How Connectivity Influences Global Shopping," *Newswire*, August 28, 2012, <http://www.nielsen.com/us/en/insights/news/2012/how-connectivity-influences-global-shopping.html>.
7. "8 Massive Benefits of Using YouTube For Business," Grow Team, <http://www.wearegrow.com/8-massive-benefits-of-using-youtube-for-business/#sthash.JcGPwAo6.dpuf>.
8. Stephanie Beck, "How One Little Symbol (#) Gets You More Clients," *Massage Today* 14 04, April 2014.
9. Stephanie Beck, "The Importance of having a Strategy for Hashtags on Social Media" (from the Social MisAlignments: Laptop Workshop).
10. Jason Mander, "Daily time spent on social networks rises to 1.72 hours," *GlobalWebIndex*, January 26, 2015, <https://www.globalwebindex.net/blog/daily-time-spent-on-social-networks-rises-to-1-72-hours>.
11. Stephanie Beck, *Social MisAlignments: The Chiropractor's Guide to Marketing Online* (SRB Solutions, 2014), 16.

Chapter 28

1. Daniel Starch, *Advertising: Its Principles, Practice, and Technique* (Nabu Press, 2010), 7.
2. Brad Fay, "Return on Word of Mouth," *Word of Mouth Marketing Association*, December 2014, 18.
3. Thomas Smith, *Successful Advertising: Its Secrets Explained* 9th Edition (1888), <https://books.google.com/books/about/Successful_Advertising.html?id=sB7yQAAACAAJ>.
4. Kathi Kruse, "The Rule of 7: How Social Media Beats Other Forms of Marketing," *Kruse Control, Inc*, January 20, 2014, <http://www.krusecontrolinc.com/how-social-media-beats-other-forms-of-marketing-rule-of-7/>.
5. Stefan Hampel, Daniel Heinrich, and Colin Campbell, "Is An Advertisement Worth the Paper It's Printed on? The Impact of Premium Print Advertising on Consumer Perception," *Journal of Advertising Research* Vol. 52 No. 1 (2012), <http://cn.cnstudiodev.com/uploads/document_attachment/attachment/197/41cb1fdc-68b4-44a3-bd6c-fb7f2befdeba.pdf>.
6. Demian Farnworth, "10 Ways to Write Damn Good Copy," *Copyblogger* Media, 2013, <http://www.copyblogger.com/good-copywriting/>.
7. Cahners Advertising Research Report," *Accountability Information Managament, Inc.*, <http://www.a-i-m.com/docs/reports/carr-reports.pdf>.
8. "10 Tips to Successful Print Advertising," *Metroland Media*, <http://www.advertising.tcnmicrosites.com/adtips.html>.
9. Allie Mundy, "The Psychology of Color in Marketing," *Prime Design Solutions Learning Center* February 2, 2015; Podcast: <http://www.primedesignsolutions.com/learning-center/psychology-color-marketing/>.
10. Jill Morton, "Why Color Matters," *Colorcom*, 2010, <http://www.colorcom.com/research/why-color-matters>.
11. Michael Link, "How U.S. Adults Use Radio and Other Forms of Audio: Results from the Council for Research Excellence," *The Nielsen Company*, October 29, 2009, <http://www.nielsen.com/content/dam/corporate/us/en/newswire/uploads/2009/11/VCM_Radio-Audio_Report_FINAL_29Oct09.pdf>.
12. David Hinkley, "Average American watches 5 hours of TV per day, report shows," *NEW YORK DAILY NEWS*, March 5, 2014, <http://www.nydailynews.com/life-style/average-american-watches-5-hours-tv-day-article-1.1711954>.

Chapter 29

1. Olivia Polger, "Webinar Recap: 500 Writers and Editors on How to Pitch," *BuzzStream*, July 17, 2014, <http://www.buzzstream.com/blog/how-to-pitch-for-pr.html>.
2. Allison Stadd, "59% of Journalists Worldwide Use Twitter, Up from 47% in 2012," *SocialTimes*, June 26, 2013, <http://www.adweek.com/socialtimes/journalists-twitter/486900>.

Chapter 30

1. James Digby, "50 Facts about Customer Experience Return," *Behavior Magazine*, October 26, 2010, <http://returnonbehavior.com/2010/10/50-facts-about-customer-experience-for-2011/>.
2. Diane Helbig, "Sixty Eight Percent Is Yours To Keep," *Small Business Trends*, May 2, 2010, <http://smallbiztrends.com/2010/05/sixty-eight-percent-is-yours-to-keep.html>.
3. Tony Hsieh, *Delivering Happiness: A Path to Profits, Passion, and Purpose* (Grand Central Publishing, June 7, 2010).
4. "Zappos Core Values," *Zappos*, <http://www.zappos.com/d/about-zappos-culture>.
5. Irene Diamond, "Make Your Appointments Stick," *Massage & Bodywork*, September/October 2012, 84.

Index

F

G

H

I

J

K

L

U

V

W

Y

Z

Other Offerings

Free Resources

SMA Community Site: sohnenmoe.customerhub.net

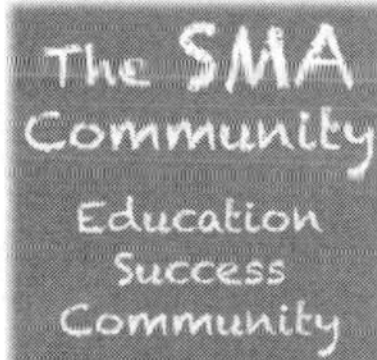

The SMA Community site contains free ebooks, posters, reproducible forms, and other practice-building resources. Your personal FileBox is available 24 hours a day. It maintains all the free files you download, as well as any digital products you purchase from our online store.

SMA Blog: sohnen-moe.com/blog

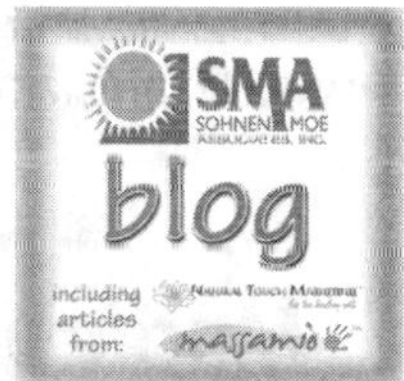

Our blog contains hundreds of free, informative articles written by experts and successful practitioners in the wellness fields. Topics include marketing, technology, treatment planning, overall success strategies, and more.

Marketing Mastery: sohnen-moe.com/marketingmastery

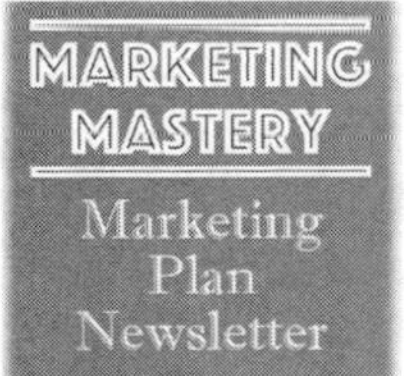

The *Marketing Mastery Newsletter* is a free subscription service to a year-long overall marketing plan. The plan includes monthly goals and weekly activity reminders delivered directly to your inbox. Use all or part of this plan to expand your marketing efforts, elevate your visibility in the community, and increase your client base.

Consulting Services

Coaching with Cherie Sohnen-Moe: sohnen-moe.com/services

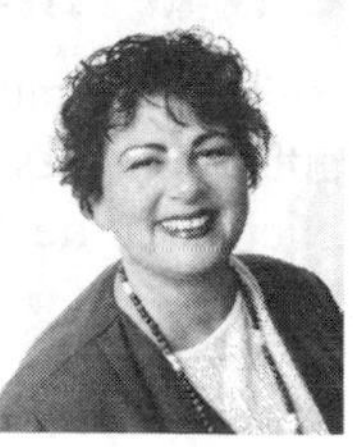

Coaching provides support for you in resolving problems and provides suggestions to implement change for a more efficient, vital, and flourishing practice. Being as consummate in business as you are in technique requires learning an entirely different set of skills. Mastering these skills can take a long time, particularly if you work alone. Direction in acquiring these skills and knowledge, along with consistent support and encouragement, can help you create the business/career you envision.

Publications

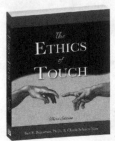

In this comprehensive work on ethics, Ben Benjamin and Cherie Sohnen-Moe address the difficult, confusing, and seldom discussed dilemmas often confronting touch therapy practitioners. By describing the issues honestly, identifying clear principles and concepts, providing specific resources, and using stories straight from the treatment room, they have written a book to guide, support, and inspire both students and seasoned practitioners. Throughout this book you'll find thought-provoking examples, models, points to ponder, practical applications, and activities that make this information personally relevant. **www.TheEthicsOfTouch.com**

Retail Mastery

This innovative book is written by two highly respected educators in the massage and bodywork profession, Cherie Sohnen-Moe and Lynda Solien-Wolfe. The information and resources in *Retail Mastery* helps you successfully incorporate product sales into your practice. **www.RetailMastery.com**

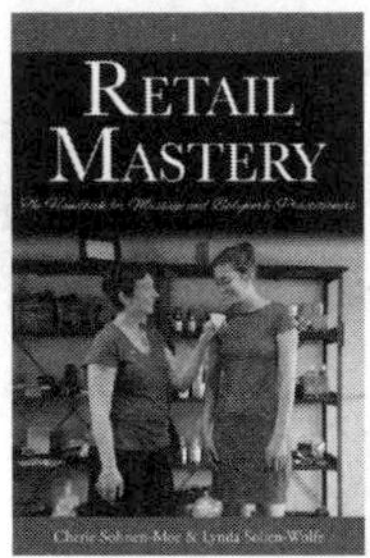

Present Yourself Powerfully

Public speaking is one of the best ways to build your business. *Present Yourself Powerfully* is a digital presentation kit that makes it easy for practitioners to give talks, workshops, and demonstrations, by providing a toolbox of ideas, techniques, and reproducible materials.

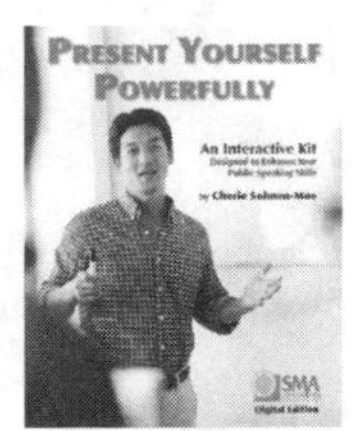

Marketing Communications

Marketing Communications for Massage Therapists provides over 100 professionally written examples of marketing emails, letters, announcements, and press releases. The pages of this PDF can be copied and pasted into your preferred word processing or email application for easy editing.

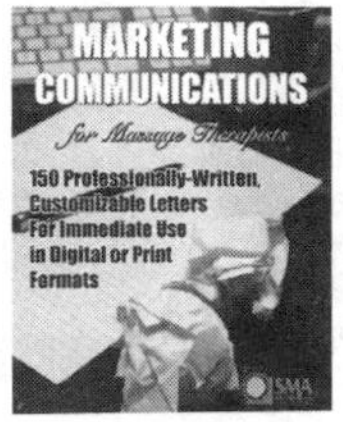

Build Your Business Plan

A business plan is an essential road map for a successful practice. *Build Your Business Plan* simplifies the planning, writing, and finalizing of this process. This kit is a PDF that includes a business plan outline, worksheets, and a 72-page sample massage therapy business plan to use as your guide.

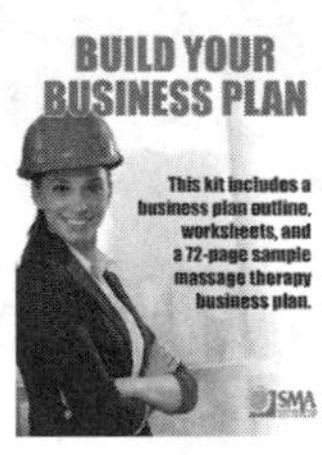

Marketing Tools

Presentation Planning Kits

Making a public presentation or teaching a class is one of the best ways to let people get to know you and what you can offer. In a single event you build your reputation, attract new clients, and even create an additional source of income all while providing a service to your community. These three A-Z planning kits make it easy!

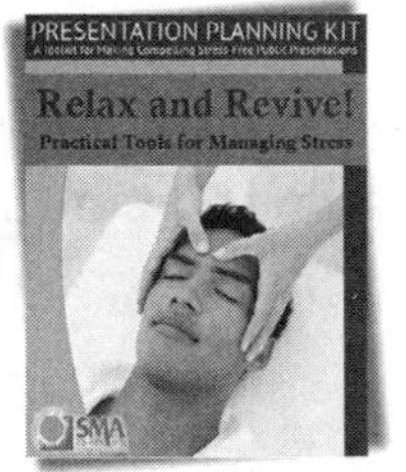

Gift Certificates

Richly illustrated, customizable gift certificates templates to offer your clients for their friends, family, and any one else.

Client Education Brochures

Educate your clients about a variety of products, modalities, and specialties available in your practice. These elegantly written and illustrated brochures have extensive information on a large number of subjects.

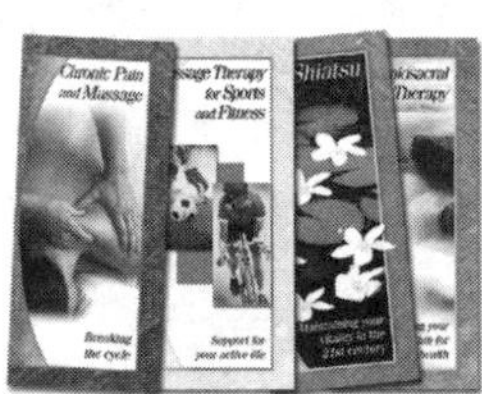

Business Card and Postcard Artwork

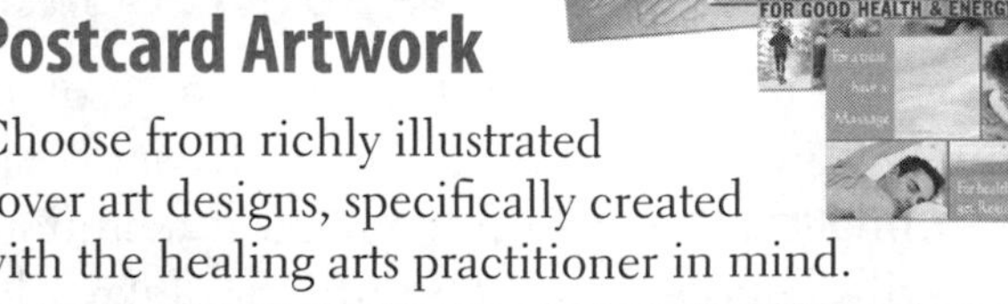

Choose from richly illustrated cover art designs, specifically created with the healing arts practitioner in mind.

www.Sohnen-Moe.com/products

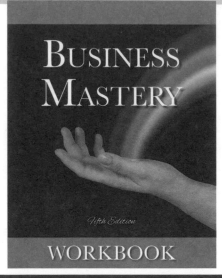